# The Communication Disorders Casebook

## Learning by Example


Shelly S. Chabon
Portland State University

Ellen R. Cohn
University of Pittsburgh


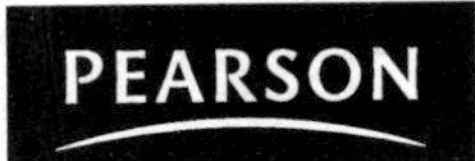


Boston Columbus Indianapolis New York San Francisco Upper Saddle River
Amsterdam Cape Town Dubai London Madrid Milan Munich Paris Montreal Toronto
Delhi Mexico City São Paulo Sydney Hong Kong Seoul Singapore Taipei Tokyo

**Vice President and Editor in Chief:** Jeffery W. Johnston
**Executive Editor and Publisher:** Stephen D. Dragin
**Editorial Assistant:** Jamie Bushell
**Vice President, Director of Marketing:** Margaret Waples
**Senior Marketing Manager:** Christopher D. Barry
**Senior Managing Editor:** Pamela D. Bennett
**Senior Project Manager:** Linda Hillis Bayma
**Senior Operations Supervisor:** Matthew Ottenweller
**Senior Art Director:** Diane C. Lorenzo
**Text Designer:** Integra Software Services
**Cover Designer:** Ali Mohrman
**Full-Service Project Management:** Thistle Hill Publishing Services, LLC
**Composition:** Integra Software Services
**Printer/Binder:** Edwards Brothers Malloy
**Cover Printer:** Edwards Brothers Malloy
**Text Font:** New Aster

Credits and acknowledgments borrowed from other sources and reproduced, with permission, in this textbook appear on appropriate page within text.



**Part opener photo credits:** Krista Greco/Merrill, pp. 7, 63; Courtesy of AbleNet, Inc., pp. 171, 328

---



**Library of Congress Cataloging-in-Publication Data**

Chabon, Shelly S.
The communication disorders casebook : learning by example / Shelly S. Chabon, Ellen R. Cohn.
p. cm.
Includes bibliographical references and index.
ISBN-13: 978-0-205-61012-9 (pbk.)
ISBN-10: 0-205-61012-9 (pbk.)
1. Speech disorders in children—Case studies. 2. Language disorders in children—Case studies. 3. Children with disabilities—Development—Case studies. 4. Speech Disorders—in infancy & childhood—Case studies. I. Cohn, Ellen R. II. Title.
RJ496.S7C45 2011
618.92'855—dc22

2010010382

10 9 8 7 6

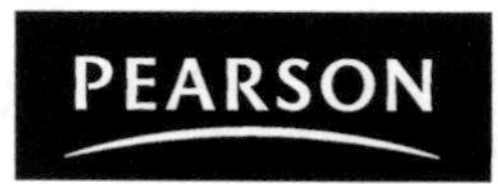


www.pearsonhighered.com

ISBN-13: 978-0-205-61012-9
ISBN-10: 0-205-61012-9

*We dedicate this work to the children and adults with communication disorders represented in this book who inspire us to do our best, and to our students whose wisdom is reflected on each page.*

# CONTENTS

## Part II
## Preschool Child Cases 63

## PART III
## School-Age Child Cases 171

# About the Authors

## The Editors

**Shelly S. Chabon**, PhD, CCC-SLP, is a Professor and Chair-Elect in the Department of Speech and Hearing Sciences at Portland State University. She was formerly the Executive Director/CEO of Children's TLC and the founder and Chair of the Department of Communication Sciences and Disorders (CSD) at Rockhurst University. She also served as Acting Chair of the CSD Department at Howard University and was Clinic Director and Clinical Coordinator at the University of Pittsburgh. She earned a BA from Brooklyn College, an MS in speech-language pathology from Penn State University, an MS in audiology from Towson State University, and a PhD from the University of Pittsburgh. Dr. Chabon is a Fellow of the American Speech-Language-Hearing Association (ASHA). She was a member of the ASHA Council for Clinical Certification, served as the Chair of the ASHA Board of Ethics, and is the ASHA 2011 President-Elect. She has written a number of articles and chapters and has co-authored four books, including a text on clinical practice in SLP and one titled *Ethics Education*. She has received several honors for her leadership and service including a Certificate of Recognition from ASHA for Special Contributions in Higher Education, an Apple Award for appreciation to an outstanding teacher, and the Dorothy Dreyer Award for volunteerism.

**Ellen R. Cohn**, PhD, CCC-SLP, is Associate Dean for Instructional Development, School of Health and Rehabilitation Sciences, and Associate Professor, Department of Communication Science and Disorders at the University of Pittsburgh. She previously served as Director of the University of Pittsburgh's Speech and Hearing Clinic and as a speech-language pathologist/research associate at the Cleft-Palate Craniofacial Center. Cohn earned a BA from Douglass College of Rutgers University, an MS from Vanderbilt University, and a PhD in speech-language pathology from the University of Pittsburgh. She has co-authored books on the topics of videofluoroscopy for persons with cleft palate, diversity in higher education, and communication as culture and co-developed a disability law degree at the School of Law. Cohn is a member of the American Speech-Language-Hearing Association, American Cleft Palate-Craniofacial Association, and American Telemedicine Association. In 2009 she was named an ASHA Diversity Champion, and she received the 2006 Honors of the Southwestern Pennsylvania Speech-Language-Hearing Association. Cohn has contributed to the *Cleft Palate-Craniofacial Journal, Educause Quarterly, Journal of Speech-Language and Hearing Disorders, Plastic and Reconstructive Surgery,* and *Radiology,* and she is the founding editor of the *International Journal of Telerehabilitation*. She serves on the Rehabilitation Engineering Research Center on Telerehabilitation, NIDRR, U.S. Department of Education.

## The Contributors

**Noma Anderson**, PhD, CCC-SLP, is Dean of the College of Allied Health Sciences at the University of Tennessee Health Science Center, Memphis. Dr. Anderson received her BA from Hampton University, her MS from Emerson College, and her PhD from the University of Pittsburgh. She taught at Hampton University and Howard University. Dr. Anderson served as ASHA Vice President for Academic Affairs, Deputy Director of the National Black Association of Speech, Language and Hearing and was elected to the Executive Board of the Council of Graduate Programs in Communication Sciences and Disorders. Dr. Anderson is a Fellow and Past President of the American Speech-Language-Hearing Association.

**Cheryl Andrews** has 27 years of experience in specialist treatment of stuttering in children and adults. Her master's degree in speech-language pathology is from the University of Northern Colorado, Greeley. Cheryl has worked in Australia since 1979 and specializes in the treatment of adults and children who stutter. Her core research interests include the development of stuttering interventions for school-age children. She is a doctoral student at the University of Sydney.

**Steven M. Barlow**, PhD, is a Professor of Speech-Language-Hearing Programs in Neuroscience, Human Biology and Bioengineering at the University of Kansas. He is also the Director of Communication Neuroscience Laboratories and Director of the Digital Electronics and Engineering Core for the Center for Biobehavioral Neuroscience Communication Disorders. He has published 80 articles on the neuroscience and biomechanics of speech and oromotor control in health and disease and a text on speech physiology. Dr. Barlow received the Keck Outstanding Scientist Award (1985), Zemlin Speech Science Award (2003, ASHA), and is principal investigator for two NIH R01 research projects concerned with early human development, sensorimotor control of the orofacial system, and brain plasticity. Recent work (Barlow, Finan, Chu, & Lee, 2008, *Journal Perinatology*) led to the development of a medical device known as the NTrainer®, which provides therapeutic patterned orocutaneous stimulation to tube-fed preterm infants to accelerate nonnutritive suck and prefeeding skills.

**Jacqueline Bauman-Waengler**, PhD, CCC-SLP, has been a university professor for over 30 years and is presently Director of Speech Consulting Services of Southern California. Her main teaching and clinical emphases have been in the areas of phonetics and phonology, including disorders of articulation and phonology in children. She has published and presented in these areas both nationally and internationally. She is the author of two textbooks, *Articulatory and Phonological Impairments: A Clinical Focus*, which is in its third edition, and *Introduction to Phonetics and Phonology: From Concepts to Transcription*.

**Christina A. Baumgartner**, MS, CCC-SLP, has been a practicing medical speech-language pathologist since 1992, working in both hospitals and universities as a clinician, speech pathology department manager, and adjunct faculty member teaching graduate dysphagia classes. Areas of clinical interest include differential diagnosis and evidence-based management of neurogenic communication disorders and dysphagia. Christina has been involved in program development in dysphagia, utilizing a multidisciplinary approach including physicians, respiratory therapists, and nurses at several medical centers throughout the country. She also spent several years establishing, developing protocols for, and managing mobile videofluoroscopy clinics around the country.

**Mindy Sittner Bridges**, PhD, CCC-SLP, is a clinical speech-language pathologist. She received her doctorate from the University of Kansas. Her research interests include the connection between language and reading disorders, early identification of children at risk for disabilities, and the use of response to intervention practices in school settings.

**Paul M. Brueggeman**, AuD, CCC-A, FAA, has been working in the field of audiology for over 10 years, with the last 9 at the University of South Dakota. In this capacity, his clinical work has continued to focus on early intervention, children with developmental disabilities (including FASD and autism), and working with the children and families who reside on tribal lands in South Dakota. His research interests involve the supervision of AuD students, adult education principles as they apply to rehabilitative processes, pediatric hearing issues in the Native American population, and psychosocial counseling in communication disorders. Throughout his career, Paul has helped children with hearing loss as well as their families.

**Louise M. Cahill**, BSpThy, PhD, is a speech-language pathologist with over 25 years of experience in clinical pediatric rehabilitation and 10 years of experience in clinical research. Her PhD, awarded in 2003, was the first to investigate speech disorders in children post-TBI. She has published over 20 peer-reviewed papers. In addition to her work on the physiological basis of speech disorders post-TBI, her most recent work has focused on treatment of these problems, in particular in the use of instrumentation and biofeedback techniques. She currently holds the position of Senior Speech Pathologist at the QLD Paediatric Rehabilitation Unit, Brisbane, Australia.

**Michael Campbell**, MS, MBA, CCC-SLP, received his master's degree from the University of Arkansas at Fayetteville and is currently Associate Professor in the UNCG Department of CSD and Director of the Speech and Hearing Program at Gateway University Research Park. Mr. Campbell has over 25 years of work experience in medical settings and has a strong background in voice rehabilitation.

**Terese Conrad**, MA, CCC-SLP, is a Clinical Educator in the Communication Sciences and Disorders Department at Wichita State University in Wichita, Kansas. She provides supervision to undergraduate and graduate students working with clients with limited language and/or with a diagnosis of ASD. Terese has over 17 years of experience providing assessment, treatment, support, and training for children and adults presenting communication disorders related to autism spectrum disorders and other developmental disabilities.

**Petrea L. Cornwell**, BSpPath, PhD, is a speech-language pathologist with 13 years of clinical and research experience in the area of brain injury rehabilitation. Her PhD, awarded in 2003, focused on examining the impact of posterior fossa and brainstem tumors on motor speech and swallowing function in children. She currently holds the position of Research Fellow (Speech Pathology) at the University of Queensland and Princess Alexandra Hospital, Brisbane, Australia. Petrea's primary areas of research interest are acquired brain injury and treatment efficacy in speech-language pathology, and she has published over 20 peer-reviewed papers in these fields.

**Deborah Cron**, ME, CCC-SLP, is a member of the Clinical Faculty in the Department of Communication Sciences and Disorders at Missouri State University. She has worked in a variety of settings, including acute care and rehabilitation, home health, public schools, and private consulting, and has practiced in small towns and major metropolitan areas, treating patients across the life span. Prior to returning to her native Ozarks, she was Administrator of Speech Language Pathology and Assistive Technology Services for a non-profit agency in New York City.

**Sena Crutchley**, MA, CCC-SLP, a graduate of UNCG, is currently an Assistant Professor in the UNCG Department of CSD and a speech-language pathologist with the Speech and Hearing Program at Gateway University Research Park. She brought to the transgender communication intervention group a background in theater and voice, expertise in multicultural issues in speech-language pathology, and 9 years of experience as a speech-language pathologist in a variety of clinical settings.

**Michael de Riesthal**, PhD, CCC-SLP, received his MS and PhD in Hearing and Speech Sciences from Vanderbilt University. Currently, he is an Assistant Professor in the Department of Hearing and Speech Sciences at Vanderbilt University School of Medicine and teaches courses on the management of aphasia and traumatic brain injury. He is a clinician at Pi Beta Phi Rehabilitation Institute at Vanderbilt University Medical Center with expertise in the management of neurogenic cognitive-communicative disorders resulting from stroke, tumor, degenerative neurological disorders, and traumatic brain injury. He has presented at numerous professional meetings and has published papers and book chapters on the topics of aphasia and dysphagia.

**Jodelle Deem**, PhD, CCC-SLP, is Associate Professor and Director of Graduate Studies in the Division of Communication Sciences and Disorders and in the Rehabilitation Sciences Doctoral Program at the University of Kentucky. She also holds a joint appointment in the Division of Otolaryngology, Head and Neck Surgery. Dr. Deem received her PhD from the University of Memphis. She is co-author with Dr. Lynda Miller of *Manual of Voice Therapy* (2nd ed.).

**Aimee Dietz**, PhD, CCC-SLP, earned her doctorate in speech-language pathology from the University of Nebraska-Lincoln. Currently, she is an assistant professor at the University of Cincinnati. She teaches courses and conducts research that focuses on aphasia and augmentative and alternative communication.

**Leo Dunham**, MS, CCC-SLP, is currently providing speech-language therapy for Hallmark Rehabilitation at Liberty Terrace Care Center in Liberty, Missouri. He obtained his master's degree in 2006 from Rockhurst University in Kansas City, Missouri. Speech-language pathology is his second career, as he spent almost 30 years working in mechanical design and engineering. Leo earned a law degree from the University of Kansas in 1987.

**Colette Edwards**, MA, CCC-SLP, received her master's degree from the University of Tennessee at Knoxville and is currently an Assistant Professor and Clinical Educator at UNCG. Ms. Edwards worked as an SLP in the public schools for 18 years. In 2004 and 2005, she supervised transgender clients in individual and group therapy at UNCG.

**Lea Helen Evans**, PhD, CCC-SLP, is a speech-language pathologist and an Assistant Professor at Vanderbilt Bill Wilkerson Center (VBWC) at Vanderbilt University. Having taught previously at the University of Mississippi and Mississippi University for Women, she is currently serving as the Preschool Team Leader at VBWC. In addition to her work with student education, she provides services to preschool children with speech and language disorders. She received her bachelor's degree from Lambuth University, her master's degree from the University of Mississippi, and her doctorate from the University of Tennessee.

**Michelle M. Ferketic**, MA, CCC-SLP, is Director, Special Interest Divisions and International Liaison Programs of the American Speech-Language-Hearing Association. Prior to joining ASHA, she was a speech-language pathologist at the University of Pittsburgh Cleft Palate-Craniofacial Center. Ms. Ferketic received her bachelor and master's degrees from the University of Pittsburgh.

**John Ferraro**, PhD, is the Doughty-Kemp Chairman and Professor of the Hearing and Speech Department, KUMC, Co-Director of the KU Intercampus Program in Communicative Disorders, and Associate Dean for Research, School of Allied Health. Prior to his appointment at KU, he served on the faculty at The Ohio State University and also as a Clinical Neurophysiologist at Swedish Medical Center in Englewood, Colorado. He received his BS in biology from Southern Colorado State College and his MS in biology and PhD in speech and hearing sciences at the University of Denver. Dr. Ferraro also completed 2 years of postdoctoral research in the Auditory Physiology Laboratory of Northwestern University under the direction of Peter Dallos.

**Diane Garcia**, MS, CCC-SLP, is an Assistant Professor at the University of Redlands where she supervises the children's speech sound disorders clinic and teaches graduate courses in phonology, diagnostics, and cultural/linguistic diversity. Diane also worked as a speech-language pathologist in the public schools. Her clinical and academic interests include assessment and remediation of articulation and phonological disorders, multicultural issues, and service delivery in the public schools. She has presented on these topics both regionally and nationally.

**Brian Goldstein**, PhD, CCC-SLP, is an Associate Professor in the Department of Communication Sciences at Temple University. He received a BA in linguistics from Brandeis University and an MA and PhD in speech-language pathology from Temple University. Dr. Goldstein is well published in the area of communication development and disorders in Latino children, focusing on phonological development and disorders in monolingual Spanish and Spanish-English bilingual children. Dr. Goldstein is the author of *Cultural and Linguistic Diversity Resource Guide for Speech-Language Pathologists*, the editor of *Bilingual Language Development and Disorders in Spanish-English Speakers*, and was the editor of *Language, Speech, and Hearing Services in Schools* from 2004–2006. He has served on numerous state and national committees including the Multicultural Issues Board, the Publications Board, and the Council of Editors of the American Speech-Language-Hearing Association. He is a Fellow of the American Speech-Language-Hearing Association.

**Howard Goldstein**, PhD, CCC-SLP, is Research Director at the Schoenbaum Family Center at The Ohio State University. He is an ASHA Fellow. His research interests include early intervention and the development of instructional approaches for teaching generalized language, literacy, and social skills to children with developmental disabilities.

**Roxann Diez Gross**, PhD, CCC-SLP, is the Director of the University of Pittsburgh Medical Center Swallowing Disorders Center and Assistant Professor of Otolaryngology at the University of Pittsburgh. She holds a secondary appointment as an Assistant Professor in the Department of Communication Science and Disorders. Her primary area of research involves a multidisciplinary team that examines the interaction between breathing and swallowing in individuals with indwelling tracheostomy tubes, Parkinson's disease, and chronic obstructive pulmonary disease (COPD). In addition, her research group is investigating an agent that has the potential to reduce the local and systemic inflammatory effects of radiation and chemotherapy on swallowing function. Dr. Gross has over 22 years of clinical experience in a variety of settings.

**Ellen Hagerman**, MA, CCC-SLP, is a Clinical Assistant Professor in the Division of Communication Sciences and Disorders at the University of Kentucky. She received her BA at the University of Kentucky and her MA at the University of Northern Colorado. She has provided evaluation and treatment in the Department of Otolaryngology's Speech & Hearing Clinic and for the University's Chandler Medical Center since 1994. She began working with laryngectomy patients in 1979 and was trained in TEP placement in 1989.

**Susan T. Hale**, MS, CCC-SLP, is Director of Clinical Education and Assistant Professor in the Department of Hearing and Speech Sciences at Vanderbilt University. An ASHA fellow, she served as the 2009 President of the American Speech-Language-Hearing Association. She has extensive previous ASHA service on councils and committees in the areas of clinical standards and professional ethics. She served as ASHA Vice President for Quality of Service in Speech-Language Pathology from 2002–2004. She teaches and lectures in the areas of professional ethics, counseling, and clinical supervision. She received her bachelor's and master's degrees from the University of Mississippi.

**Gail Harris-Schmidt**, PhD, CCC-SLP, is a Professor and Chair of the Department of Communication Sciences and Disorders at Saint Xavier University in Chicago. She received her BA in psychology and MA in speech-language pathology from Vanderbilt University and her PhD in learning disabilities from Northwestern University. She is a member of the Scientific and Clinical Advisory Committee of the National Fragile X Foundation, for which she wrote sections of the Foundation website (www.fragilex.org). She is the co-author, with Dr. Dale Fast, of *The Source for Fragile X Syndrome* and "Fragile X Syndrome: Genetics, Characteristics, and Educational Implications" (in *Advances in Special Education*, Vol. 11, 1998). She has co-presented numerous workshops at the national, state, and local levels on the causes and characteristics of and intervention for children with fragile X syndrome.

**Pam Hart**, PhD, CCC-SLP, speech-language pathologist, is a faculty member at Rockhurst University in Kansas City, Missouri where she teaches a variety of classes in child language and augmentative and alternative communication (AAC). Investigation of literacy skill acquisition for individuals who use AAC is a focus of Dr. Hart's research. Clinically, Dr. Hart provides AAC assessment and intervention services with the Adaptive Computer and Communication Technology program at The Rehabilitation Institute of Kansas City.

**Brooke Hatfield**, MS, CCC-SLP, is a Senior Speech-Language Pathologist at the National Rehabilitation Hospital in Washington, DC. She works primarily with patients with acquired neurogenic communication disorders. She has published and/or presented in the areas of best practices in inpatient stroke rehabilitation, advocacy, group aphasia treatment, and augmentative communication. She received her bachelor's degree in speech pathology and audiology from Miami University in 1996 and her master's degree from Vanderbilt University in 1998.

**Barbara W. Hodson**, PhD, CCC-SLP, is a Professor in the Department of Communication Sciences and Disorders at Wichita State University. An ASHA Fellow, she is a Board Recognized Specialist in Child Language and received the Frank Kleffner Clinical Career Award in 2004 and ASHA Honors of the Association in 2009. Her major professional interests include clinical phonology, metaphonology, and early literacy.

**Tiffany P. Hogan**, PhD, CCC-SLP, is a clinical speech-language pathologist and Assistant Professor in the Department of Special Education and Communication Disorders at the University of Nebraska–Lincoln. Her research focuses broadly on the connection between language development and reading acquisition with an aim at improving early identification and treatment of language-based reading disabilities.

**Emily M. Homer**, MA, CCC-SLP, is Assistant Coordinator of the Speech/Language/Hearing Therapy Program in St. Tammany Parish Schools in Louisiana. She is the 1999 recipient of the Louis M. DiCarlo Award for the establishment of an interdisciplinary dysphagia team in her school district. The majority of her 33 years in the field of speech-language pathology have been in the public school setting. Ms. Homer served as Chairman of ASHA's working committee on dysphagia in the schools. She has presented at ASHA Conventions and offered teleconferences on dysphagia in the schools. She contributed to the Language, Speech and Hearing Services in the Schools forums on dysphagia in the schools and Seminars in Speech and Language and several Division 13 newsletter articles.

**Karen Hux**, PhD, CCC-SLP, received her doctorate in speech-language pathology at Northwestern University. Currently, Dr. Hux is an Associate Professor at the University of Nebraska–Lincoln. She has extensive clinical, research, and teaching experience relating to the language and cognitive challenges of people with acquired brain damage.

**Carla Wood Jackson**, MS, CCC-SLP, is an Assistant Professor in Communication Disorders at Florida State University. She received her doctoral degree at the University of Kansas and has been a certified speech-language pathologist since 1994. Her research and teaching interests include family-centered early intervention with special populations, child language disorders, and dual language learners. Currently she directs a personnel preparation project funded by the Department of Education for training speech-language pathologists to provide early intervention services to children with severe disabilities.

**Cynthia Jacobsen**, PhD, CCC-SLP, ASHA Fellow, is the Director of the Hearing and Speech Clinics and the Cleft Palate Clinic at Children's Mercy Hospital and Clinics, Kansas City, Missouri. She serves on the board of the KS-MO chapter of the International Dyslexia Association and is interested in reading problems of children with and without cleft palate.

**Kathy J. Jakielski**, PhD, CCC-SLP, is Associate Professor and Chair of the Department of Communication Sciences and Disorders at Augustana College in Rock Island, Illinois. Dr. Jakielski worked full time as a clinical speech-language pathologist for 9 years prior to returning to graduate school to pursue her doctorate in the area of normal and disordered speech acquisition, with a focus on children with childhood apraxia of speech (CAS). She has worked with children with CAS for 25 years. Dr. Jakielski is particularly interested in adolescents with CAS and their long-term outcomes as well as intervention efficacy. She is a professional advisory board member for the Childhood Apraxia of Speech Association of North America and has presented and published her findings in the area of CAS and non-CAS speech impairment in children and teens.

**Pat Kearns**, MS, CCC-SLP, is Vice President of Clinical Services at Quality Living, Inc., Omaha, Nebraska. She completed undergraduate studies at Doane College and received her master's degree in physical therapy from the University of Nebraska Medical Center. Ms. Kearns has many years of experience working with adult neurologically based rehabilitation, with specialty areas including gait and biomechanics.

**Sandra Keener**, AuD, CCC-A, is a Clinical Assistant Professor in the Hearing and Speech Department at the University of Kansas Medical Center. She received her BA, MA, and AuD from the University of Kansas. Her clinical interests are pediatric hearing assessment and intervention and cochlear implants. She teaches a graduate course in cochlear implants and hearing assistance technologies. She serves on the Advisory Committee for Sound Beginnings (Kansas Early Hearing Detection and Intervention [EHDI] program).

**Dorothy Kelly**, MS, CCC-SLP, is a speech-language pathologist specializing in assistive technology in St. Tammany Parish Schools in Louisiana. She is on the interdisciplinary dysphagia team where she serves as case manager at several schools. She has participated in presentations on dysphagia, oral motor, and augmentative communications in her district as well as in the community. Prior to working in the school system she was employed at a hospital where she performed numerous bedside and video fluoroscopic swallowing evaluations on infants, children, and adults in the intensive care, acute, skilled nursing, and outpatient environments. She also performed video fluoroscopic swallow studies on all patients in the study titled "Benefits of Thickened Feeds in Previously Healthy Infants with Respiratory Syncytial Viral Bronchiolitis" (in *Pediatric Pulmonology,* Vol. 31, 2001).

**Gail B. Kempster**, PhD, CCC-SLP, is an Associate Professor in the Department of Communication Disorders and Sciences at Rush University in Chicago and the Program Director in Speech-Language Pathology. She received her bachelor's degree from Valparaiso University. Her master's degree was completed at Purdue University and her PhD at Northwestern University. Currently, she teaches courses in anatomy and physiology, research methods, and voice disorders and maintains active clinical and research interests in voice and voice disorders. Her most recent scholarly efforts are associated with the Consensus Auditory Perceptual Evaluation of Voice, the instrument known as the CAPE-V, developed for documenting perceived quality features of voice.

**Teresa Kennalley**, AuD, CCC-A, is a Clinical Assistant Professor at KUMC, where she is a clinical supervisor and course instructor. She earned her BA and MA degrees from Wichita State University and her AuD from the Pennsylvania School of Optometry. She has practiced for 25 years as a pediatric audiologist and was an active advocate for passing legislation mandating universal newborn hearing screening in the state of Kansas. She chaired the original task force establishing guidelines for newborn screening in Kansas and served on the original Advisory Committee for Sound Beginnings.

**Ann W. Kummer**, PhD, CCC-SLP, is Senior Director of the Division of Speech Pathology at Cincinnati Children's Hospital Medical Center, one of the largest pediatric speech pathology programs in the country. She is also Professor of Clinical Pediatrics at the University of Cincinnati and an ASHA Fellow. Dr. Kummer has presented workshops on both national and international levels on resonance disorders and velopharyngeal dysfunction and business practices in speech-language pathology. She is the author of many professional articles, 12 book chapters, and an author of the text entitled *Business Practices: A Guide for Speech-Language Pathologists*, published by ASHA. She is co-author of the SNAP test for the Nasometer (KAYPentax), an inventor of the Oral & Nasal Listener, and author of the text *Cleft Palate and Craniofacial Anomalies: The Effects on Speech and Resonance.*

**Joanne P. Lasker**, PhD, CCC-SLP, is currently an Associate Professor in the Department of Communication Disorders at Florida State University. She has published numerous papers and chapters related to assessment and treatment of adults living with acquired neurogenic communication disorders who may benefit from augmentative and alternative communication (AAC) techniques. In collaboration with Dr. Kathryn L. Garrett, Dr. Lasker created an online assessment tool entitled the *Multimodal Communication Screening Test for People with Aphasia* (MCST-A), designed for people with aphasia who may be suitable for AAC intervention. She is investigating a treatment technique combining speech generating devices and speech practice for adults with apraxia of speech. In 2000, Dr. Lasker was invited to participate in the Medicare Implementation Team panel—a group of professionals who advocated successfully for Medicare funding of AAC speech-generating devices for adults with acquired communication disorders.

**Dorian Lee-Wilkerson**, PhD, CCC-SLP, is an Associate Professor and also serves as the Coordinator of the Graduate Program in Communicative Sciences and Disorders at Hampton University in Hampton, Virginia. She has presented and published in the areas of diversity, HIV and substance abuse, academic preparation, and clinical training.

**Erin Brooker Lozott**, MS, CCC-SLP, received her master's in communication sciences and disorders at Nova Southeastern University. She worked as a speech language pathologist in the Broward County School System and at Miami Children's Hospital–Dan Marino Center. Erin travels internationally as an autism consultant, conducting trainings, speaking at conferences, and developing programs for families of children with autism spectrum disorders. Erin is a graduate-level adjunct professor at the University of Central Florida Department of Communication Sciences and Disorders. She also works at UCF Center for Autism and Related Disabilities (UCF-CARD) and also has her own speech and language private practice.

**Nidhi Mahendra**, PhD, CCC-SLP, is an Assistant Professor and directs the Aging and Cognition Research Clinic in the Department of Communicative Sciences and Disorders at California State University, East Bay. She is a certified bilingual speech language pathologist with expertise in adult neurogenic language disorders and multicultural issues influencing speech pathology service delivery. She has worked in skilled nursing, hospitals, and private practice settings. She is a member of a committee convened by the American Speech-Language-Hearing Association and the Academy of Neurologic Communicative Disorders and Sciences (ANCDS), charged with developing evidence-based practice guidelines for speech language pathologists serving clients with dementia.

**Eileen Marrinan**, MS, MPH, CCC-SLP, is the Director of the Central New York Cleft and Craniofacial Center at Upstate Medical University in Syracuse, New York. She has dedicated her 20-plus-year career to the care of children with cleft-related speech disorders. Eileen has an academic background in speech pathology and public health. She has focused her research activities in the area of outcome studies and has authored peer-reviewed papers and chapters on cleft and craniofacial–related topics. She is an Adjunct Professor at Syracuse University and has lectured nationally and internationally.

**Julie J. Masterson**, PhD, CCC-SLP, is a Professor of Communication Sciences and Disorders at Missouri State University, where she teaches courses in phonology, language-learning disabilities, and research design. Dr. Masterson is a Fellow of the American Speech-Language-Hearing Association and has served as ASHA Vice President for Research and Technology and President of the Council of Academic Programs in Communication Sciences and Disorders. She was Co-Chair of the 1999 Convention of the American Speech-Language-Hearing Association. Dr. Masterson has over 100 publications and presentations at professional conferences in the areas of spelling, child language, phonology, and technology. She has been an associate editor for the *American Journal of Speech-Language Pathology* and has served as a guest associate editor for *Journal of Speech and Hearing Research; Language, Speech, and Hearing Services in Schools; Topics in Language Disorders;* and *Seminars in Speech and Language*.

**Vicki McCready**, MA, CCC-SLP, received her master's degree from Western Reserve University and is currently Professor and Director of the Speech and Hearing Center in the Department of Communication Sciences and Disorders at The University of North Carolina at Greensboro (UNCG). Ms. McCready has over 30 years of experience in supervision and clinical education and has supervised transgender clients since 2004. She became an ASHA Fellow in 1998.

**Miechelle McKelvey**, PhD, CCC-SLP, completed her doctoral degree in speech-language pathology at the University of Nebraska–Lincoln. She is currently an assistant professor at the University of Nebraska–Kearney, where she teaches courses and conducts research in the area of adult acquired neurogenic disorders.

**Deanna K. Meinke**, MS, CCC-A, is an Associate Professor of Audiology at the University of Northern Colorado in Greeley, CO. She is board certified in audiology by the American Board of Audiology, clinically certified by the American Speech-Language-Hearing Association, and is a Fellow of the American Academy of Audiology. Presently, she serves as past-president for the National Hearing Conservation Association and chairs the "Safe-in-Sound" expert committee for the National Institute of Occupational Safety and Health. She is involved in hearing loss prevention as a clinician, a consultant, an educator, and a researcher. Her current research interests include distortion product otoacoustic emissions and the prevention of noise-induced hearing loss across the life span.

**Ross G. Menzies**, PhD, is a clinical psychologist and head of the Anxiety Disorders Clinic at the University of Sydney. He is an Associate Professor and member of the research team at the Australian Stuttering Research Centre. He has developed cognitive behavior therapy packages for the treatment of obsessive-compulsive disorders and published theories of the origins of phobias. He has an interest in anxiety with those who stutter.

**Brookes Metzler-Barrack**, MS, CCC-SLP, graduated from Rockhurst University in 2003 with a master's degree in communication sciences and disorders. She began her work with children with autism spectrum disorders in 1999, providing home-based respite care and behavioral intervention. She has been employed both in the public school systems and outpatient clinics and served as an early intervention speech-language pathologist in the natural environment with infants and toddlers with special needs. She currently runs an early childhood relationship-based classroom for children with autism spectrum disorders in Kansas City, Missouri.

**Deborah Moncrieff**, PhD, CCC-A, researches auditory disorders across the life span, with particular emphasis on the negative impact of auditory disorders on communication, language, learning, and reading. She has developed and gathered normative data on new tests for clinical assessment of APD. She has also developed a therapeutic approach for remediating children with a binaural integration type of APD (sometimes referred to as an integration deficit), characterized by a unilateral ear deficit during tests of dichotic listening.

**Teri H. Munoz**, MS, CCC-SLP, is a Clinical Instructor in the Department of Communication Sciences and Disorders at Florida International University and the Executive Director of the Pediatric Center for Communication & Feeding Deficiencies, Inc. in Miami. She received her master's degree in speech-language pathology from Nova Southeastern University in 1997. Her bachelor's degree is in special education and was obtained from Florida International University in 1991. Ms. Munoz is the owner/director of a private pediatric practice.

**Sue O'Brian**, PhD, is a Postdoctoral Fellow with the Australian Stuttering Research Centre at The University of Sydney. She has over 20 years of experience treating and conducting clinical trials for adults and children who stutter. Her interests include treatment of anxiety in those who stutter, developing new treatment models for the control of stuttering in adults, and developing methods to measure stuttering in adults and children.

**Mark Onslow**, PhD, is a Professor and the Foundation Director of the Australian Stuttering Research Centre at The University of Sydney. He is also a Principal Research Fellow of the National Health and Medical Research Council of Australia. His core research interests include stuttering treatment research, measurement of stuttering, anxiety in stuttering, and causal theory about stuttering.

**Jean Pedigo**, MA, is the Preschool Program Director at the Children's Center for the Visually Impaired in Kansas City, Missouri. She began working with blind and visually impaired children as a staff speech-language pathologist in 1998 and has worked with toddlers and preschoolers with a wide range of ocular conditions and cortical visual impairment as well as with children who have multiple impairments. In addition to speech and language interventions, she has particular interest in the feeding and oral-sensory needs of this population. She received a BA in French from the University of Missouri-Columbia and an MA in speech-language pathology from California State University, Los Angeles.

**Kristin Pelczarski**, PhD, CCC-SLP, earned her doctorate in the Department of Communication Science and Disorders at the University of Pittsburgh in 2008. Her research explores phonological awareness, phonological encoding, and other linguistic aspects of stuttering in children and adults. Pelczarski also conducts clinical outcomes research at Children's Hospital of Pittsburgh and the Stuttering Center of Western Pennsylvania where she practices as a certified speech-language pathologist. Pelczarski works with preschool, school-age, and adolescent children who stutter and their families. She formerly served as the National Professional Relations Administrator for the National Stuttering Association.

**Beate Peter**, PhD, CCC-SLP, obtained her clinical and academic training at the University of Washington, Seattle, where she graduated from the Department of Speech and Hearing Sciences with BS, MS, and PhD degrees. Mentored by Carol Stoel-Gammon, PhD, she developed an interest in subtypes of childhood speech sound disorders. Her dissertation research showed that some children with severe speech sound disorders have difficulty with timing accuracy in oral as well as hand tasks. During the last year of her doctoral studies, she began working as a speech-language pathologist in the public schools, and it is there that she served the preschooler described in the chapter in this book. She is currently pursuing postdoctoral research in medical genetics to explore the role of processing speeds in communication disorders from a molecular and quantitative genetics perspective.

**Meredith A. Poore**, MA, is a doctoral student in speech physiology and neuroscience at the University of Kansas. Her extensive work with premature infants in the neonatal intensive care unit concerns the relations between patterned orocutaneous stimulation (via NTrainer® technology), development of suck and oral feeding skills, and the emergence of babbling. Ms. Poore and colleagues have recently published an original data-based study on the effects of patterned orocutaneous stimulation on the stability of the suck central pattern generator in tube-fed premature infants (Poore et al., *Acta Paediatrica*, 2008), and she is co-author of several articles in pediatric oromotor development and speech production and perception in adults.

**Sheila Pratt**, PhD, CCC-A/SLP, is a faculty member in the Department of Communication Science and Disorders at the University of Pittsburgh and a researcher on the Geriatric Research Education and Clinical Center at the VA Pittsburgh Healthcare System. She teaches courses in auditory rehabilitation and speech perception. Her research focuses on the diagnosis and treatment of communication disorders that occur secondary to hearing loss in children and adults.

**Jill E. Preminger**, PhD, CCC-A, is an Associate Professor of Audiology at the University of Louisville School of Medicine. She coordinates the research program for the Doctor of Audiology Program and is a past winner of the Program in Audiology Teaching Award. Her research interests are in adult rehabilitative audiology. She is involved in measuring the efficacy of group audiologic rehabilitation programs, the role of spouses in the rehabilitation process, and techniques to validate hearing aid fittings. Dr. Preminger is an associate editor for the *Journal of Speech, Language, and Hearing Research* as well as an assistant editor for the *Journal of the American Academy of Audiology*. She is a past president of the Academy of Rehabilitative Audiology.

**Erin Redle**, PhD, CCC-SLP, is a speech-language pathologist and Research Coordinator at Cincinnati Children's Hospital Medical Center and an Adjunct Assistant Professor at the University of Cincinnati. Dr. Redle specializes in pediatric feeding, swallowing disorders, and early motor development for both speech and swallowing. She has presented nationally on these topics. Dr. Redle and Dr. Carolyn Sotto are currently conducting a longitudinal study of fricative development in children between the ages of 9 months and 3 years.

**Suzanne Coyle Redmond**, MA, CCC-SLP, is a Senior Speech-Language Pathologist at the National Rehabilitation Hospital in Washington, DC. She works primarily with patients with acquired neurogenic communication disorders. She has published and/or presented in the areas of aphasia, traumatic brain injury, voice, and ethics. She received her bachelor's degree in speech pathology and audiology from Miami University in 1997 and her master's degree from Miami University in 1999.

**Jenny A. Roberts**, PhD, CCC-SLP, is an Associate Professor in the Department of Speech-Language-Hearing Sciences at Hofstra University. She is a developmental psychologist and ASHA-certified speech-language pathologist. She became interested in the language development of internationally adopted children while working as an SLP in the late 1990s. At that time, there was little published research available for determining typical language development in the population of internationally adopted children. In 2000, she began collaborating with colleagues, some of whom had adopted children of their own, and together they conducted several studies on the language development of children adopted from China. She is the proud aunt of two beautiful nieces adopted from China.

**Richard A. Roberts**, PhD, CCC-A, is the Director of Vestibular Services for Alabama Hearing & Balance Associates, a private audiology practice. He received his PhD from the University of South Alabama. Dr. Roberts has previously held positions on the faculty at the University of Mississippi and the University of South Florida, where he continues to teach as an adjunct professor. Dr. Roberts also held the position of Director of Clinical Studies at The American Institute of Balance. He is well published in the leading peer-reviewed scientific journals of the field and serves as an editorial consultant to many of these. Dr. Roberts has been an assistant editor for the *Journal of the American Academy of Audiology* since 2002. He is frequently invited to lecture on various vestibular topics at the national and international level.

**Elaine S. Sands**, PhD, CCC-SLP, is an Associate Professor in the Department of Communication Sciences and Disorders at Adelphi University, Garden City and New York. Dr. Sands has served as Department Chair and Dean of the School of Education and holds the rank of Associate Professor of Communication Sciences and Disorders. She received her BA from Brooklyn College, MS from the University of Michigan, and PhD from New York University. At Michigan she trained in the nationally recognized Residential Aphasia program. Dr. Sands is a Fellow of the American Speech-Language-Hearing Association and a charter member of the Academy of Aphasia. She is past president of the Long Island Speech Language and Hearing Association and has received the Distinguished Service Award of the New York State Speech Language and Hearing Association. In 1999 she received the Honors of the Long Island Speech-Language-Hearing Association. She is a past member of ASHA's Professional Services Board and the ASHA Board of Ethics.

**Michele Schmerbauch**, MS, CCC-SLP, received her master's degree in speech-language pathology at the University of Nebraska–Lincoln. She is currently practicing at Luther Midelfort, a Mayo Clinic affiliate hospital in Eau Claire, Wisconsin. She has clinical experience in acute care and rehabilitation settings with individuals with acquired brain injuries.

**Jamie B. Schwartz**, PhD, CCC-SLP, is Associate Professor in the Department of Communication Sciences and Disorders at the University of Central Florida. She teaches graduate courses in language development and disorders, emergent literacy acquisition, developmental reading and writing disorders, and research methods. She is a consultant for the University of Central Florida's Center for Autism and Related Disabilities (UCF-CARD). She has published her research in a variety of peer-reviewed journals as well as the Campbell Collaboration Library, an electronic repository of peer reviews in education, crime and justice, and social welfare.

**Diane M. Scott**, PhD, CCC-A, is the Associate Dean of Graduate Studies in the School of Education at North Carolina Central University (NCCU). She is also a faculty member in the Department of Communication Disorders at NCCU. Dr. Scott has taught at Hampton University, Michigan State University, and Howard University. She served as the Director of Multicultural Affairs at the American Speech-Language-Hearing Association. Her areas of interest in audiology include pediatric audiology, diagnostic audiology, genetics, and multicultural issues. She has presented at conferences and published articles and book chapters on the audiological effects of sickle cell disease.

**Kathleen A. Scott**, PhD, CCC-SLP, is an Assistant Professor in the Department of Speech-Language Hearing Sciences at Hofstra University. Her doctoral dissertation was on the spoken and written language skills of school-age children adopted from China. She has made several presentations and written articles concerning the language development of internationally adopted children. She is the proud aunt of two beautiful nephews adopted from Guatemala.

**Kathleen Scaler Scott**, PhD, CCC-SLP, is a speech-language pathologist and Board Recognized Specialist in Fluency Disorders and has practiced clinically for 15 years in school, hospital, and private practice settings. Ms. Scaler Scott has lectured nationally and internationally on fluency and social communication disorders. She is currently Coordinator of the International Cluttering Association.

**Jeff Searl**, PhD, CCC-SLP, is an Associate Professor in the Hearing and Speech Department at the University of Kansas Medical Center. Dr. Searl obtained his master's and PhD degrees in speech-language pathology from this same department in 1991 and 1999. He currently teaches and performs clinical work related to voice disorders, communication issues associated with cleft lip/palate, and swallowing disorders. Dr. Searl's research interests are in voice disorders, motor speech production in both normal and disordered speech, and head and neck cancer rehabilitation, particularly aerodynamic and articulatory changes in alaryngeal speech.

**Trisha L. Self**, PhD, CCC-SLP, is an Assistant Professor in the Communication Sciences and Disorders Department at Wichita State University in Wichita, Kansas, and is a Board Recognized Specialist in Child Language. She teaches a graduate course in autism spectrum disorders and undergraduate courses in genetics and organic anomalies and introduction to clinical practices. She also supervises students working with clients who have been diagnosed on the autism spectrum. Trisha has 22 years of experience working with children with severe speech-language disabilities, including those diagnosed on the autism spectrum.

**Amee P. Shah**, PhD, CCC-SLP, is an Assistant Professor in the Speech and Hearing Department at Cleveland State University. She has extensive clinical experience as a speech-language pathologist, specializing in working with the bilingual population and clients with foreign-accents. Her research at the Speech Acoustics & Perception Laboratory at CSU involves cross-language speech perception and production, with a focus on understanding variables and processes underlying foreign accentedness. She has numerous presentations and publications related to her research.

**Robert J. Shprintzen**, PhD, CCC-SLP, is the director of several programs at Upstate Medical University in Syracuse, New York, including the Communication Disorder Unit, The Velo-Cardio-Facial Syndrome International Center, and the Center for Genetic Communicative Disorders. He is Professor of Otolaryngology and Professor of Pediatrics. He authored or co-authored more than 190 peer-reviewed papers and chapters and is the author of six books, including *Velo-Cardio-Facial Syndrome: Diagnosis and Evaluation*. He is widely credited for delineating four genetic disorders, all of which bear his name in the medical literature. He is an ASHA Fellow and he received ASHA's Outstanding Clinical Achievement Award in 1992. In 1995, Dr. Shprintzen founded The Velo-Cardio-Facial Syndrome Educational Foundation, Inc. and served as that organization's Executive Director from 1995 through 2003. He has been the President of two international professional societies and served as editor for two, as well.

**Jeffry Snell**, PhD, completed a master's degree in Psychometrics Psychology at Northeast Louisiana University and a doctoral degree in psychology at the University of Southern Mississippi with a specialization in clinical psychology. Dr. Snell currently serves as Director of Research and Psychology Services at Quality Living, Inc., Omaha, Nebraska.

**Carolyn Sotto**, PhD, CCC-SLP, is Assistant Clinical Professor and Undergraduate Director in the Department of Communication Sciences and Disorders at the University of Cincinnati. She teaches graduate and undergraduate courses in child language, literacy, and phonology. She has presented to pediatricians, teachers, administrators, and speech-language pathologists at numerous state and national conferences.

**Tamsen St Clare**, BA, is a clinical psychologist with extensive experience in cognitive behavior therapy. She was involved in a recent randomized controlled trial of cognitive behavior therapy for social anxiety in those who stutter, and this led to her interest in this disorder. She currently works at the Department of Medical Psychology at Westmead Hospital in Sydney.

**Kenneth O. St. Louis**, PhD, CCC-SLP, is a Professor of speech-language pathology at West Virginia University. A Board Recognized Specialist in Fluency Disorders, he has contributed widely to the literature on cluttering and stuttering for 35 years. St. Louis was the first recipient of the Deso Weiss Award for Excellence in Cluttering.

**Julie A. G. Stierwalt**, PhD, CCC-SLP, is an Associate Professor of Communication Disorders at Florida State University, where she teaches courses in anatomy and physiology, dysphagia, acquired communication disorders, structural-based communication disorders, and medical speech pathology. Dr. Stierwalt received her BA and MA from the University of Northern Iowa, and her PhD from the University of Iowa. She has published numerous articles and chapters in the areas of neurogenics and dysphagia. Dr. Stierwalt is an ASHA Fellow, serves on the Executive Council for NSSLHA, and frequently serves on the ASHA Convention Program Committee as Topic Chair and reviewer in the areas of adult language, motor speech, and dysphagia.

**Kathy H. Strattman**, PhD, CCC-SLP, is an Associate Professor in the Department of Communication Sciences and Disorders at Wichita State University. She is a Board Recognized Specialist in Child Language and a past recipient of the Kansas Speech-Language Pathologist of the Year Award. Her teaching, clinical, and research interests are in the areas of language and literacy development and intervention.

**Natasha Trajkovski**, PhD, is an SLP who specializes in the treatment of preschool children who stutter. Her core research interests include the development of stuttering interventions for preschool children. She earned her PhD at the Australian Stuttering Research Center, University of Sydney.

**Rebecca Volk**, BS, is a graduate student in speech-language pathology at the University of Arizona. Her clinical interests include language-literacy disorders across the life span. After finishing her master's degree, she plans to obtain a PhD, focusing on brain functioning, language, and literacy.

**David Ward**, PhD, is a Lecturer and Director of the Speech Research Laboratory at the University of Reading, UK. A qualified speech-language pathologist, he has lectured widely on fluency disorders and has written a number of research papers, book chapters, and recently a textbook on stuttering and cluttering.

**Janelle Ward**, MA, CCC-SLP, graduated from the University of Missouri–Columbia with a bachelor's degree in communication sciences and disorders and a master's degree in speech-language pathology. Mrs. Ward has previously worked as a speech-language pathologist in the public schools and is currently the Director of Clinical Services at Quality Living, Inc., Omaha, Nebraska.

**Amy L. Weiss**, PhD, CCC-SLP, is a Professor in the Department of Communicative Disorders at the University of Rhode Island. She is a Fellow of the American Speech-Language-Hearing Association and currently serves as the Chair of its Board of Division Coordinators. A Board Recognized Specialist in Child Language (ASHA), Dr. Weiss teaches courses in child language disorders that focus on infancy through adolescence as well as courses in speech sound disorders, fluency disorders, and cultural and linguistic diversity as related to assessment and intervention. Her research has investigated the interface between pragmatic language use and the presence of language disorders in children who stutter as well as children diagnosed with SLI or hearing impairment. She is currently editing a book that will explore the relationship between the individual differences that young clients bring to the clinical table and the success of their speech-language intervention.

**Kristy Weissling**, SLP.D., CCC-SLP, received her professional doctorate from Nova Southeastern University and is currently a lecturer at the University of Nebraska–Lincoln. Dr. Weissling has clinical, research, and student supervisory experiences in the areas of adult acquired communication disorders and augmentative and alternative communication.

**Laurie Wells**, AuD, FAAA, is a board-certified audiologist and manager of audiology for Associates In Acoustics, Inc., a consulting firm specializing in the prevention of noise-induced hearing loss. She currently serves as the American Academy of Audiology representative on the Council for Accreditation in Occupational Hearing Conservation and is a past president of the National Hearing Conservation Association.

**Jonathon P. Whitton** is a doctoral candidate in the Division of Communicative Disorders at the University of Louisville School of Medicine where he is a past winner of the AuD Spirit Award. He has worked in the Audiologic Rehabilitation lab at the university for over a year. His research interests are related to the plasticity of the central auditory nervous system (CANS) and in particular understanding the changes that occur in the CANS in response to atypical development and to what degree perceptual training can normalize CANS function. He is conducting funded research in perceptual training–induced malleability of multisensory circuits. Jonathon is also involved in research at Vanderbilt University and the University of Kentucky. Jonathon has served at the local and national levels as a board member of the National Association of the Future Doctors of Audiology.

**Judith Widen**, PhD, CCC-A, is an audiologist and Associate Professor in the Department of Hearing and Speech at the University of Kansas Medical Center (KUMC). She has a BA from Washington State University, an MS from Portland State University, and her PhD from the University of Washington. Much of her career has focused on hearing screening and assessment of infants and children. She participated in three national multicenter grants and has served on working groups for the National Institute of Deafness and Other Communication Disorders (NIDCD) and the American Speech-Language Hearing Association (ASHA). Most recently she was an ASHA representative to the Joint Committee on Infant Hearing.

**Suzie Wiley**, OTR, is an occupational therapist at The Rehabilitation Institute of Kansas City where she specializes in access strategies related to assistive technology for computer access, AAC, and environmental control. She co-founded the institute's Adaptive Computer and Communication Technology Program in 1989. Over the past 13 years, Suzie has served as an adjunct faculty member responsible for the assistive technology curriculum in the Occupational Therapy programs at Rockhurst University in Kansas City and the University of Missouri–Columbia.

**Diane L. Williams**, PhD, CCC-SLP, is an Assistant Professor in the Department of Speech-Language Pathology at Duquesne University. She has over 30 years of clinical experience with children and adults with a range of developmental language disorders including both low- and high-functioning autism. Dr. Williams studies cognition, language processing, and learning in high-functioning older children, adolescents, and adults with autism using behavioral measures and functional magnetic resonance imaging. She is the Co-Director of the NIH-funded Autism Center for Excellence at the University of Pittsburgh and is affiliated with the Center for Cognitive Brain Imaging at Carnegie Mellon University. Dr. Williams has published and presented extensively on the neurodevelopmental disorder of autism. A primary focus of her research program is the design of intervention based on an understanding of how individuals with autism process information.

**Judith Maige Wingate**, PhD, CCC-SLP, is an Assistant Clinical Professor at the University of Florida, Department of Communication Sciences and Disorders and serves as Director of Clinical Education. She holds a bachelor's degree in music therapy from Charleston Southern University. She received a master's in speech pathology from the University of South Florida in 1983 and her PhD in speech pathology from the University of Florida in 2004. Dr. Wingate is an active member of the Voice Care Team at the University of Florida Ear, Nose, and Throat Clinic. She specializes in the treatment of occupational voice disorders and the singing voice. She is the author of *Healthy Singing*, a vocal health book for singers. She is a member of the Continuing Education Board of the American Speech-Language-Hearing Association.

**Carole Wymer**, MS, CCC-SLP, is a clinical speech language pathologist and clinical instructor in the Department of Speech, Language and Hearing Sciences at the University of Arizona. Her experience includes evaluation and treatment of preschool speech and language disorders in the public schools and pediatric clinics.

**J. Scott Yaruss**, PhD, CCC-SLP, is an Associate Professor in the Department of Communication Science and Disorders at the University of Pittsburgh and the Associate Director of the Department of Audiology and Communication Disorders at Children's Hospital of Pittsburgh. A Board Recognized Specialist in Fluency Disorders, Dr. Yaruss has served on the board of directors for the National Stuttering Association and as Associate Coordinator for the American Speech-Language-Hearing Association Special Interest Division for Fluency Disorders. His research examines linguistic, motoric, and temperamental factors that contribute to the development of stuttering in young children as well as methods for evaluating treatment outcomes in children, adolescents, and adults who stutter. Dr. Yaruss is an ASHA Fellow.

**Scott R. Youmans**, PhD, CCC-SLP, is an Assistant Professor in the Department of Communication Sciences and Disorders at Long Island University's Brooklyn Campus. He obtained his BS from the College of Saint Rose, his M.Ed. from North Carolina Central University, and his PhD from Florida State University. Dr. Youmans has had clinical experience in schools, rehabilitation centers, outpatient clinics, nursing homes, consulting, and private practice; however, the majority of his clinical career has been spent as an acute care, hospital-based speech-language pathologist. His clinical specializations include adults with acquired neurogenic communication and swallowing disorders and status postlaryngectomy. Dr. Youmans teaches in the areas of research, anatomy and physiology, dysphagia, voice, and motor speech disorders. His research publications and presentations are in the area of adult acquired neurogenic communication disorders and, in particular, swallowing and swallowing disorders.

**Emily A. Zimmerman**, MA, CFY-SLP, is a doctoral student (speech physiology and neuroscience) at the University of Kansas. Her work in the neonatal intensive care unit concerns the relations between patterned orocutaneous stimulation (via NTrainer® technology) and the development of suck and oral feeding skills in tube-fed preterm infants who are also at risk for brain injury and neurodevelopmental outcomes. Ms. Zimmerman has recently published an original data-based study on the effects of pacifier stiffness on ororhythmic pattern production in infants (Zimmerman et al., *J. Neonatal Nursing*, 2008), and is co-author of several articles in pediatric oromotor development.

**Robyn A. Ziolkowski**, PhD, CCC-SLP, is on the research faculty at The Ohio State University. Her research interests include literacy and language development/disorders, socioeconomic differences in achievement, and evidence-based practice. She has over 14 years of clinical experience working with children and adults with communication disorders.

# PREFACE

## *Casebook Songs*

### Introducing Our Book

*The Communication Disorders Casebook: Learning by Example* is intentionally different from most textbooks in communication sciences and disorders in both breadth and depth. The book includes an unusually broad examination of individuals with a variety of communication disorders. In-depth case reports describe real-life examples of clinical encounters between clinicians and the clients they serve, with references to current literature and discussion of scientific evidence, clinicians' experiences, and clients' preferences.

We hope that the book will serve many audiences, including students, practicing clinicians, colleagues from other health care professions, and consumers of speech-language pathology and audiology services. An accompanying **Instructor's Manual,** led in authorship by our dear friend and colleague Dr. Dorian Lee-Wilkerson, poses provocative questions concerning each case, offers additional resources, and includes a test bank.

This book brings together a remarkably diverse and gifted group of scholars and clinicians. The cases themselves involve individuals across the age range. The text contains 61 cases divided into four sections by age group (infant/toddler, preschool, school age, and adult). Each situation depicts a unique relationship between at least two partners: a client and a clinician. Each author shares his or her story so that readers can learn about individuals with communication disorders and how they are evaluated and treated from the perspectives of those who provide services. The first chapter describes the common elements of each case study.

Our collective approach is decidedly client centered and challenges readers to give weight to both the art and science of our profession. We trust you will agree that the therapeutic relationship that develops between a clinician and client (and/or the client's family) is enhanced by a spirit of mutual respect and collaboration and a focus on solutions and quality of life.

### Reaching Back—Before We Look Ahead

To set the stage for your reading of the case studies, we ask you to think back to the first person you met with atypical speech and/or hearing. Can you recall the details of that interaction, the individual's communication characteristics, and how you felt? How did this person function within his or her day-to-day environment? What impact did this person have on your decision to enter or interact with our profession? We will each share one of our stories.

**Shelly:** I have a number of clients whom I remember with affection and gratitude. I will begin at the beginning, with my first client as a new graduate student. My "clinical assignment" (I will call him Bill) was a college freshman who stuttered. This young man was a basketball star and was over 6'6" tall. As someone who is not quite 5' and who had never worked with a person who stuttered, I felt intimidated by his height and the severity of his speech disorder and concerned about how I could help, given my limited experience. Each time Bill spoke he diverted his eye contact, his face turned red, and he started to perspire, apparently because of the effort required to communicate. It seemed as if he stuttered on every word. I wanted to politely excuse myself, but his gentleness and his determination "to get rid of 'this' before it ruins everything" changed my mind and my life. I read all I could find on stuttering, talked with professors and supervisors, and observed my fellow student clinicians. I also decided to accompany Bill to some of his classes and even a few basketball game practices so I could see and hear his communication outside of the clinic room. He worked hard and seemed extremely motivated to change. We shared in the success of his becoming stutter-free and of the partnership that led him down a new path. During treatment, he spoke of the pain and frustration he felt as a person who stuttered. He continually expressed his appreciation to me for what had been achieved. I am not sure I ever told him just how much he meant to me. Perhaps I didn't know. So, "thank you, Bill. You had a profound and lasting impact on me as a person and a professional."

**Ellen:** My first memories of a person with an atypical speech disorder date to the late 1950s, when I was no more than 3 years old. Like Shelly, I am profoundly grateful for the lessons learned. Walking hand-in-hand with my dad on the way to buy a new toy at the five-and-ten store, we passed by a man whose loud voice and appearance truly startled me. My father whispered, "Don't be scared, that's Cookie." He warmly acknowledged Cookie and introduced me to him.

Cookie, as he was affectionately known by almost all who lived in our small New Jersey seaside town, was a man with multiple disabilities. He was largely edentulous and had a very hoarse voice and limited, difficult-to-understand speech. By traditional clinical standards, Cookie's speech and expressive language would indeed be considered disordered. In addition, Cookie walked with a severe gait disturbance and one arm appeared contracted. Cookie's vocal quality attracted attention and was jarring to listen to—initially frightening small children. That is, however, only part of the story. Cookie was known by first name and was beloved and since remembered by many of the residents. Cookie held a full-time job in which he used his voice to sell a product. With a smile for all, each day Cookie stood near the five-and-ten store on Broadway Avenue and called out "aper, aper" to sell *The Daily Record*.

U.S. Poet Laureate (1997–2000) Robert Pinsky, PhD, also a native of Long Branch, New Jersey, immortalized Cookie in his collection of poetry, *The Figured Wheel: New and Collected Poems, 1966–1996*. Pinsky vividly celebrated Cookie and his hoarse voice within the fabric of a small town's "song" in the title of his poem, "A Long Branch Song."

First, Pinsky presented the environment within which Cookie lived:

*Some days, in May, little stars.*
*Winked all over the ocean. The blue*
*Barely changed all morning and afternoon:*

And then, as in any good case report, Pinsky succinctly described Cookie's voice, unique communication style, and employment:

*The chimes of the bank's bronze clock;*
*The hoarse voice of Cookie, hawking*
The Daily Record *for thirty-five years.**

Later, U.S. Representative Frank Pallone entered "A Long Branch Song," additional Pinsky poems, and his own recollection of Cookie in the 1997 U.S. Congressional Record (H.R.R., 1997-05-06).

How many of us can say that we are affectionately remembered by our first name (and a distinctive voice) by several generations of one small town, were celebrated by both a U.S. Poet Laureate and a U.S. congressman, and featured in the preface of a book on communication science and disorders? Cookie's story embodies our commitment to the importance of looking

* "A Long Branch Song" from *The Figured Wheel: New and Collected Poems 1966–1996* (p. 148), by Robert Pinsky. 

beyond a diagnosis. We must always interpret the impact of our clients' communication capacities on their hopes and dreams as they relate to their family and friends, workplaces, and communities. It is important to create the possibilities for joyful human communication in the context of accepting environments that de-emphasize the prefix *dis* in the term *disability*.

Remembering Cookie and Bill and the thousands of clients we have collectively had the privilege to know, we have written this book to underscore the importance of putting the person first. We trust you will enjoy meeting the clients and gifted clinicians within these 61 case studies and that you will be enriched by their collective "songs."

Shelly S. Chabon, PhD, CCC-SLP
Ellen R. Cohn, PhD, CCC-SLP

## Authors' Note

Cookie is referred to by his real name, as the author did not engage in a clinical interaction with him. He has been previously publicly named in newspapers, a book, and the U.S. Congressional Record.

## Reference

Pallone, F. (May 5, 1997). America's 39th Poet Laureate Robert Pinsky, C-SPAN Congressional Chronicle, http://www.c-spanarchives.org/congress/?q=node/77531&id=6819033

# ACKNOWLEDGMENTS

***To our authors:*** Thank you for entrusting your outstanding work to this project. As co-editors of this text, we recognize we may be biased in our assessment, but even our high hopes did not prepare us for the level of quality of content and the degree of cooperation we received from you, our colleagues.

***To our project assistants:*** We could not have asked for two better project assistants: Natasha Hanova (in Kansas) and Clare Sabatini (in Oregon).

***To a treasured colleague:*** We thank Dr. Dorian Lee-Wilkerson for her contributions as first author of the Instructor's Manual.

***To our publisher:*** Thank you to Stephen D. Dragin, Executive Editor and Publisher, Pearson Education; Editorial Assistant Anne Whittaker; Senior Project Manager Linda H. Bayma; Angela Urquhart at Thistle Hill Publishing Services; and many others who provided the guidance and support needed to bring this book to press.

***To our dear families and friends:*** We are immensely grateful for your sustaining love, encouragement, and understanding. You are our true sources of strength, laughter, and pride.

# Making the Case for Case-Based Learning

Ellen R. Cohn and Shelly S. Chabon

## An Overview

> *For three decades as a physician, I looked to traditional sources to assist me in my thinking about patients; textbooks and medical journals, mentors and colleagues with deeper or more varied clinical experience; students and residents who posed challenging questions. But after writing this book, I realized that I can have another vital partner who helps improve my thinking, a partner who may, with a few pertinent and focused questions, protect me from the cascade of cognitive pitfalls that cause misguided care. That partner is present in the moment when flesh-and-blood decision-making occurs. That partner is my patient or her family member or friend who seeks to know what is in my mind, how I am thinking. And by opening my mind I can more clearly recognize its reach and its limits, its understanding of my patient's physical problems and emotional needs. There is no better way to care for those who need my caring.* (Groopman, 2007, p. 269)

*The Communication Disorders Casebook: Learning by Example* is a book about a few of the many special people with communication problems and those who are privileged to serve them. It provides students, faculty, and practicing clinicians with relevant "real-life" examples of clinical encounters between clinicians and clients. Why did we perceive a need for this text? Although there are many excellent resources in communication sciences and disorders, few books present rich, "student-friendly" case studies across a broad spectrum of settings, client ages, and communication disorder types. These cases illustrate the importance of asking "pertinent and focused questions" (Groopman, 2007), seeking to reconcile the perspectives of all involved, and accepting that there are likely to be "multiple truths" (L. Fox, group presentation, June 3, 2009).

We envisioned several audiences for this book with a shared interest in the use of case studies as an experiential education strategy that provides both foundational knowledge and awareness of its utility in clinical work.

1. *Prospective students* who are considering undergraduate and/or graduate study in communication sciences and disorders might read this book to expand their views of the discipline by gaining the perspectives of practicing clinicians.
2. *Undergraduate and graduate students* in communication sciences and disorders might apply these "real-life" cases to their classroom studies.
3. *New clinicians* might use this book to assist them in developing a framework for clinical decision making.
4. *University faculty members and practicing clinicians* may wish to acquire new understanding of parts of the field they might not typically encounter and gain new perspectives from experienced clinicians related to their current practice.

We also expect that some *persons with communication disorders and their families* may read specific cases to gain insights concerning their personal communication challenges.

The cases described in this book are intentionally varied in terms of the client's age, complexity and type of communication disorders, diagnostic and treatment approaches, and length of treatment. The body of work, however, is unified as follows. Consistent with our clinical philosophies, we have adopted a "client"-centered approach, wherein a real or fictional person (sometimes a composite of individuals seen over an author's years of clinical practice) is the central focus of each chapter. Of course, one chapter on the topic of a speech or hearing disorder cannot represent the entire universe of people with that particular disorder. There are no "textbook cases." Two individuals who share a common diagnosis are not likely to be otherwise identical. We do expect, however, that the background information and clinical reasoning the authors present will elucidate each topic area, and that questions generated and methods considered may be relevant to the treatment of other individuals.

Readers of the book may use it to expand their knowledge of a wide range of communication disorders in both children and adults as well as their skill in applying that knowledge to solve a clinical problem. They may relate to the individuals described on the following pages on an affective level, resulting in empathy and a quality of understanding and caring about the individuals featured. We believe that this combination of facts and feelings may well increase readers' application, retention, and generalization of the content. We also hope that review of these cases will encourage readers to "think like clinicians." That is, reading about the experiences of the clients and clinicians featured in this text will provide an appreciation for the opportunities and the challenges involved in the practice of speech-language pathology and audiology.

Some of these cases describe treatment approaches that are supported empirically. Others reflect the wisdom of practice and insights accumulated from clinical careers filled with tested and reasoned discoveries. All provide a balanced, multidimensional context in which the complexities and ambiguities of the clinical relationship are evident and clinical decisions are realized. In short, we believe that readers will benefit from the lessons learned and shared by the authors.

The text is divided into four sections by client age group (infant/toddler, preschool, school age, adult). It contains 61 cases selected to exemplify both the diversity of our services and the uniqueness of those we serve. A broad review of all of these cases will uncover a variety of methodological approaches to the treatment of individuals with communication disorders. Some of these approaches could not have been foreseen a decade ago. Others have a long tradition in our profession. An examination of a single case will reveal the practical application of an array of methodological possibilities. Each individual case is presented in depth and, as appropriate, includes the following common elements:

- Conceptual knowledge: contains information needed to adequately interpret and resolve the case
- Short introductory paragraph: establishes the problem to be considered
- Background information: provides the historical information necessary to understand the case, summarizes recent developments and significant milestones leading to the clinical problem, and identifies the pertinent facts
- Evaluative findings: allows authors to discuss a professional hypothesis and possible courses of treatment, in consideration of best data, clinical judgment, and individual patient needs
- Description of course of treatment: details the procedures followed for the chosen treatment option, including analysis of patients' responses to the intervention
- Further recommendations: allows for clinician "wrap-up" and review of treatment results as well as reworking of the initial hypothesis and/or suggestions for maintaining positive effects of treatment
- Reference section: lists all sources used within the case for the interest and aid of the reader and for close or further study

## What Is a Case Study?

Each case study in this text is a comprehensive, realistic account of a person with a communication problem that illustrates the decision-making process used to develop, implement, and evaluate clinical services provided by a speech-language pathologist or audiologist. Each case offers a narrative description of the facts, beliefs, feelings, and experiences of the people involved.

## How to Use This Book

*Simply put, good thinkers are good questioners.* (King, 1995, p. 13)

This text is based on the observation that speech-language pathologists and audiologists need strong theoretical knowledge in combination with scientific and clinical skill to make culturally relevant and ethically responsive clinical judgments. It can provide a forum for both the theoretical and the practical aspects, the art and science, of clinical work. Ideally, readers will be moved by a particular case to challenge its theoretical foundation, to ask questions about their own and others' clinical positions, to examine the contexts for the clinical actions, and to consider all of the possible consequences of the professional decisions. One way that this can be accomplished is through the use of questions designed to assess understanding of concepts and theories, their relationship to previous knowledge and experience, and their application to future work. How and why were particular hypotheses formulated? How were evaluation results interpreted, and how were the interpretations applied? How and why did the authors choose particular approaches to intervention? As professionals, we are often distinguished by these types of questions as they inform our scholarship as well as our practices.

Questioning is at the core of science and thus is also central to our clinical success. Asking the right questions guides us to make well-reasoned clinical decisions. So how do you, the reader, know what questions to ask? What types of questions will help you to "realize your potential to learn" (Bain, 2004) from these case studies and lead to an approach of clinical decision making that is clear and understandable? Chabon and Lee-Wilkerson (2006) described a learning framework, adapted from Fink (2003), that offers a prospective organization for such questions. King (1995) provided some "generic question stems," or exemplars, and the level of thinking reflected in each. Lemoncello (2009, unpublished) adapted King's work and created a "Critical Thinking Template" to facilitate case analyses. The following are a few examples of questions relevant to the clinical decision-making process that were formulated based on these earlier writings and incorporated into the learning stages proposed by Fink (2003). When we ask ourselves these questions, we can use them as a mechanism for applying acquired knowledge and skills in new contexts. They foster an ethic of inquiry that shapes the clinical decision-making process reflected by the clinicians and writers included in this text.

## Question Framework

- ***Foundational Knowledge:*** *What do you know about the client in the case study you read?* These questions involve the recall of information, facts, and concepts at a level that invites explanation:
  - What are all of the relevant facts?
  - What are the key physical/emotional/neurological factors that are impaired?
  - Who are the key people involved?
  - What activities are limited for the client because of his or her communication abilities or inabilities?
- ***Skill in Application of Knowledge:*** *How can the information you read be used?* These questions lead to making decisions, solving problems, and performing clinical tasks:
  - Did the client's communication or swallowing improve with treatment, and if so, in what ways?
  - How did the clinician know that the treatment approach was or was not successful?
  - What was measured?
- ***Skill in the Integration of Knowledge:*** *How does the information you read relate to what you knew before?* These questions involve analysis and synthesis, and they reflect connections with previous learning and experiences:
  - What are the strengths and weaknesses of the treatment approach(es) used and assessment methods selected?

   - What are some of the differences between this disorder and other similar or related disorders?
   - What are the differences between the treatment approach(es) used and other similar or related approaches?
   - Was there consensus between the client/family's and clinician's account of the case?
   - Is adequate use made of previous research and observations?
   - Are the inferences drawn clear, sound, and appropriate?
   - How does the information compare with your previous knowledge about or experience with this disorder and/or the treatment of this disorder?
- ***Skill in Acknowledgment of the Human Dimension:*** *Why is what you read important to you and to those you serve? How does what you read confirm or alter your attitudes about the client, family, and yourself as a clinician?* These questions lead to increased insight about self and others:
   - In considering the family's account of the case:
      - What do they believe caused the problem?
      - What were their hopes/fears about the progression and length of the treatment?
      - What are their expectations about the outcome?
      - How might the client's perceptions affect the outcomes of the case?
   - Who will be the client's supports throughout and following treatment?
      - How might the clinician's perceptions of family support affect his or her choice of treatment approach?
   - How did the problems described affect the client's and the client's family's daily life and the interaction between the client and his or her significant others?
   - How will cultural/social factors support or inhibit the treatment?
   - How will personal traits of the clinician support/inhibit the treatment?
   - Whose interests were served and whose were ignored?
   - Does the approach selected reflect an objective attitude? Does the approach take the client's perspective into account?
- ***Skill in Assessing the Relevance of Knowledge:*** *Why is what you read important?* These questions examine the reasons that underlie or support methods or actions and result in meaningful reflection and self-assessment:
   - How does the action taken reflect current criteria, standards, and theory?
   - Why do you believe the clinician selected the particular treatment/assessment method?
   - What are some alternative treatment options/assessment methods?
   - What are the primary reasons for the current outcome?
   - Would you use the same treatment/assessment method? Why or why not?
   - What factors might have led to a different outcome? Why?
- ***Skill in Self-Directed Learning:*** *How do you plan to use what you read about in this case?* These questions lead to active engagement in independent scholarship and reflective practice that continues beyond the reading of a particular case or cases:
   - How could the information provided in the case be applied to other clients?
   - Are there unanswered questions/concerns?
   - How can the treatment program be duplicated and continued by other clinicians/researchers?
   - How can you or other professionals evaluate the treatment described in your own practice?
   - How do the outcomes in the current case study compare to other related cases reported in the literature?
   - What evidence is available to refute or confirm the approaches taken?

These questions are offered as examples and are designed to represent different levels of critical thinking. They will encourage readers to think deeply about and beyond each case. Readers are encouraged to pose other questions or make interpretations of the level or complexity of the learning process, even if they differ from the framework outlined here. Our goal is to ensure that each reader can approach a case with an "inquiring mind" (King, 1995). The use of case studies is based on academic research on learning and the best practices that encourage it. Although the environment and culture in which speech-language pathologists and audiologists practice assign justifiable importance to behavioral outcomes, evidence-based practice, and data collection, we must never forget that it is the person whom we serve who is our partner in the clinical process. We must honor each person's attitudes, aspirations, and quality of life in a competent and ethical manner, as they reside duly at the center of our efforts.

> *The secret of the care of the patient is in caring for the patient.* (Peabody, 1925)

## References


Bain, K. (2004). *What the best college teachers do*. Cambridge: Harvard University Press.

Chabon, S., & Lee-Wilkerson, D. (2006). Instructor's manual and test bank for Anderson and Shames. *Human communication disorders: An introduction* (7th ed.). Boston: Pearson Education.

Fink, L. D. (2003). *Creating significant learning experiences*. San Francisco: Jossey-Bass.

Groopman, J. E. (2007). *How doctors think*. Boston: Houghton Mifflin.

King, A. (1995). Designing the instructional process to enhance critical thinking across the curriculum. *Teaching of Psychology*, *22*(1), 13–17.

Lemoncello, R. (2009). *Critical thinking template* [handout]. Portland, OR: Author.

Peabody, F. W. (1927). The care of the patient. *JAMA*, *88*, 877–882.

PART I

# Infant or Toddler Cases

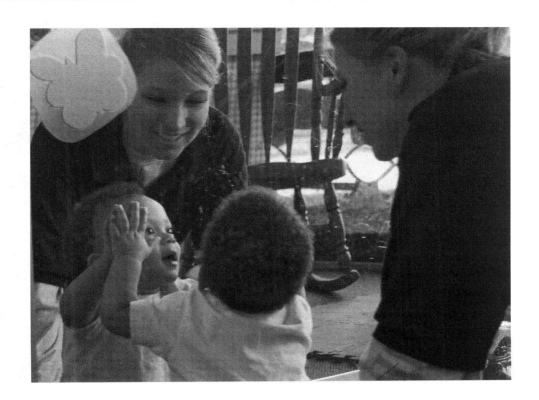

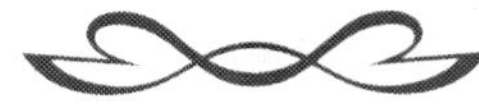

# Autism

CASE 1

# Anne: Developing a Communication Assessment and Treatment Plan for a Toddler Diagnosed with Autism Spectrum Disorders: Special Considerations

*Trisha L. Self and Terese Conrad*

## Conceptual Knowledge Areas

This case study challenges readers to consider their knowledge of development from birth to age 3 years in the specific areas of cognition, receptive/expressive language, play, oral-motor and sensory-motor skills, self-regulation, and nutrition.

Most infants have an innate drive to learn language and socialize with others (Janzen, 2003). In fact, when children's learning systems are developing typically, these skills are acquired automatically without being taught. For children on the autism spectrum, however, early learning strategies, communication skills, and early social skills typically do not develop without intervention.

Early in the developmental process, children on the autism spectrum demonstrate difficulties attending to people. They tend to avoid interactions with others and thus experience fewer opportunities to hear language and practice reciprocal communication. Additionally, because children with an autism spectrum disorder (ASD) typically are not intrinsically motivated to participate in and/or initiate social interactions, they do not engage in the conventional play activities toddlers often use to learn about their environment and the early rules for social engagement (Janzen, 2003).

Children on the autism spectrum often demonstrate difficulties with modulating, processing, and integrating sensory information. These sensory challenges often affect a child's desire to engage in social interactions, and thus affect his or her ability to benefit from naturally occurring learning situations.

The following case study involves a young female child who was referred to a university-based speech-language-hearing clinic by a developmental pediatrician. The child was reported to have delayed speech, language, cognitive, and social skills. She had a history of ear infections and her nutrition intake was poor. The developmental pediatrician had informed the parents that the child was demonstrating early signs of an autism spectrum disorder.

## Description of the Case

### Background Information

At age 1 year 10 months, Anne was referred to a university speech-language-hearing clinic (SLHC) by a developmental pediatrician. The pediatrician was concerned, as were the child's parents, that Anne's receptive and expressive language skills were significantly delayed. The pediatrician also recommended the family seek a highly structured early intervention program within the community.

Upon referral to the university SLHC, the family was asked to complete a case history prior to being scheduled for a speech-language evaluation. Review of the case history and other evaluations provided by the family revealed the following developmental information.

#### Past Medical History

Anne was born to a 25-year-old female at 40 weeks gestation. There was no reported use of alcohol, tobacco, and/or drugs during the pregnancy. At birth, Anne weighed 7 lb 10 oz and was 19 in. long. She responded immediately to breastfeeding and continued to do so without difficulty.

Her mother reported that Anne had chronic ear infections, which were not responsive to antibiotic treatment. Prior to receiving pressure equalization (PE) tubes at approximately 17 months of age, Anne had stopped responding to most sounds, her balance was generally poor, and she had not yet started walking. After receiving the PE tubes, she responded more readily to certain sounds and her balance quickly improved. Not long after the tubes were placed, she began walking.

Anne had otherwise been a healthy child. She had no known drug allergies, and her immunizations were current.

#### Developmental History

Anne began to roll over at approximately 6 months of age, sat independently at 7 months, crawled at about 9 months, and began walking at 17 months (almost immediately after PE tubes had been placed). Anne's mother reported that Anne began to imitate "mama" and "dada" at about 15 months, but would not say those words spontaneously until she was approximately 19 months old. Her mother also reported that Anne babbled at times and imitated a few other words (car, dog).

To communicate her wants/needs, Anne's mother indicated that her daughter would walk to the desired object and stand near it; sometimes she would knock on it and/or attempt to obtain the item on her own. Anne did not use any distal pointing, nor did she use other typical gestures to obtain a desired item/activity.

Her mother reported that Anne was able to respond appropriately to simple questions, such as "Where's your cup?" "Where's your shoe?" and "Where's your brother?" by moving to and/or retrieving the labeled object/person. Additionally, when someone said, "Ready to go outside?" she moved to the door, or when someone said, "Let's go for a ride," she moved toward the garage door. Anne followed an individual's gestural line of regard when items of interest were pointed out and accompanied by information such as "There's a bird" or "There's a cat." But, if she was not interested in the object, she was nonresponsive.

Anne liked to assemble puzzles, roll cars, stack Duplos™, and flip through magazines. She was able to roll a car back and forth with an adult. Anne did not initiate her own play, but would "play" if an adult initiated it. If Anne got excited during play, she would flap her hands and rock back and forth.

Anne was able to feed herself and drank from an open-mouthed cup. She reportedly ate a variety of foods, as long as the foods did not require much chewing.

At bedtime, Anne allowed someone to brush her teeth and tolerated being given a bath, but would not independently wash herself. She did not resist being dressed and, at times, would attempt to assist her parents during this process.

Anne's mother reported that a particular blanket was the greatest source of comfort for her daughter. When Anne held her blanket, it seemed as though she was in another world. She did not respond to activity and/or sound. Because of this, Anne's mother limited the time she was able to access the blanket. She was only allowed to have it during nap times, at bedtime, and when they went out of the house for errands and appointments.

When Anne was approximately 16 months of age, her mother became concerned that she was not walking and her communication skills appeared to be delayed. She took her daughter to a local hospital for an evaluation of her communication and motor skills. At the time of the evaluation, Anne's skills were considered well below normal limits. Her speech and language skills were, reportedly, 7–10 months delayed. Her eye contact and joint attention skills were observed to be poor. She was essentially nonverbal. She demonstrated repetitive hand and finger movements and did not tolerate change. She did not play appropriately with toys (often mouthing them or engaging in perseverative movements back and forth). Following the evaluation, Anne began to receive physical therapy and speech-language treatment until her insurance would no longer support payment.

### Family History/Social History

Anne lived with her mother, father, and brother. Her mother, Amy, was 27 years old, had a college degree, and stayed at home with Anne during the day. Anne's father, Jerrod, was 36 years old and was employed as a computer technician. Anne's brother was 3 years old, and appeared to be developing typically. The parents indicated that there had been a history of developmental differences on both sides of their family. Amy reported that she had a 16-year-old cousin who had been diagnosed with high-functioning autism. Jerrod reported having a sister who was socially challenged, but who had no formal diagnosis.

### Medical Diagnostic History

At age 1 year 8 months Anne was evaluated by a developmental pediatrician. The child's mother reported that she continued to be concerned that Anne was not expressing her needs, had delays in her speech, and did not respond consistently to her name.

During the evaluation Anne did not separate easily from her mother. A neurodevelopmental evaluation revealed that Anne had low muscle tone in both her upper and lower extremities. She was, however, walking independently at the time of the evaluation.

Anne did not want to participate in many activities with the examiner as she demonstrated stranger anxiety during most of the examination. She did respond favorably when cars were presented and moved from her mother's lap to roll them back and forth repeatedly across the floor. She also enjoyed moving a ball back and forth while lying on the floor to watch the rolling movement. She demonstrated excitement when the examiner blew bubbles by flapping her hands. She did not, however, make any attempts to request more. Anne would not respond when the examiner repeatedly called her name and would not establish joint attention with activities presented by her mother or the examiner.

## Reason for Referral

At the time of evaluation, the developmental pediatrician indicated that Anne had significant speech and language delays and poor joint attention and social interaction skills. She was also reported to have stereotypic behaviors. Although the mother was told that Anne demonstrated early signs of an autism spectrum disorder, the doctor indicated that a specific diagnosis might not be reliable prior to 2 years of age.

Based on the findings of the diagnostic evaluation, the developmental pediatrician recommended that the parents seek early intervention services along with individual speech-language treatment. Additionally, he recommended that Anne be tested for fragile X syndrome and have high-resolution chromosome testing completed. After her second birthday, it was recommended that the family return to his office in consultation with a psychologist to reassess the status of the autism spectrum disorder characteristics using the Autism Diagnostic Observation System (Lord, Rutter, DiLavore, & Risi, 1999).

Following the completion of this examination, the parents contacted the local university SLHC for an evaluation with the intent to schedule Anne to receive speech-language intervention.

## Findings of the Evaluation

At age 1 year 9 months, Anne was first brought to the university SLHC by her mother. Based on the information reported in the case history and the medical documentation received from the developmental pediatrician, it was determined that it would be beneficial to design Anne's sessions to provide diagnostic therapy. The purpose for pursuing this plan was to develop a baseline for Anne's receptive and expressive skills and to determine an appropriate communication system based on her abilities and her communication needs (Prelock, 2006).

### Diagnostic Therapy Findings

Anne's ability to initially participate in treatment sessions was inconsistent. She demonstrated a great deal of difficulty transitioning from the waiting room to the treatment room, even when her mother provided her physical support and remained in the treatment room throughout the session.

Anne tended to have more success during treatment when she was reinforced with highly motivational toys (toys with wheels) that she could operate independently while lying on the floor and watching the wheels move back and forth. When she was presented with toys that required assistance from an adult to appropriately activate them (open containers, turn knobs), she would engage in the following behaviors: turn/move away from the adult, refuse to participate, drop to the floor, whine, cry, crawl under furniture, and hide her face. Additionally, Anne would throw items (that were not intended to be thrown) in an apparent attempt to protest engaging with that particular item. Typically, when Anne was frustrated, she would cry, retrieve her blanket, and attempt to get her mother to pick her up. When her mother immediately picked her up, Anne's crying subsided quickly. If her mother did not readily respond and pick her up, the behavior would escalate and the crying continued for several minutes. When Anne came to treatment without her blanket, her ability to participate functionally in any portion of the session decreased and the whining and crying behaviors increased.

## Treatment Options Considered

### Initial Treatment Plan

Prior to completing the diagnostic treatment period, it had been anticipated that Anne's treatment goals would include encouraging her to tolerate hand-over-hand assistance during play activities, spontaneously indicating preferences by choosing 1 item out of a field of 3, and spontaneously requesting an item by exchanging an object/symbol/representation of the item with an adult. Based on the results of the diagnostic therapy sessions as described above, her goals were revised. More importantly, the following modifications were incorporated in an attempt to decrease excess stimulation, reduce stress created by the environment, and encourage Anne to focus and participate.

### Physical Modifications

Current evidence for children with an ASD (Division TEACCH, n.d.) suggests that, when necessary, the physical environment of the treatment room be modified so that unnecessary visual stimulation (decorations on the walls, excess furniture) is eliminated; sensory stimulation that might be distracting/irritating (bright lights, extra treatment materials) is reduced; and preferred motivators to assist with transitions between and within treatment activities are incorporated, thus creating a structured, positive working/playing atmosphere for the child.

To create this type of environment for Anne, the following modifications were implemented. To assist with Anne's transition from the waiting room to the treatment room, a "texture walk" (path of differing textures) was created. This path, approximately 30 feet long, contained a variety of textured pieces (bubble wrap, carpet mats, smooth/silky textures) lined up along the carpeted hallway. Anne was encouraged and assisted to remove her shoes and socks prior to proceeding down the path. Often, Anne stopped and rubbed her feet on certain textures. These textures were also incorporated into the session so she could access them as needed during treatment. Typically, Anne did not need physical assistance to transition down the hallway; only occasional verbal encouragement was needed to keep her moving forward.

The lights in this hallway were turned off; only natural lighting was used as Anne moved from the waiting room to the treatment room. Additionally, her sessions were conducted without overhead fluorescent lighting. The room was lit by the lighting that came through the window naturally in the treatment room.

The furniture in the treatment room was limited. Needed chairs were placed against the walls and only a large tub that was approximately table height for Anne was placed in the center of the room. Other tubs containing additional treatment items were placed near the wall and out of the direct visual line. The large tub contained two to three highly preferred items. Anne was encouraged to choose one toy and engage in functional play for a period of time. When she was finished with the toy, she was encouraged to place it in a finished basket (with a lid), rather than throwing it when she was frustrated and/or wanted to switch activities.

Anne's blanket was available for her to access, when needed, at each session. She often carried it into the therapy room and dropped it when she became interested in activities in the treatment room. The blanket was left in an area that was visible to her throughout the session. The amount of time she spent holding, touching, and/or cuddling in the blanket was tracked (Kranowitz, 2005).

## Course of Treatment

With type of environment established, Anne's goals were revised to encourage her to participate in therapy activities without exhibiting off-task behavior (crying, dropping to the floor) while interacting with the clinicians; to choose 1 preferred item (with minimal prompting) from a field of 2; and to spontaneously request an item by touching a container, which held a desired item, or a digital picture representing that item.

## Analysis of Client's Response to Treatment

Once the physical environment was modified and Anne's treatment goals were revised, her inappropriate behaviors (crying, whining, throwing, hiding, etc.) were reduced. After approximately 2.5 months, Anne was participating and interacting appropriately during 90% of the session (45-minute sessions were scheduled 2 times per week; baseline, 9%). She was making choices from a field of 2 items (one preferred, one foil) with 83% accuracy (baseline, 0%). She began to request an item by touching a container or a representational digital picture with 66% accuracy (baseline, 0%).

The following semester, the modifications used previously were incorporated into Anne's treatment. Although Anne's off-task behaviors had decreased from the past semester, they continued to disrupt her ability to participate at maximal levels throughout treatment sessions. She continued to demonstrate a "need" to hold preferred toys throughout an entire session and would cry/whine during some transitions between activities. After several sessions, the clinicians began to identify additional motivators for Anne. Soon, she began to work without needing to hold her preferred toys. Additionally, she began to respond favorably to a visual work schedule and was eventually able to transition from the waiting room to the treatment room and between activities without incident (Division TEACCH, n.d.).

Anne's goals for this semester included touching an object/color photo to request a preferred item; selecting a picture and choosing the appropriate corresponding item when presented with a choice of two color pictures/photos representing preferred items/activities; and finally, exchanging a picture/photo with a communication partner to request a preferred item/activity (Frost & Bondy, 2002). Initially, Anne's baseline score was 0% for all targeted objectives; by the end of the semester (approximately 3 months; two 45-minute sessions/week), she achieved 90% accuracy or above on all three objectives. Anne also began to spontaneously produce some intelligible and approximated verbalizations (e.g., "no"; "ball"; "block"; /bu/; /mo/) during various activities.

Because Anne achieved her targeted goals, an additional goal was added to improve her turn-taking skills during play-based activities. Initially, Anne was not able to take turns; by the end of the semester, she was able to take her turn at the appropriate time with minimal verbal prompts 96% of the time during highly preferred activities.

## Further Recommendations

It was recommended that future treatment focus on developing appropriate communicative means/acts to assist Anne with making requests and indicating protest/rejection. Additionally, it was recommended that Anne be encouraged to use and practice appropriate means/acts, via a Picture Exchange Communication System (PECS), to communicate with different communication partners in a variety of contexts/activities.

## Author Note

This information was based on a hypothetical case.

## References


Division TEACCH. (n.d.). Educational Approaches. Retrieved November 12, 2007, from www.teacch.com

Frost, L., & Bondy, A. (2002). *The Picture Exchange Communication System training manual* (2nd ed.). Newark, DE: Pyramid Educational Products.

Janzen, J. E. (2003). *Understanding the nature of autism: A guide to the autism spectrum disorders* (2nd ed.). San Antonio, TX: PyschCorp.

Kranowitz, C. S. (2005). *The out of sync child: Recognizing and coping with sensory processing disorder* (2nd ed.). New York: Perigee.

Lord, C., Rutter, M., DiLavore, P., & Risi, S. (1999). *Autism Diagnostic Observation System*. Los Angeles, CA: Western Psychological Services.

Prelock, P. (2006). *Autism spectrum disorders: Issues in assessment and intervention*. Austin, TX: PRO-ED.

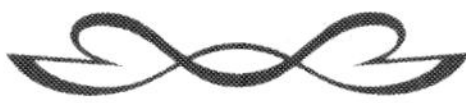



# CASE 2

# Nancy: A Toddler with Cleft Lip and Palate: Early Therapy

*Cynthia Jacobsen*

## Conceptual Knowledge Areas

Speech-language pathologists (SLPs) working with families of children with cleft lip and palate may provide counsel and support when a child is born and convey optimism regarding a child's future while teaching parents how to implement a home program to stimulate early communication development.

In our cleft palate clinic, the SLP typically meets with the family within a few months after a child's birth. During initial visits, the SLP discusses the impact of cleft lip and palate on hearing, speech, and language development. The Cleft Palate Foundation publishes several brochures designed to educate parents regarding cleft lip and palate. Using these materials, the SLP explains the effect of a cleft on speech, provides suggestions to parents to encourage oral sound play and to ignore speech sounds that are made in the nose or throat, and teaches parents how to reinforce sounds and to systematically increase sound variety through playful structured parent-child interaction. The SLP selects sounds that are easy to produce such as /w/, /m/, /n/, /l/, and /b/, teaches parents to practice consonant vowel syllables such as "baba," "lala," and "wewe," and discusses warning signs for hearing loss. Detailed therapy suggestions for infants and toddlers with cleft lip and palate are described in Peterson-Falzone, Trost-Cardamone, Karnell, and Hardin-Jones (2006).

The SLP listens to parent concerns and observes parent-child interaction. One goal in the first months is to reflect on family concerns in "living room language," maintaining a nonjudgmental attitude. There will be many opportunities to observe the family to discern how well the family is coping with the many demands placed on them. The SLP addresses questions such as: Is the family bonding with the baby? Is the family coping well with the child's medical condition and facial deformity? Does the family know what to say to strangers who ask pointed questions about the cleft? Is the child feeding efficiently in order to conserve calories, grow, and be ready for surgery? Are there other health concerns? The SLP tries to answer these questions, and if necessary, encourages the family to talk to the primary care physician and cleft team members.

Because a child with cleft lip and palate has an oral structure that affects speech in specific ways, the SLP needs to know the effects of cleft lip and palate on speech production. Children with cleft palate have speech errors that may be due to several sources, including deviant oral structure and function, deviant phonology, and conductive hearing loss. It is essential for the SLP to diagnose problems accurately to provide correct treatment. This case describes a child who had speech errors due to both velopharyngeal insufficiency and deviant phonology.

## Cleft Palate

A cleft is an abnormal opening in an anatomical structure. Clefts occur when tissues fail to fuse during early embryologic development. A cleft lip is an opening in the lip and can occur on one or both sides of the mouth, often involving the alveolar ridge. A cleft palate is an opening in the palate, which functions as the roof of the mouth and the floor of the nose.

When a baby has a bilateral cleft lip and palate, the lip and maxillary alveolar process are cleft under both nostrils and the central portion of the lip is misaligned. The columella, the central structure of the nose, is usually absent or displaced. There are clefts through the alveolar ridge, affecting dentition. The soft and the hard palate are cleft on both sides of the nasal septum (Shprintzen, 1995).

A child with a cleft lip and palate is best treated by a team of specialists who have expertise in the care of children with cleft lip and palate. "Affiliated" cleft palate teams are recognized by the American Cleft Palate–Craniofacial Association as meeting specific parameters of care. A team allows for systematic and comprehensive planning in the long-term care of a child. A cleft palate team has at least three specialists and often 6 to 10 members. The plastic surgeon manages the reconstruction of facial defects, such as those of the nose, lip, and palate. The otolaryngologist concentrates on the ears and larynx. There is at least one and possibly several dental specialists. Dental health professionals provide consultation at team visits and make recommendations to community dentists and orthodontists. A pediatric dentist cares for teeth; an orthodontist corrects the placement and positioning of the teeth; a prosthodontist constructs oral appliances if needed; and an oral/maxillofacial surgeon might operate on the upper and/or lower jaws and mouth. Team SLPs diagnose and often treat children with speech disorders and sometimes assist with feeding instruction. Audiologists evaluate hearing and manage hearing loss. A genetic counselor or geneticist explains hereditary links to a child's cleft. A dietician monitors growth and development and instructs parents on feeding a child efficiently and with sufficient calories. Nursing staff serve as the liaison between parents and surgeons and provide education before and after surgery. Mental health specialists and social workers help families to access resources and deal with the adjustment to the birth of a child with facial differences. The child's pediatrician or primary care physician provides ongoing medical care. There are other specialists such as occupational therapists and lactation nurses.

A cleft palate affects tongue position in the mouth. In an infant with normal anatomy, the tongue makes a seal against the palate and elevates to squeeze the nipple against the hard palate as the lips create a seal. The tongue then sweeps backward and increases the space in the anterior oral cavity. The milk is expressed from the nipple by a combined action of the tongue squeezing out the contents of the breast or bottle nipple with negative pressure created in the oral cavity by sucking the milk into the mouth (Sidoti & Shprintzen, 1995). When there is a cleft palate, the oral cavity and the nasal cavity are continuous, preventing the infant from creating negative pressure. Because the infant with a cleft palate needs to interrupt sucking in order to take breaths, she cannot coordinate breathing and drinking and there is often nasal regurgitation. Most infants with clefts are able to feed and gain weight with simple adjustments to bottle feeding.

Repair of the palate occurs at approximately 1 year of age. Prior to the repair the baby has been practicing speech with the oral and nasal cavities joined together. The tongue position of an infant with a cleft may be in the cleft or to the side, resulting in an incorrect tongue resting position from which babbling occurs. The infant lacks intraoral air pressure to play with sounds in a typical manner. Sounds may not be made in the correct locations or compensatory tongue placements and constrictions at the level of the pharynx or larynx may result as the baby attempts to close off the oral cavity from the nasal cavity. The baby may also experience conductive hearing loss, which can affect the ability to hear and say sounds (Peterson-Falzone et al., 2006).

Babies with cleft lip and palate may make fewer consonants and fewer multisyllabic productions than noncleft babies. Babies with cleft palate appear to be delayed in the onset of babbling and may avoid making sounds that require alveolar and palatal contact. They often make consonants that don't require high intraoral air pressure, such as nasals (/m/, /n/), glides (/w/, /y/), and glottals (/h/). Palatal and alveolar consonants are not heard until after palatal repair (Peterson-Falzone et al., 2006.) Although it is possible for some to catch up in speech sound usage by preschool years, many continue to have misarticulations.

## Description of the Case

### Background Information

#### History and Newborn Team Visit

Following a full-term uneventful pregnancy, Nancy was born with a bilateral cleft lip and palate. There was no prior family history of cleft palate, although a sibling had received speech therapy. The family was intact with no psychosocial concerns. Nancy was first seen in the Cleft Palate Clinic at age 9 days. Although she passed her newborn hearing screening, the otolaryngologist on the team recommended monitoring the ears for possible otitis media. A speech-language pathologist (SLP) counseled the family on the effects of a cleft palate on speech development and resonance and instructed the parents on methods for language stimulation. A dietician provided feeding instruction while a dentist fabricated a feeding appliance. Nancy was fed using a Special Needs Feeder, formerly the Haberman feeder (Medela, Inc.), a newborn feeding device that allows parents to control liquid flow. With parent education in child positioning, bottle usage, and length of time to feed, Nancy learned to feed well and she gained weight (Turner et al., 2001). The craniofacial plastic surgeon counseled the family regarding upcoming surgery to repair the bilateral cleft lip and subsequent surgery to repair the cleft palate.

#### Medical Care and Concerns: First Year

Between the first visit at 9 days and the next team visit at 12 months, Nancy was followed by the otolaryngologist and the plastic surgeon. The plastic surgeon repaired the bilateral cleft lip at 3 months. Following episodes of chronic otitis media, bilateral myringotomy and tubes were placed by the otolaryngologist at 8 months of age.

#### Second Team Visit

At 12 months of age Nancy returned for a team visit. Hearing testing was within normal limits. The dietician observed that the child was growing and gaining weight. Routine oral home care was in place. The nurse recommended that the child be weaned from the bottle in preparation for palatal surgery at age 13 months.

A formal assessment and a parent report of speech and overall development were obtained. Parents reported that the child's motor and play skills were developing nicely. The child said her first word at 8 months. Due to limited sound usage, the parents taught "baby signs." Nancy began to use sign language at 9 months. She was beginning to make two-word combinations; however, she usually combined a word with a gesture or sign to communicate. Nancy spontaneously used signs for "please," "thank you," and "more," and demonstrated pretend play. She was social, had an excellent attention span, followed verbal commands, identified pictures in books, and imitated motor requests.

Although Nancy's overall development was excellent, she had a very limited repertoire of speech sounds. Nancy said /m/, /n/, and /h/, and occasionally /p/. She could say these sounds at the beginning and ends of syllables and repeat two syllables containing the same consonant such as "mama." She made nasal consonants (/m/, /n/) for plosive sounds such as /t/, /d/, /k/, and /g/. Parent education was provided regarding compensatory speech errors. The parents were told to encourage oral sound productions and to avoid reinforcement of compensatory sounds with glottal and pharyngeal placements. It was recommended that Nancy return for a speech reevaluation in 6 months and for a complete team assessment at 2 years of age.

## Findings of the Evaluation

### 18-Month Speech and Language Evaluation

***Language Development*** Language development was assessed with the Receptive-Expressive Emergent Language (REEL) Scale (Bzoch, League, & Brown, 1978), and the Sequenced Inventory of Communication Development (Hedrick, Prather, & Tobin, 1984). Language comprehension and expression were within normal limits. Nancy had a speaking vocabulary of 20 words and engaged in two-word combinations. She usually communicated through single-word approximations, signs, and gestures.

***Speech Mechanism Examination*** Nancy closed her lips while playing, during cup drinking, and when saying words. The symmetry and continuity of lips were good. Nancy moved her lips and tongue adequately for speech sound production. She protruded and elevated the tongue tip and tongue blade in imitation. Additional observations included that the hard palate was intact with a high-arched palatal vault and the soft palate appeared to be short with minimal movement.

***Resonance*** Speech was characterized by moderate hypernasality and suspected nasal air emission. Nasal grimacing and snorting was observed. Nasal grimacing, snorting, and growls signaled that Nancy was trying to valve the velopharyngeal opening in the throat and nose.

***Articulation*** The SLP obtained a speech sample including words spoken during play and after single-word imitation. She used phonetic transcription of errors and then documented the size of the sound inventory, sound types, and constraints on producing sounds. She compared Nancy's sound development to the sound development of normal children of the same age and sex. She noted maladaptive compensatory misarticulations such as sounds made by closing the glottis (glottal stop). The SLP classified the error types, such as substitution (including compensatory), omission, distortion, or voicing. She listened for the presence and degree of hypernasality and the presence of nasal air emission, while she watched facial movements for nasal grimacing. She also related perceptual speech information with examination of the child's mouth.

Nancy produced the /m/, /n/, /l/, /h/, and /p/ sounds. The /p/ sound lacked plosion. Oral pressure for sounds was not obtained during imitation. For example, Nancy said "nani" for /Barney/, "huni" for /honey/, "mi" or "pi" for /please/, and "memi" for /baby/. Nancy showed a reduced phonemic repertoire. In 15 utterances, she marked consonants with 8 /n/ sounds, 12 /m/ sounds, 3 /h/ sounds, and one /p/ sound. Vowels were accurate. The lack of stop consonants such as /b/, /p/, and /d/ signaled a cleft-related speech disorder.

Nancy's list of sounds and sound substitutions suggested that she lacked velopharyngeal closure to produce oral sounds such as /b/, /d/, and /g/. In addition, she was omitting sounds that did not require strong intraoral pressure, such as /w/. As Nancy continued to develop, it appeared that her speech problems were due to two separate sources, one structural and one phonological in nature.

## Course of Treatment

### Speech Therapy 18–24 Months

The SLP showed Nancy's parents how to encourage oral sound play and to ignore nasal and pharyngeal sounds. Parents were told to play speech games that involved one or two consonants at a time with the goal of increasing the frequency of making or imitating sounds. During game time parents used a mirror and held toys near the mouth to help Nancy increase oral sounds and to learn that mouth movements required oral airflow. The parents paired toy use with key words containing target sounds. With systematic, frequent imitation of oral-motor movements and speech, Nancy increased imitation. For example, an oral airflow activity was puffing up the cheeks with air, and then tapping the cheek to release air through the lips in small pops. Props such as cotton balls, pinwheels, and blowing toys, though not used to improve articulation, demonstrated the movement that occurred when air came out of the mouth. Speech activities included saying words with targeted sounds combined with actions. Parents spoke key words such as "pop," "ball," and "baby" in interactive play. Gestures and speech were combined to teach the pairing of speech and action, such as feeding a doll with a spoon and saying "mmmm," or petting a toy lamb and saying "baaa." Parents identified a few key words and actions to use at home. For example, Nancy had a favorite toy puppy and she looked for it saying "puppy." She practiced a hopping game to say "hop" as she hopped to target picture cards, and she said "up" to stack cups for "up" for the final /p/ sound. Parents made a booklet of target words such as "baby," "mommy," "daddy," "bunny," and "puppy," to practice sounds and the sequencing of CVCV syllables (consonant-vowel). Parents rewarded oral sound productions even if sounds were unavoidably nasal in quality. Parents and the SLP modeled the placement for /t/ and /d/ and at times used visible and exaggerated sound productions to teach the idea that sound was made in the mouth with elevation of the tip of the tongue. The SLP instructed parents to teach the postvocalic /p/ as in /up/ in order to prevent the use of /h/ or glottal stop following the vowel. As mastery of one or two oral consonants was achieved, other consonants were taught in the syllable final position, such as /b/ or /d/ (e.g., "cub," "bed"). Parents were told that frequent, systematic practice of selected targeted sounds was essential to achieve mastery.

Nancy received 18 therapy sessions between 18 and 24 months of age with the following initial goals: to imitate /p/ and /b/ in isolation and in consonant-vowel syllables such as "bee" and "pie," and to say /b/ and /p/ in vowel-consonant combinations such as "pop" and "up." Correct placement was achieved; however, productions were made with mild to moderate nasal air emission. Subsequent goals included correct placement for /t/, /d/, /k/, and /g/ with oral airflow. A goal to use lingual-alveolar placement for /t/ and /d/ resulted in 75% correct placement for /t/. Placement for /k/ and /g/ sounds was not obtained. Correct placement was verified when Nancy's nose was occluded. Nancy could not produce any fricative sounds when stimulated (/f/, /s/, /z/) but substituted the /h/ consonant whenever a fricative was attempted.

Because Nancy had moderate hypernasality and nasal air emission, nasendoscopy was scheduled. Although nasendoscopy is typically scheduled after age 3 years, Nancy's parents were eager to know the specific nature of the velopharyngeal insufficiency to obtain early secondary surgery, and the team felt that Nancy could cooperate with the procedure. The parents helped prepare their child for scope insertion.

After Nancy suffered repeated ear infections, the otolaryngologist removed a blocked left ear tube and replaced ear tubes at 20 months.

## Analysis of Client's Response to Intervention

### Two-Year Cleft Team Visit Findings

At the 2-year team visit, hearing was normal, height and weight were normal, and there were no other health concerns. The dentist reported that there was a posterior cross-bite and an extra tooth in the area of the cleft. The speech-language pathologist documented normal language, severe articulation disorder, moderate hypernasality, and nasal air emission.

The plastic surgeon noted a bilateral alveolar cleft and a nasoalveolar fistula. Since Nancy's buccal (cheek) vestibule was small, the surgeon recommended future deepening of the buccal vestibule to have braces placed at the time of the erupting of the first molars. He observed the short palate and concurred with the need for nasendoscopy. The treatment plan was to continue speech therapy, complete nasendoscopy, and obtain routine dental care.

Nasendoscopy is an imaging technique in which a flexible fiber-optic endoscope is inserted into the nasal passages to view the velopharyngeal mechanism during speech. The scope allows visualization of the movement of the soft palate as well as movement of lateral and posterior pharyngeal walls. Nancy cried during part of the scoping, but the SLP and plastic surgeon were able to view the velopharyngeal port while Nancy was speaking. There was leakage of air into the nasal cavity across the entire palate. Slight symmetrical palatal movement and slight lateral pharyngeal wall movement were observed. The team diagnosed moderate to severe velopharyngeal insufficiency. The surgeon recommended a Furlow Z-plasty operation to lengthen the soft palate as well as a sphincter pharyngoplasty to reduce the size of the velopharyngeal space. The team also recommended that Nancy remain in once-weekly speech therapy prior to surgery to maintain correct articulatory placement and to avoid additional compensatory errors such as pharyngeal stops.

Although the goal of speech therapy prior to surgery was to maintain correct placement for sounds, Nancy also showed a severe phonological disorder. She continued to front velars so that "key" became "tea"; stopped fricatives so that "fun" became "pun"; glided liquids so that "light" became "white"; and stopped the affricate "ch" so that "chair" because "tair." She reduced consonant clusters so that "play" became "pay" and omitted final consonants.

Following four months of once-weekly therapy (18 therapy sessions), Nancy imitated all /b/ and /p/ consonants in CV syllables with the nose occluded as in "bee" and "pie," and half of /b/ and /p/ in consonant-vowel-consonant words such as "bib" or "pop." She was able to make lingual-alveolar contact for /t/ and /d/ in some positions of words as well as to produce an oral air stream for /f/ and /s/, although sound productions were /p/ for /f/ and /h/ for /s/ at 100%. Nancy still scored at the 1st percentile when retested on the Goldman-Fristoe Test of Articulation (Goldman & Fristoe, 2000).

## Team Care and Follow-Up over the Next Several Years

***Speech and Velopharyngeal Functioning*** Velopharyngeal competency was obtained following secondary palatal surgery at age 28 months. Within several months after surgery, Nancy produced syllable final consonants such as /p/, /m/, /n,/ /b/, /k/, /l/, /v/, and /z/, but continued to demonstrate a severe phonological disorder. Thus, therapy focused on the ability to produce speech sounds across syllable positions and in words, phrases, and sentences, which yielded an increase in intelligibility. Nancy continued in speech therapy for 226 sessions, and a parent home program was provided. Nancy completed therapy with a team SLP at age 5 years with a residual mild to moderate articulation disorder. School-based therapy subsequently addressed dentalized productions of lingual-alveolar sounds and lateralized /s/ on /s/ clusters. After two years of school-based speech therapy, Nancy was at age and grade level in all areas of communication and academics.

***Hearing*** Hearing was within normal limits.

***Sleep*** At age 3 years Nancy was referred for a sleep study because of nighttime awakenings, daytime naps, and a noisy sound when falling asleep. The sleep study was normal and the problems spontaneously resolved.

***Nutrition*** At age 3 years most of Nancy's calories came from liquids. With a dietician's assistance, parents changed the diet and Nancy grew and gained weight normally.

***Dental*** At age 7 years, a community dentist began expansion of the alveolar arch and the posterior cross-bite was corrected.

***Plastic Surgery*** Following dental arch expansion, the surgeon repaired a nasoalveolar fistula and completed alveolar bone grafting to provide adequate bone within the alveolar cleft. The surgeon and parents discussed additional surgeries, which would include lengthening of the columella and correction of a residual lip and nose deformity.

***Psychosocial*** Nancy had many friends and did well in school.

## Author Note

The family gave permission to share this case. Many thanks to colleague Sally Helton, M.S. CCC-SLP, for treating the patient described. This was based on a real case but the name was changed. Many thanks to members of the cleft palate team at Children's Mercy Hospital and Clinics, Kansas City, MO, who provided team care: Virender Singhal, M.D., Margo Humenczuk, R.D., Robin Onikul, D.D.S., Thomas Eyen, M.D., and Claudia Magers, M.S. CCC-SLP. Thanks also to Nancy Rosenthal, Ph.D., for suggestions regarding the manuscript.

## References

Bzoch, K., League, R., & Brown, V. (1978). *Receptive-Expressive Emergent Language Test* (2nd ed.). Austin, TX: PRO-ED.

Cleft Palate Foundation. http://www.cleftline.org

Goldman, R., & Fristoe, M. (2000). *Goldman-Fristoe Test of Articulation* (2nd ed.). Minneapolis, MN: Pearson.

Hedrick, D., Prather, E., & Tobin, A. (1984). *Sequenced Inventory of Communication Development*. Los Angeles: Western Psych Corp.

Medela. Haberman feeder. McHenry, IL. www.medela.us

Peterson-Falzone, S. J., Trost-Cardamone, J. E., Karnell, M. P., & Hardin-Jones, M. A. (2006). *The clinician's guide to treating cleft palate speech*. St. Louis, MO: Mosby.

Shprintzen, R. J. (1995). A new perspective on clefting. In R. J. Shprintzen & J. Bardach (Eds.), *Cleft palate speech management. A multidisciplinary approach*. St. Louis, MO: Mosby.

Sidoti, E. J., & Shprintzen, R. J. (1995). Pediatric care and feeding of the newborn with a cleft. In R. J. Shprintzen & J. Bardach (Eds.), *Cleft palate speech management. A multidisciplinary approach*. St. Louis, MO: Mosby.

Turner, L., Jacobsen, C., Humenczuk, M., Singhal, V., Moore, D., & Bell, H. (2001). Feeding efficiency and caloric intake in breast milk fed cleft lip and palate infants with and without prosthetic appliance and lactation education. *Cleft Palate Craniofacial Journal, 38*(5), 519–524.


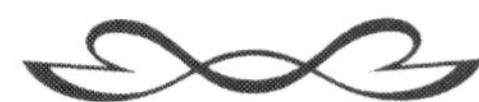

## DEVELOPMENTAL DELAY

# CASE 3

# Ben: A Toddler with Delayed Speech and Developmental Milestones


*Erin Redle and Carolyn Sotto*


## Conceptual Knowledge Areas

When evaluating young children, clinicians are frequently challenged to differentially diagnose a "late-talker" from a child who may have a true speech or language delay. The therapeutic recommendations, including a "wait and see approach" versus early enrollment in therapeutic services, are based on an accurate initial diagnosis. At this time there is not a definitive set of criteria for differential diagnosis of speech or language delay for toddlers acquiring expressive language. What appears to be limited expressive output in an otherwise typical toddler may be the result of true expressive language delay or may reflect a delay or disorder in the child's speech production/phonological system. Clinicians must observe the complex interaction of expressive language and phonological development to make an informed diagnosis.

To learn language, a child must assign representation to the lexicon and extract relevant phonological properties of such words for language production. The association between lexical and phonological development is observed in children with precocious language development as well as in children with delayed language development (Paul & Jennings, 1992). Children with large vocabularies utilize a greater variety of sounds and sound combinations, while children who generate only a few words produce a more limited number of sounds and sound combinations (Storkel & Morrisette, 2002). The relationship between phonological and lexical development is also supported by research on late talkers. In a study of children identified as late-talkers, children with 10 or more words and a larger phonemic repertoire at the initial assessment made more progress than the second group of late-talkers with fewer than 10 words and a smaller phonemic repertoire (Thal, Oroz, & McCaw, 1995). Similar findings were reported by Williams and Elbert (2003). Experimental evidence also demonstrates that the severity of a phonological delay at 2 years is predictive of the potential risk of continuing with a language delay at 3 years of age (Carson, Klee, Carson, & Hime, 2003). These particular findings, however, are limited as they are based on the reassessment of only 13 of the original 28 participants available for follow-up assessment. The number of different consonants a child uses in words is clearly associated with expressive language development (McCune & Vihman, 2001; Rescorla & Ratner, 1996). Although the magnitude of the phonetic inventory alone is not predictive when attempting to differentiate delayed from deviant language development (Williams & Elbert, 2003), it should be considered in making a clinical recommendation.

### Early Phonological Development

Early phonological development is governed by physiologic factors and reflects both speech and language development (Locke, 2004; Smith & Goffman, 2004). One of the earliest developmental speech milestones, the onset of canonical babbling (consonant-vowel elements), is linked to later language outcomes. Infants who are delayed in producing well-formed syllables in canonical babbling had smaller expressive vocabularies at 18, 24, and 30 months when compared to infants who demonstrated canonical babbling by 11 to 12 months of age (Oller, Eilers, Neal, & Schwartz, 1999). Both the placement and manner of sound production are important considerations in early phonological development. Bilabials and stops are the most prevalent sound classes reported in the early language/phonology literature, most likely due to their ease of production (Locke, 2004; McCune & Vihman, 2001). Although these are generally accepted to be the most common productions, the clinician should not ignore the presence or absence of other manners of production or variations in placement. Fricatives are generally considered a later developing sound class (Bricker, 1967; Goldman, Fristoe, & Williams, 2000; Prather, Hedrick, & Kern, 1975; Sander, 1972; Templin, 1957), but there are actual data to support observations that toddlers produce this manner of phonemes. Clinicians may want to attend to the presence or absence of fricative production in children with potential speech and language delays. Fricatives are needed for the production of several syntactical markers as children develop language and are actually motorically more difficult to produce. Therefore, when weighting factors that may make a child a late vs. a delayed talker, the presence of fricatives in the repertoire may be a marker for the motor control necessary to incorporate the phonological, morphological, and syntactical rules of language with motor components of speech production.

## Description of the Case

This case is about a child who was seen for an early speech-language evaluation at a pediatric hospital in a metropolitan city in the United States. The evaluation was conducted by a licensed and certified speech-language pathologist.

### Reason for Referral

Ben, a 22-month-old male, was referred by his pediatric neurologist for a speech and language evaluation. Ben's parents were concerned that he was not talking as much as his brother did at the same age. Additionally, some of Ben's motor development was "slow," prompting his parents to seek both an occupational and a physical therapy assessment when Ben was 8 months old.

## Background Information

### Pertinent History

Ben was accompanied to the evaluation by his mother and father, who both actively participated in the interview and assessment process.

### Neonatal History

Ben's neonatal history was unremarkable. His parents could not remember his specific Apgar scores nor recall any complications. He was discharged from a well-baby nursery within 48 hours of his birth.

### Medical History

Ben was diagnosed with congenital hypotonia. He was referred to a pediatric neurologist at 17 months of age by his physical therapist (PT) and occupational therapist (OT) because of concerns about his low tone. At that time the pediatric neurologist conducted a thorough clinical assessment as well as magnetic resonance imaging (MRI) of the brain and spine; bilateral EMG testing including the hands, arms, legs, and feet; and a 1-hour EEG. Other than presenting with mild-moderate low tone, Ben's neurological system appeared to be completely normal.

By parental report, he had one prior ear infection and was successfully treated with antibiotics. Hearing was formally assessed by a pediatric audiologist and was within normal limits. There was no history of speech and language delays in the immediate or extended family.

### Developmental History

Motor milestones were delayed with independent sitting reported at 8 months, crawling at 11 months, and walking at 17 months. Following his initial occupational and physical therapy evaluations Ben was enrolled in both physical and occupational therapy and continued these therapies on a monthly basis. His parents reported he was still a "clumsy" walker and tended to fall frequently. He did not yet display hand dominance.

Based on parental report, speech and language milestones were also delayed. The clinicians linked questions about development to major holidays to assist in determining the time frame of several developmental milestones. Since Ben's birthday was in early January, the clinician targeted speech and language milestones at his first Passover (approximately 3–4 months), summer vacations (approximately 6 months), and around Hanukah (almost 1 year). Using this technique, his parents recalled his specific speech and language skills at these times. They reported that he was cooing at 4 months and babbling from the summertime through his first birthday. Ben produced his first true word, "dada," on a summer vacation (approximately 18 months). He slowly developed a vocabulary of approximately 11 words including mama, dada, baba/bottle, uh-oh, no, wawa/water, sa/Sammie (family dog), ga/Grant (brother), i/eat, di/drink, and hi. He also frequently "jabbered" in a conversational manner, but without true words.

By report Ben understood "everything" and pointed to items named, family members when named, and to indicate something he wanted. His mother reported he sometimes became frustrated when she could not figure out what he was pointing to on the pantry shelves or in the refrigerator. He looked at books with his parents and turned the pages.

### Treatment History

Ben received occupational and physical therapy on a monthly basis. He was referred for early intervention services, but these had not yet begun.

### Social History

Ben's older brother, who was 4 years, 1 month, had no developmental delays. He played with his brother and several cousins on a regular basis and engaged well with other children of all ages.

Both parents were well educated (mother was a preschool teacher, father an attorney) and read to their children daily. The grandmother provided child care when the parents were at work.

## Findings of the Evaluation

Ben's communication was assessed using the Rossetti Infant-Toddler Language Scale (Rossetti, 2006) and through clinical observations. All other skills assessed by the Rossetti scale including interaction-attachment, gesture development, pragmatics, play, and language comprehension were within normal limits.

### Expressive Language

Expressive language skills were delayed with skills solid at 12–15 months and scattering up to 15–18 months as assessed using the Rossetti scale. These results were supported by clinical observations and an attempted conversational speech-language sample. Although Ben did not use connected words, it is always best practice for the clinician to attempt to collect, transcribe, and analyze speech and language productions within a natural context of the child's own language (vocabulary, grammar) and running speech (sounds, prosody). He imitated "mama, dada," and several utterances of connected consonant and vowel sounds with varying intonational patterns ("jabbering") and clear communicative intent. These productions were not intelligible to the examiner or Ben's family.

### Receptive Language

As measured by the Rossetti scale, Ben's receptive language was within normal limits. Additionally, he followed novel 1-step directions and simple 2-step directions. He demonstrated an age-appropriate understanding of several words expected at his age through pointing to the specified items in books and photos when they were named.

### Phonological Development

The Arizona Articulation Proficiency Scale—Third Revision (Arizona 3) (Fudala, 2000) was attempted to assess consonants and vowels in various word positions. However, the Arizona-3 could not be completed as Ben could not name or imitate names of most of the stimulus pictures. Based on parents' report and the observed limited word productions and vocalizations, Ben's phonemic repertoire included /m, d, b, n, s, g, h/. Vowel errors were not noted. His syllable shape in words was primarily consonant-vowel (CV) with some CVCV observed. He was, however, able to string together longer sequences of consonants and vowels (e.g., CVCVCV, CVCVCVC) in "jabbering."

***Gestures*** Ben used several gestures to communicate including waving, pointing, and a "thumbs-up." These observations were consistent with his use of gestures at home; his gestures score on the Rossetti scale was also within normal limits.

***Pragmatics, Interaction-Attachment, Play*** Pragmatics, interaction-attachment, and play were all found to be within normal limits on the Rossetti scale. Following a brief familiarization period he engaged well with the examiner, demonstrated both nonverbal and verbal turn-taking in play, and interacted appropriately with his parents. Consistent and appropriate eye contact was noted. He engaged in parallel and symbolic play. His parents again reported that these behaviors were consistent with their observations at home.

***Other Clinical Observations*** Vocal quality and resonance were clinically judged to be within normal limits for the limited productions observed.

### Oral Mechanism Examination

Formal and comprehensive oral mechanism assessments are extremely difficult in children of this age because of their limited ability to follow directions, as well as their apprehension of strangers approaching their oral cavity. Ben's oral-facial structures appeared symmetrical. His oral-facial tone was low-normal to mildly hypotonic and was consistent with the tone throughout his body. The strength of his articulators seemed adequate for speech production. During play he was able to imitate puckering for kissing and sticking his tongue out at someone. An intraoral assessment could not be completed, but he was able to produce pressure consonants, and his parents did not report food or liquids coming out of his nose while eating and drinking. Although these factors do not necessarily exclude the potential for velopharyngeal incompetence or a submucous cleft, they reflect adequate velopharyngeal structure and function for speech production. Overall, oral-motor skills were adequate for speech production.

### Examiners' Impressions

Based on the results of this evaluation, Ben presented with moderately delayed expressive language skills and severely delayed phonological development. The greatest difficulty was his limited ability to put sounds together into words, most likely due to his small phonemic repertoire. The clinician was faced with determining if Ben was potentially a late-talker or actually had a true expressive language delay.

The following factors were considered:

1. With the exception of expressive language and phonology, all other essential linguistic foundations including receptive language, pragmatics, and play were within normal limits. This suggests he had the foundation for language (late-talker) but was not producing age-appropriate expressive language.
2. Ben produced sounds utilizing almost all articulatory placements (bilabial, alveolar, velar, glottal) and different manners (stop, glide, fricative) yet the number of consonants he produced was very limited. Additionally, his syllable shapes in word production were not age-appropriate (no CVC, CVCVC) and no final consonants were observed.
3. During the discussion of the results, Ben's mother questioned the diagnosis of childhood apraxia of speech (CAS). Although the examiner did not mention CAS, the family was aware of this terminology from a family friend. The examiner discussed the difficulty with a correct differential diagnosis of CAS in very young children. Ben did demonstrate a few characteristics that may be consistent with CAS, including limited syllable shapes and an overall motor coordination problem. However, Ben's vowel repertoire was varied and vowel errors were not noted in his spontaneous productions. Additionally, prosodic variation was noted in longer utterances and consonant errors were consistent. Ben also correctly produced a fricative, which is believed to require more advanced speech motor control. Differential diagnosis of CAS in children under 3 years of age is difficult, especially if these children exhibit very limited expressive language (American Speech-Language-Hearing Association, 2007).

### Parental Counseling

The family was counseled regarding the results of the evaluation and their options for treatment. They expressed understanding of the results and discussed both the diagnosis and the efficacy of the proposed treatment approaches with the clinician. Ben's mother, a preschool teacher, was concerned about his future literacy development. Additionally, he was to start at a new day care facility in a few weeks and the parents wanted to ensure a smooth transition.

## Treatment Options Considered

The speech-language pathologist presented the family with a continuum of treatment options. The first choice was a "wait and see" approach in which Ben would not receive any direct speech or language therapy. If his parents chose this option, they could continue to provide general language stimulation in the home, but without the direct guidance or supervision of a speech-language pathologist. Another option for the family was speech-language therapy.

Direct intervention for language-delayed toddlers could improve both linguistic complexity and speech sound productions (Girolametto, Pearce, & Weitzman, 1997; Robertson & Weismer, 1999). His parents chose to begin direct speech and language treatment sessions.

## Course of Treatment

The long-term goal for Ben's speech and language therapy was to improve his expressive language skills to an age-appropriate level. The short-term goals included:

1. Increasing the number of different words and word approximations that he was producing
2. Increasing the number of different phonemes and the complexity of the syllable shapes produced

## Analysis of the Client's Response to Intervention

Ben made consistent progress in treatment. After approximately 6 months of therapy, his vocabulary grew to approximately 75 words, including some rote multi-words phrases such as "thank you," "what's that," and "I don't know." He was not yet producing true spontaneous two-word combinations but could imitate these with a direct model (e.g., "want cookie"). His spontaneous phonemic repertoire increased to include: /n, m, d, b, g, k, p, t, s, z, w, h/ and his syllable shapes included CV, VC, CVCV, VCVC, CVC, and CVCVC. All other language skills, including receptive language, play, and pragmatics, continued at least at age-level. Additionally, his parents reported he was consistently using spoken language to interact with his brother during play. Ben's parents consistently implemented speech- and language-building strategies recommended by their treating therapist in the home, greatly improving the rate of his language development.

## Further Recommendations

Ben should continue with speech-language pathology services to continue to improve his speech sound development and expressive language skills, including vocabulary development and spontaneous use of multi-word combinations. Improving his phonological development is also targeted to improve literacy development in the future.

## Author Note

This was a fictional case based upon the performance of several children the authors had evaluated.

## References


American Speech-Language-Hearing Association. (2007). *Childhood apraxia of speech* [Technical Report]; http://www.asha.org/docs/html/TR2007-00278.html

Bricker, W. (1967). Errors in the echoic behavior of preschool children. *Journal of Speech and Hearing Research, 10*, 67–76.

Carson, C., Klee, T., Carson, D., & Hime, L. (2003). Phonological profiles of 2-year-olds with delayed language development: Predicting clinical outcomes at age 3. *American Journal of Speech-Language Pathology, 12*, 28–39.

Davis, B., & Velleman, S. (2008). Establishing a basic speech repertoire without using NSOME: Means, motive, and opportunity. *Seminars in Speech and Language 29*, 312–319.

Fudala, J. (2000). *The Arizona Articulation Proficiency Scale, Third Revision*. Los Angeles: Western Psychological Services.

Girolametto, L., Pearce, P. S., & Weitzman, E. (1997). Effects of lexical intervention on the phonology of late talkers. *Journal of Speech and Hearing Research, 40*, 338–348.

Goldman, R., Fristoe, M., & Williams, K. (2000). *Goldman-Fristoe Test of Articulation, Second Edition: Supplemental Developmental Norms*. Circle Pines, MN: American Guidance Service.

Locke, J. L. (2004). How do infants come to control the organs of speech. In B. Maasen, R. Kent, H. Peters, P. van Lieshout, & W. Hulstijn (Eds.), *Speech motor control in normal and disordered speech* (pp. 175–190). Oxford: Oxford University Press.

McCune, L., & Vihman, M. M. (2001). Early phonetic and lexical development: A productivity approach. *Journal of Speech, Language, and Hearing Research, 44*(3), 670–684.

Oller, D. K., Eilers, R. E., Neal, A. R., & Schwartz, H. K. (1999). Precursors to speech in infancy: The prediction of speech and language disorders. *Journal of Communication Disorders, 32*(4), 223–245.

Paul, R., & Jennings, P. (1992). Phonological behavior in toddlers with slow expressive language development. *Journal of Speech and Hearing Research, 35*, 99–107.

Prather, E., Hedrick, D., & Kern, C. (1975). Articulation development in children aged two to four years. *Journal of Speech and Hearing Disorders, 40*, 179–191.

Rescorla, L., & Ratner, N. (1996). Phonetic profiles of toddlers with specific expressive language impairment (SLI-E). *Journal of Speech, Language, and Hearing Research, 39*, 153–156.

Robertson, S. B., & Weismer, S. E. (1999). Effects of treatment on linguistic and social skills in toddlers with delayed language development. *Journal of Speech, Language, and Hearing Research, 42*, 1234–1248.

Rossetti, L. (2006). *The Rossetti Infant-Toddler Language Scale*. East Moline, IL: LinguiSystems.

Sander, E. K. (1972). When are speech sounds learned? *Journal of Speech and Hearing Disorders, 37*, 55–63.

Smith, A., & Goffman, L. (2004). Interaction of motor and language factors in the development of speech production. In B. Maasen, R. Kent, H. Peters, P. van Lieshout, & W. Hulstijn (Eds.), *Speech motor control in normal and disordered speech*. Oxford: Oxford University Press.

Storkel, H., & Morrisette, M. (2002). The lexicon and phonology: Interactions in language acquisition. *Language, Speech, and Hearing Services in Schools, 33*, 24–37.

Templin, M. C. (1957). *Certain language skills in children*. Minneapolis: University of Minnesota Press.

Thal, D., Oroz, M., & McCaw, V. (1995). Phonological and lexical development in normal and late-talking toddlers. *Applied Psycholinguistics, 16*, 407–424.

Williams, A. L., & Elbert, M. (2003). A prospective longitudinal study of phonological development in late talkers. *Language, Speech, and Hearing Services in the Schools, 34*, 138–153.

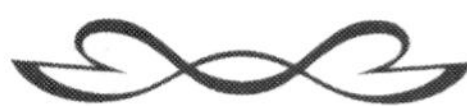



CASE 4

# Lily: An Infant with a Sensorineural Hearing Loss

*Judith Widen, Sandra Keener, Teresa Kennalley, and John Ferraro*

## Conceptual Knowledge Areas

For decades professionals in speech, hearing, and deaf education fields have provided anecdotal claims that children with hearing loss achieve the best language and speech outcomes when hearing loss is identified and treatment begun early in life. It was not until the 1990s that research data were published showing just *how early* intervention should begin. Yoshinaga-Itano, Sedey, Coulter, and Mehl (1998) showed that when intervention was begun by 6 months of age, language outcomes often fell within the normal range, but later intervention resulted in delays in receptive and expressive language outcome regardless of degree of hearing loss, mode of communication, or socioeconomic status. These findings were supported by a subsequent study by Moeller (2000), who documented that best outcomes were related to intervention within the first year of life as well as intervention that actively involved the family.

Hearing loss is one of the most prevalent birth defects. It is estimated that 2 or 3 out of every 1,000 children in the United States are born deaf or hard of hearing (NIDCD, 2008). It is much more prevalent than the metabolic disorders for which newborn screening has been available since the 1960s (Mehl & Thomson, 1998). Since hearing loss is rarely apparent via physical examination and the majority of cases present no risk factors (Mauk, White, Behrens, & Vohr, 1991), the need for universal screening of all newborns is necessary to identify those who may need early diagnosis and treatment.

As the data of Yoshinaga-Itano et al. (1998) and Moeller (2000) were accumulating, advances were being made in the physiologic measurement of hearing that did not require the baby's active participation. Assessment of auditory brainstem responses (ABR) came into widespread use in the 1980s (Gorga, Kaminski, Beauchaine, Jesteadt, & Neely, 1989) and otoacoustic emissions (OAEs) in the 1990s (Kemp, Ryan, & Bray, 1990). Screening versions of these measurements were automated so that hearing screening might be affordable (Hermann, Thornton, & Joseph, 1995; Maxon, Vohr, & White, 1996). State mandates for universal newborn hearing screening and federal support of state efforts rose dramatically from the mid-1990s until today when nearly 95% of babies in the United States are screened for hearing loss before hospital discharge (NCHAM, 2008).

Programs of screening, plus the necessary follow-up resulting in diagnosis and treatment, have been termed EHDI, for Early Hearing Detection and Intervention (CDC, 2008). Its goals include identification of hearing loss by 1 month of age, diagnosis by 3 months, and intervention no later than 6 months of age. Pediatric audiologists are able to confirm hearing loss and define its type, severity, and configuration within the first months of life (Widen & Keener, 2003). Hearing aids can be fitted and early intervention begun within the first half year of life.

## Description of the Case

This case describes an infant with congenital profound sensorineural hearing loss detected via universal newborn hearing screening at birth, diagnosed via audiologic measures appropriate for young infants by 3 months of age, referred for otologic diagnosis, fitted with amplification, and referred to early intervention within the first 6 months of life.

### Background Information and Reason for Referral

Lily was the firstborn child of 19-year-old parents who lived in the metropolitan Kansas City area. She was born in a Kansas City, Kansas, hospital, which provided newborn hearing screening to every newborn according to the State of Kansas law, regulations, and guidelines (www.soundbeginnings.org). This particular hospital's protocol was to refer babies who did not pass the hearing screen to the Audiology Clinic, Department of Hearing and Speech, University of Kansas Medical Center. This clinic was equipped to provide comprehensive audiologic services to infants and young children and was staffed by audiologists with experience testing very young children. The clinic also included the administrative offices of the Hartley Family Center, a program for families with infants and toddlers (birth to age 3 years) who are deaf or hard of hearing, and children of deaf parents.

Lily's parents are high school graduates. The father worked for a lawn service company; the mother worked in a local music store until the baby was born. The pregnancy progressed normally without complications. The baby was born three weeks before the due date, weighed 2,600 grams, and was considered a full-term newborn. Delivery was uncomplicated. There was no evidence of prenatal or perinatal infections. The baby failed its newborn otoacoustic emissions (OAE) hearing screen when it was first administered in the hospital nursery. A second repeat screen was done just before hospital discharge at 2 days of age. The baby did not pass the repeat screen in either ear. The nursery staff made an appointment for Lily to come to the Audiology Clinic for a hearing rescreen, and diagnostic evaluation if needed.

The appointment was set for 4 weeks after birth, but the family did not appear. It was later learned that the parents did not know about the appointment made by the hospital staff. After numerous phone calls to parents, the baby's primary care physician, and the hospital, another appointment was made. Based on family income and the lack of health insurance, Lily was eligible for a one-time diagnostic hearing test through Kansas Special Health Care Needs.

### Findings of the Evaluation

#### Diagnostic Audiologic Evaluation

When Lily was 2 months, 2 weeks old, her mother brought her to the Audiology Clinic. She reported that the baby had had no illnesses since birth. The baby was uncongested on the day of the evaluation. The mother reported that there was no history of childhood hearing loss on either side of the family. She indicated that she and her husband thought the baby was inconsistent in her response to sound; sometimes she seemed to respond, other times not.

The evaluation began with otoacoustic emissions testing (OAE). OAEs were not present in either ear, so the audiologist proceeded with a full diagnostic evaluation. At such a young age, physiologic measures are performed to estimate hearing status. An auditory brainstem response (ABR) test using 500 Hz and 2,000 Hz tone bursts at varying intensities was administered to approximate threshold. In the right and left ear, no response was measured at 500 Hz at a level of 95 dBnHL, and no response was measured at 2,000 Hz at a level of 100 dBnHL. There was no response to click stimuli at 95 dBnHL. These levels are the maximum levels allowable by the equipment. Both transient and distortion product OAEs were absent in each ear. Tympanometry was performed to evaluate middle ear status. Results were consistent with normal middle ear function on each side. Acoustic reflex testing, performed on each ear, revealed absent acoustic reflexes at all frequencies.

In summary, the audiologic evaluation indicated severe-to-profound sensorineural hearing loss. Although the ABR is not a hearing test per se, its thresholds correlate with hearing sensitivity. The absence of recordable responses at 500 Hz at 95 dBnHL and 2,000 Hz at 100 dBnHL were consistent with the presence of profound hearing loss. Normal tympanometry and absent acoustic reflexes were consistent with sensorineural hearing loss. The lack of OAEs corroborated these findings.

## Treatment Options Considered

The results of the exam were explained to the mother, who was in contact with the baby's father via cell phone at various times throughout the evaluation. It was explained that without intervention, this degree of hearing loss would have a negative impact on development of receptive and expressive language, and speech skills, which, in turn, might affect personal, social, and academic skills. The audiologist indicated that early intervention services and hearing aids might help to minimize the negative impact and optimize development of growth in these areas. Given the degree of hearing loss estimated today, cochlear implant candidacy could be considered in the future, following trial with hearing aids.

The final report, which went to the parents, hospital, primary care physician, Infant Toddler Services, and the Kansas Sound Beginnings program, listed the following recommendations, which are explained in further detail later in this case:

- Recommendation 1: Contact Infant Toddler Services to develop an individualized Family Service Plan (IFSP) to include hearing loss.
- Recommendation 2: Referral for otologic examination for two purposes: (a) for otologic evaluation to diagnose ear pathology and determine etiology, and (b) to obtain medical clearance for hearing aid fitting. [This recommendation was directed to the baby's pediatrician, who would then share the responsibilities with the otologist of his or her choice.]
- Recommendation 3: Ongoing audiologic testing to confirm today's results, further define amount of residual hearing, and monitor changes in hearing status. Behavioral testing should begin when baby reaches 6 months of age.
- Recommendation 4: Return to clinic within a month for hearing aid fitting with binaural amplification. (Earmold impressions to be taken during visit for confirmatory testing.)
- Recommendation 5: Lily's mother was given the Kansas Department of Health and Environment (KDHE) Sound Beginnings information booklet, which explains hearing testing, hearing testing results, and provides guidance for parents when determining what they need to do for their child with hearing loss.

### Additional Testing

Two weeks later Auditory Steady State Response (ASSR) testing was undertaken to determine whether there was residual hearing in the 90–110 dB HL range. The ASSR was elicited using 1,000, 2,000, and 4,000 Hz stimuli at varying intensities to approximate thresholds. Levels of 110 dB (dial reading) were not exceeded. No response was recorded for 1,000 and 4,000 Hz in either ear. At 2,000 Hz a threshold of 105 dB was recorded for the right ear and 95 dB for the left ear (these values correlate with thresholds of 95 dB HL and 85 dB HL on the audiogram for right and left ears, respectively). The ASSR results were consistent with the ABR results indicating profound hearing loss bilaterally. During the recording, clinicians noted behavioral reactions to high levels of sound, which were supported by the ASSR at 2,000 Hz.

### Otologic Examination

The otologist included the following statements in the Impression section of the medical record: "Healthy appearing 4-month-old with profound sensorineural hearing loss. . . . It appears to be non-syndromic. . . . There is no evidence of skin lesions, no renal abnormalities, or other associated problems."

Further recommendations were made: an EKG to rule out prolonged Q-T syndrome, ophthalmologic evaluation, and genetic evaluation, especially for connexin 26 disorders.

The otologist discussed Lily's candidacy for a cochlear implant (CI) with the parents. At an 8-month visit, he planned to obtain a magnetic resonance imaging (MRI) scan of the brain and internal auditory canals with computerized tomography (CT) scans to rule out malformations in the inner ear and study the course of the auditory nerve. Pending those results, cochlear implantation would be scheduled for 12 months of age.

### Amplification

At the second visit to the Audiology Clinic, when the ASSR test was done, earmold impressions were taken and sent to an earmold laboratory with instructions for a helix-style, soft vinyl mold, using the full length of the impression. For babies, we request a "double dip" for extra-secure fit. Digital compact very-high-power behind-the-ear aids were ordered through the Sertoma HEARRT program, which loans hearing aids to families who are considering cochlear implantation. The output of the hearing aids was verified with the Desired Sensation Level protocol using the Verifit system with simulated real-ear measurements. Output levels of the hearing aids did not exceed the projected uncomfortable level and targets were appropriate.

Parents were given instruction about how to use and care for the hearing aids. They were directed to return for follow-up when new earmolds were needed or in 2 months, whichever occured first. With rapid growth in the infant period, earmolds must be changed frequently.

## Course of Treatment

The Infant Toddler Services (ITS) mentioned in Recommendation 1 above is a comprehensive, statewide system of community-based, family-centered early intervention services for young children (birth through age 2 years) with disabilities and their families. The services are provided through the implementation of Part C of the Individuals with Disabilities Education Act (IDEA), U.S. Department of Education, Office of Special Education Programs. In Kansas ITS is administered through the Kansas Department of Health and Environment, which also administers the Newborn Hearing Screening Program. ITS should be staffed with personnel who have a background in hearing loss and know the resources that are available to the parents within their locale, so that all families who have infants or children with hearing loss will receive information about a full range of options regarding amplification and technology, communication and intervention, and accessing appropriate counseling services. In Lily's case, her parents chose to enroll in the Hartley Family Center (www.kumc.edu/hfc/). They chose to receive direct services in their home where early interventionists (speech-language pathologists, early childhood special educators, and teachers of the deaf and hard of hearing) would work with them to provide auditory stimulation and language stimulation. They also enrolled in the Baby Steps parent group described on the HFC website. Lily's early interventionist supported the audiologists' recommendations for full-time use of amplification and offered to accompany the family to later appointments with audiology and otology.

## Analysis of Client's Response to Intervention

Lily's cognitive and motor development proceeded on course. Given her parents' interest and persistence in providing language and auditory stimulation in this first year of life, and given the likelihood for early cochlear implantation, Lily's prognosis for language development that proceeds on a normal course is good, as is her eventual verbal speaking ability.

## Author Note

This is a fictional patient based on features of several babies and their families in our collective history.

## References


Centers for Disease Control and Prevention (CDC). (2008). www.cdc.gov/ncbddd/ehdi/

Gorga, M. P., Kaminski, J. R., Beauchaine, K. L., Jesteadt, W., & Neely, S. T. (1989). Auditory brainstem responses from children three months to three years of age: Normal patterns of response II. *Journal of Speech and Hearing Research, 32*, 281–288.

Hermann, B. S., Thornton, A. R., & Joseph, J. M. (1995). Automated infant hearing screening using ABR: Development and validation. *American Journal of Audiology, 4*, 6–14.

Kemp, D. T., Ryan, S., & Bray, T. (1990). A guide to the effective use of otoacoustic emissions. *Ear and Hearing, 11*(2), L 93–105.

Mauk, G. W., White, K. R., Behrens, T., & Vohr, B. R. (1991). The effectiveness of screening programs based on high-risk characteristics in early identification of hearing impairment. *Ear and Hearing, 12*, 312–319.

Maxon, A. B., Vohr, B. R., & White, K. R. (1996). Newborn hearing screening: Comparison of a simplified otoacoustic emissions device (ILO1088) with the ILO88. *Early Human Development, 45*(1-2), 171–178.

Mehl, A. L., & Thomson, V. (1998). Newborn hearing screening: The great omission. *Pediatrics, 101*(1), e4.

Moeller, M. P. (2000). Early intervention and language development in children who are deaf and hard of hearing. *Pediatrics, 106*(3), 1–9.

National Institute of Deafness and Other Communication Disorders (NIDCD). (2008). www.nidcd.nih.gov/health/hearing/

National Center for Hearing Assessment and Management (NCHAM). (2008). www.infanthearing.org

Widen, J. E., & Keener, S. K. (2003). Diagnostic testing for hearing loss in infants and young children. *Mental Retardation Research Reviews, 9*, 220–224.

Yoshinaga-Itano, C., Sedey, A. L., Coulter, D. K., & Mehl, A. L. (1998). Language of early- and later-identified children with hearing loss. *Pediatrics, 102*, 1161–1171.


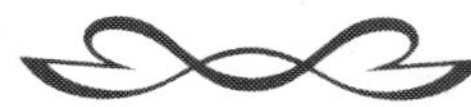

# FRAGILE X SYNDROME

CASE **5**

# Jake: The Move from Early Intervention to Early Childhood Education for a Child with Fragile X Syndrome


*Gail Harris-Schmidt*


## Conceptual Knowledge Areas

This case is designed for those with both some knowledge of and interest in young children with speech and language disorders due to genetic syndromes, such as fragile X syndrome. Some knowledge of Early Intervention (EI) and Early Childhood Education (ECE) is helpful, but not required, to fully appreciate the complexities of this case. Understanding and awareness of interdisciplinary service provision is also useful. Fragile X syndrome is the most common inherited cause of intellectual disabilities. Women may be carriers of the abnormal X chromosome, but the syndrome only appears clinically in their male offspring. Boys with the full mutation typically have cognitive impairments. These can range from mild learning disabilities to severe cognitive disabilities. Boys with fragile X also often have speech, language and developmental delays, attention and behavioral issues, and sensory overload problems. Most boys with fragile X have some autistic-like characteristics, and some are diagnosed with autism (Hagerman & Hagerman, 2002).

## Description of the Case

The Early Intervention (EI) and Early Childhood Education (ECE) teams in a suburban public school began working with Jake and his parents, as Jake was about to turn 3 years of age and transition into Early Childhood Special Education. The ECE team consisted of Jake's parents, a school psychologist, school social worker, speech-language pathologist (SLP), physical therapist (PT), and occupational therapist (OT).

### Background Information

Jake was the first child of a suburban, middle-class, college-educated couple. His father (Will) was a high school history teacher, and his mother (Jenny) a part-time school nurse. Jake's mother was pregnant with a second child at the time of the initial ECE evaluation.

Jake was born full-term without complications after an uneventful pregnancy. He weighed 7 pounds, 5 ounces at birth and was 21 inches long. There were no initial concerns about Jake's medical status, and he was discharged after one day in the hospital. Jake's mother had difficulty nursing him, as he had a weak sucking reflex. She began bottle feeding when he lost weight during his first few weeks and tried a variety of nipples to aid his sucking. Jake was a somewhat "floppy" baby (with low muscle tone), but his parents assumed that he would gain more muscular control as he developed. He had prominent ears, which the parents found endearing.

As Jake approached his first birthday, his parents became more concerned about his development. He was very "high strung" and irritable, and he had problems sleeping and eating. His parents tried soy milk, thinking that he might have lactose intolerance, but Jake remained fussy both as he ate and afterward. He was late in holding his head up and sitting, and he had not yet begun to crawl. He rarely cooed or babbled and made no attempts to imitate syllables.

Jake had already had three ear infections before his first birthday; consequently, throughout his second year, the pediatrician monitored his ears carefully and finally referred the family to an ear, nose, and throat specialist. Jake's hearing was tested periodically from 12 months on. Tympanometry performed at 15 and 18 months of age revealed bilateral fluid. Pressure equalization tubes were inserted at 18 months. One tube was subsequently replaced, while the other (original) tube was still intact at the time he entered ECE. Jake's parents attributed some of his speech and language delays to the ear infections, and the pediatrician assured them that Jake would "catch up."

During his second year, Jake had difficulty making eye contact and did not display the joint attention to books and toys that his parents saw with other children his age. He often fixated on TV shows or toddler DVDs and screamed until they were shown repeatedly. He continued to be "high strung" and flapped his hands when overstimulated. He chewed on his clothing and occasionally on his hand. Jenny and Will expressed concerns to their pediatrician about Jake's lack of sociability and raised the possibility that Jake might be displaying some symptoms of autism. The pediatrician did not think that Jake displayed autistic characteristics and stated that it was far too early to be considering such a diagnosis.

Jake began to walk at 19 months and said his first word at 23 months ("Bu" for "Burt" of *Sesame Street*). He had not slept through the night during his first two years. He was an extremely picky and messy eater; he often stuffed food into his mouth until it was overly full, and then spit it out. He continued to drink from a bottle. Often the only way his parents could get him back to sleep at night was by giving him a bottle of juice.

### Reason for Referral

By his second birthday, Jake's parents were concerned enough about his developmental delays to seek a referral from their pediatrician for a developmental evaluation with the Early Intervention

(EI) providers in their area. The EI team conducted a play-based evaluation in Jake's home when he was 24 months old. Jake's mother completed the interview and the MacArthur-Bates Communicative Development Inventories: Words and Gestures (Fenson et al., 2006a); the SLP at first considered giving the parents the more age-appropriate MacArthur-Bates Words and Sentences (Fenson et al., 2006b) inventory to complete, but decided against it once she saw how limited Jake's language was. Even with the questions designed for those 8 to 16 months old, his mother indicated concerns in all areas.

Jenny reported that Jake's receptive language skills were better than his expressive skills. He could recognize and point to pictures in books and characters in TV shows and movies and could recognize family names (e.g., Mommy, Daddy, Grandma, Grandpa) and find the appropriate person. He knew and could point to a variety of animals and match their sounds to the animal's name. The SLP attempted some play-based interactions, but had difficulty getting Jake to cooperate. She observed oral-motor skills, but neither she nor the occupational therapist could conduct a complete oral-motor exam, due to his resistance. The occupational therapist observed his overall low muscle tone, hypersensitivity to touch, and strong reactions to loud sounds.

## Early Intervention

Jake qualified for EI services based upon developmental delays of more than 30% in at least two areas (the requirements of the state in which the family lived). Since he qualified on the basis of speech-language and fine motor delays, with some less severe gross motor delays, an Individual Family Service Plan (IFSP) was developed.

A home-based and center-based program was initiated. The SLP and OT provided therapy simultaneously at home once weekly and worked with the parents on language stimulation, oral-motor activities, and sensory integration/calming techniques. Jenny and Will also attended a series of parent education programs based upon the "It Takes Two to Talk" Hanen Program (Manolson, 1992) designed for parents of children with language delays.

Once each week, Jake and his mother attended a center-based EI class at a local Easter Seals agency, where a small group of parents and children met for language and motor stimulation activities. The SLP used picture cues with Jake to help him learn the routines of the sessions. She found that he responded very well to visual cueing and to routines. He began to anticipate and cooperate with the sequence of activities in the center-based program. If routines and schedules changed, he became agitated. During some sessions, he became extremely overstimulated and uncooperative and tried to bite or hit other children.

The SLP tried a Picture Exchange Communication System (PECS; Frost and Bondy, 2002) and attempted to teach Jake sign language to help him make his wants and needs known; however, as he approached his third birthday, Jake had not made much progress. His parents were somewhat resistant to the use of any type of augmentative or alternative communication (AAC) system, as they continued to hope that Jake would become more verbal. Jake made some gains throughout the year, increasing his expressive vocabulary to five words and improving his receptive vocabulary and understanding of simple one-step commands.

When Jake was 33 months old (2 years, 9 months), his parents received a letter from Jenny's cousin Sara. Her 5-year-old son, who had many developmental delays, had recently been diagnosed with fragile X syndrome. Sara had tested positive as a carrier of fragile X, with the premutation of the syndrome. Both of her parents were tested, and Sara's father (Jenny's uncle) was found to be a carrier, with a premutation and no effects. As a man cannot inherit the X chromosome from his father (fathers pass the Y chromosome, but not the X, to all sons), the fragile X gene was traced back to Sara's and Jenny's grandmother. This meant that any of the grandmother's children (including Jenny's father) might also be a carrier of the fragile X gene.

Jenny and Will were devastated to learn the news of the genetic mutation in the family and sought testing for Jake and themselves. Since a father cannot pass the fragile X gene to his son, Will realized that he did not need to be tested. Jake and Jenny were tested through a blood sample sent to a large medical center with a genetic testing facility. Jake was found to have the full mutation of fragile X syndrome; Jenny was found to be a carrier, a person with the genetic repeat pattern in premutation range.

At the time of the testing, Jenny was pregnant with their second child. She learned that she had a 50-50 chance of passing the fragile X gene to her unborn child, as she had both eggs with the fragile X marker and unaffected eggs. She elected to have genetic testing and learned that her second child, a girl, did not carry the fragile X gene.

At the time of the transition to Early Childhood Education, Will and Jenny were still reeling from news of the fragile X diagnosis. They had thought that Jake's numerous, recurring ear infections or other factors might be causing his difficulties and hoped that intervention would help him "grow out" of his delays. Jenny was feeling extremely guilty for being a "silent carrier" of a genetic disorder, although her husband was very supportive and assured her that it was no one's "fault." It was at this time that Jake began the evaluations for ECE programming, and his parents faced choices about the most appropriate setting for Jake's needs and goals.

## Findings of the Evaluation: Early Childhood Education Evaluation

Jake was first assessed in his home with his mother and father present. Observations, language sampling, checklists, the Peabody Picture Vocabulary Test-4 (Dunn and Dunn, 2007), and the Rossetti Infant-Toddler Language Scale (Rossetti, 2006) were used to complete the assessment. The Preschool Language Scale-Fourth Edition (Zimmerman, Steiner, & Pond, 2002) was attempted, but Jake's attention was minimal, and little was gained from the items sampled. He was unable to comprehend many of the tasks, nor to complete the expressive tasks.

On the Peabody Picture Vocabulary Test-4, Form B (PPVT-4), Jake received a raw score of 5, which converted to a standard score of 65, more than two standard deviations below the mean. Even with the first few pictures, he had some difficulty comprehending what to do and maintaining attention to the task, and the SLP often had to point to each of the four pictures in order to get him to scan them all. She believed that inattention interfered enough that the test score might have been quite minimal and not totally valid.

On the Rossetti Infant-Toddler Language Scale (Rossetti, 2006), Jake demonstrated receptive language skills in the 9–12 month range, with some scatter skills at the 12–15 month range. Most language comprehension items were either reported or observed in those ranges.

The SLP and OT observed Jake in play with his parents and attempted to interest him in some of the toys they had brought. Observations of play and nonverbal communication skills revealed strong attachment skills to familiar people, but great difficulty with unfamiliar people. His joint attention to objects with both his parents and the SLP and OT was poor, and they often had to move an object in front of his face to get him to attend to it. He used some intentional gestures to get objects that he wanted, and he showed some functional use of objects in play, especially in imitation. He did not play with objects in a creative way, but sometimes banged or shook them. Results of developmental testing placed Jake below his age range for play, when compared to his peer group. His short attention span and frequent outbursts contributed to his difficulty in play skills.

Expressive scores fell in the 6–9 month range, with some scatter skills in the 9–12 and 12–15 month ranges. Jake used five words expressively (no, me, do/go, mo/more, bu [Burt]), and his mother reported five additional words that she had heard. Informal play-based assessment revealed no two-word combinations. Jake imitated words in play scripts, such as bop/pop, bi/big, and boo/book. These were limited to his current phonetic inventory (/p/, /b/, /m/, /n/, /t/, /d/). He vocalized in order to express his desire to change tasks. He expressed frustration when he was not understood by refusing to attempt the word again. The SLP noted that Jake had very poor eye contact and problems with joint attention.

It was difficult to conduct a thorough oral-motor exam, as Jake demonstrated much resistance to being touched around the face and mouth. The SLP had asked his mother to bring in a variety of food and drinks and attempted to get him to eat pudding, chew a cookie or bagel, and drink from various cups. The SLP noted that he had a high, narrow palate and low muscle tone in his oral musculature. Related to poor mouth closure, lip competence, including rounding and retraction, was weak. Jaw strength and grading for chewing and feeding were also affected. Jake demonstrated an immature feeding pattern consisting of munching and sucking foods, as well as swallowing without chewing to completion. According to his parents, Jake was picky about the foods he would eat. In the evaluation, he preferred crunchy and soft foods. Jake's parents reported that he still drank from a bottle at bedtime and a sippy cup during the day. At the time of the evaluation, Jake could not drink from a juice box. Observation of Jake's use of a straw revealed a sucking pattern resting the straw on the tongue blade, rather than using lip rounding and closure to seal and move the liquid up and into the oral cavity for swallowing. No choking was observed in the evaluation, but his parents reported some choking when he stuffed his mouth with too much food.

The occupational therapist concurred with the sensory concerns and found Jake to be a child with hyperarousal, sensory overload issues, and an extremely short attention span. Fine motor skills were found to be well below his age range, with some sensory issues noted. Gross motor skills were found to be below the range for his age, with most difficulty seen in motor planning. Jake demonstrated motor planning difficulties in his speech, as well as with his body in space. His parents reported that he tripped a lot at home.

The social worker interviewed both of Jake's parents and found a very loving, resilient, and caring couple, who were deeply concerned about their little boy and his development. She sought out materials from the National Fragile X Foundation, both for the school team and for Jake's parents. She referred them to a local Fragile X Resource Group, so that they would be able to talk with other parents and find support there.

The school psychologist attempted to administer a preschool intelligence test at the special education center, but had great difficulty given Jake's short attention span and anxiety. She believed there were cognitive delays, but could not report any scores or results.

## Findings of the Evaluation: Results and Diagnostic Hypothesis

Jake was determined to have speech, language, and oral-motor delays consistent with fragile X syndrome. He was also diagnosed with sensory and motor delays affecting his level of arousal, eating and sleeping patterns, and fine motor skills. A report of his cognitive abilities was not included in the summary. Jake was diagnosed with "developmental delay" with speech-language delay as a secondary diagnosis.

## Treatment Options Considered

The team worked to develop an appropriate Individualized Educational Plan (IEP) for Jake's move to an ECE program. His goals clearly required collaborative programming, utilizing the expertise of a variety of professionals. The team immediately ruled out speech-language and occupational therapy services as a nonattending student (that is, one with no other daily program) as inappropriate. They also ruled out a program designed for young children with profound disabilities, as Jake's IEP goals could not be met appropriately in a setting designed for children with much more involved needs.

Two different settings were discussed. There was some disagreement among team members about the most appropriate placement for Jake. One of the settings was in a "blended" classroom in a local public school; the classroom included some at-risk children (not diagnosed with special education classifications) along with children who had a variety of special education classifications (Down syndrome, hearing loss, language delay, phonological delay, autistic spectrum disorders). An early childhood special education teacher taught the half-day class with twice-a-week services from a speech-language pathologist and occupational therapist, and two classroom paraprofessionals. The SLP and OT were present on opposite days and did not provide services together. They did attempt to collaborate by phone and e-mail and help each other with appropriate language/sensory activities. The classroom was very "language rich," lively, and busy. The walls were all decorated in bright colors, and the noise level was often high.

The second placement discussed was a half-day, more structured special education class designed for children who had moderate-to-severe disorders. The program was housed in a special education center with other classes for children in special education from age 3 years through grade 8. All eight children in the class had multiple needs. Some were nonverbal and used augmentative communication (AAC) devices. Others had physical disabilities with cognitive delays. A nurse was on staff, along with an early childhood special education teacher, speech-language pathologist, occupational therapist, and physical therapist. The SLP, OT, and PT were in attendance for an hour each day of the four-day a week program. Their services overlapped, and they often coordinated lessons that targeted integrated movement and language activities. On Friday of each week, staff members made home visits to work with parents and children in their own homes. An expert in AAC was a program consultant and visited weekly. The classroom was also language-rich, but more structured and calm than the first one. The room contained a "quiet area," with a small pop-up tent, beanbag chairs, picture books, and calming music on tapes. There was a small gym nearby, with a ball pit, swings, mats, and a trampoline for sensory activities.

Will and Jenny visited both classrooms and determined that the "blended" classroom provided opportunities for Jake to interact with and imitate more verbal peers and to have good role models for play. The speech-language pathologist agreed and also recommended the blended classroom. She believed that Jake would benefit from the stimulating language environment there. She also felt that the SLP and OT could design some calming activities for Jake, which could be implemented even when they were not in the classroom at the same time. She believed that the SLP in the blended classroom could consult with the AAC specialist at the special education center to design more helpful ways to augment Jake's expressive language.

The occupational therapist had concerns about the "blended" classroom, as he considered it to be overwhelming to the senses. He believed Jake might have more behavioral problems because of the visual and auditory hyperstimulation. He thought that Jake would get more individual attention in a quiet, structured setting, with easy access to calming spaces and activities. He stated that with more staff available and more opportunities for collaborative programming, Jake would make better progress. He felt that Jake could be included in other settings later.

The school psychologist agreed with the OT as she had seen Jake's behavioral and anxiety issues in her attempts to complete an assessment. She believed that if some of the attention and behavior issues could be treated, then Jake might be able to move out of the special education center into a setting that offered more mainstreaming.

## Description of Course of Treatment

Ultimately, the team decided to place Jake in the blended classroom with access to more verbal children. He turned 3 years of age in July and began the program in late August. Jake's baby sister had been born in the prior spring, and Jenny took a maternity leave. At home, she followed up on suggestions from the school faculty, sent a notebook back and forth each day to communicate, and was a very collaborative member of Jake's ECE team.

## Analysis of Client's Response to Intervention

Jake had great difficulty at first with the transition to the new setting and a longer morning, particularly without his mother present. He was scheduled to take the special education bus to school. However, Jenny drove him, as his resistance to the transportation was so strong. He had several "meltdowns" during the first weeks and had to be taken by his one-on-one aide for walks to a quiet place. His behavior continued to be an issue throughout the year, as sensory overload often preceded an aggressive outburst. The staff became better at noticing the antecedents to a behavioral crisis (e.g., becoming red in the face, flapping his hands, or chewing on his clothing) and tried to intercede before Jake would hit or bite another person or himself.

The staff gradually found various ways to calm Jake and help him make it through the morning. The early childhood teacher was excellent at using visual cues for the entire class, and she made sure to go through the picture schedule each day. If there were changes in the schedule, she discussed them with Jenny in advance, so that both of them could work with picture cues to prepare Jake for the day. She provided many visual cues in her teaching, and Jake responded well to them. With both Jake and a child diagnosed with autism in her class, she became more sensitive to the noise level and overload issues in the classroom.

The occupational therapist designed a "sensory diet," which included a variety of deep-pressure activities (e.g., wall pushups, rolling in a blanket). She also provided him with a weighted vest during some activities, which seemed to provide the sensory input he needed to calm him. She and the SLP communicated by e-mail and tried to design some activities that would help Jake meet multiple goals in both speech/language and sensory motor areas. She found that Jake enjoyed puzzles and was very good with putting 10–20-piece puzzles together. She worked to integrate language into his puzzle time, as she labeled pieces and made comments about their placements (e.g., "Oh, it's under the swing").

The SLP integrated sensory activities into her goals and activities, as she worked in four different areas: (1) Receptive goals included a focus on increasing Jake's comprehension of vocabulary in thematic units and completion of one-step directions. (2) Expressive goals in language and articulation were aimed at increasing his phonetic inventories and his expressive vocabulary. She used many pictures, storyboards, and low-tech AAC devices to help him develop additional ways to express himself. (3) Oral-motor and feeding goals centered on increasing Jake's awareness of and strengthening his oral musculature. (4) Social-pragmatic goals included fostering turn-taking, requesting items, and initiating play. A few simple signs (such as "more") helped him to communicate some wants and needs.

At the end of the school year, his standard score on the Peabody Picture Vocabulary Test-4 (Dunn and Dunn, 2007) increased by 7 points. He did especially well with words that included his interests (transportation and animals) and added receptive vocabulary from all the thematic units of the year. He also comprehended directions utilizing simple prepositions.

His progress in expressive speech was not as good. He added 20 single words, but did not increase his sound repertoire. For example, he labeled five new items as "ba": ball, baby, bottle, big, and bear. He could differentiate the items and clearly knew what they were receptively, but his pronunciation was very unclear. Jake made gains in using gestures more expressively and meaningfully.

Jake made some progress in oral-motor areas. He began to drink from a straw that had been cut in half (he could not use the narrow juice box straws), and he could blow bubbles. His eating was still messy. However, his family and the school staff worked on controlling how much he should have on his plate, so that he would not overstuff his mouth and choke.

Social-pragmatic and play skills remained difficult, although Jake would cooperate in structured interactions. He preferred the adult teachers to his classmates and did not make overtures to play unless prompted with very specific directions. He would cooperate in routines, such as going around the snack table to hand out napkins, but continued to have difficulty with eye contact or any verbalization while accomplishing such tasks. He preferred to play alone and often stacked blocks or scooped sand repetitively. During center times, the SLP tried to work with him by playing in a parallel way with comments (self-talk) about what she was doing. She also worked to have another child play near him, while she engaged them both in an activity.

## Further Recommendations

At the end-of-the-year annual review and IEP update, the team again discussed the option of moving Jake to the special education classroom housed in the special education center. Jake's parents were pleased with the blended setting and believed that he was making progress. They still hoped that more expressive language and calmer behavior was possible.

The SLP believed that some aspects of the alternative classroom might be beneficial for Jake, including the consultation of the AAC technology expert and the amount of time that the SLP and OT were simultaneously in the classroom. However, she and the others agreed that Jake was making progress, and the team decided to keep Jake in the same placement for another year.

### Author Note

The client, "Jake," is fictional, based upon a number of children with fragile X syndrome seen by the author.

### References


Dunn, L., & Dunn, D. (2007). *Peabody Picture Vocabulary Test* (4th ed.). Minneapolis: AGS Corporation.

Fenson, L., Marchman, V., Thal, D., Dale, P., Reznick, S., & Bates, E. (2006). *MacArthur-Bates Communicative Development Inventories: Words and Gestures* (2nd ed.). Baltimore: Brookes Publishing.

Fenson, L., Marchman, V., Thal, D., Dale, P., Reznick, S., & Bates, E. (2006). *MacArthur-Bates Communicative Development Inventories: Words and Sentences* (2nd ed.). Baltimore: Brookes Publishing.

Frost, L., and Bondy, A. (2002). *The Picture Exchange Communication System training manual* (2nd ed.). Newark, DE: Pyramid Educational Products.

Hagerman, R., & Hagerman, P. (2002). *Fragile X syndrome: Diagnosis, treatment, and research* (3rd ed.). Baltimore: Johns Hopkins University Press.

Manolson, A. (1992). *It takes two to talk: The Hanen program for parents*. Toronto: The Hanen Centre.

Rossetti, L. (2006). *The Rossetti Infant-Toddler Scales*. East Moline, IL: LinguiSystems.

Zimmerman, I., Steiner, V., & Pond, R. (2002). *Preschool Language Test-4*. San Antonio, TX: The Psychological Corporation.


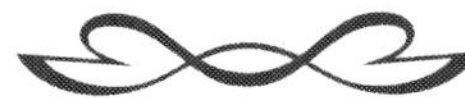

## PRENATAL ALCOHOL/DRUG EXPOSURE

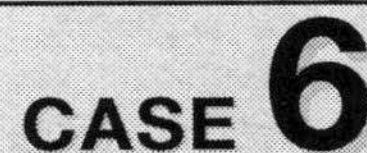

# CASE 6 Sybil: Alcohol and/or Prenatal Drug Exposure


*Dorian Lee-Wilkerson*


## Conceptual Knowledge Areas

Each year, more than 4 million babies are born in the United States. One million of those babies are reportedly born with prenatal exposure to alcohol and/or other drugs (National Center for Health Statistics, 2007). The *2006 National Survey on Drug Use and Health* in the United States estimates that 8.3 million children ages 0 to 17 years are currently living with the effects of prenatal exposure to alcohol and/or drugs; that 12% of pregnant women between the ages of 15–44 years report drinking during their pregnancy; and that 4% report using illicit drugs at some time during their pregnancy (SAMHSA, 2007). May and Gossage (2001) report that 40,000 babies are born annually with fetal alcohol spectrum disorder. The numbers of babies born with prenatal exposure to other drugs is unknown, because it is estimated that the majority of these infants, 75–95%, go home undiagnosed (Young, 2006).

For over 30 years researchers have investigated the effects of prenatal alcohol and drug exposure on child development. Yet more is known about the prenatal effects of alcohol than about the prenatal effects of drug use. For additional information about the challenges of identifying children with prenatal drug exposure as well as the known effects of prenatal drug exposure, see Arendt, Singer, Minnes, and Salvator (1999).

Fetal alcohol spectrum disorders (FASDs) include a wide range of physical, mental, and behavioral characteristics that are associated with maternal use of alcohol during pregnancy. The most severe form of FASD is fetal alcohol syndrome (FAS). The Centers for Disease Control (CDC, 2006) reports that FAS occurs in 0.2–1.5 per 1,000 live births. Children with FAS usually present with abnormal facial features and growth deficiencies. Children with FAS may also exhibit attention deficits, memory impairments, learning disability, visual disturbances, hearing impairment, and/or speech and language impairment. In addition to FAS, FASDs include alcohol-related birth defects (ARBDs) and alcohol-related neurodevelopmental disorders (ARNDs). The reported prevalence rate for ARBD and ARND combined is three times higher than the rate of FAS. Children with ARBD may have defects of the skeletal and major organ systems along with some behavioral and cognitive problems. Children with ARND may experience neurological impairments affecting vision, hearing, motor movements, balance, cognition, behavior, and sensory integration (CDC, 2006; SAMHSA, 2007). According to the Centers for Disease Control, a child with FASD may experience one or more of the characteristics listed in Figure 6.1.

SAMHSA cites results of a University of Washington study by Streissguthand and others (2004) showing that FASD places a child at risk for school failure, substance abuse, mental illness, poor employment history, and involvement in the criminal justice system.

The National Institute on Drug Abuse (NIDA) has supported numerous studies and has compiled a summary of 24 current investigations that have or are presently examining the long-term effects of prenatal drug exposure (NIDA Notes, 2004), including cocaine, marijuana, opiates, ecstasy, methamphetamine, and tobacco. One of the largest in this group is the Maternal Lifestyle Study (Lester et al., 2004) that reported the outcomes of 1,388 1-month-old infants born with prenatal drug exposure. These infants were found to experience poor quality of movement and regulation, lower arousal, higher excitability, hypertonia, and nonoptimal reflexes.

Rivkin and his associates (2008) used volumetric MRI to image the brains of 35 adolescents and found that the effects of prenatal drug exposure may persist beyond early childhood. These researchers found reductions in the cortical gray matter of participating adolescents. Moreover, the researchers found evidence of an additive effect. That is, the adolescents who were exposed to a greater variety of drugs and alcohol prenatally had greater

- Small for gestational age
- Small stature
- Facial abnormalities
- Poor coordination
- Mental retardation
- Lower than average IQ scores
- Learning disabilities
- Hyperactivity
- Sleep disturbances
- Poor reasoning and judgment
- Speech-language delays

FIGURE 6.1 Characteristics of FASD

- Low birth weight
- Premature birth
- Small for gestational age
- Failure to thrive
- Infectious diseases
- Sudden infant death syndrome
- Fetal alcohol syndrome

FIGURE 6.2 Medical Outcomes of Prenatal Drug Exposure

- Delayed speech and language development
- Atypical social interactions
- Feeding difficulties
- Poor fine motor development
- Poor gross motor development
- Irritability
- Unpredictable sleep patterns
- Minimal play strategies
- Hyperactivity
- Attention deficits
- Poor self regulation
- Difficulty transitioning from one activity to the next
- Auditory processing deficits
- Visual processing deficits

FIGURE 6.3 Developmental Outcomes of Prenatal Drug Exposure

reductions in brain volume when compared with their peers who were reportedly exposed to a single drug. The research of Scher, Richardson, and Day (2000) revealed that women who drink or use drugs during pregnancy often use multiple substances that can include combinations of alcohol, marijuana, tobacco, cocaine, and/or other illicit drugs. Figures 6.2 and 6.3 list the medical and developmental outcomes of children with prenatal drug exposure as reported by the ARCH National Resource Center (1997).

There is also research showing that the effects of intrauterine alcohol and drug exposure is compounded by the association of additional risk factors such as poor nutrition, inadequate prenatal care, limited social supports, unsafe home environments, and unstable lifestyles (Pulsifer, Radonovich, Belcher, & Butz, 2004; Watson & Westby, 2003). Coggins, Timler, and Olswang (2007) note that children with a history of alcohol and drug exposure live in a state of "double jeopardy." Children suffering with the effects of prenatal drug and alcohol exposure are more likely to be born to single mothers living in poverty. They are more likely to be born to mothers who did not complete high school and to mothers and fathers who are or have been involved in the criminal justice system.

For many children, drug exposure and its associated risks do not end at birth. In a study by Pulsifer et al. (2004), 66% of the 104 participating mothers reported continued use of drugs after the birth of their child. Children with prenatal drug and alcohol exposure, born to parents who continue use after the child's birth, are placed at greater risk for developmental delay because of adverse environmental factors such as poor parenting and/or multiple foster care placements (Brown, Bakeman, Coles, Platzman, & Lynch, 2004). Children with histories of alcohol and drug exposure living with parents who continue use are also more likely to experience neglect, verbal abuse, physical abuse, and/or involvement with Child Protective Services than their nonexposed counterparts (Rogers-Adkinson & Stuart, 2007).

It is difficult to predict the developmental outcomes of children born with prenatal exposure to drugs and alcohol. Some children will present with pronounced signs and symptoms of exposure at birth (e.g., children with FAS). Others may not exhibit signs until they enter school and are faced with cognitively demanding tasks. Researchers have shown that biological factors such as frequency of exposure, amount and type of exposure, and genetic susceptibility will interact with environmental factors such as family income, family lifestyle, employment history, and educational background to produce the disparate clinical profiles that define this population (Watson & Westby, 2003). The following case presents an opportunity to examine the speech and language patterns of a child in light of her history of prenatal exposure to drugs and alcohol, her social and developmental history, and her present status, and to use this information to plan for follow-up care as she progresses in school.

## Description of the Case

### Background Information

#### Relevant Facts

Sybil's maternal grandparents applied for participation in the university's 6-week summer clinic session. At the time of the application, she was 7 years and 9 months old, enrolled in a public school in the second grade, and receiving speech therapy services. The school-based speech-language pathologist made the referral to the summer program.

#### History

Sybil lived with her maternal grandparents. At the time of the assessment, neither the grandparents nor Sybil had contact with her biological parents. The grandparents stated that they had no knowledge of where their daughter, Sybil's mother, was living or how she was doing. They believed Sybil's biological father was 40 and had completed high school, but did not know what he did for a living. The grandparents also stated that they were deeply concerned about their daughter because they had not heard from her in over 2 years. Their daughter began experimenting with drugs in high school, became pregnant, and dropped out of school in the 10th grade. The child from this first pregnancy was raised by his paternal grandparents and is currently attending a local community college. The grandparents also reported that their daughter had been treated for cocaine addiction at least twice before Sybil's birth. Unfortunately, she was not able to maintain recovery. Their daughter became pregnant with Sybil, her second child, when she was 28 years of age and experiencing a relapse. Their daughter reportedly stopped drinking alcohol, taking cocaine and marijuana, and stopped smoking when she discovered that she was pregnant with Sybil. This occurred during the second trimester of the pregnancy. She gave birth to Sybil when she was 29 years of age. Sybil, however, tested positive for exposure to cocaine, marijuana, and tobacco at birth.

The grandparents also indicated that their daughter and her boyfriend, Sybil's father, enrolled in drug and alcohol treatment after Sybil's birth and cared for her for two years, with their help. Both parents subsequently experienced a relapse and lost custody of Sybil. The grandparents became Sybil's legal guardians when she turned 3 years of age.

Sybil's grandmother works as a housekeeper and her grandfather works as a long-distance truck driver. They described their income level as low-to-middle SES and they own their home. They have raised four children and continued to despair over the plight of their oldest child, Sybil's mother. Their other three children are doing well with family and careers. Besides Sybil, the grandparents have five other grandchildren who live out of state with their parents.

The grandparents reported that Sybil's medical history was unremarkable with the exceptions of prenatal poly-drug exposure and typical cases of tonsillitis and bronchitis at ages 3 and 4, respectively. They could not accurately report about Sybil's attainment of developmental milestones, but noted that they enrolled her in a special preschool program because of a referral made by Sybil's pediatrician at age 3 years, 3 months. Sybil's pediatrician made the referral because of delays in gross motor skills and speech development.

Sybil had experienced school failure in spelling, reading, and mathematics. She liked school and enjoyed reading. She was an active child and demonstrated difficulty in managing her moods when she experienced frustration. Sybil often responded poorly to parental discipline.

### Reason for Referral

Sybil was referred to the 6-week summer clinic by her school speech-language pathologist to help her maintain the skills she had achieved during the school year and to facilitate additional growth.

## Findings of the Evaluation

Sybil's speech and language skills were evaluated 1 week prior to the start of the 6-week summer session. She was age 7 years, 10 months at the time of testing. Sybil demonstrated speech delay for the sounds / ʧ, r, l/ and for consonantal blends. The Goldman-Fristoe Test of Articulation 2 (2000) revealed the following errors: ʃ/ʧ, w/r substitutions in blends, and omission of / l / in blends. Stimulability for all errors was noted at word level.

Sybil demonstrated specific language impairment at the time of testing. She obtained a listening comprehension score of 6 years, 7 months and an oral expression score of 5 years, 4 months on the Oral and Written Language Scales (OWLS; Carrow-Woolfolk, 1995). Informal testing revealed difficulty with following 1-part, 2-part, and 3-part directions, responding appropriately to "wh" questions, and incorrect use of verb tenses in phrases and sentences. Sybil also did not maintain attention to all language tasks and showed behavioral signs of frustration when the examiner attempted to return her attention to the tasks.

Sybil's hearing was screened in an audiometric booth at 20 db HL, bilaterally for the frequencies of 500, 1,000, 2,000, 4,000, and 8,000 Hz. She passed the screening. The oral mechanism screening examination produced unremarkable findings with the exception of the diadochokinetic tasks. Rapid movements for single syllables, two syllables, and three syllables were all below age-expected rates.

## Treatment Options Considered

Treatment options for speech delay included use of Minimal Pairs Contrast Training (Bernthal & Bankson, 2004) to target sounds using a linguistic approach and Van Riper's traditional (Bernthal & Bankson, 2004) approach to target sounds using a motor approach. Minimal Pairs Contrast Training was considered because Sybil demonstrated stimulability, suggesting that her errors were linguistic in nature. Stimulability was confined, however, to word level. Baseline testing revealed that as the complexity of the phonetic context increased, Sybil's motor control and stimulability for correction decreased. Van Riper's traditional approach proved to be a better choice of treatment because it provided practice in syllables and nonsense words to enhance motor control. Also, baseline testing showed that Sybil was able to detect errors in the clinician's speech and her own speech. These data suggested minimal need for perceptual training.

Treatment options for the language impairment included use of drill play and modeling, focused stimulation, facilitative play, and script therapy. Drill play and modeling were used to teach verb tense targets, response to "wh" questions, and following directions. Drill play was used briefly (5–10 minutes) at the beginning of sessions, because Sybil preferred to be engaged in physical activities that involved small groups of people. Facilitative play was used to provide practice for targets taught through drill, but was discontinued because Sybil had difficulty transitioning from one activity to the next. Focused stimulation and script therapy were more effective in providing practiced use of language and speech targets, because the start and end points of each activity could be clearly established by the clinician. The techniques of modeling, utterance expansion, and utterance extension were incorporated during focused stimulation and whenever the opportunity occurred.

## Course of Treatment

The goals for the 6-week summer session included:

1. To spontaneously produce /ʧ/ in all word positions at sentence level while engaged in play and structured activities at an 80% accuracy level
2. To spontaneously produce /r/ and /l/ blends in words while engaged in play and structured activities at an 80% level of accuracy

3. To spontaneously respond to "wh" questions while engaged in play and structured activities at a 90% accuracy level
4. To spontaneously respond to 1-step and 2-step instructions while engaged in play and structured activities at a 90% accuracy level
5. To spontaneously express present, past, and future tenses of irregular verbs while engaged in play and structured activities at an 80% accuracy level

Treatment was provided 3 hours a day for 4 days a week for a period of 6 weeks during the summer session, yielding a total of 72 hours of therapy. Each goal was targeted every day and included in periods of individual and group treatments. Forty-five minutes of each day were devoted to individual speech training using Van Riper's traditional approach. Forty minutes of each day were devoted to individual language training using drill play and modeling, focused stimulation, script therapy, and free play. Forty-five minutes were used for group practice of speech and language targets using focused stimulation, modeling, and utterance expansion and utterance extension techniques. In the group sessions, 4–5 clients along with their student clinicians targeted speech and language goals using art projects, dramatic play, preliteracy and literacy tasks, and field trips. The remaining 45 minutes were used for parent training, free play, rest and bathroom breaks, transitioning from one session to the next, and snacks. Figures 6.4, 6.5, and 6.6 detail the treatment steps.

Daily tallies of performances were kept and formal progress measures were gathered at the end of 3 weeks and at the end of 6 weeks. A semester progress report was written based on the formal data collected at the end of the 6-week session.

## Analysis of the Client's Response to Intervention

Sybil made progress in treatment. Post-therapy testing at the end of the 6-week session showed that Sybil spontaneously produced /ʧ/ in all word positions in sentences with 85% accuracy and /r/ and /l/ blends in words with 95% accuracy. She responded to "wh" questions with 75% accuracy. Sybil responded to 1-step commands with 100% accuracy and to 2-step commands with 80% accuracy. Her accuracy for use of present, past, and future tenses of irregular verbs was also good. She used the present, past, and future tenses of the verb "to be" with 90% accuracy, the verb "to have" in the present and future tenses with 75% accuracy and the past tense with 60% accuracy, and the verb "to go" in the present and future tenses with 80% accuracy and in the past tense with 70% accuracy.

## Further Recommendations

Sybil will most likely continue to benefit from speech-language pathology services to improve speech intelligibility, language comprehension, and language expression. The impact of these benefits will most likely be seen in academic performance and self-regulation.

FIGURE 6.4 Treatment Steps for Individualized Speech Session (Van Riper's Approach)

- Perceptual training
- Production in isolation
- Production in nonsense syllables
- Production in words
- Production in phrases
- Production in sentences
- Production in conversation

FIGURE 6.5 Treatment Steps for Individualized Language Training

- Drill play and modeling
- Focused stimulation
- Script therapy
- Free play along with modeling, utterance expansion, and utterance extension techniques

*Source*: Information from *Introduction to Clinical Methods in Communication Disorders* (2nd ed.), by R. Paul and P. Cascella, 2007, Baltimore: Paul H. Brookes Publishing.

- Focused stimulation along with modeling, utterance expansion, and utterance extension techniques
- Script therapy
- Free play using modeling, utterance expansion, and utterance extension techniques

FIGURE 6.6 Treatment Steps for Group Practice of Speech and Language Skills

*Source*: Information from *Introduction to Clinical Methods in Communication Disorders* (2nd ed.), by R. Paul and P. Cascella, 2007, Baltimore: Paul H. Brookes Publishing.

## Author Note

Sybil's case represents a compilation of several cases seen in the Hampton University Speech-Language-Hearing Clinic. The author thanks Mrs. Cheryl H. Freeman for assisting with the development of the case profile.

## References

ARCH National Respite Network and Resource Center. (1997, April). *Children with prenatal drug and/or alcohol exposure*, Factsheet No. 49. Retrieved May 30, 2008, from http://www.archrespite.org

Arendt, R., Singer, L., Minnes, S., & Salvator, A. (1999). Accuracy in detection of prenatal drug exposure. *Journal of Drug Issues, 29*(2), 203–214.

Bernthal, J., & Bankson, N. (2004). *Articulation and phonological disorders* (5th ed.). Boston: Pearson.

Brown, J., Bakeman, R., Coles, C., Platzman, K., & Lynch, M. (2004). Prenatal cocaine exposure: A comparison of 2-year-old children in parental and nonparental care. *Child Development, 75*(4), 1282–1295.

Carrow-Woolfolk, E. (1995). *Oral and Written Language Scales (OWLS)*. Circle Pines, MN: American Guidance Service.

Centers for Disease Control (CDC). (2006). *Fetal alcohol spectrum disorders*. Retrieved June 2, 2008, from www.cdc.gov/ncbddd/fasd/index.html/

Coggins, T., Timler, G., & Olswang, L. (2007). A state of double jeopardy: Impact of prenatal alcohol exposure and adverse environments on the social communicative abilities of school-age children with fetal alcohol syndrome. *Language, Speech and Hearing Services in Schools, 38,* 117–127.

Goldman, R., & Fristoe, M. (2000). *Goldman-Fristoe Test of Articulation 2*. Circle Pines, MN: American Guidance Service.

Lester, B., Tronick, E., LaGrasse, L., Seifer, R., Bauer, C., & Shankaran, S., et al. (2004). Summary statistics of neonatal intensive care unit network neurobehavioral scale scores from the maternal lifestyle study: A quasinormative sample. *Pediatrics, 113*(3), 668–675.

May, P., & Gossage, J. (2001). Estimating the prevalence of fetal alcohol syndrome: A summary. *Alcohol Research & Health, 25*(3), 159–167.

National Center of Health Statistics. (2007). *Births/natality*. Retrieved June 2, 2008, from http://www.cdc.gov/nchs/fastats/births.htm

NIDA Notes. (2004). *Conference provides overview of consequences of prenatal drug exposure.* Retrieved May 29, 2008, from http://www.drugabuse.gov/NIDA_notes/Nnvol19N3/Conference.html

Paul, R., & Cascella, P. (2007). *Introduction to clinical methods in communication disorders* (2nd ed.). Baltimore: Paul H. Brookes Publishing.

Pulsifer, M., Radonovich, K., Belcher, H., & Butz, A. (2004). Intelligence and school readiness in preschool children with drug exposure. *Child Neuropsychology, 10,* 89–101.

Rivkin, M., Davis, P., Lemaster, J., Cabral, H., Warfield, S., & Mulkern, R. et al. (2008). Volumetric MRI study of brain in children with intrauterine exposure to cocaine, alcohol, tobacco, and marijuana. *Pediatrics, 121*(4), 741–750.

Rogers-Adkinson, D., & Stuart, S. (2007). Collaborative services: Children experiencing neglect and the side effects of prenatal alcohol exposure. *Language, Speech and Hearing Services in Schools, 38,* 149–156.

Scher, M., Richardson, G., & Day, N. (2000). Effects of prenatal cocaine/crack and other drug exposure on electroencephalographic sleep studies at birth and one year. *Pediatrics, 105*(1), 39–48.

Streissguth, A., Bookstein, F., Barr, H., Sampson, P., O'Malley, K., & Young, J. (2004). Risk factors for adverse life outcomes in fetal alcohol syndrome and fetal alcohol effects. *Journal of Developmental and Behavioral Pediatrics, 25*(4), 228–238.

Substance Abuse and Mental Health Services Administration (SAMHSA). (2007). *Results from the 2006 National Survey on Drug Use and Health: National Findings* (Office of Applied Studies, NSDUH Series H-32, DHHS Publication No. SMA 07-4293). Rockville, MD: Author.

Watson, S., & Westby, C. (2003). Strategies for addressing the executive function impairments of students prenatally exposed to alcohol and other drugs. *Communication Disorders Quarterly, 24*(4), 194–204.

Young, N. (2006). *Substance-exposed infants: Policy and practice*. Presentation to the Substance Abuse and Mental Health Services Administration, Center for Substance Abuse Treatment and the Administration on Children, Youth and Families Children's Bureau, Office on Child Abuse and Neglect, June 20, 2006. Retrieved May 31, 2008, from http://www.ncsacw.samhsa.gov

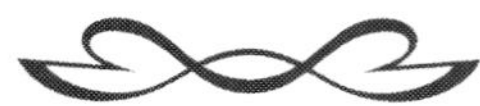

## SICKLE CELL DISEASE

CASE 7

# Nicole: Auditory and Neurocognitive Impact of Sickle Cell Disease in Early Childhood

*Diane M. Scott*

## Conceptual Knowledge Areas

Sickle cell disease (SCD) is a genetically inherited abnormality of the hemoglobin molecule, which is responsible for carrying oxygen in red blood cells (RBCs). Normal RBCs are always soft and flexible and have no problems squeezing through capillaries. Inside normal RBCs, hemoglobin is dissolved in a watery solution and remains dissolved under all conditions. Inside the RBCs of a person with SCD, hemoglobin stays dissolved under some conditions and not under others. Instead of remaining liquid, hemoglobin forms crystals that twist the RBCs out of shape. The RBC is no longer soft and flexible. Crystallized hemoglobin has the following consequences:

1. RBCs clog blood vessels and blood flow backs up. Oxygen is not delivered to organs that need it.
2. When an organ's oxygen supply is cut off, it is damaged and produces pain. Damage can be serious and pain severe (referred to as painful episodes or crises).

3. When RBCs are damaged, the body destroys them. These RBCs cannot be reproduced as rapidly as normal RBCs. So many RBCs are damaged and destroyed in people with SCD that they suffer from chronic anemia. An adequate diet and folic acid are utilized in treating the chronic anemia.
4. People with SCD are not hardy. They are in danger of getting infections; they are frequently incapacitated; they do not grow and develop as well as their peers; and they are not likely to live as long (Bloom, 1995).

SCD refers to sickle cell anemia, sickle cell trait, and sickle cell variants, which are combinations of the sickle cell gene and another gene responsible for hemoglobin production. The sickle gene (Hb S) is present in approximately 8% of African Americans. More than 2 million people in the United States, nearly all of them of African American ancestry, carry the sickle gene. The incidence of sickle cell anemia (HbSS) in the United States is 1 in 500 persons at birth. More than 70,000 patients have homozygous Hb S disease (Distenfeld, 2007; *Prevalence and incidence*, 2008). In 1973, the average lifespan for a person with SCD was 14 years. Based on data from 1995, the average lifespan now is 42 years for men and 48 years for women (Bloom, 1995; Distenfeld, 2007).

Universal newborn screening programs for sickle cell disease (which also identify sickle cell trait) exist in all 50 states and the District of Columbia and in Puerto Rico and the Virgin Islands. At birth 50% to 95% of hemoglobin is fetal hemoglobin (Hb F). After birth the percentage drops off at a rate of 3% to 4% each week, changing to Hb A, Hb S, or another hemoglobin. Thus, by 4 to 5 months of age, RBCs in children with SCD are capable of sickling.

Children with SCD routinely are given prophylactic (preventive) antibiotics and a pneumococcal vaccination to prevent infections. They are especially susceptible to *Streptococcus pneumoniae* (which can cause septicemia or meningitis) and *Hemophilus influenzae* (which can cause nose, throat, and ear infections). Penicillin is generally begun at 2 months of age, while the pneumococcal vaccine is given at 2 years of age.

The only drug currently approved by the Food and Drug Administration (FDA) for the treatment of SCD is hydroxyurea. Hydroxyurea increases the production of Hb F, which retards sickling. As the Hb F level rises, the frequency and severity of vasoocclusive crises declines.

After birth, Hb F production is replaced by Hb S production in babies with SCD. During early infancy, the baby is usually without symptoms. Infections start after 2–3 months, but many children remain symptom-free for a year or more. In the absence of prophylactic antibiotics, children may die of infections between the ages of 1 and 3 years. In early childhood, hand-foot syndrome (blocked blood flow in the bones of the hands and feet causes local swelling accompanied by pain and fever) is often the first presenting problem. Infections, especially of the lungs and kidneys, begin at the same time, though their incidence can be modified by the administration of prophylactic antibiotics. Infections are often associated with painful episodes or crises. Painful episodes can produce organ damage.

The presence of SCD may affect hearing, speech, and language skills. One of the clinical manifestations of sickle cell disease is that sickle-shaped cells tend to occlude smaller veins and capillaries, possibly including those supplying blood to the cochlea. Data from various studies indicate that permanent peripheral hearing loss is most likely to manifest itself as a high-frequency sensorineural hearing impairment (Scott, 2000). The incidence of conductive hearing impairment may vary because children with SCD are more susceptible to infections, yet at the same time they are taking prophylactic antibiotics to prevent infections (Scott, 2000).

In addition, central nervous system (CNS) manifestations, which include the auditory pathways, are frequent in SCD. It is postulated that CNS involvement affecting auditory perception could be due to small-vessel obstruction, although angiographic studies have revealed people with SCD who have partial or complete occlusion of such major intracranial vessels as the internal carotid, middle, and anterior cerebral arteries (Sarniak et al., 1979). Children with SCD may present with higher rates of peripheral and central auditory impairment compared to children with normal hemoglobin.

Central nervous system involvement is most prevalent in childhood and adolescence. Manifestations of CNS involvement include ischemic and hemorrhagic stroke, transient ischemic attacks, seizures, headache, altered mental status, cognitive difficulties, and silent infarctions. Stroke is a destructive complication of sickle cell anemia, manifesting itself clinically in 10% of patients by age 20 years (Ohene-Frempong et al., 1998) and as silent cerebral infarction by magnetic resonance imaging (MRI) in another 17% to 22% (Kinney et al., 1999; Pegelow et al., 2002). Wang et al. (1998) studied infants with SCD whose mean age was 18 months using MRI and found that 11% of 39 infants had evidence of a silent infarct. Studies have found that 36% of children ages 2 to 5 years with SCD had significant ectasia of the basilar artery, and vasculopathic changes were observed by magnetic resonance angiography in the cranial arteries of several patients under 1 year of age (Steen, Hu, et al., 2002). The etiology of stroke in sickle cell anemia remains unclear (Hoppe et al., 2004). All children with SCD should be screened with transcranial Doppler ultrasound because the propensity for stroke is associated with abnormal blood flow velocity in large arteries (Adams et al., 1998). Strokes are managed with general support and transfusion. The aim in managing strokes is to lower the concentration of Hb S to less than 30%, and an exchange blood transfusion may be required (Distenfeld, 2007).

## Description of the Case

### Background Information

Nicole J. was a 21-month-old African American female who was brought to the University Speech, Language and Hearing Clinic because of concerns regarding her hearing abilities, given her history of middle ear infections. She was referred by her pediatrician. Nicole was accompanied to the clinic by her mother, Ms. J. She was scheduled for a complete audiologic assessment. Student clinicians conducted the assessment with supervision by the audiologist.

Nicole was the youngest of three children who lived with both of her parents and her two brothers. Her mother, who was 28 years old, was an elementary school teacher, while her father, who was 32 years old, was a social worker. Nicole's brothers were 5 and 8 years of age. Nicole had sickle cell anemia (HbSS) of moderate severity. Both Nicole and an older brother had been identified with sickle cell anemia at birth. The oldest sibling had normal hemoglobin. The parents were not screened for the sickle cell gene until the birth of their second son. Nicole attended day care but was absent from time to time when she was having a crisis. She had been hospitalized once during a crisis. She had her first bout of otitis media at 8 months of age and had had three more since then. Nicole's regular medications at that time included penicillin and folic acid. Although she was small for her age, her developmental milestones were within normal limits except for her speech and language skills. She was somewhat unintelligible and had not started communicating in two-word utterances. Ms. J. described Nicole as a "happy child," though she was becoming frustrated when unable to communicate her wants and needs. Ms. J. believed that Nicole did not hear normally when she had a middle ear infection. The audiologist noted that Ms. J. seemed to be handling the chronic health problems of two of her children well. She had extended family to call for assistance. Ms. J. had educated herself about SCD. The audiologist noted that Nicole was an amiable child. She sounded congested on the day of testing.

### Findings of the Evaluations

The otoscopic examination revealed clear ear canals, though it was difficult to visualize the tympanic membrane due to small ear size. Immittance testing revealed negative middle ear pressure with rounded peaks in both ears. Acoustic reflex testing revealed elevated contralateral thresholds for both ears.

Given the constraints based on Nicole's age and attention span, audiological testing was abbreviated. Testing revealed that Nicole had air conduction thresholds of 15–20 dB HL across the speech frequencies bilaterally. The Speech Reception Thresholds (SRTs) were obtained using a picture-pointing response with a limited set of choices; the SRTs agreed with the pure tone averages. Bone conduction testing could not be completed.

The results of the evaluation indicated borderline normal to mild hearing impairment across the speech frequencies bilaterally. SRTs agreed with pure tone thresholds. Negative middle ear pressure was found in both ears suggesting eustachian tube dysfunction.

History information and observations clearly showed that Nicole was unintelligible at times and delayed in language development. Ms. J. stated that Nicole never had a transcranial Doppler ultrasound or MRI, and the pediatrician had not suggested one. Nicole's brother with SCD had shown no delays in his speech and language development, and no concerns were noted when he was tested at the same age with an established test of skills appropriate to kindergarten.

## Representation of the Problem at the Time of Evaluation

Are Nicole's delays in speech and language skills due to her recurrent bouts of otitis media alone, or is the presence of sickle cell disease more directly affecting both the occurrence of the otitis media and her speech and language delays?

Nicole had a documented history of otitis media, a common disorder of childhood. Though otitis media is less prevalent in African Americans, that does not necessarily make Nicole less susceptible to otitis media; however, the presence of SCD may have made her more susceptible to ear infections. Nicole's speech and language skills were delayed. Was the history of otitis media the reason for the delays in Nicole's speech and language skills, or does the presence of SCD and the speech and language delays indicate the possibility of a silent infarct?

## Treatment Options Considered

Recommendations were as follows:

- Nicole should be retested in 3 weeks to determine her middle ear status and her pure tone thresholds. In the interim, Nicole's communication partners were encouraged to modify their communication with her. Recommendations included getting her attention before speaking, speaking with her at her height (level), and turning down or removing background noise or other distractions. This recommendation would be made regardless of the cause of the otitis media. The status of Nicole's auditory system should be monitored.
- Nicole should receive audiological reevaluations every 3 months, given her history of otitis media and the developmental level of her speech and language skills. This recommendation would be made regardless of the cause of the recurrent ear infections. The test battery should consist of pure tone thresholds (air and bone conduction), speech reception thresholds, word recognition testing, immittance testing including (multifrequency) tympanometry and acoustic reflex testing, and electrophysiologic tests including auditory brainstem response (ABR) and otoacoustic emissions (transient and distortion product). Tests should be added as she ages and her attention span lengthens. Some of these tests were chosen because Nicole has sickle cell anemia. For example, changes in Wave I of the ABR may reflect the modulation of cochlear blood flow. Otoacoustic emissions provide an objective measure of hair cell function independent of retrocochlear activity (confirming a cochlear origin of hearing impairment associated with SCD) (Burch-Sims & Matlock, 2005).
- Another question related to the long-term monitoring of Nicole's hearing once the bouts of otitis media disappeared. Given the presence of SCD, would Nicole develop a sensorineural or central auditory hearing impairment as she aged? A higher incidence of hearing impairment in children with SCD compared to children with normal hemoglobin has been observed (Scott, 2000); however, those with SCD who are 25 years and older are more likely to have sensorineural hearing loss than younger patients (Piltcher, Cigana, Friedriech, Quintanilha Ribeiro, & Selaimen da Costa, 2000). Possible long-term effects of SCD on the central nervous system were a concern. Steen, Hu, et al. (2002) tested the

hypothesis that young children with SCD and no history of stroke are at risk for cognitive impairment. The scores of kindergarten children in the Memphis schools on the Developing Skills Checklist (Wennerholm et al., 1990a, 1990b) were examined. These children had no history of stroke. Children with SCD scored lower than controls in auditory discrimination, and there was a trend toward lower scores in language.

- Nicole should receive a speech and language assessment, thus a referral was made to a speech-language pathologist. This recommendation would be made regardless of the cause of the speech and language delays. However, cerebrovascular disease is a common cause of morbidity in patients with sickle cell anemia. Ten percent have strokes by the age of 20 and up to an additional 22% have silent infarcts. Nicole's speech and language skills may need to be monitored even if she is dismissed from therapy. Some neurobehavioral testing suggests that children with SCD who are completely normal by magnetic resonance imaging (MRI) can still be cognitively impaired. Steen, Fineberg-Buchner, et al. (2005) found that among 30 patients who were normal by MRI there were substantial deficits in Wechsler (1991) Full-Scale IQ, Verbal IQ, and Performance IQ compared to a group of their peers. These findings suggest that there is diffuse brain injury in children with SCD. This diffuse brain injury could affect attention and executive skills as well as spatial skills.
- Nicole's pediatrician should be contacted, with the permission of Ms. J. to discuss research recommending a transcranial Doppler ultrasound as a predictor of the possibility of stroke and/or MRI as a means to determine the presence of silent infarcts. One or both tests should be scheduled for Nicole.

## Course of Treatment

Nicole returned for audiological retesting in 4 weeks and her pure tone thresholds had improved to 5–10 dB HL across the speech frequencies. Tympanograms indicated normal middle ear pressure and compliance. Acoustic reflex thresholds were within normal limits. She had been seen by a speech-language pathologist for a speech and language diagnostic. Nicole had begun receiving therapy twice a week at day care.

It took time to get Ms. J. to agree to allow the audiologist to discuss the issue of a transcranial Doppler ultrasound with Nicole's pediatrician. Ms. J. felt it was unnecessary given her son's normal development, even though he also had sickle cell anemia. The pediatrician recommended the transcranial Doppler ultrasound. The velocities of the large artery blood flow indicated low risk for stroke.

## Analysis of the Client's Response to Intervention

Nicole's speech and language skills improved while she was in therapy. Ms. J., a teacher, worked with all of the children on their language and mathematical skills. Nicole continued to have audiological reevaluations on a regular basis. No permanent peripheral or central hearing loss has been noted.

## Author Note

This case is not based on an actual patient.

## References


Adams, R. J., McKie, V. J., Hsu, L., Files, B., Vichinsky, E., & Pegelow, C., et al. (1998). Prevention of first stroke by transfusion in children with sickle cell anemia and abnormal results on transcranial Doppler. *New England Journal of Medicine, 339*, 5–11.

Bloom, M. (1995). *Understanding sickle cell disease*. Jackson, MS: University of Mississippi.

Burch-Sims, G. P., & Matlock, V. R. (2005). Hearing loss and auditory function in sickle cell disease. *Journal of Communication Disorders, 38*, 321–329.

Distenfeld, A. (2007). *Sickle cell anemia*. Retrieved January 30, 2008, from http://www.emedicine.com/MED/topic2126.htm

Hoppe, C., Klitz, W., Cheng, S., Apple, R., Steiner, L., Robles, L., et al. (2004). Gene interactions and stroke risk in children with sickle cell anemia. *Blood, 103*(6), 2391–2396.

Kinney, T. R., Sleeper, L. A., Wang, W. C., Zimmerman, R. A., Pegelow, C. H. M., & Ohene-Frempong, K., et al. (1999). Silent cerebral infarcts in sickle cell anemia: A risk factor analysis. *Pediatrics, 103*, 640–645.

Ohene-Frempong, K., Weiner, S. J., Sleeper, L. A., Miller, S. T., Embury, S., & Moohr, J. W., et al. (1998). Cerebrovascular accidents in sickle cell disease: Rates and risk factors. *Blood, 91*, 288–294.

Pegelow, C. H., Macklin, E. A., Moser, F. G.,Wang, W. C., Bellow, J. A., & Miller, S. T., et al. (2002). Longitudinal changes in brain magnetic resonance imaging findings in children with sickle cell disease. *Blood, 99*, 3014–3018.

Piltcher, O., Cigana, L., Friedriech, J., Quintanilha Ribeiro, F. A., & Selaimen da Costa, S. (2000). Sensorineural hearing loss among sickle cell disease patients from southern Brazil. *American Journal of Otolaryngology, 21*(2), 75–79.

*Prevalence and incidence of sickle cell anemia*. (2008). Retrieved March 10, 2008, from http://wrongdiagnosis.com/s/sickle_cell_anemia/prevalence.htm

Sarniak, S., Soorya, D., Kim, J., Ravindranath, V., & Lusher, J., et al. (1979). Periodic transfusions for sickle cell anemia and CNS infarction. *American Journal of the Diseased Child, 133*, 1254–1257.

Scott, D. M. (2000). Managing hearing impairment in culturally diverse children. In T. J. Coleman (Ed.), *Clinical management of communication disorders in culturally diverse children* (pp. 271–294). Boston, MA: Allyn and Bacon.

Steen, R. G., Fineberg-Buchner, C., Hankins, G., Weiss, L., Prifitera, A., & Mulhern, R. K. (2005). Cognitive deficits in children with sickle cell disease. *Journal of Child Neurology, 20*(2), 102–107.

Steen, R. G., Hu, X. J., Elliott, V. E., Miles, M. A., Jones, S., & Wang, W. C. (2002). Kindergarten readiness skills in children with sickle cell disease: Evidence of early neurocognitive damage? *Journal of Child Neurology, 17*(2), 111–116.

Wang, W. C., Langston, J. W., Steen, R. G., Wynn, L. W., Mulhern, R. K., Wilimas, J. A., et al. (1998). Abnormalities of the central nervous system in very young children with sickle cell anemia. *Journal of Pediatrics, 132*, 994–998.

Wechsler, D. (1991). *Manual for the Wechsler Intelligence Scale for Children-Third Edition*. San Antonio, TX: The Psychological Corporation.

Wennerholm, T. R., Taylor, C., McGarvey-Levin, L., et al. (1990a). *Developing Skills Checklist: Administration and Score Interpretation Manual*. Monterey, CA: CTB/McGraw-Hill.

Wennerholm, T. R., Taylor, C., McGarvey-Levin, L., et al. (1990b). *Developing Skills Checklist: Norms Book and Technical Bulletin*. Monterey, CA: CTB/McGraw-Hill.

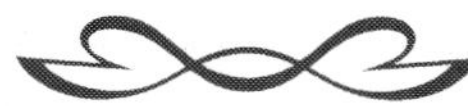



CASE 8

# Leona: Oromotor Entrainment Therapy to Develop Feeding Skills in the Preterm Infant

*Steven M. Barlow, Meredith A. Poore, and Emily A. Zimmerman*

## Conceptual Knowledge Areas

Suck is a precocial ororhythmic motor behavior in humans and is integral to competent oral feeds. However, premature infants often demonstrate oromotor dyscoordination and are unable to suck and feed orally (Bu'Lock, Woolridge, & Baum, 1990; Comrie & Helm, 1997). This represents a frequent and serious challenge both to the neonatal intensive care unit (NICU) survivors and the physician-provider-parent teams. The potential causes for delayed or impaired suck development are numerous and may result from neurologic insult to the developing brain, feeding intolerance, postsurgical recovery, diabetes, or as a result of ventilator interventions, which interfere with ororhythmic pattern formation. For example, lengthy oxygen supplementation procedures in the NICU cost the preterm infant precious sensory and motor experiences during a critical period of brain development when the central patterning of suck and prefeeding skills are being refined. Even the presence of a nasogastric (NG) feeding tube has negative effects on sucking and breathing (Shiao, Youngblut, Anderson, DiFiore, & Martin, 1995). Trussing the lower face with poly tubes and tape also restricts the range and type of oral movements and limits cutaneous experiences with the hand and fingers. Interruption of these experiences may impair fragile syntheses of how the brain maps these functions (Bosma, 1970; Hensch, 2004). For some preterm infants, poor suck and oromotor dyscoordination persists well into early childhood and may lead to significant delays in the emergence of other oromotor behaviors, including feeding, babbling, and speech-language production (Adams-Chapman, 2006; Ballantyne, Frisk, & Green, 2006). Moreover, failure to establish oral feeding skills in the NICU may result in the infant being sent home on gavage or G-tube feedings, and hinder the development of coordinated oromotor behavior. The difficulties associated with establishing oral feed competence along with the additional costs for extended hospitalization underscore the need for assessment and therapeutic tools to facilitate the development of normal oromotor skills (da Costa, van den Engel-Hoek, & Bos, 2008; Fucile, Gisel, & Lau, 2002, 2005; Lau & Hurst, 1999).

Feeding readiness is often evaluated by an infant's display of non-nutritive sucking and oromotor patterning (Bingham, Thomas, Ashikaga, & Abbasi, 2008; Lau, 2006). Suck appears in utero between 15 and 18 weeks gestational age (GA) and is remarkably stable and well patterned by 34 weeks postmenstrual age (PMA) (Hack, Estabrook, & Robertson, 1985). The non-nutritive suck (NNS), defined as any repetitive mouthing activity on a blind nipple or pacifier that does not deliver a liquid stimulus (Goldson, 1987; Wolff, 1968), typically consists of a series of compression bursts and pause intervals. Each burst contains 6–12 suck cycles that manifest an initial deceleration phase of frequency modulation over the first 5 cycles to a steady state of approximately 2 Hz (Urish, Barlow, & Venkatesan, 2007). The maturation and coordination of the NNS precedes the suck-swallow-breathe pattern associated with the slower 1 Hz pattern characteristic of the nutritive suck (Gewolb, Vice, Schweitzer-Kenney, Taciak, & Bosma, 2001; Lau & Schanler, 1996; Medoff-Cooper, 2005).

Establishing a patterned NNS for the developing infant benefits growth, maturation, and gastric motility, while decreasing stress (Abbasi, Sivieri, Samuel-Collins, & Gerdes, 2008; DiPietro, Cusson, Caughy, & Fox, 1994; Field, 1993; Lau & Hurst, 1999; Lau & Schanler, 1996; Pickler, Frankel, Walsh, & Thompson, 1996; Pickler, Higgins, & Crummette, 1993), improving state control prefeed (DiPietro et al., 1994; Gill, Behnke, Conlon, & Anderson, 1992; Gill, Behnke, Conlon, McNeely, & Anderson, 1988; McCain, 1992; Pickler et al., 1996) and postfeed (Pickler et al., 1993), and enhancing oral feeds (Barlow, Finan, Chu, & Lee, 2008; McCain, 1995; Poore, Zimmerman, Barlow, Wang, & Gu, 2008). Use of a pacifier for NNS appears to decrease the frequency of apnea and cyanosis and to improve breastfeeding scores (Volkmer & Fiori, 2008). The NNS accelerates the transition from tube to independent oral feeding and is presumed to enhance the maturation of neural systems responsible for ororhythmic activity (Bernbaum, Pereira, Watkins, & Peckham, 1983; Field et al., 1982; Measel & Anderson, 1979). The sensory consequences associated with the production of NNS appear to provide beneficial effects on oral feeding performance and the development of specific sucking skills (Fucile et al., 2002, 2005). Accurate assessment of oromotor dyscoordination in the preterm infant extends beyond the immediate issues surrounding the transition to oral feed competency, and may serve as a potent clinical marker for brain development and neurodevelopmental outcomes (Mizuno & Ueda, 2005). Infants with perinatal distress and neurologic impairments demonstrate a significantly slower mean rate and greater variability of non-nutritive suck (Dreier & Wolff, 1972). Children with severe neurodevelopmental problems at 18 months tend to have arrhythmic nutritive expression/suction patterns as premature infants (Mizuno & Ueda, 2005).

## Suck Central Pattern Generator

The mammalian suck is the earliest-appearing somatic motor rhythm and is primarily controlled by a neural network known as the suck central pattern generator (sCPG). The sCPG consists of bilateral, linked internuncial circuits within the brainstem pontine and medullary reticular formation (Barlow & Estep, 2006; Iriki, Nozaki, & Nakamura, 1988; Tanaka, Kogo, Chandler, & Matsuya, 1999). Based on animal models, the minimal circuitry for ororhythmic activity resides between the trigeminal motor nucleus and the facial nucleus in the brainstem (Tanaka et al., 1999), situated to function as premotor inputs to lower motor neurons. The sCPG is centrally modulated by multiple inputs, including descending pathways from the sensorimotor cortex and reciprocal connections with the cerebellum (Boughter et al., 2007; Bryant et al., 2007), which serve to modulate ororhythmic activity. Thus, it is important to assist human infants to regulate their behavioral "state" through careful posturing and orientation during clinical testing as this will affect the nature of descending inputs to the sCPG. The sCPG can also be modified by sensory input arising from oral mechanoreceptors that encode the consequences of oral movements and external stimulation (i.e., breast, pacifier or bottle nipple, touch) along central pathways of the trigeminal system. Suck entrainment has been demonstrated in term infants through 6 months of age using a patterned orocutaneous stimulus delivered to perioral and intraoral tissues (Finan & Barlow, 1998). Entrainment is defined as the phase locking of centrally generated suck motor patterns to an applied external stimulus, and represents a powerful method of achieving neural synchrony among sensorimotor pathways. Therefore, it is not surprising that stimulation of the lips and tongue are common methods used to evoke sucking behaviors (Fucile et al., 2002, 2005; Rocha, Moreira, Pimenta, Ramos, & Lucena, 2007).

## Oromotor Entrainment: NTrainer®

The neuroscientific principles underlying sensorimotor entrainment of ororhythmic motor activity have been translated to a new clinical application for preterm infants who exhibit poor suck and feeding difficulties. A new biomedical device known as the NTrainer® system was developed in the authors' laboratory and is coupled to a popular silicone pacifier (Soothie®, Children's Medical Ventures/Respironics, Inc.) common to many NICUs worldwide. The NTrainer® transforms the Soothie® pacifier into a pressurized orocutaneous stimulator suitable for use with premature infants. This motorized pacifier is presented to the infant for alternating 3-minute stimulus epochs during nasogastric (NG) tube feeds in the NICU. The novel orosensory experience afforded by the NTrainer® mimics the spatiotemporal dynamics of non-nutritive suck and has been correlated to rapid organization of suck in infants who exhibit poor feeding skills (Barlow et al., 2008; Poore et al., 2008).

The NTrainer® system consists of a servo-controlled pneumatic actuator and microprocessor to dynamically modulate intraluminal pacifier pressure, and two software modules: (1) NeoSuck RT®, designed to perform automated real-time digital sampling and assessment of the infant's non-nutritive suck and ororhythmic patterning at cribside in the NICU, and (2) NTrain®, engineered to synthesize and deliver patterned orocutaneous stimulation to the infant either during NG feeds or immediately before a scheduled feed (breast/bottle).

## NNS Assessment

The NNS compression pressure waveforms are digitized periodically (daily recommended) from each infant at cribside 15 minutes prior to a scheduled feed using the mobile NTrainer® system running the NeoSuck RT® software. Infants remain connected to the pulse-oximetry monitors at all times to ensure that respiration, heartbeat, and oxygen saturation levels are adequate to support oromotor activity. An infant-preferred Soothie® silicone pacifier serves as the interface to a specially designed receiver (see Figure 8.1), which incorporates a lubricated spherical acetyl head coupled to a Luer cannula and instrumented with a Honeywell pressure transducer (DC-coupled, low-pass Butterworth @ 50 Hz, 3,000 samples/sec @ 16-bits voltage resolution).

Infants are held in a developmentally supportive semi-inclined posture (Figure 8.2). Background/overhead lighting is dimmed in the immediate area to promote eye contact with the developmental specialist (neonatal nurse, neonatologist, developmental speech-language pathologist, physical therapist). (The personnel who administer the NTrainer® in the NICU vary by hospital site and may or may not be affiliated with the feeding team). Sampling of NNS behavior is initiated when the infant achieves an optimal behavioral state, that is, drowsy to active alert (state 3, 4, or 5 as described by the Naturalistic Observation of Newborn Behavior,

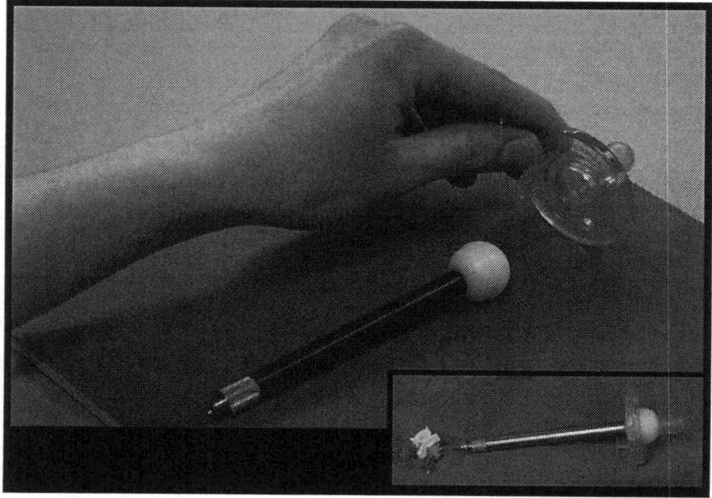

FIGURE 8.1 Soothie Silicone Pacifier and Receiver with Luer Cannula for Intraluminal Pressure Transduction

*Source*: Communication Neuroscience Laboratories, University of Kansas.

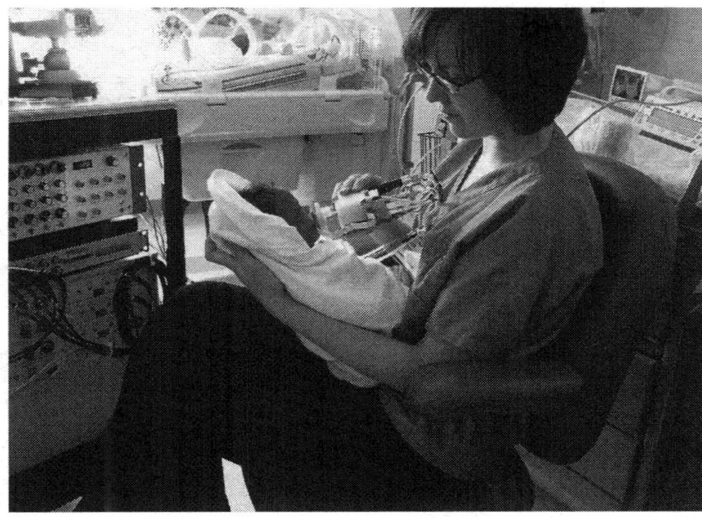

FIGURE 8.2 Cribside in the NICU, Testing NNS in a Premature Infant with the NTrainer

*Source*: Communication Neuroscience Laboratories, University of Kansas.

Newborn Individualized Developmental Care and Assessment Program; NIDCAP) (Als, 1995). Three minutes of NNS behavior is typically digitized for each infant per session, with the most productive 2-minute epoch subjected to formal quantitative and statistical analysis.

A sample output from the NeoSuck RT® is shown for a healthy preterm infant at 35 weeks PMA (Figure 8.3) and a tube-fed RDS preterm infant at 35 weeks PMA (Figure 8.4). The real-time display provides the clinician with the NNS compression waveform and associated histogram updates for suck amplitude ($cmH_2O$), inter-NNS burst-pause periods (sec), and intra-NNS burst-suck cycle periods (sec). For the healthy preterm infant, well-organized NNS bursts with peak pressures averaging approximately 25 $cmH_2O$ alternate with pause periods. The nipple compression cycle count for the 3.5 minute sample is 108. In contrast, the dissolution of the NNS burst

FIGURE 8.3 Screenshot of NeoSuck RT® Graphical User Interface for Sampling Non-nutritive Suck in a Healthy Preterm Infant

Well-organized NNS burst-pause sequence shown in lower left panel. Histograms shown (clockwise) for suck cycle amplitude ($cmH_2O$), NNS burst-pause periods (sec), and a cluster of within-burst NNS cycle periods (sec).

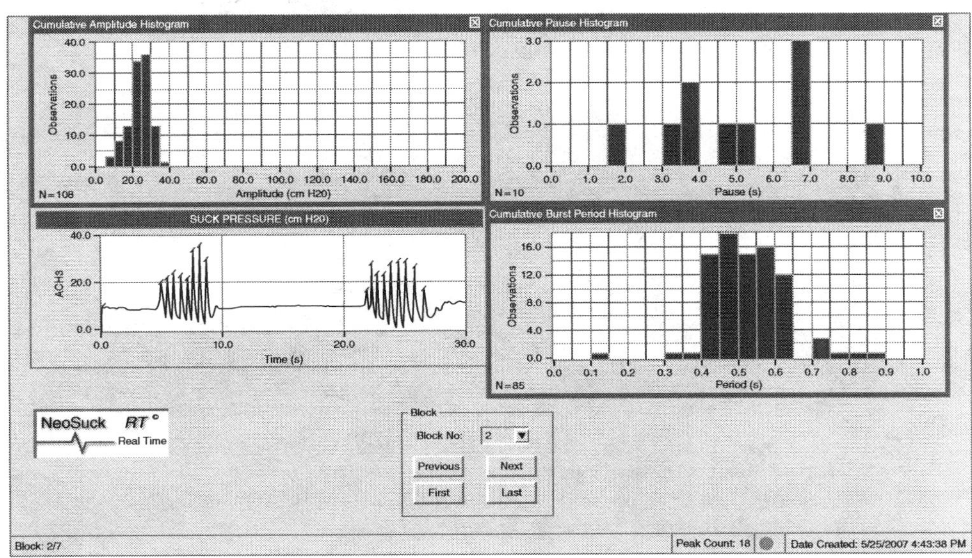

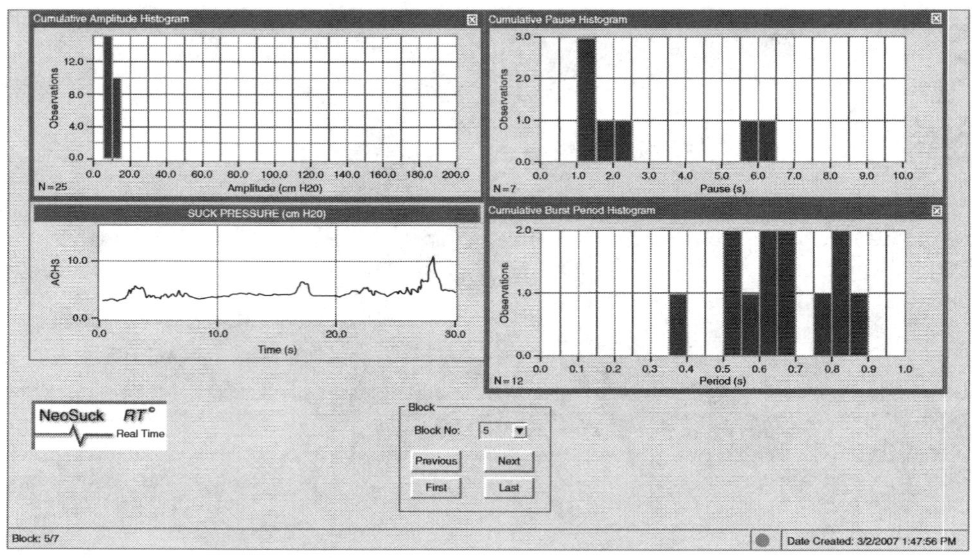


FIGURE 8.4 Screenshot of NeoSuck RT® Graphical User Interface for Sampling Non-nutritive Suck in an RDS Preterm Infant

Lack of a developed NNS burst- pause is apparent in lower left panel. Histograms shown (clockwise) reveal attenuated suck cycle amplitude ($cmH_2O$), NNS burst-pause periods (sec), and degraded within-burst NNS cycle periods (sec).

structure for the tube-fed RDS infant corresponds to a disorganized nipple compression pattern and indistinguishable NNS bursts. The amplitude of oral compression output is likewise reduced to approximately 5 $cmH_2O$, with only 25 compression cycles identified in the 3.5-minute sample of digitized records.

Infants assigned to the NTrainer® intervention receive alternating 3-minute epochs of patterned orocutaneous stimulation, typically during gavage feeds. This helps the infant develop an association between pleasurable oral stimulation and satiation from liquid nutrient entering the stomach. The NTrainer® stimulus train currently used has been programmed to mimic the temporal features of NNS. As shown in Figure 8.5, precise stimulus control is

FIGURE 8.5 The Servo-Controlled Pneumatic Linear Actuator Engineered in our Laboratory for the NTrainer® System to Synthesize Patterned Orocutaneous Stimulation in Preterm Infants

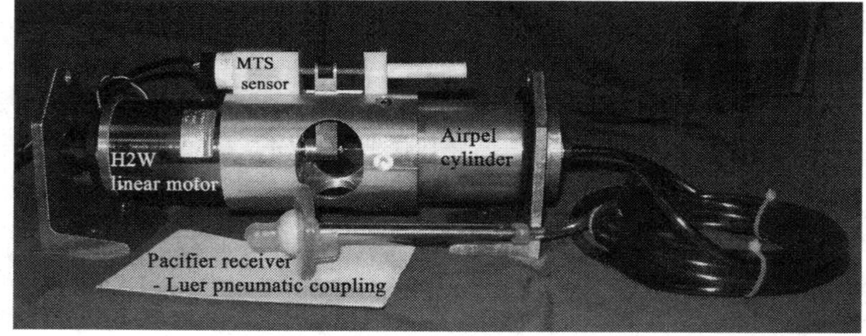


*Source*: Adapted from "Patterns for the Premature Brain: Synthetic Orocutaneous Stimulation Entrains Preterm Infants with Feeding Difficulties to Suck," by S. M. Barlow, D. S. Finan, S. Chu, and J. Lee, 2008, *Journal of Perinatology*, 28, pp. 541–548. Photo by Steven M. Barlow.

achieved with a custom-designed servo linear motor (H2W Technologies, Inc.) operating under position feedback and coupled in series with a pneumatic Airpel® glass cylinder actuator and the pacifier receiver. An MTS® displacement sensor is used for position feedback control in order to deliver a repeatable stimulus to the infant's mouth. A 16-bit digital-to-analog converter is used to synthesize an orocutaneous pneumatic pulse train, which consists of a series of 6-cycle bursts and 2-second pause periods. Individual cycles within-burst are presented at 1.8 Hz. This synthetic pulse train is used to drive the servo motor to modulate the intraluminal pressure and shape of the infant's Soothie® pacifier. The changes in intraluminal pressure yield a radial expansion of the pacifier nipple of approximately 135 microns with a 25 millisecond rise/fall time (Barlow et al., 2008). This novel instrumentation transforms the infant's pacifier into a "pulsating nipple" that resembles the temporal pattern of a well-formed NNS burst. A total of 34 synthetic NNS burst-pause trains are presented to the infant during a single 3-minute NTrain® session. Infants are typically treated with the NTrainer® stimulus three to four times per day Monday through Friday during scheduled gavage feeds over a 10-day period, or until the infant attains 90% oral feeds for two consecutive days.

## Advanced NNS Digital Signal Processing

In studies of NNS fine structure (Estep, Barlow, Vantipalli, Lee, & Finan, 2008; Poore et al., 2008; Stumm et al., 2008; Zimmerman & Barlow, 2008), 2-minute samples reflecting the most active period of NNS behavior generated by the preterm infant are selected from each raw data file for analysis. These are identified based on a waveform discrimination and pressure threshold detection algorithm in the NeoSuck® software program, which indexes pressure peaks at a user-defined pressure threshold. Identification of the time-amplitude intercepts for individual pressure peaks is achieved by calculation of the first derivative of the pressure signal. Zero-crossings in the pressure derivative function along with a pressure recruitment rate and hysteresis function are used to index nipple compression pressure peaks in the digitized waveforms. This algorithm permits objective identification of NNS burst activity as distinct from nonorganized mouthing compressions. Six objective measures can be extracted from indexed records of suck, including the following minute-rate variables: (1) *Total Compressions*, defined as the sum of all pressure events per minute, (2) *Non-NNS Events*, defined as nipple compression pressure events not associated with an NNS burst sequence, (3) *NNS Cycles*, defined as suck compression cycles with cycle periods less than 1,000 milliseconds and occurring within the NNS burst structure per minute, and (4) the number of *NNS Bursts* that consisted of two or more nipple compression cycles. The remaining NNS performance measures are (5) mean number *NNS Cycles/Burst*, and (6) a ratiometric calculation known as *NNS Cycles%Total*, defined as NNS Cycles expressed as a percentage of total nipple compressions ([Burst-related NNS cycles/Total Mouthing Events] x 100).

## NNS Spatiotemporal Index

The physiological approach to the assessment and habilitation of suck in the NICU includes a functional assessment of the integrity of the neural circuitry driving the suck central pattern generator through an analysis of suck pattern structure and stability (Poore et al., 2008). Coordinated NNS that is minimally variable from burst to burst indicates motor system integrity and is an important foundation for coordination with other emergent behaviors, such as swallow and respiration. A highly promising digital signal processing technique known as the Non-Nutritive Suck Spatiotemporal Index (NNS STI) has been developed to quantify the emergence of stable non-nutritive suck in preterm infants. The mathematical tenets underlying this computational technique have been used successfully to assess kinematic variability and pattern formation in limb (Atkeson & Hollerbach, 1985; Georgopoulos, Kalaska, & Massey, 1981) and speech (Smith, Johnson, McGillem, & Goffman, 2000; Smith & Zelaznik, 2004) motor subsystems. The NNS STI provides the clinician with a single numerical value, calculated from the cumulative sum of the standard deviations of an amplitude- and time-normalized set of suck pressure waveforms, and represents the stability of the infant's oromotor sequence. In essence, this measure provides a quantitative composite index of non-nutritive suck pattern stability. This metric eliminates the need to count suck pressure peaks or measure individual cycle periods. Instead, the Non-Nutritive Suck Spatiotemporal Index is designed to quantify the infant's suck over a selected burst pattern epoch, thereby providing NICU clinicians with a summative index or "gestalt" of oromotor pattern formation and stability. Obtaining a 2-minute sample of NNS behavior daily in the NICU with the NTrainer® cribside system is sufficient to chart an infant's progress toward stable suck production (Poore et al., 2008).

The NNS STI measure has also been used successfully to document the effects of the NTrainer® patterned orocutaneous therapy on suck development among tube-fed premature infants with respiratory distress syndrome who have endured, on average, 40 days of oxygen supplementation therapy (Poore et al., 2008).

## Description of the Case

Leona is a preterm infant, the first child of a 25-year-old mother who received prenatal care. Leona was born at 31 weeks GA by cesarean section with a birth weight of 1,300 g, birth length of 39 cm, and head circumference of 28 cm. Soon after birth, she received a diagnosis of respiratory distress syndrome (RDS) and was prescribed 26 days of oxygen therapy. Like many preterm infants, she exhibited poor oromotor skills and a delayed suck pattern. This was evident in both her NeoSuck RT® assessments and resultant NNS STI scores. At 36 weeks PMA, Leona had an NNS STI of 89 (Figure 8.6). Thus, her poor suck output and delayed transition to oral feeds made her an ideal candidate for the NTrainer®. The NTrainer® was initiated at 36 weeks PMA. One week after pairing the NTrainer® stimulus with gavage feeds 3 to 4 times per day, she had her first PO feed at 37 weeks PMA. During this feed she took 62.5% of her bottle. Following this initial PO feed, she took 100% of all of her bottles and was discharged a week later. At 37 weeks PMA, her NNS STI score had improved to 50, demonstrating the potent effect of the NTrainer® therapy on improving NNS and feeding outcomes.

For comparison, a preterm control infant, Harrison, is included in this report. He was born the third of triplets by cesarean section at 31 weeks GA, birth weight of 1540 g, birth length of 42 cm, and head circumference of 28 cm. His mother was 48 years old at the time of delivery and received prenatal care. Harrison received 11 days of oxygen therapy and also was diagnosed with RDS. He received weekly NeoSuck RT ®assessments. The nursing staff offered him a pacifier on a regular basis; however, the NTrainer® patterned orocutaneous intervention was not provided. At 36 weeks PMA, he had an STI of 71 (Figure 8.6). Feeding by mouth was a significant challenge, requiring 44 days to attain a modest 36% oral feed level. His final STI score was completed at 38 weeks PMA and increased slightly to 72, indicating that he regressed on his ability to suck. Due to the difficulty Harrison had with transitioning successfully to oral feeds, he was sent home on gavage feed. During his scheduled 6-month NICU follow-up clinic at Stormont-Vail Medical Center, Harrison was starting to eat cereal and fruit by spoon but still relied mostly on his tube feeds for all liquid nourishment.

### Summary and Conclusions

Human brain development is a dynamic process that continues throughout gestation (Adams-Chapman, 2006). A critical period of brain growth and development occurs in late gestation (Bosma, 1970; Hensch, 2004) that is vital for the development of various neural structures and pathways involved in oromotor control and coordination of suck, swallow, and breathe to support safe nutritional feeds. The premature infant is predisposed to multiple factors related to developmental immaturity, which mediates the risk for brain injury and subsequent abnormal neurologic sequelae, including the risk for development of intraventricular hemorrhage (IVH), periventricular leukomalacia (PVL), hypoxic respiratory failure, hyperbilirubinemia, and infection. Importantly, the late preterm brain is only a fraction of the full-term brain weight and a significant proportion of brain growth, development, and

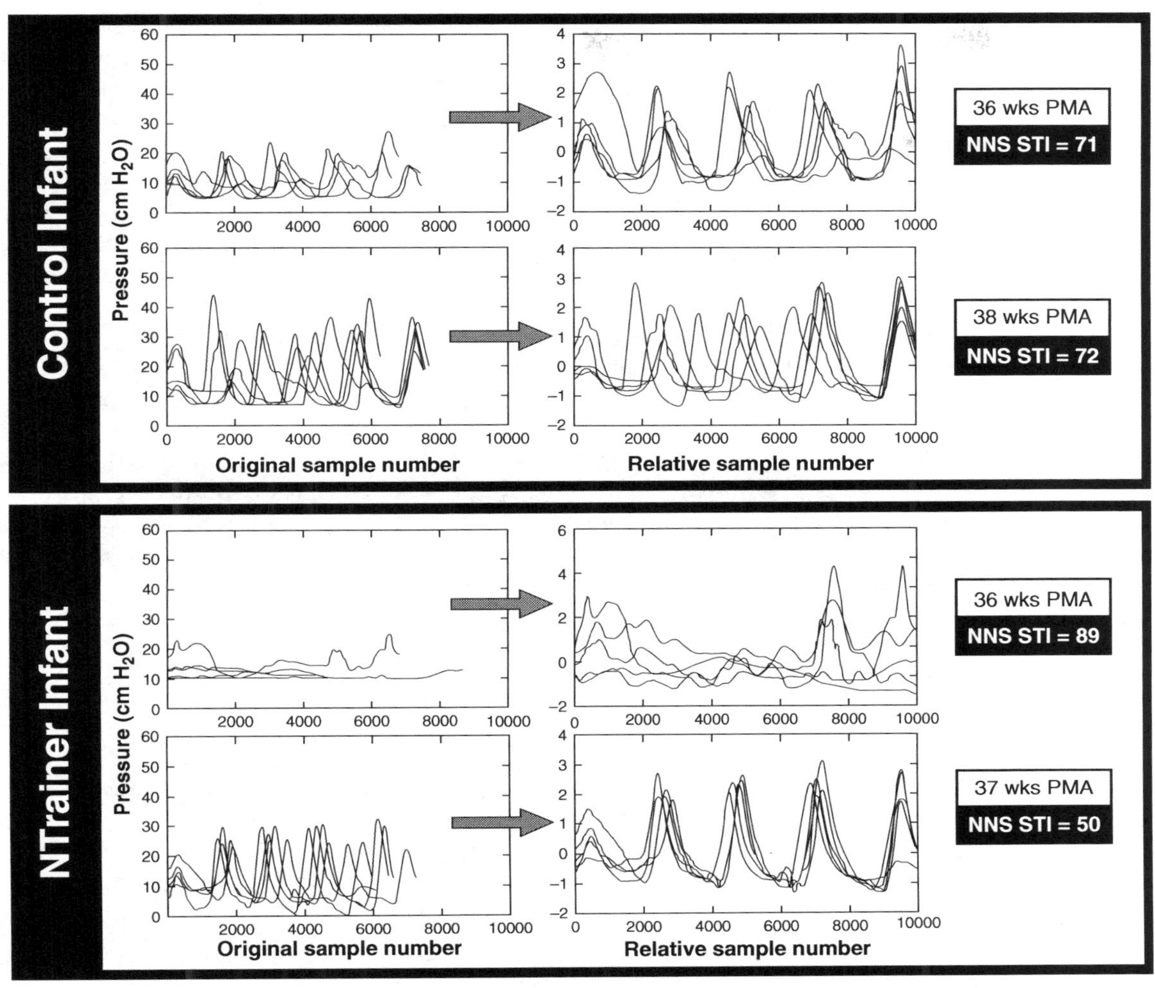


FIGURE 8.6 Upper Panel Block Depicts the Non-nutritive Suck Spatiotemporal Index (NNS STI) Digital Signal Processing Results for a Control (No Intervention) Tube-Fed Infant with RDS at 36 Weeks Postmenstrual Age (PMA) and Again at 38 Weeks PMA

Five superimposed raw NNS records (left) are transformed to normalized records (right) to demonstrate pattern formation resulting from suck CPG activity with the NNS STI scores. The bottom panels show the normalized NNS records and resultant STI values. The lower panel block depicts the NNS STI results for the present case report, a tube-fed RDS preterm infant at 36 weeks PMA before intervention (36 weeks PMA) and following NTrainer® patterned orocutaneous intervention (37 weeks PMA).

networking occurs during the last 6 weeks of gestation. These tissues are vulnerable to injury during this critical time period of development. Disruption of critical pathways needed for neuronal or glial development may result from sensory deprivation and/or motor restriction associated with respiratory distress syndrome and interventions that truss the infant's face with tubing and tape to support oxygen therapies.

Fortunately for the human infant, the brainstem sCPG responds to peripheral input (Barlow et al., 2008; Finan & Barlow, 1998; Rocha et al., 2007) and adapts to changes in the local oral environment (Zimmerman & Barlow, 2008). Collective results from studies in neonatal intensive care units demonstrate the potent effects of a motorized silicone pacifier nipple on the development of NNS in preterm infants. The patterned orocutaneous experience is physiologically salient and spectrally patterned to resemble the "burst-pause" structure of the NNS. This form of stimulation serves to entrain the activity patterns of populations of mechanoreceptor afferents located in the lips, tongue, and jaw of the neonate, which in turn influence firing patterns of the respective orofacial lower motor neurons. This is a central tenet of one of the basic principles of pathway formation, "neurons that fire together, will wire together" (Löwel & Singer, 1992).

The application of mechanosensory entrainment as a habilitation strategy has ecological validity in assisting the infant to produce appropriate oromotor output. This approach is consistent with contemporary ideas on the role of sensory-driven neural activity in pathway formation (Marder & Rehm, 2005; Penn & Shatz, 1999) and the notion that appropriate oral experiences may be critical in the final weeks of gestation for the formation of functional central neural circuits.

The richness of the patterned orocutaneous experience offered by the NTrainer® presents a new neurotherapeutic application for the habilitation of suck in premature infants in the NICU (Barlow et al., 2008; Poore et al., 2008). The regimen includes repeated exposure to patterned orocutaneous events, distributed over 3 or 4 feeds totaling approximately 45 minutes per day in the NICU. Intervention is delivered concurrent with NG tube feeds over 7 to 10 days. It provides the preterm infant with a neural entrainment experience that facilitates the development of central neural pathways that regulate suck. Use of an orocutaneous entrainment stimulus has the advantage of being safe and pleasurable for the neonate and easily administered by the physician-provider-parent teams in the NICU, including developmental speech-language pathologists.

## Author Note

This work was supported by grants NIH R01 DC003311 (S. M. Barlow), NIH P30 HD02528, and NIH P30 DC005803. Special thanks to the physicians, nurses, and staff in the NICU at Stormont-Vail HealthCare, Topeka, KS. The IRB at Stormont-Vail HealthCare approved the use of the NTrainer® protocol prior to the testing of all infants, and informed consent was obtained from all parents of infants enrolled in the study. The infants described in this case study are real and were actively involved in the NTrainer® study. All names have been changed to protect the infants' identities.

## References

Abbasi, S., Sivieri, E., Samuel-Collins, N., & Gerdes, J. S. (2008). Effect of non-nutritive sucking on gastric motility of preterm infants. *Pediatric Academic Society*, 5840.22, 213.

Adams-Chapman, I. (2006). Neurodevelopmental outcome of the late preterm infant. *Clinical Perinatology, 33*, 947–964.

Als, H. (1995). A manual for naturalistic observation of the newborn (preterm and full term infants). In E. Goldson (Ed.), *Nurturing the premature infant: Developmental interventions in the neonatal intensive care nursery* (pp. 77–85). New York: Oxford University Press. Atkeson, C. G., & Hollerbach, J. M. (1985). Kinematic features of unrestrained vertical arm movements. *The Journal of Neuroscience, 5*, 2318–2330.

Ballantyne, M., Frisk, V., & Green, P. (2006). Language impairment in extremely-low-birth-weight infants. *Pediatric Academic Society*, 5532.178.

Barlow, S. M., & Estep, M. (2006). Central pattern generation and the motor infrastructure for suck, respiration, and speech. *Journal of Communication Disorders, 39*, 366–380.

Barlow, S. M., Finan, D. S., Chu, S., & Lee, J. (2008). Patterns for the premature brain: Synthetic orocutaneous stimulation entrains preterm infants with feeding difficulties to suck. *Journal of Perinatology, 28*, 541–548.

Bernbaum, J. C., Pereira, G. R., Watkins, J. B., & Peckham, G. J. (1983). Nonnutritive sucking during gavage feeding enhances growth and maturation in premature infants. *Pediatrics, 71*, 41–45.

Bingham, P. M., Thomas, C. S., Ashikaga, T., & Abbasi, S. (2008). Non-nutritive sucking measure predicts feeding skills in tube-fed premature infants. *Pediatric Academic Society*, 3778.1, 93.

Bosma, J. F. (1970). Summarizing and perspective comments: Part V. Form and function in the infant's mouth and pharynx. In J. F. Bosma (Ed.), *Second symposium on oral sensation and perception* (pp. 550–555). Springfield, IL: Charles C. Thomas.

Boughter, J. D., Bajpai, T., St. John, S. J., Williams, R. W., Lu, L., & Heck, D. H. (2007). Genetic analysis of oromotor movements in inbred and BXD recombinant inbred mice. *Society for Neuroscience*, 407.12.

Bu'Lock, F., Woolridge, M. W., & Baum, J. D. (1990). Development of coordination of sucking, swallowing and breathing: Ultrasound study of term and preterm infants. *Developmental Medicine and Child Neurology, 32*, 669–678.

Byrant, J. L., Roy, S., Boughter, J. D., Goldowitz, D., Swanson, D., Morgan, J. I., et al. (2007). A proposed new function of the mouse cerebellum: Temporal modulation of brain stem pattern generator activity. *Society for Neuroscience*, 78.17.

Comrie, J. D., & Helm, J. M. (1997). Common feeding problems in the intensive care nurseries, maturation, organization, evaluation, and management strategies. *Seminars in Speech and Language, 18*, 239–261.

da Costa, S. P., van den Engel-Hoek, L., & Bos, A. F. (2008). Sucking and swallowing in infants and diagnostic tools. *Journal of Perinatology, 28*, 247–257.

DiPietro, J. A., Cusson, R. M., Caughy, M. O., & Fox, N. A. (1994). Behavioral and physiologic effects of nonnutritive sucking during gavage feeding in preterm infants. *Pediatric Research, 36*, 207–214.

Dreier, T., & Wolff, P. H. (1972). Sucking, state, and perinatal distress in newborns. *Biology of the Neonate, 21*, 16–24.

Estep, M., Barlow, S. M., Vantipalli, R., Lee, J., & Finan, D. (2008). Non-nutritive suck burst parametrics in preterm infants with RDS and oral feeding complications. *Journal of Neonatal Nursing, 14*(1), 28–34.

Field, T. (1993). Sucking for stress reduction, growth and development during infancy. *Pediatric Basics, 64*, 13–16.

Field, T., Ignatoff, E., Stringer, S., Brennan, J., Greenberg, R., Widmayer, S., et al. (1982). Nonnutritive sucking during tube feedings: Effects on preterm neonates in an intensive care unit. *Pediatrics, 70*, 381–384.

Finan, D. S., & Barlow, S. M. (1998). Mechanosensory modulation of non-nutritive sucking in human infants. *Early Human Development, 52*, 181–197.

Fucile, S., Gisel, E., & Lau, C. (2002). Oral stimulation accelerates the transition from tube to oral feeding in preterm infants. *Journal of Pediatrics, 141*, 230–236.

Fucile, S., Gisel, E., & Lau, C. (2005). Effect of an oral stimulation program on sucking skill maturation of preterm infants. *Dev Med Child Neurol, 47*, 158–162.

Georgopoulos, A. P., Kalaska, J. F., & Massey, J. T. (1981). Spatial trajectories and reaction times of aimed movements: Effects of practice, uncertainty and change in target location. *Journal of Neurophysiology, 46*, 725–743.

Gewolb, I. H., Vice, F. L., Schweitzer-Kenney, E. L., Taciak, V. L., & Bosma, J. F. (2001). Developmental patterns of rhythmic suckle and swallow in preterm infants. *Developmental Medicine and Child Neurology, 43*, 22–27.

Gill, N. E., Behnke, M., Conlon, M., & Anderson, G. C. (1992). Nonnutritive sucking modulates behavioral state for preterm infants before feeding. *Scandinavian Journal of Caring Sciences, 6*, 3–7.

Gill, N. E., Behnke, M., Conlon, M., McNeely, J. B., & Anderson, G. C. (1988). Effect of nonnutritive sucking on behavioral state in preterm infants before feeding. *Nursing Research, 37*, 347–350.

Goldson, E. (1987). Nonnutritive sucking in the sick infant. *Journal of Perinatology, 7*(1), 30–34.

Hack, M., Estabrook, M. M., & Robertson, S. S. (1985). Development of sucking rhythm in preterm infants. *Early Human Development, 11*, 133–140.

Hensch, T. (2004). Critical period regulation. *Annual Review of Neuroscience, 27*, 549–579.

Iriki, A., Nozaki, S., & Nakamura, Y. (1988). Feeding behavior in mammals: Corticobulbar projection is reorganized during conversion from sucking to chewing. *Developmental Brain Research, 44*, 189–196.

Lau, C. (2006). Oral feeding in the preterm infant. *Neoreviews, 7*, 19–27.

Lau, C., & Hurst, N. (1999). Oral feeding in infants. *Current Problems in Pediatrics, 29*, 105–124.

Lau, C., & Schanler, R. J. (1996). Oral motor function in the neonate. *Clinics in Perinatology, 23*, 161–178.

Löwel, S., & Singer, W. (1992). Selection of intrinsic horizontal connections in the visual cortex by correlated neuronal activity. *Science, 255*, 209–212.

Marder, E., & Rehm, K. J. (2005). Development of central pattern generating circuits. *Current Opinion in Neurobiology, 5*, 86–93.

McCain, G. C. (1992). Facilitating inactive awake states in preterm infants: A study of three interventions. *Nursing Research, 41*, 157–160.

McCain, G. C. (1995). Promotion of preterm infant nipple feeding with nonnutritive sucking. *Journal of Pediatric Nursing, 10*, 3–8.

Measel, C. P., & Anderson, G. C. (1979). Nonnutritive sucking during tube feedings: Effect upon clinical course in preterm infants. *Journal of Obstetric, Gynecologic, and Neonatal Nursing, 8*, 265–271.

Medoff-Cooper, B. (2005). Nutritive sucking research: From clinical questions to research answers. *The Journal of Perinatal and Neonatal Nursing, 19*, 265–272.

Mizuno, K., & Ueda, A. (2005). Neonatal feeding performance as a predictor of neurodevelopmental outcome at 18 months. *Developmental Medicine and Child Neurology, 47*, 299–304.

Penn, A. A., & Shatz, C. J. (1999). Brain waves and brain wiring: The role of endogenous and sensory-driven neural activity in development. *Pediatric Research, 45*, 447–458.

Pickler, R. H., Frankel, H. B., Walsh, K. M., & Thompson, N. M. (1996). Effects of nonnutritive sucking on behavioral organization and feeding performance in preterm infants. *Nursing Research, 45*, 132–135.

Pickler, R. H., Higgins, K. E., & Crummette, B. D. (1993). The effect of nonnutritive sucking on bottle-feeding stress in preterm infants. *Journal of Obstetric, Gynecologic and Neonatal Nursing, 22*, 230–234.

Poore, M., Barlow, S. M., Wang, J., Estep, M., & Lee, J. (2008). Respiratory treatment history predicts suck pattern stability in preterm infants. *Journal of Neonatal Nursing*, doi:10.1016/j.jnn.2008.07.006, *epub* ahead of print.

Poore, M., Zimmerman, E., Barlow, S. M., Wang, J., & Gu, F. (2008). Patterned orocutaneous therapy improves sucking and oral feeding in preterm infants. *Acta Paediatrica, 97*, 920–927.

Rocha, A., Moreira, M., Pimenta, H., Ramos, J., & Lucena, S. (2007). A randomized study of the efficacy of sensory-motor-oral stimulation and non-nutritive sucking in very low birth weight infants. *Early Human Development, 83*, 385–389.

Shiao, S.-Y. P. K., Youngblut, J. M., Anderson, G. C., DiFiore, J. M., & Martin, R. J. (1995). Nasogastric tube placement: Effects on breathing and sucking in very-low-birth-weight infants. *Nursing Research, 44*, 82–88.

Smith, A., Johnson, M., McGillem, C., & Goffman, L. (2000). On the assessment of stability and patterning of speech movements. *Journal of Speech Language Hearing and Research, 43*, 277–286.

Smith, A., & Zelaznik, H. N. (2004). Development of functional synergies for speech motor coordination in childhood and adolescence. *Developmental Psychobiology, 45*, 22–33.

Stumm, S., Barlow, S. M., Estep, M., Lee, J., Cannon, S., & Gagnon, K. (2008). The relation between respiratory distress syndrome and the fine structure of the non-nutritive suck in preterm infants. *Journal of Neonatal Nursing, 14*(1), 9–16.

Tanaka, S., Kogo, M., Chandler, S. H., & Matsuya, T. (1999). Localization of oral-motor rhythmogenic circuits in the isolated rat brainstem preparation. *Brain Research, 821*, 190–199.

Urish, M. M., Barlow, S. M., & Venkatesan, L. (2007). Frequency modulation of the sCPG in preterm infants with RDS. Abstracts for the *American Speech-Language-Hearing Association*, Boston, MA. Session 1993.

Volkmer, A. S., & Fiori, H. H. (2008). Non-nutritive sucking with a pacifier in preterm infants. *Pediatric Academic Society*, 3535.1, 75.

Wolff, P. H. (1968). The serial organization of sucking in the young infant. *Pediatrics, 42*, 943–956.

Zimmerman, E., & Barlow, S. M. (2008). Pacifier stiffness alters the dynamics of the suck central pattern generator. *Journal of Neonatal Nursing, 14*(3), 79–86.

# PART II
# Preschool Child Cases

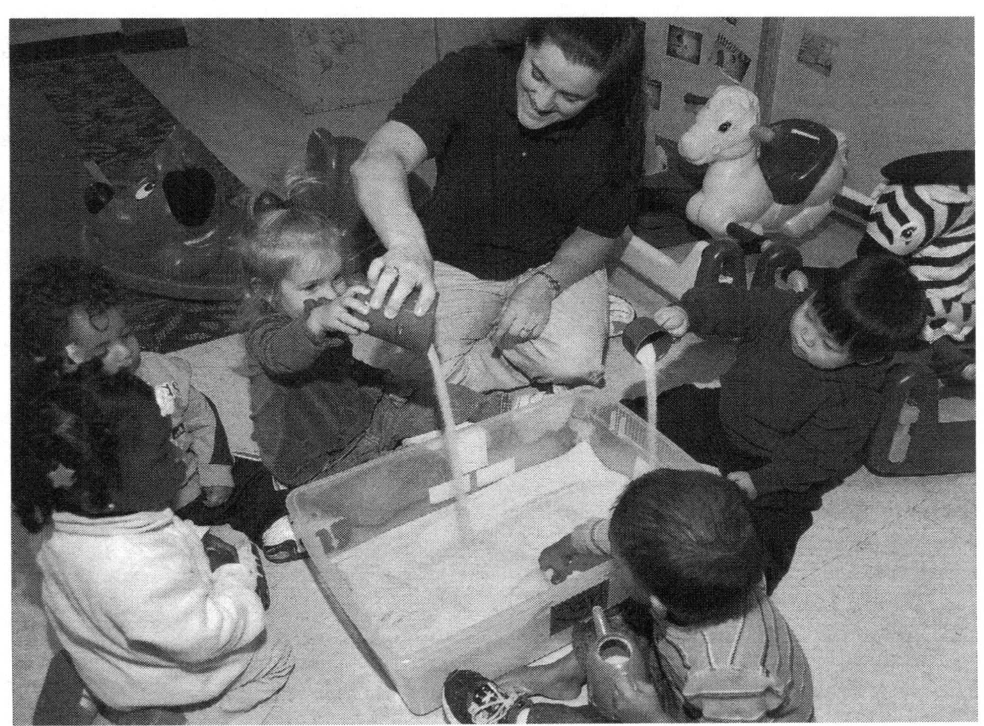

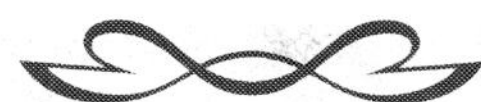

# Ankyloglossia

## Case 9

# Kyle: To Clip or Not to Clip . . . What Is the Answer?

*Ann W. Kummer*

## Conceptual Knowledge Areas

### What Is Ankyloglossia?

*Ankyloglossia* is commonly referred to simply as "tongue-tie." Ankyloglossia is a relatively common congenital anomaly that is usually detected soon after birth. It is characterized by partial fusion—or in rare cases, total fusion—of the tongue to the floor of the mouth due to an abnormality of the lingual frenulum, sometimes called the lingual frenum.

A *frenum* is a narrow fold of mucous membrane connecting a moveable body part to a fixed part. Its purpose is to stabilize and check undue movement of that body part. A *frenulum* is a small frenum. The *lingual frenulum* is a fold of mucous membrane that arises from the floor of the mouth and attaches to the mid-portion of the tongue. Its function is to stabilize the tongue, without interfering with tongue tip movement. Ankyloglossia is a condition in which the lingual frenulum has an atypically anterior attachment near the tip of the tongue (see Figure 9.1). The frenulum may also be unusually short. This can result in restricted tongue tip movement to some extent.

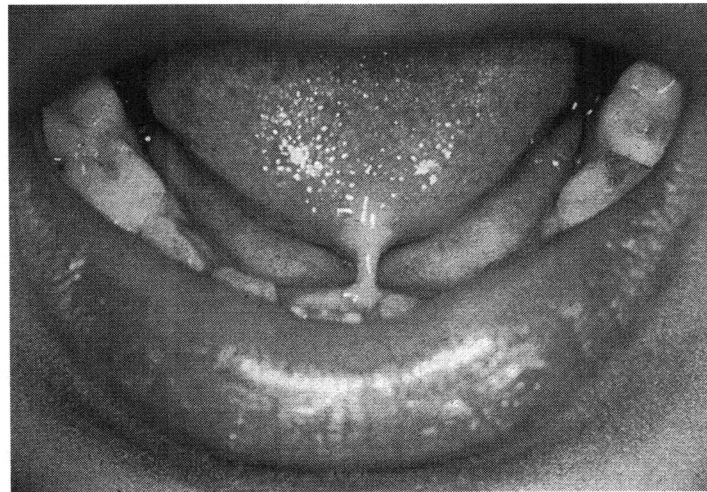

FIGURE 9.1 Ankyloglossia with the Lingual Frenulum Attached to the Tongue Tip

*Source:* From Kummer. *Cleft Palate and Craniofacial Anomalies*, 2E. © 2008 Delmar Learning, a part of Cengage Learning, Inc. Reproduced by permission. www.cengage.com/permissions

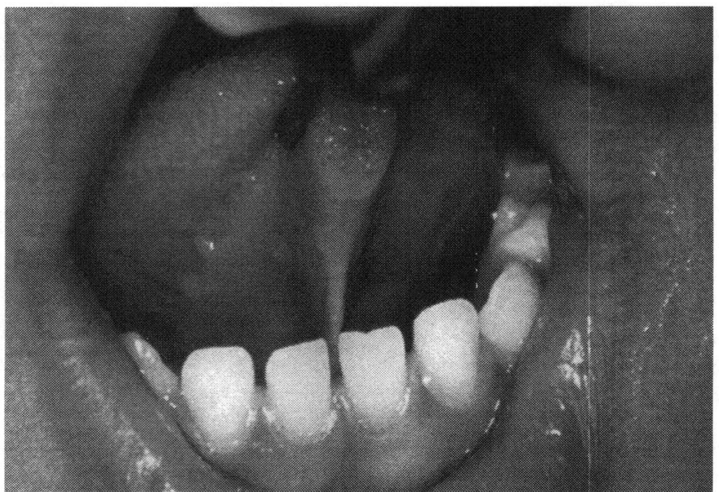

FIGURE 9.2 Ankyloglossia with a Short Lingual Frenulum

## How Common Is Ankyloglossia?

The reported figures of the prevalence of ankyloglossia vary significantly—from less than 1% to as frequent as 97% in newborns. The variation in reported prevalence has to do with the fact that "normal" and ankyloglossia are at opposite ends of a continuum. Where the line is drawn between normal and abnormal affects the reported prevalence figures. Most reports place the prevalence in newborns at about 4% to 10% however (Segal, Stephenson, Dawes, & Feldman, 2007).

## How Is Ankyloglossia Diagnosed?

Diagnosing ankyloglossia is usually simple. With protrusion attempts, the tongue tip appears notched in midline, resulting in a heart-shaped edge. The individual with ankyloglossia may be unable to protrude the tongue past the edge of the lower gingiva or mandibular incisors. In addition, the individual may be unable to touch the alveolar ridge with the tongue tip when the mouth is open (see Figure 9.2).

## What Are the Functional Effects of Ankyloglossia?

The functional effects of ankyloglossia depend on the severity of the lingual restriction. Most individuals have little or no effect. In addition, the lingual restriction tends to decrease over time, because with growth in the first 4 to 5 years of life, there is a significant change in oral cavity structures. The alveolar ridge grows in height, the teeth begin to erupt, and the tongue grows and narrows at the tip. At the same time, the lingual frenulum recedes, stretches, and may even rupture spontaneously. Therefore, with time, the severity of the ankyloglossia lessens, the initial restrictions of lingual movement diminish, and the functional effects improve or are eliminated.

Some individuals do experience functional difficulties as a result of the ankyloglossia. These are generally in the following areas:

- ***Feeding problems.*** Approximately 25% of newborns with ankyloglossia have trouble latching onto a nipple for sucking, thus affecting their feeding. Older individuals with ankyloglossia may have difficulty moving a bolus around in the oral cavity and clearing food from the sulci and molars with the tongue. This problem could result in chronic halitosis and contribute to dental decay.
- ***Dentition.*** If the lingual frenulum is attached high on the gingival ridge behind the lower mandibular incisors, it can pull the gingiva away from the teeth and even cause a mandibular diastema. This is usually not a problem until the child is 8–10 years old.

- ***Cosmetics.*** There is no doubt that ankyloglossia may look abnormal when protruding the tongue. It has even been described as a forked or "serpent" tongue.
- ***Kissing.*** There can be difficulty with "French" kissing.
- ***Speech.*** Through the centuries, it has been a common folk belief that if the tongue tip cannot move well due to ankyloglossia, it must affect speech. However, there is no evidence in the literature to support this belief. On the contrary, many authors over the last few decades have disputed the belief that there is a causal relationship between ankyloglossia and speech. A review of the literature results in very few articles that even mention ankyloglossia as a possible contributor to speech problems.

## What Sounds Could Be Affected by Ankyloglossia?

Theoretically, ankyloglossia might affect tongue tip speech sounds that require lingual elevation or protrusion. It would never affect the production of sounds that do not require the tongue tip, such as bilabial, labiodental, or velar sounds.

Although lingual articulation against the alveolar ridge is a problem with ankyloglossia, this is usually true only when the mouth is fully open. It may not be a problem when the mouth is partially closed for speech. In addition, many lingual-alveolar sounds (/t/, /d/, /n/) are produced with the top of the tongue tip so that very little tongue elevation or mobility is required. The /s/ and /z/ sounds are usually produced with the tongue tip elevated slightly, but these sounds can also be produced normally with the tongue tip down. The English /r/ sound can be produced with the tongue tip up or down, as long as the back of the tongue is elevated on both sides. Ankyloglossia is more likely to affect the production of the Spanish /r/ because it requires lingual vibration.

The sound that requires the most lingual elevation is /l/, and therefore it is the most likely to be affected by ankyloglossia. However, even the /l/ sound can be produced with the tongue tip down so that the dorsum of the tongue articulates against the alveolar ridge.

Protrusion of the tongue past the mandibular incisors is often a problem with ankyloglossia. However, speech requires only minimal lingual protrusion. The most the tongue needs to protrude is against the back of the maxillary incisors for the /th/ sound.

## How Can You Determine If Ankyloglossia Is Affecting Speech?

The examiner should determine if the child is able to achieve relatively normal placement for the /l/ and /th/ sounds, which are the English sounds that are most likely to be affected by ankyloglossia. If the child cannot achieve normal placement in isolation, yet there are multiple other articulation errors, the problem may be an articulation disorder rather than lingual restriction due to ankyloglossia.

Ankyloglossia could be considered a *contributing* factor to a speech problem if the child cannot produce the /l/ and /th/ sounds, even with the alternate placement just noted, yet all other speech sounds are produced normally. Ankyloglossia may also be a complicating factor if there is oral-motor dysfunction.

## How Is Ankyloglossia Treated?

If ankyloglossia is noted at birth, but it is not causing problems with feeding, nothing needs to be done. It can always be treated in the future if problems arise.

If the child demonstrates one or more of the problems previously noted, however, a *frenulectomy* (surgical release of the tongue) can be done. In past times, midwives used a sharpened fingernail to slit the frenulum immediately after birth. Currently, frenulectomies are performed by surgeons or pediatricians. Frenulectomies can be done in the office for adults, but children usually require anesthesia to ensure adequate cooperation.

The procedure takes only a few minutes to perform. The frenulum is divided with scissors or with electrocautery. Sutures are usually not required.

The risks of frenulectomy are minimal, but they include pain, minor bleeding, or infection. In most cases, the mobility of the tongue after frenulectomy prevents scarring from occurring during the healing process. In rare cases, however, scarring occurs and can further limit the mobility of the tongue. The scar tissue is excised and a series of flaps are created on the floor of the mouth to close the defect. This "Z-plasty" procedure minimizes the risk of additional scar formation.

### Summary

Both ankyloglossia and speech problems commonly occur in children. Therefore, it is not surprising that these conditions are often seen together. A co-occurrence of these two findings does not mean that there is a causal relationship between the two. There is very little in the literature that even addresses ankyloglossia and speech—perhaps because a causal relationship is not commonly seen. Most experienced speech-language pathologists would suggest that ankyloglossia is unlikely to cause speech problems. Therefore, frenulectomy is rarely indicated for speech-related reasons, unless it is very severe or there are concomitant oral-motor problems. Although frenulectomy is a minor procedure with a low risk of morbidity, the true danger is the disappointment that can result when parents are led to believe that this will correct speech problems that are actually due to other causes. Frenulectomy may be warranted for problems with early feeding, bolus manipulation, dentition, or aesthetics.*

## Description of the Case

The following case report describes a child who was diagnosed with ankyloglossia and underwent a frenulectomy for treatment.

### Background Information and Reason for Referral

Kyle, age 4 years, 10 months, was seen for a speech evaluation at the request of an attorney. Kyle had a history of ankyloglossia and speech problems. When he was about 4 years old, one of his speech-language pathologists told the parents that Kyle's "tongue-tie" was contributing to his speech problems. She therefore referred Kyle back to his otolaryngologist for a frenulectomy. The frenulectomy had been done 8 months previously. The parents were suing the child's pediatrician for not recommending a frenulectomy earlier, preferably before Kyle started talking.

#### Pertinent History

Both parents accompanied Kyle to the evaluation and served as informants. They provided the following information:

***Neonatal History*** Kyle was the product of a full-term pregnancy and normal delivery. The only neonatal problem reported was difficulty with breast feeding. Once the mother switched from breast feeding to bottle feeding, the feeding difficulties resolved.

***Medical History*** Kyle's medical history included chronic middle ear effusion with infections, requiring the insertion of PE tubes on three occasions. As noted, Kyle underwent a frenulectomy at the age of 4 years, 2 months. Additional medical history was unremarkable.

***Developmental History*** According to his mother, Kyle's motor milestones were accomplished within normal limits. However, his speech development was somewhat delayed (due to the tongue-tie, in her opinion). Kyle seemed to understand speech as well as other children his age and started putting words together well before his second birthday, but his speech was always hard to understand.

---

*Text on pages 65–68 from "Ankyloglossia: To Clip or Not To Clip? That's the Question," by A. Kummer, 2005, Dec. 27), *The ASHA Leader,* 10(17), pp. 6–7, 30. Copyright 2005 by the American Speech-Language-Hearing Association. Adapted with permission.

***Treatment History*** Kyle began speech therapy just before the age of 3 years. He was still receiving speech therapy at a local hospital and also at his preschool. His mother noted that although his articulation had improved as a result of therapy, progress had been very slow. She admitted that the frenulectomy did not seem to have the positive effect on Kyle's speech that they had expected.

## Findings of the Evaluation

The following is a summary of the evaluation results:

### Language

Kyle was communicating with complete sentences. An informal screening revealed normal syntax and morphology.

### Speech/Articulation

Articulation was characterized by the following errors on the single word level: bilabials for labiodentals (p/f, b/v); fronting of velars (t/k, d/g); stopping of sibilants (t/s, d/z, t/sh, t/ch, d/j); substitution of /w/ or /y/ for /l/; f/th; reduction of blends; and inconsistent voiced/voiceless substitutions. Stimulability testing revealed the ability to produce most misarticulated phonemes in isolation, including /l/ and /th/. When asked to repeat words such as "money," "baby doll," "teddy bear," and "buddy," Kyle did reasonably well because these words contain mostly the bilabial and lingual-alveolar plosives—the phonemes that he could produce. However, when asked to produce one of these words repetitively, his articulation completely broke down. In connected speech, there was a significant increase in inconsistent errors and frequent phoneme omissions. Intelligibility of connected speech was poor.

### Resonance

Resonance was variable. During the production of single words, resonance was normal. In conversational speech, however, there was inconsistent hypernasality, and sometimes even hyponasality on nasal consonants.

### Voice

Voice quality was normal.

### Intraoral Examination

An intraoral examination revealed an intact velum. The tonsils were moderately enlarged. Occlusion was in a normal Class I relationship. The frenulum had been split and therefore was not restricting. Kyle was able to protrude, lateralize, and elevate the tongue without difficulty.

### Examiner Impressions

Kyle demonstrated a severe speech disorder characterized by the use of primarily early developmental sounds, such as nasals and plosives (bilabial and lingual-alveolar); inconsistent voiced/voiceless substitutions; inconsistent nasal/oral and oral/nasal substitutions; and an increase in inconsistent errors and omissions with increased utterance length and/or phonemic complexity. These are characteristic of apraxia of speech. The irony is that Kyle had learned to produce lingual-alveolar sounds (tongue-tip sounds) as a substitution for other sounds, including velars (which involve the back of the tongue). Also, Kyle was able to produce the /l/ and /th/ sounds in isolation without difficulty. It was suspected that this was the case even prior to the frenulectomy.

### Parent Counseling

The parents were counseled regarding the results of the evaluation. They were told that apraxia is a motor speech disorder that has a neurological basis. There was no evidence that this history of ankyloglossia was a contributing factor in Kyle's case. In fact, there was evidence to the contrary.

## Treatment Options Considered

Further speech therapy was recommended, but with increased involvement of the family. It was explained that speech therapy is like taking piano lessons—if you don't practice between the lessons, you never develop the motor memory and motor skills to play the piano. Because apraxia is a motor speech disorder and speech is something that is done continuously throughout the day, daily speech practice is particularly important and should be done several times a day. The parents were instructed on methods of incorporating speech practice into their daily routine.

### Follow-Up

The parents seemed to understand the explanations regarding Kyle's speech disorder. A few weeks after the evaluation, they chose to drop the lawsuit against the pediatrician and even sent him a letter of apology.

## Further Recommendations

*This case illustrates the critical importance of evidence-based practice.*

Because there was the co-occurrence of ankyloglossia and a speech disorder, the speech-language pathologist made the assumption that there was a causal relationship. This was done without considering the evidence.

Due to this misdiagnosis, there were several negative consequences. The child underwent unnecessary (albeit minor) surgery. The parents expended time and money for the procedure and were given false hope that it would help to correct Kyle's speech. Finally, the parents and pediatrician went through months of unnecessary angst and expense related to the lawsuit.

A lesson in this case is that health care practitioners (including speech-language pathologists) need to be cautious of jumping to conclusions, particularly those that can have significant consequences. Instead, they should examine the evidence prior to making a referral for treatment, particularly one that involves surgery. In cases like this, the speech-language pathologist should study the literature and use appropriate evaluation procedures to come to the best conclusion regarding diagnosis, etiological factors, and appropriate treatment.

## Author Note

This information was taken from an actual case.

## Reference

Segal, L. M., Stephenson, R., Dawes, M., & Feldman, P. (2007). Prevalence, diagnosis, and treatment of ankyloglossia: Methodologic review. *Canadian Family Physician, 53*(6), 1027–1033.

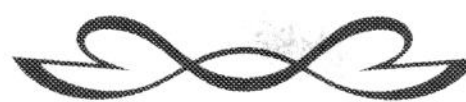

## Apraxia

# Case 10

# Matthew: The Changing Picture of Childhood Apraxia of Speech: From Initial Symptoms to Diagnostic and Therapeutic Modifications

*Jacqueline Bauman-Waengler and Diane Garcia*

## Conceptual Knowledge Areas

Conceptual knowledge relevant to this case study includes, first, a basic understanding of phonological development in preschool children. The time frame, from 3 to 6 years old, is an important one in the acquisition of speech sounds, syllable shapes, and phonotactic possibilities. It is important that the clinician have a well-founded conceptual framework of normal acquisition patterns versus those that are considered deviant.

Second, the clinician should have a working knowledge of the symptom complex known as *childhood apraxia of speech* (CAS). Although the exact characteristics associated with this diagnostic label have changed and still remain controversial, this case study draws on resources such as the American Speech-Language-Hearing Association (ASHA) position statement and technical report on childhood apraxia of speech (ASHA, 2007a, b) and other current resources, which are found throughout the case study and in the references section.

Third, the clinician should be acquainted with three treatment approaches: the *cycles approach* (Hodson, 1997; Hodson & Paden, 1991), *integral stimulation techniques* (Strand & Skinder, 1999), and the *multiple oppositions approach* (Williams 2000a, b). The cycles approach has been used to treat unintelligible children for decades regardless of the etiology. Although it was not specifically designed for children with motor-planning difficulties, this method has been successfully combined with integral stimulation to specifically address those motor-planning problems (Berman, 2001; Berman, Garcia, & Bauman-Waengler, 2007). The multiple oppositions approach directly addresses the collapse of multiple phonemes within a child's phonemic inventory. These three approaches were utilized during different phases of the treatment program. Integral stimulation and the multiple oppositions approach are explained in some detail in the following case study.

## Description of the Case

### Background Information

Matthew was originally seen at age 3 years, 1 month at a university clinic for a 2-hour diagnostic evaluation. He was accompanied by his mother. He was a rather serious child with a pleasant smile, sandy-colored hair, and freckles, who was intent on pleasing the clinicians. He cooperated throughout the entire diagnostic session; thus, the results that were obtained were considered to be representative of his skills at that time.

## Reason for Referral

Matthew was referred to the clinic by his mother, who was concerned about his speech skills. She stated that he was hard to understand and that, although he enjoyed talking to people, his speech was often unintelligible. She had become proficient at interpreting his utterances and thought that she understood him approximately 50% to 70% of the time. Other people, however, typically could not understand Matthew and he became occasionally frustrated.

### Family History

Matthew lived with his biological parents and one younger sister, who was 17 weeks old at the time of the initial evaluation. The family was considered upper middle class; the mother was a teacher who was staying home with the two children and the father was a lawyer. All family members were Caucasian, and English was the only language spoken at home. It was noted that Matthew's father, paternal aunt, and paternal uncle had experienced speech difficulties, and that his father and aunt had received speech services as children.

### Medical History

Matthew was born full-term with no complications during the pregnancy or labor and delivery. He had no current medical concerns, although he did have mild allergies and was considered to have occasional mild asthmatic symptoms. Both vision and hearing were evaluated and were within normal limits.

### Developmental History

His mother described Matthew's development as "average" during the first 3 years. He sat alone at 4 to 5 months, walked alone at 11½ months, drank from a cup at 1 year, dressed himself at 2 years, said his first word at 9 to 10 months, and put two words together at 18 months. His verbalizations were considered very difficult to understand from the beginning of his speech attempts, and no dramatic changes had occurred in his speech development over the past 2 years.

### Educational History

Matthew was not enrolled in school. He had attended speech therapy since the age of 2 years, 3 months. However, the family moved several times and therapy was of short duration and inconsistent.

## Findings of the Evaluation

The results of the Goldman-Fristoe Test of Articulation-2 (GF-2) (Goldman & Fristoe, 2000) are summarized in Table 10.1. Matthew exhibited vowel substitutions and frequent substitutions of [b], [d], and [n] for other consonants. His speech was characterized by the diagnostic team as being "highly unintelligible." Results of the oral peripheral exam indicated possible oral apraxia. For example, Matthew had difficulty executing volitional oral motor movements

TABLE 10.1 Goldman-Fristoe Test of Articulation-2 Scores from Initial Evaluation

| Test, Date, Age of Child | Error Score | Standard Score | 95% Confidence Interval | Percentile Rank |
|---|---|---|---|---|
| Goldman-Fristoe-2, 12-05-07, Age 3;1 | 65 | 66 | 60–72 | 3 |

after a model; he could not pucker his lips or move his tongue from side to side when a model was provided. He also had difficulty moving his tongue without moving his head.

Although a language test was not given, Matthew's pragmatic skills and language comprehension were judged as being within normal limits. He was able to follow directions and answer questions age appropriately. However, his speech was so unintelligible that a formal assessment of expressive semantics and morphosyntax was not attempted and a language sample could not be completed.

It was hypothesized that Matthew demonstrated childhood apraxia of speech (CAS). Thus the primary contributor to his speech production difficulties was thought to be impairment in planning or programming movement sequences (ASHA, 2007b). Matthew exhibited many characteristics of CAS identified in the literature (Caruso & Strand, 1999; Flahive, Velleman, & Hodson, 2005; Smit, 2004). During the initial evaluation, Matthew exhibited signs of oral apraxia, a severely limited consonant inventory, and his intelligibility was minimal. Assimilation errors were common (for example, "mum" for "gum"), as were vowel substitutions. Matthew had difficulty imitating speech sounds in the absence of any oral motor weakness, and the frequency of his errors increased in longer words and utterances. He also demonstrated occasional initial consonant deletion (for example, "up" for "cup") and epenthesis, particularly insertion of the schwa vowel at the end of words. Although his mother remarked about the consistency of his productions, Matthew often produced the same word several different ways during the initial evaluation. This inconsistency contributed to the hypothesis of apraxia of speech.

## Treatment Options Considered

Individual speech therapy was recommended for Matthew, twice weekly for 50-minute sessions. This case study spans the course of three semesters of treatment, each semester consisting of approximately 12 weeks. A different pair of student clinicians was assigned each semester to implement Matthew's remediation program under the close guidance of a university supervisor. Upon initiation of therapy, approximately 1 month after the diagnostic evaluation, further assessment of Matthew's expressive phonology and articulation was conducted using the Goldman-Fristoe Test of Articulation-2—GF-2, the Hodson Assessment of Phonological Patterns-3—HAPP-3 (Hodson, 2004), the Receptive One-Word Picture Vocabulary Test—ROWPVT (Brownell, 2000), and intelligibility measures. These results are summarized in Table 10.2.

## Course of Treatment

The cycles approach (Hodson, 1997; Hodson & Paden, 1991) was selected as an appropriate therapy program for Matthew. It is specifically designed for young children with multiple error patterns and highly unintelligible speech. The authors provide clear guidelines for target selection and implementation, as well as specific directions on how to structure remediation sessions—distinct advantages for student clinicians with little expertise in developing therapeutic protocols. In addition, the cycles approach includes a home program component that is easy and quick to administer, allowing Matthew's parents to be active participants in his treatment without placing unrealistic demands upon their time. Studies supporting the effectiveness of pattern-based

TABLE 10.2 Results of Testing at Beginning of Therapy

| Test | Score | Standard Score | Percentile Rank/ Percentage |
|---|---|---|---|
| GF-2 | Error Score = 60 | 68 | 5 |
| HAPP-3 | Total Occurrence of Major Phonological Deviations = 131 | Ability Score = <55 | <1 = Severe |
| ROWPVT | Raw Score = 34 | 96 | 39 |
| Speech Sample | 6/25 completely intelligible responses | | 24% completely intelligible responses |

| | |
|---|---|
| 1. Review | Child reviews previous session's word cards. |
| 2. Auditory Bombardment | Amplified stimulation for 1–2 minutes of clinician reading approximately 12 words with target sound. |
| 3. Target Word Cards | Three to five target word cards are prepared. Client repeats words modeled by the clinician. |
| 4. Production Practice | Games are used as the clinician and child take turns naming the pictures. Clinician provides models and/or tactile cues so that the child achieves 100% success on target patterns. |
| 5. Stimulability Probes | Child's stimulability is assessed for potential targets for the next session. Child should be able to accurately model selected words. |
| 6. Auditory Bombardment | Step 2 is repeated. |
| 7. Home Program | Parent or school aide participates in a 2-minute per day home program. Words are read from the week's auditory bombardment (Step 2) and the child names word cards from Step 3. |

FIGURE 10.1 Overview of Cycles Therapy Session

approaches are primarily case studies (Kamhi, 2006). Despite the absence of large clinical trials, the cycles approach has been used to successfully treat highly unintelligible children for decades, regardless of etiology (Hodson, 1997; Hodson & Paden, 1991).

An initial cycle of targets was developed for Matthew following Hodson's recommendations (Hodson, 1997), with minor modifications. Error patterns that occurred with more than 40% frequency were targeted, including specific initial and final consonant deletions, anterior-posterior contrasts, s-clusters, and liquids. The initial consonants /m/ and /w/ were targeted in order to address class deficiencies in the categories of nasals and glides, as well as to decrease initial consonant deletion. Stimulability for each exemplar was probed the week prior to implementation. Initial /k/, /l/, /r/, and final s-clusters were deleted from the first cycle because Matthew was unable to produce these sounds, (or, with /r/, modify the production) despite maximum cueing.

Therapy sessions were structured according to guidelines developed by Hodson (1997) for the cycles approach and incorporated auditory bombardment, production practice, and a home program (as outlined in Figure 10.1). Each week a small set of words was carefully selected containing the target sound (e.g., initial /w/). Remediation sessions were designed to maximize productions of the target words while keeping Matthew actively engaged and motivated. His favorite activities proved to be bowling and fishing—in fact, he wore his fishing hat to every session in hopes that a fishing rod might appear.

An initial cycle of targets was developed for Matthew following Hodson and Paden's guidelines. See Tables 10.3 and 10.4 for a summary of the target patterns.

Although the cycles approach was not specifically designed for children with motor-planning difficulties, experts have suggested that it may be an appropriate program when combined with remediation techniques proved effective for childhood apraxia of speech (Berman, 2001; Flahive et al., 2005). Therefore, based upon the initial provisional diagnosis of CAS, aspects of integral stimulation therapy were incorporated into Matthew's therapy program: (1) Mass practice (many repetitions of a few targets) was emphasized initially, moving to (2) more distributed practice (repetitions of more targets with a common gestural basis) as productions improved. (3) A continuum of temporal relationships between the clinician's presentation of stimulus and Matthew's response was utilized, including simultaneous production, immediate repetition, and delayed repetition. (4) During imitation tasks, a slow rate was initially employed and the rate was slowly increased until Matthew could successfully imitate at a normal rate (Flahive et al., 2005; Gildersleeve-Neumann, 2007; Strand & Skinder, 1999).

Other therapeutic adaptations that have been recommended for children with motor-planning difficulties were also utilized. Selection of target words involved careful attention to phonetic complexity (Bauman-Waengler, 2008; Hodson & Paden, 1991). Words with simple syllable

TABLE 10.3 Primary Target Patterns—Early Cycles

| Error Pattern | HAPP-3 | Potential Target |
|---|---|---|
| **EARLY DEVELOPING PATTERNS** | | |
| Syllableness | Could produce vowel nuclei of multisyllabic words | No |
| Initial consonants /p, b, m, w/; /t, d, n/ | Could produce /b, d, n/ Class deficiencies—difficulties with initial glides & nasals (including initial /w/ & /m/) | Yes, initial glides or nasals |
| Final consonants /p, t, k/ | Consistently deleted | Yes |
| **ANTERIOR-POSTERIOR CONTRASTS** | | |
| Velars /k, g/ or glottal /h/ | Consistently was unable to produce /h/, deleted or replaced /k/ and /g/ | Yes |
| Alveolars /t, d/ (possibly alveolar /n/ or labials /p, b/ if lacking) | Could produce these sounds | No |
| **/S/ CLUSTERS** | | |
| Word-initial /sp, st, sm, sn, sk/ | Consistently deleted or replaced word-initial s-clusters | Yes |
| Word-final /ts, ps, ks/ | Consistently deleted or replaced word-final s-clusters | Yes |
| **LIQUIDS** | | |
| Word-initial /l/ | Consistently deleted or replaced word-initial /l/ | Yes |
| Word-initial /r/ | Consistently deleted or replaced word-initial /r/ | Yes |

shapes were chosen initially. For example, when targeting initial /m/, words with a consonant-vowel (CV) syllable shape were used, such as "me," "my," and "mow." Coarticulatory effects were considered, including the movements necessary to achieve transitions between consonants and vowels. Thus, "mop" was chosen as a target to represent the CVC syllable shape because it included two bilabials and a final consonant (/p/) that was already present in Matthew's inventory, whereas "mug" was eliminated as a potential target word because it involved movement from the front to the back of the mouth and included a phoneme (/g/) not yet produced by Matthew.

Another adaptation of the cycles approach that was implemented was increasing the number of sessions devoted to each exemplar. Hodson recommends one hour of therapy for each target sound, yet Matthew received 3 hours of therapy for each exemplar identified in his cycle. The extra time allowed Matthew more success. The initial session for each sound was usually quite difficult and tiring for both Matthew and his clinicians as he required intensive

TABLE 10.4 Targets for Cycle Approach with Matthew

| Pattern | Exemplar |
|---|---|
| Initial glide deficiency | Initial /w/ |
| Initial nasal deficiency | Initial /m/ |
| Final consonant deletion | Final /p/ |
| Final consonant deletion | Final /t/ |
| Final consonant deletion and anterior-posterior contrasts | Final /k/ |
| Anterior-posterior contrasts | Initial /k/ |
| s-clusters | Initial /sn/ |
| s-clusters | Initial /st/ |
| Liquids | Initial /l/ |

cueing and instruction to learn a new sound. The use of multimodality cueing, another recommended technique for children with CAS (ASHA, 2007b; Smit, 2004), was instrumental in achieving the correct manner and placement of new targets. The clinicians utilized visual, auditory, tactile, and kinesthetic cues. Although some cueing strategies were deemed ineffective (Matthew found the use of a mirror very distracting), continued experimentation usually resulted in the identification of effective prompts. Gestural cues, with tactile and kinesthetic elements, were the most facilitative. Matthew enjoyed throwing his arms up when producing a /w/ and sliding one hand down the other arm for /s/. As therapy progressed, he spontaneously used learned gestures to self-cue correct productions.

## Progress

After Matthew had participated in speech therapy at the university clinic for approximately 1 year, his parents expressed concerns regarding their son's progress. Although they had noted some improvement, Matthew's speech was still highly unintelligible to most people; they were hoping for a faster rate of progress and wanted to explore other therapy options. A careful review of Matthew's progress and current status was conducted in response to his parents' concerns. Results of the HAPP-3 indicated a pattern of slow, but steady progress over the two semesters of treatment. Matthew's severity rating had improved from "severe" to "moderate" and the "Total Occurrences of Major Phonological Deviations" (the TOMPD score) had decreased from 131 to 95. His improved scores were attributable to an increase in production of /s/ blends in the initial and final positions of words, /k/ in the final position, and /w/ and /j/ in the initial position. However, the HAPP-3 results did not reflect the continued presence of voicing errors and a strong preference for alveolar sounds (particularly /d/) that resulted in frequent assimilation errors. Tables 10.5 and 10.6 summarize the Hodson Assessment of Phonological Patterns-3 and the Goldman-Fristoe Test of Articulation-2.

TABLE 10.5 Test Results from Hodson Assessment of Phonological Patterns-3

| Date of Testing, Age | Total Occurrences of Major Phonological Deviations | Severity Interval | Consonant Category Deficiencies Sum | Ability Score | Percentile |
|---|---|---|---|---|---|
| Initial<br>Date: 1–07<br>CA: 3–2 | 131 | Severe | 87 | <55 | <1 |
| End of 1st Sem.<br>Date: 5–07<br>CA: 3–6 | 118 | Severe | 81 | <55 | <1 |
| End of 2nd Sem.<br>Date: 12–07<br>CA: 4–0 | 95 | Moderate | 64 | <55 | <1 |

TABLE 10.6 Test Results from the Goldman-Fristoe Test of Articulation-2

| Date, Age | Error Score | Standard Score | Percentile |
|---|---|---|---|
| Initial<br>Date: 1–07<br>CA: 3–2 | 60 | 68 | 5 |
| End of 1st Sem.<br>Date: 5–07<br>CA: 3–6 | 58 | 58 | 4 |
| End of 2nd Sem.<br>Date: 12–07<br>CA: 4–0 | 53 | 64 | 4 |

It was time to revisit the question of childhood apraxia of speech. Matthew had just turned 3 years old when he was originally evaluated. It is difficult to diagnose CAS in young children (ASHA, 2007a), and sometimes early indicators of apraxia may resolve into patterns that are more consistent with a phonological disorder or other idiopathic developmental speech disorders (McCauley & Strand, 1999). Reviewing the initial list of characteristics demonstrated by Matthew, several changes were evident. He no longer demonstrated initial consonant deletion or epenthesis. The occurrence of vowel errors had significantly decreased and was now largely restricted to difficulties with rhotic vowels. His ability to imitate both nonspeech motor movements and speech sounds had dramatically improved. In fact, his consonant inventory in imitative contexts had expanded to include most age-appropriate phonemes, although in spontaneous speech he continued to demonstrate frequent sound substitutions.

After therapy began, ASHA released a technical paper and position paper on childhood apraxia of speech identifying three characteristics of apraxia that had "gained some consensus among investigators" (ASHA, 2007b, p. 4). These segmental and suprasegmental features included (1) inconsistency of errors, (2) difficulty transitioning between sounds and syllables, and (3) prosodic difficulties. Matthew did not demonstrate these features at the end of his second semester of therapy. His accurate production of words during therapy sessions was attributed to attempts at self-correction. Error patterns were consistent at both the word and sentence level, so the frequency of his errors no longer increased with the length of utterances. Difficulties transitioning between sounds were occasionally noted when Matthew was learning a new sound, but not during spontaneous productions. In addition, his prosody (including lexical and phrasal stress) was appropriate. Matthew was now telling elaborate stories to his clinicians, with his mother acting as interpreter. Her uncanny ability to interpret Matthew's speech might be attributed to the consistency of his productions and his adult-like prosody.

As Matthew's language developed, the lengths of his utterances increased, yet were riddled with homonyms. In the case of children with phonological-based errors, the substitution and omission of sounds may result in the production of the same phonetic form (e.g., /du/) for multiple lexical items (e.g., /tu/, /stu/, /flu/). The term *homonymy*, as used here, thus refers to the substitution of a preferential consonant (e.g., /d/) for many potential phonemes (e.g., /t/, /st/, /fl/), resulting in one phonetic string produced for many lexical items.

Although his receptive vocabulary continued to grow (as evidenced by his performance on the Receptive One-Word Picture Vocabulary Test), his expressive vocabulary development was hindered by his restricted phonemic inventory. By frequently collapsing many different sounds to the /d/ phoneme, Matthew created homonyms that do not exist in the adult lexicon. For example, he pronounced the words "two," "shoe," "flu," and "stew" as "do". He intended to produce different words, yet they all sounded the same to an unfamiliar listener, resulting in low speech intelligibility and considerable frustration during therapy.

## Treatment—Revised

The inability to utilize the contrastive features of sounds to create meaning (i.e., new words) is the hallmark of a phonological disorder. As the occurrence of homonyms in Matthew's speech increased and the characteristics of a motor planning disorder (CAS) diminished, a shift in both diagnostic and intervention strategies was needed. Therapy that emphasized the linguistic function of sounds, rather than their motor production, seemed appropriate. The multiple oppositions approach, as described by A. Lynn Williams (2000b), seemed a perfect fit for Matthew. The purpose of this approach is to reduce homonymy in a child's system by increasing phonemic contrasts.

Multiple oppositions therapy involves larger treatment sets than traditional minimal pair therapy. Rather than targeting one contrast pair (e.g., "do" and "shoe"), a whole family of homonyms is targeted simultaneously (e.g., "do," "shoe," "two," "flu," "stew"). Each child's unique phonological system is analyzed to identify phonemic collapses, and targets are developed to systematically expand, contrast, and reduce homonymy. Analysis of Matthew's speech revealed that the following phonemes were substituted by /d/: /w/, /b/, /p/, /t/, /f/, /k/, /g/, /v/, /l/, /s/, "sh," "ch," "j" (as in "judge"), and "th" (voiced and unvoiced). In addition, almost all consonant blends were produced as a singleton /d/, including /bl/, /br/, /dr/, /fl/, /fr/, /gl/, /gr/, /kl/, /kr/, /kw/, /sk/, /sl/, /sm/, /sn/, /st/, /sw/, /skw/, and /tr/.

Williams (2005) recommends the selection of target phonemes that are maximally distinct from the preferred sound and represent maximal classification—that is, the target sounds represent different categories of place, manner, and voicing. Focusing on the collapses created by substitution of the /d/ phoneme, /p/, /k/, /st/, and "sh" were initially chosen. Each of the chosen sounds contrasted with the /d/ phoneme across two or more distinctive features. For example, "sh" differs from /d/ because it is voiceless as opposed to voiced, and it is a continuant strident, not a stop. The four phonemes also represented a variety of places and manners of production in addition to including both singleton phonemes and a cluster. The selection of targets representing maximal distinctions and maximal classifications is designed to facilitate phonological reorganization and generalization to untreated phonemes (Williams, 2000a, 2005).

The next step was to create families of words that were produced by Matthew as homonyms and contained these target sounds. The first attempts to identify groups of words that contained /p/, /k/, /st/, and "sh" yielded mixed results. Here are some examples:

- day pay K stay shay?
- die pie kie? sty shy
- doe poe? koe? stow show

As illustrated, some combinations produced words that did not exist in American English (e.g., "kie" and "koe") and in other instances, the word did not occur in Matthew's lexicon (e.g., "sty" and "stow"). The decision was made to revise the list of target sounds beyond the initial four that were identified, in order to create word families that included functional, age-appropriate vocabulary. The singleton consonants "s," "l," and "w" were added to the list and /k/ was replaced by /g/, yielding homonym families such as these:

- day pay way say lay
- die pie why lie shy
- doe go low sew show

Initial consonant blends were also expanded beyond the initial selection of /st/ to include other /s/ blends as potential targets:

- day pay way say lay *stay*
- die pie why lie shy *sky*
- doe go low sew show *snow*

Attention was given to the function of syllable shapes in the creation of homonym families due to Matthew's restricted phonotactic inventory—his preferred syllable shape was CV (consonant-vowel). By deleting a consonant from a blend, Matthew changed the syllable shape of CCV words to CV. Thus, "stay" was produced as "day." In a similar fashion, by deleting the final consonant of words in connected speech, Matthew reduced CVC words to CV. Thus, CVC words such as "wait" and "late" were also produced as "day" as Matthew changed the initial phonemes to /d/ and deleted the final phonemes. Even CCVC words (e.g., "skate") became CV words (e.g., "day") as several processes occurred within a single word. Therefore, word families were expanded to include various word shapes, including CV, CCV, CVC, and CCVC, as illustrated:

- day (CV) pay (CV) way (CV) say (CV) lay (CV) stay (CCV)
- date (CVC) wait (CVC) late (CVC) gate (CVC) skate (CCVC)

The multiple oppositions approach is primarily a target selection approach. Unlike the cycles approach, it does not provide specific guidelines for the structuring of therapy sessions or the amount of time spent with each target. In this regard, it requires more independent decision making by clinicians. Matthew's clinicians chose to target one group of homonyms each week (for two 50-minute sessions), alternating between words with open syllables (CV and CCV) and words with closed syllables (CVC and CCVC). For example, one week the target words included day, pay, way, say, lay, and stay; the following week the target words included day, date, wait, late, gate, and skate. Each week the previous week's targets were reviewed before proceeding to new words. Twice during the 4-month treatment period, a week was devoted to reviewing all of the word families that had been introduced so far.

Target words were represented by pictures. Therapy activities were similar to those utilized during implementation of the cycles approach, including matching and hunting games, as well as (of course!) fishing. This semester, though, the clinicians emphasized the meaning of words and the semantic consequences of misproductions—similar to recommendations for minimal pair therapy (Barlow & Gierut, 2002). Thus, opportunities were created for Matthew to produce the target words while directing the clinicians to carry out an activity. For example, Matthew might be required to tell the clinician which fish to catch. If he intended the clinician to catch the fish with a picture of "pay" on it, yet he said "day," he would experience the semantic consequence of his error as she chose the wrong fish.

Matthew's mother successfully employed similar strategies when reviewing the pictures sent home each week. She reported that she would lay the pictures on a table and ask Matthew to tell her which picture to pick up, thus requiring accuracy on his part. If she displayed pictures of "pie," "shy," and "sky" on the table and Matthew said "die," she would emphasize the semantic differences between his actual production and his intended production. She noted that the word families helped her son understand that he was producing different words as the same word. Over the course of this final semester of treatment, she witnessed Matthew exerting more effort to produce words correctly and increased self-awareness of both errors and progress. "He feels like he's getting somewhere," Mrs. C stated. "He is feeling success."

## Progress—Final

Overall, Matthew's mother expressed greater satisfaction with the multiple oppositions approach than the cycles approach. Discussing the third semester of treatment, she reported that once Matthew learned a target word, he did not forget it; she often observed him using the new words at home in various speaking contexts. In addition, as Matthew's expressive lexicon expanded, his mother noticed that sounds that had been targeted within the homonym families (e.g., initial /w/, /p/, /s/, etc.) were spontaneously produced in new vocabulary words that had not been worked on in therapy. Her only concern was that the new sounds were not carrying over to words that had been in Matthew's vocabulary since a young age. For example, Matthew tended to produce the "sh" sound as /d/, so one of his families of homonyms included "show" as a target word. Matthew learned the word "show"—a new vocabulary word for him—and produced it correctly in various contexts. He also demonstrated accurate production of the "sh" sound in new words that he learned at home. However, the word "shoe," which was a word he had used for over a year and had not been included in any word families, continued to be produced as "do."

Matthew's parents, clinicians, and supervisor all reported great progress during the third semester, so results of the standardized assessment were surprising and a bit disappointing. Although test results indicated some improvement (a reduction of the TOMPD on the HAPP-3 from 95 to 84 and the error score on the GF-2 from 53 to 48—see Tables 10.7 and 10.8), they did not seem to reflect the subjective perception of progress shared by the adults in Matthew's environment. His mother stated that while watching the administration of the HAPP-3, she thought to herself, "Oh no, it [the improvement] is not showing up." Why? Perhaps the items on the tests included many "old" words that he was continuing to produce as he always had and did not reflect his new phonological knowledge. Or perhaps the tests were not measuring the specific skills that Matthew had gained.

Item analysis of Matthew's responses indicated that many areas of improvement were not scored on the HAPP-3 and/or the GF-2, thus preventing significant numerical gains. For example, Matthew demonstrated remarkable improvement in his production of vowel sounds, and yet neither test includes vowel errors in the calculations for standardized scores. HAPP-3 scores also do not include voicing errors, and, therefore, Matthew's increased ability related to prevocalic voicing was not noted. Although the GF-2 results did reflect the improvement in voicing, they did not numerically account for the significant increase in substitution errors with a corresponding decrease in omission errors. For example, "cup" was produced as "up" on the initial GF-2, whereas Matthew produced it as "tup" during the final administration of this test.

TABLE 10.7 Test Results after the Third Semester of Therapy

| HAPP-3, Date, Age | Total Occurrences of Major Phonological Deviations | Severity Interval | Consonant Category Deficiencies Sum | Ability Score | Percentile |
|---|---|---|---|---|---|
| End of 3rd Sem.<br>Date: 4–08<br>CA: 4–5 | 84 | Moderate | 56 | <55 | <1 |

| GF-2, Date, Age | Error Score | Standard Score | Percentile |
|---|---|---|---|
| End of 3rd Sem.<br>Date: 5–08<br>CA: 4–6 | 48 | 65 | 5 |

Both productions were scored as errors, yet the latter production demonstrates significant progress—in intelligibility, production of the CVC word shape, reduction of initial consonant deletion, and expansion of his phonemic inventory to include initial /t/. In addition, many of Matthew's other productions during the final assessment were much closer approximations of the target word or sound than they had been a year earlier. Consonant clusters now often contained at least one of the target sounds; "truck" was now produced as "tuck" rather than "dud," and "spoon" was produced as "poon" rather than "boon." Atypical substitution patterns were in many instances replaced by typical phonological patterns. For example, /r/ was now substituted by a /w/ and not a /d/, and an initial b/k substitution was replaced by a t/k substitution, representing the emergence of gliding and velar fronting—common error patterns exhibited by many young children.

These improvements in vowel production and voicing, along with decreases in omission errors and atypical patterns, likely explain the improvement in overall speech intelligibility reflected in the analysis of spontaneous speech samples (see Table 10.8). When Matthew started treatment, slightly over half of his utterances were completely unintelligible to an unfamiliar listener. By the end of the third semester of treatment, none of his utterances were completely unintelligible—all of them were either partially or completely understood. This method of assessing Matthew's speech production abilities provided a better representation of the progress described by his parents and clinicians than the formal articulation and phonological assessments that were administered.

TABLE 10.8 Intelligibility of Speech Samples Throughout Treatment

| | Completely Intelligible | Partially Intelligible | Unintelligible | Completely or Partially Intelligible |
|---|---|---|---|---|
| Initial<br>Date: 1–07<br>CA: 3–2 | 6/25<br>24% | 6/25<br>24% | 13/25<br>52% | 12/25<br>48% |
| End of 1st Sem.<br>Date: 5–07<br>CA: 3–6 | 12/25<br>48% | 6/25<br>24% | 7/25<br>28% | 18/25<br>72% |
| End of 2nd Sem.<br>Date: 12–07<br>CA: 4–0 | 11/25<br>44% | 9/25<br>36% | 5/25<br>20% | 20/25<br>80% |
| End of 3rd Sem.<br>Date: 5–08<br>CA: 4–6 | 16/25<br>64% | 9/25<br>36% | 0/25<br>0% | 25/25<br>100% |

## Analysis of Client's Response to Intervention

It appears that Matthew experienced more progress than was reflected by the formal assessment results. Yet the question remains: Did Matthew achieve more progress during the final semester of treatment than during each of the preceding semesters? That is, was the multiple oppositions approach more effective than the combination of the cycles approach and integral stimulation? The data collected over the course of the three semesters indicate a steady expansion of Matthew's sound and syllable structure inventories. Acquisition of vowels, velars, glides, and stridents, as well as CVC and CCVC word shapes, occurred over the entire course of treatment. There was a steady decline in omission errors, accompanied by a corresponding increase in substitutions. However, a qualitative change occurred during the third semester in the nature of the substitutions. Previously, Matthew had substituted a /d/ phoneme, and occasionally a /b/ or /n/ phoneme, for almost all initial consonants. Upon completion of 4 months of multiple opposition therapy, he demonstrated a significant increase in the variety of initial consonants that he produced, thus reducing the occurrence of homonyms—the exact effect hoped for. The decrease of homonymy and increase in more typical substitution patterns contributed to larger gains in overall speech intelligibility during the last semester. Other advantages of the multiple oppositions approach reported by Matthew's mother were generalization to untreated targets, better retention of learned skills, and more self-awareness of both errors and successful productions.

In conclusion, Matthew demonstrated significant progress over the course of his three semesters of treatment, thanks in large part to the dedication of his clinicians and the active participation of his parents. The catalyst for his accelerated growth during the final semester may have been multifaceted. A shift in diagnosis, the implementation of the multiple oppositions approach, greater client maturity, and attention to parental concerns—all may have played a role in Matthew's improved speech production abilities.

## Author Note

The authors would like to acknowledge all those who contributed to Matthew's therapy, including his parents, his clinicians (Nancy Alyssa McFall, Larissa Lapine, Gina Tashjian, Lisa Iland, and Nicole Clark), and his other clinical supervisor, Cynthia Wineinger. This project was reviewed and accepted by the IRB board at the University of Redlands, IRB # 21-06.

## References

American Speech-Language-Hearing Association. (2007a). *Childhood apraxia of speech: Position Statement*. Retrieved April, 2007, from http://www.asha.org/docs/html/PS2007-00277.html.

American Speech-Language-Hearing Association. (2007b). *Childhood apraxia of speech: Technical Report*. Retrieved January 5, 2008, from http://www.asha.org/docs/html/TR2007-00278.html.

Barlow, J., & Gierut, J. (2002). Minimal pair approaches to phonological remediation. *Seminars in Speech and Language, 23*(1), 57–67.

Bauman-Waengler, J. (2008). *Articulatory and phonological impairments: A clinical focus* (3rd ed.). Boston: Allyn & Bacon.

Berman, S. (2001). *Phonology targets: More patterns and themes for groups*. Austin, TX: PRO-ED.

Berman, S., Garcia, D., & Bauman-Waengler, J. (November, 2007). *Cycles approach and integral stimulation: Outcome measures for unintelligible children*. Poster session. American Speech-Language-Hearing Association. Boston, MA.

Brownell, R. (Ed.). (2000). *Receptive One-Word Picture Vocabulary Test*. Novato, CA: Academic Therapy Publications.

Caruso, A., & Strand, E. (1999). Motor speech disorders in children: Definitions, background, and a theoretical framework. In A. Caruso & E. Strand (Eds.), *Clinical management of motor speech disorders in children* (pp. 1–28). New York: Thieme.

Flahive, L., Velleman, S., & Hodson, B. (November, 2005). *Apraxia and Phonology*. Seminar. American Speech-Language-Hearing Association. San Diego, CA.

Gildersleeve-Neumann, C. (2007, Nov. 6). Treatment for childhood apraxia of speech: A description of integral stimulation and motor learning. *The ASHA Leader, 12* (15), 10–13, 30.
Goldman, R., & Fristoe, M. (2000).*Goldman-Fristoe Test of Articulation* (2nd ed.). Circle Pines, MN: American Guidance Service.
Hodson, B. (1997). Disordered phonologies: What have we learned about assessment and treatment? In B. Hodson & M. Edwards, *Perpectives in applied phonology* (pp. 197–224). New York: Aspen.
Hodson, B. (2004). *Hodson Assessment of Phonological Patterns (HAPP-3)*. Greenville, SC: Super Duper.
Hodson, B., & Paden, E. (1991). *Targeting intelligible speech: A phonological approach to remediation*. San Diego: College-Hill Press.
Kamhi, A. (2006). Treatment decisions for children with speech-sound disorders. *Language, Speech, and Hearing Services in Schools, 37*, 271–279.
McCauley, R., & Strand, E. (1999). Treatment of children exhibiting phonological disorder with motor speech involvement. In A. Caruso & E. Strand (Eds.), *Clinical management of motor speech disorders in children* (pp. 187–208). New York: Thieme.
Smit, A. (2004). *Articulation and phonology resource guide for school-age children and adults*. New York: Thomson Delmar Learning.
Strand, E., & Skinder, A. (1999). Treatment of developmental apraxia of speech: Integral stimulation methods. In A. Caruso & E. Strand (Eds.), *Clinical management of motor speech disorders in children* (pp. 109–147). New York: Thieme.
Williams, A. (2000a). Multiple oppositions: Case studies of variables in phonological intervention. *American Journal of Speech-Language Pathology, 9*, 289–299.
Williams, A. (2000b). Multiple oppositions: Theoretical foundations for an alternative contrastive intervention approach. *American Journal of Speech-Language Pathology, 9*, 282–288.
Williams, A. (2005). From developmental norms to distance metrics: Past, present, and future directions for target selection practices. In A. G. Kamhi & K. E. Pollock (Eds.), *Phonological disorders in children: Clinical decision making in assessment and intervention* (pp. 101–108). Baltimore: Brookes.

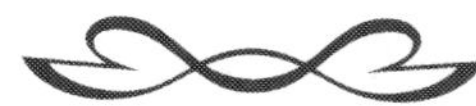

## Augmentative Communication

# Case 11

# Katie: Pediatric AAC: Katie's Journey

*Carla Wood Jackson*

## Conceptual Knowledge Areas

Cerebral palsy (CP) is a disorder that affects the ability to move and maintain balance and posture. It is the result of an injury to or developmental problem with parts of the brain (Centers for Disease Control, 2008). Persons with CP present with a motor impairment characterized by hyper (stiff), hypo (floppy), or mixed muscle tone that may range in severity from mild clumsiness to not walking at all. Difficulty with precise muscle movements for speech leads to complex communication challenges. Children with CP often have normal cognition or a mild to moderate intellectual disability. They generally require support from a number of different professionals including physical therapists, speech-language pathologists, occupational therapists, special education teachers, and personal aides. Due to their complex communication challenges and physical constraints, children with cerebral palsy commonly require augmentative and alternative communication systems.

Augmentative and alternative communication (AAC) refers to all forms of communication supplementing verbal speech that are used to express thoughts, needs, wants, and ideas. An AAC system is an integrated group of components including the symbols, aids, strategies, and techniques used by individuals to enhance communication (ASHA, 1991, p. 10). Binger and Light (2006) reported that approximately 12% of preschoolers receiving special education services required augmentative or alternative communication. This suggests a pressing need for speech-language pathologists to be knowledgeable about providing services for children who require AAC. Recent studies indicate a growing demand for pediatric augmentative and alternative communication in response to medical advances and improved neonatal care. Children with a variety of disabilities may require AAC including children with developmental disabilities, autism, apraxia, and multiple disabilities.

An individual's augmentative communication system may involve multiple components including unaided and aided forms. Unaided communication forms such as gestures, sign language, eye gaze, and facial expressions do not require any external aids separate from the individual. Aided communication systems include those that are external to the person's body such as picture communication boards, voice output devices, and switches. Selecting appropriate assistive technology supports entails individualized assessment to determine appropriate characteristics of the system tailored to the individual's strengths and needs. Considerations include selection technique (direct or scanning), display (lexical items, representations, organization), and presentation such as number of items, size, spacing, location, and color.

There is growing evidence that early use of AAC facilitates or enhances communicative exchanges in young children with complex communication challenges (Campbell, Milbourne, Dugan, & Wilcox, 2006). Switch activation has been shown to be effective in increasing the frequency of environmental control, switch interface, and in supporting cause-effect understanding in children with severe motor disabilities as young as 11 months of age (Behrmann & Lahm, 1983; Hanson & Hanline, 1985; Horn, Warren & Reith, 1992; Light, 1993; Meehan, Mineo, & Lyon, 1985; Sullivan & Lewis, 2000). Additionally, research findings suggest increased communicative interaction following integration of voice output communication aids in naturalistic preschool classroom routines (Schepis, Reid, Behrmann, & Sutton, 1998).

## Description of the Case

### Background Information

Katie is the youngest child in her family, a bright-eyed little girl, diagnosed with severe cerebral palsy at 9 months old. Katie is nonambulatory, presenting with both hyper- and hypotonic muscle tone and limited range of motion. Katie initially communicated primarily through crying and body language, prompting her family and service providers to consider assistive technology to support her communication development. Throughout her early years, Katie's augmentative communication system evolved in response to changes in her interests and preferences, communication demands, skill development, environment, and communication partners. Aside from her challenges, Katie is a typical young child. Her parents exemplified this in stating, "Katie enjoys all the things other kids do (ice cream, swinging, wagon rides, swimming, listening to music, having a book read to her). We just have to assist her in the enjoyment of these activities."

### Reason for Referral

#### Family and Child History

Katie was born to a middle-class family in the suburbs of a midwestern university community. She was referred to the local Part C Infant-Toddler Coordinating Council at 6 months of age due to delays in her acquisition of developmental milestones. Although she was drinking formula through a bottle, she was not gaining weight at the expected rate. Her parents were concerned that she was not holding her head up or rolling over independently. They also noticed that she was not babbling or vocalizing as often as her older sister did at that age. Katie was referred to a local infant-toddler agency and a developmental pediatrician who confirmed the diagnosis of severe cerebral palsy.

### Desired Outcomes

Katie's family wanted her to vocalize more frequently to foster development of speech. They hoped she would adapt socially and acquire a means to communicate her wants and needs at home and day care. It was important to her parents that Katie play and engage in interactions with her peers and her sister. They wanted Katie to interact with peers and be accepted by them. Goals in the area of motor development, such as sitting upright so that she could interact with her environment, were also a high priority to Katie's parents. They wanted to foster her muscular strength, tone, and control for later walking. Katie's parents were also concerned about her growth and nutrition, noting that she became fatigued easily with bottle feedings and wasn't gaining weight at the rate they expected.

## Findings of the Evaluation

### Teaming

Teaming was integral to service provision beginning with the initial evaluation. Katie's initial service team consisted of Katie's parents and her sibling, a speech-language pathologist, a physical therapist, the lead teacher at Katie's child care center, a consulting family resource specialist, and the early childhood resource specialist who served a dual role as the family service coordinator. The therapists were employed by different agencies in the community that contracted with the local Infant-Toddler Coordinating Council (ICC). The family resource specialist was directly employed by the local ICC and consulted with the therapists and family to assist in providing access to desired resources and supports. For example, if the physical therapist recommended specific equipment for physical support and positioning, the family service coordinator and family resource specialist worked together with the team to secure access through lending agencies, local funding sources, and/or the family's insurance.

The team members co-treated in pairs to maximize cross-training and provide consultation to caregivers. When reflecting on services, Katie's parents wrote, "It is critical that all the providers communicate effectively. We want the providers to communicate more with the paras (i.e., paraeducators), because they spend the most time with her. We often learn the paras are left out of the discussions with the providers." All therapists alternated the setting for sessions between the family's home and the child care setting. Sessions consisted of conversing with caregivers, discussing and demonstrating strategies, and facilitating opportunities for Katie to progress toward achieving desired outcomes. Her parents recently reflected on the service delivery, stating: "Having services come to our home was extremely beneficial."

## Treatment Options Considered

Intervention for Katie was determined by the family's priorities and desired outcomes, available evidence, clinical experiences, and Katie's preferences. Therapists worked together with the family to identify appropriate supports and implement evidence-based strategies to promote desired outcomes.

## Course of Treatment

Katie's parents desired that she have a means to express herself and that she gain weight. The speech-language pathologist provided informational resources to the staff at the child care center regarding encouraging vocalizations. The team determined that underlying cognitive milestones of object permanence and cause-and-effect understanding could be targeted during playtime routines. A BIGmack switch was proposed as a low-tech support for requesting "more." A high-caloric flavored PediaSure formula was provided to encourage weight gain. Since the nipple on the bottle required great effort for Katie, a sippy cup was introduced as well as a special-order feeding cup with a preloadable straw. The physical therapist worked with the family resource specialist to support seating and positioning. Katie responded well to the use of thermoform in the center of a booster seat or donut-shaped pillow, which allowed her to play on the floor in an upright position with her sister. This seating made Katie more accessible for inclusion in play with dolls with her sister at home, as well as play with other children at the child care center. Other positioning supports for Katie varied by routine. At home she acquired a lap tray for a booster seat for mealtimes and an adapted bath seat to assist with upright seating in the bathtub.

One of her parents' highest priorities was to ensure that Katie be integrated with peers, adapt socially, and have a way to communicate in those environments, as they believed this would facilitate her learning. Research findings suggest increased communicative interaction following integration of voice output communication aids in naturalistic preschool classroom routines (Schepis et al., 1998). To promote Katie's communicative exchanges, service providers discussed communication opportunities with Katie's family and teachers at the child care center and preschool. Mealtime was challenging because they wanted Katie to increase her caloric intake with the least amount of exertion, so choice making or requests were not seen as feasible. Floor play and bathtime were determined to be the best times to regularly focus on Katie's communicative exchanges at home. Katie would be encouraged to request more desired items and indicate a preference or choice through any means.

In addition to identifying communicative opportunities and demands, the team was challenged to identify appropriate assistive technologies to meet Katie's communication demands. While the BIGmack was initially attempted, it was quickly apparent that Katie had an aversive reaction to the "click" of the switch. Activating the device often startled and agitated her. To accommodate her dislike of the "click" selection feedback, a flat plate switch was used to activate a small voice output device with up to 8 switch ports. Multiple plate switches of bright contrasting colors could be presented on her tray at one time with the voice output device positioned under the tray. Utilizing direct selection appeared to be appropriate for Katie since scanning required her to have more precise timing and control of her selection timing.

Other considerations for assistive technologies for Katie included lexical items (vocabulary), representations (symbols), organization, and presentation. Katie's team brainstormed to ensure the items were concrete, appealing or motivating, and personalized to Katie's unique interests, opportunities, and communication partners. Designing her system involved consideration of social play opportunities in her environment, Katie's visual access to items, and motor access or positioning. Free play activities with peers in the child care setting were the initial choices. During free play, the children had an opportunity to select specific toys or activities. Katie appeared to enjoy playing with peers using cheerleading pom-poms, having books read to her, and having the children play with toys on her laptray. As a toddler, Katie demonstrated hypersensitivity to light. Her vision was negatively affected by glare. In an effort to optimize her visual access, the lexical items on the brightly colored plate switches were represented with both a picture and a miniature object (miniature book) or remnants (e.g., strings of the pom-pom). Due to Katie's motor constraints, the plate switches were placed at least 6–8 inches apart across Katie's tray 2–3 at a time. Katie was given time to explore and play with the items that were presented. Katie's selections were spontaneous and unsupported physically, but generally involved stiff arm movements, and therefore her choices appeared most successful when items were presented with "swinging room" between them. When positioned with trunk support and her feet in contact with the floor or seating equipment, Katie reached across midline to activate a colorful plate switch without verbal prompting.

A visual scene display (VSD) organizational layout was also considered for Katie's AAC technology options. VSDs refer to the use of a digital photo or picture scene in which vocabulary items are embedded as "hot spots" (defined areas with speech output) within the picture. VSDs offer the potential advantage of facilitating lexical access (Drager et al., 2004). In a recent study, preschool-age typically developing children performed significantly better in locating vocabulary items on AAC technologies when the vocabulary was presented in a contextual scene format rather than a grid format (Drager et al., 2004). It was suggested that referents may be more comprehensible or recognizable in a visual scene that preserves the item's contextual relevance, coherence, and size integrity. VSDs were not utilized during Katie's early years. Katie's access to pictures and photos was limited by visual and motor constraints in physically accessing items. Hot spots on the VSD needed to be large, preferably with three-dimensional remnants, and 6–8 inches apart. Due to potential benefits, visual scene displays could be considered in the future as Katie's physical access improves.

## Analysis of Client's Response to Intervention

As Katie advanced to preschool her sensitivity to appropriate auditory selection feedback ("click") became less apparent. BIGmack switches were better tolerated, although at times Katie still blinked and startled upon activation. Service providers consulted with the preschool teacher and paraeducators to identify social communication opportunities within daily routines. Her parents noted that Katie enjoyed exchanges with peers. For example, she had a tray on her wheelchair and delivered milk to classmates. Assistive technology supports were identified to enhance communicative exchanges with peers. During recess, the paraeducator held the green BIGmack switch while supporting Katie at the top of the slide. She activated the voice output "Go down the slide! Wee!" when she was ready to launch. Caregivers also encouraged Katie to vocalize simultaneously using an open vowel such as /o/ for "go" or /i/ for "wee." Katie quickly began to anticipate this activity, and peers began to enjoy participating in the game as well. The interaction with peers provided natural reinforcement for her use of voice output while giving her increased control over her environment.

A dynamic display device was considered to facilitate Katie's access to a large number of pages with stored vocabulary, while only needing a few items on each display page at a time. Because Katie's choices had to be large and spaced apart, static displays or object choices limited the number of items she could select from at any time. A dynamic display allows multiple pages of vocabulary to be linked together electronically, so a single selection may result in a new array of choices. Drager, Light, Speltz, Fallon, and Jeffries (2003) examined young children's ability to learn to use dynamic display systems. Young children (2½-year-olds) were able to learn to use the AAC technologies, but were reported to have great difficulty learning to locate vocabulary on dynamic display systems. Given the potential advantages for Katie's access to linked pages of vocabulary, a SpringBoard AAC device was explored with Katie when she was in preschool. At the time, Katie's physical access to the device was compromised by the glare and limited visual contrast of a dynamic display screen. Additionally, motor constraints prohibited Katie from using direct selection when choices were positioned within 6–8 inches of each other. As often observed secondary to cerebral palsy, Katie did not have precise or anticipatory control of the timing of motor movements needed to facilitate the use of a scanning selection technique with the dynamic display device. Although the dynamic display system was initially favored due to potentially superior access to a larger number of lexical items, it was concluded that it was not an efficient option for Katie's physical access at that time but could be reconsidered in the future as her motor control improved.

Katie's parents reflected positively on their experiences during her early years. They expressed gratitude for positive outcomes and their support systems, including family, friends, and faith-based community. They stated, "Katie has taught us a lot about patience, compassion, and not to take anything for granted." When asked for their advice to other parents of children with complex communication challenges, her parents wrote:

> Take advantage of support services as soon as you can. Learn as much as you can from those services and resources. Learn to be patient. You must advocate for your child. It is indeed a balancing act to make sure your child receives proper services. Build positive relationships early on. Also, be vocal in the development of the IEP and make sure goals are met or adjusted accordingly.

Finally, when asked about advice they would share with service providers, Katie's parents advised, "They need to realize that every situation is different. There is no one-size-fits-all."

## References


American Speech-Language-Hearing Association. (1991). Report: Augmentative and alternative communication. *ASHA, 33* (Suppl. 5), 9–12.

Behrmann, M., & Lahm, E. (1983). *Critical learning: Multiple handicapped babies get on-line*. Paper presented at the meeting of the Council for Exceptional Children National Conference on the Use of Microcomputers in Special Education, Harford, CT.

Binger, C., & Light, J. (2006). Demographics of preschoolers who require AAC. *Language, Speech, and Hearing Services in Schools, 37*, 200–208.

Campbell, P., Milbourne, S., Dugan, L., & Wilcox, J. (2006). A review of evidence on practices for teaching young children to use assistive technology devices. *Topics in Early Childhood Special Education, 26*(1), 3–13.

Centers for Disease Control National Center on Birth Defects and Developmental Disorders. (2008). *Learn the signs. Act early*. Retrieved November, 2008, from http://www.cdc.gov/CDCTV/BabySteps/

Drager, K., Light, J., Carlson, R., D'Silva, K., Larsson, B., Pitkin, L., et al. (2004). Learning of dynamic display AAC technologies by typically developing 3-year-olds: Effect of different layouts and menu approaches. *Journal of Speech, Language, and Hearing Research, 47*, 1133–1148.

Drager, K., Light, J., Speltz, J., Fallon, K., & Jeffries, L. (2003). The performance of typically developing 2½–year-olds on dynamic display AAC technologies with different system layouts and language organizations. *Journal of Speech, Language, and Hearing Research, 46*, 298–312.

Hanson, M., & Hanline, M. (1985). An analysis of response-contingent learning experiences for young children. *Journal of Americans with Severe Handicaps, 10*, 31–40.

Horn, E., Warren, S., & Reith, H. (1992). Effects of a small group microcomputer-mediated motor skills instructional package. *Journal of the Association for the Severely Handicapped, 17*, 133–144.

Light, J. (1993). Teaching automatic linear scanning for computer access: A case study of a preschooler with severe physical and communication disabilities. *Journal of Special Education Technology, 12*, 125–134.

Meehan, D., Mineo, B., & Lyon, S. (1985). Use of systematic prompting and prompt withdrawal to establish and maintain switch activation in a severely handicapped student. *Journal of Special Education Technology, 7*, 5–10.

Schepis, M., Reid, D., Behrmann, M., & Sutton, K. (1998). Increasing communicative interactions of young children with autism using a voice output communication aid and naturalistic teaching. *Journal of Applied Behavior Analysis, 31*, 561–578.

Sullivan, M., & Lewis, M. (2000). Assistive technology for the very young. Creating responsive environments. *Infants and Young Children, 12*, 34–52.

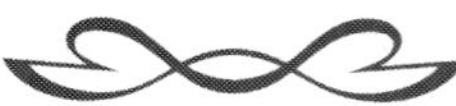



# CASE 12

# Christopher: Speech and Language Intervention for a Child with Autism: A Relationship-Based Approach

*Brookes Metzler-Barrack*

## Conceptual Knowledge Areas

Knowledge of typical development and developmental milestones, including speech, language, motor, cognitive, and social-emotional development, is important in understanding this case. An infant as young as 3 months old is able to self-regulate by sucking on a pacifier or being rocked by a caregiver and is able to smile and show pleasure. By the age of 9 to 12 months an infant is able to understand names of familiar objects and people and say a few words. Between the ages of 1 and 2 years a neuro-typical toddler is able to scribble and walk alone and backwards. Between the ages of 2 and 3 years a neuro-typical child is able to use concrete symbolic play as well as explore his or her environment in order to learn. Children with special needs often demonstrate uneven social-emotional, speech, language, physical, and cognitive development. Understanding these differences as well as observing uneven developmental patterns can be beneficial in the diagnosis and treatment of children with autism spectrum disorders (Greenspan & Wieder, 2006). Experience in working with both neuro-typical children as well as children with special needs is therefore vital in understanding this case study.

## Description of the Case

In the spring of 2004 Sherry and Craig J. took their son, Christopher, to his pediatrician. They had noticed that at the age of 25 months he was using very few words, became easily upset, and would not play with them for long periods of time. Their two older children had been "late bloomers," not talking until well after what was typical. At Christopher's age his siblings had expressive vocabularies of at least 100 words, and they could use words to ask for food, drink, and preferred toys, could build block towers and play movement games, and could calm easily with the help of familiar people.

### Background Information

Christopher had never been an "easy" infant. He often cried when he was not rocked, and his mother noted that he did not seem able to calm without movement. Christopher had reflux and his parents presumed that he was uncomfortable and therefore difficult to quiet. His father noticed that Christopher never enjoyed playing "peek-a-boo" and seemed content only if he was held, rocked, or was in his motorized swing. As Christopher grew and still was not talking, his mother was encouraged by her Parents as Teachers parent educator to talk to his pediatrician. Knowing the family background, his pediatrician assured her that Christopher was most probably a "late bloomer" and would begin talking soon. His parents noticed that he did not engage with toys in the same way as their other children.

Christopher often examined all parts of toys before playing with them. He sometimes let familiar people play with him, although he typically moved from toy to toy or activity to activity. Christopher enjoyed roughhousing games and smiled and laughed when he was being chased or tickled. He could roll a car back and forth and loved looking through books as well as doing the same puzzle over again. Winters were long and hard on the family. Being in the Midwest meant staying indoors. Christopher loved nature and would often go to the door and cry until someone let him out. He took his parents' or older sisters' hands and pulled them toward the door to indicate that he wanted to go outside. His oldest sister tried to play with him but often complained that he would not follow the rules and was not fun to play with. He had an easier time playing with his sister Kally, who was 10 months older than him. Kally and Christopher would play chase games for long periods of time, but she too would get frustrated when he would take her toys and not listen when she asked him to return them.

## Reason for Referral

By the spring of 2004, Christopher's parents were worried about his lack of speech. He seemed to learn quickly and could identify all the letters of the alphabet as well as five different colors. His pediatrician had also become more concerned. He noted that although Christopher's eye contact was immediate when mom and dad were roughhousing and tickling him, he had no eye contact when he had a favorite toy in his hand or when he was flipping through books. His mother told the pediatrician that Christopher would not play with his older sisters and did not like going to the store or other crowded or noisy places. It had become difficult for the family to go to restaurants unless there was a play area. The pediatrician observed Christopher's lack of speech and his undeveloped play skills, and saw that while he loved flipping through books, he would not point to pictures. The parents were devastated when the pediatrician explained that these were early warning signs of autism. As recommended, they immediately made an appointment with the university clinic and researched autism via the Internet.

When the parents brought Christopher to the clinic they were met by a psychologist, speech-language pathologist, occupational therapist, and social worker. The team began with questions about developmental milestones. The mother reported that Christopher was a product of a full-term pregnancy and there were no complications at birth or after. Christopher passed his newborn hearing screening. His medical history was significant for chronic otitis media and gastro-esophageal reflux disease (GERD). He had pressure equalization (PE) tubes placed at 18 months and had not had an ear infection since that time. Shortly after he began eating baby food his reflux lessened, although he continued to avoid a few foods. He had achieved some developmental milestones within normal limits; for example, he rolled over at 4 months, crawled at 9 months, and walked at 13 months. Speech and language milestones were delayed; for example, he did not say his first real word until 18 months and his expressive vocabulary was limited.

## Findings of the Evaluation

The clinic team administered the Vineland Adaptive Behavior Scales (Sparrow, Balla, & Cicchetti, 1984), the Childhood Autism Rating Scales (CARS) (Schopler, Reichler, & Ro, 1986), and the Rossetti Infant-Toddler Language Scale (Rossetti, 1986). The team observed Christopher in play with his family and also took turns playing with him themselves. The team observed that although he would roll cars back and forth, he would typically lie on his side to watch the wheels on the cars move. Christopher was able to pretend to feed a doll, but only after his mother did it. He did not add any ideas to pretend play with dolls. He indicated his wants and needs by using contact gestures and some limited speech. The speech-language pathologist noted that Christopher typically used jargon with a few real words. He did not imitate during the evaluation, but his mother reported he would sometimes imitate songs he had heard or parts of cartoons. The team also noted that Christopher would look at books, but appeared to be flipping the pages in order to self-stimulate rather than look at words or pictures.

Christopher did have some skills that were above age expectations. He could identify, by pointing, all the letters of the alphabet, five colors, and three shapes. His mother reported he enjoyed watching *The Magic School Bus* video (Scholastic, 2001), and she believed he had learned several pre-academic skills from this video. The clinic team also noted that Christopher demonstrated the most natural eye contact and social reciprocity during sensory motor play. He also demonstrated more attention to task when sensory motor input was added. His parents reported that he enjoyed swinging outside, jumping on the bed, playing chase games, and roughhousing. When the parents left the room, Christopher immediately cried and ran toward the door. His parents were told to come back into the room. He did not calm until his father gave him a book to flip through. The team also noted that although Christopher enjoyed roughhousing and tickle games with his parents, he did not let the clinic team touch him without crying and moving toward his parents.

On the Vineland Adaptive Behavior Scales (Sparrow, Balla, & Cicchetti, 1984), Christopher received low scores in the areas of communication, daily living skills, and socialization. The team noted that although Christopher's reflux had lessened, he had many food aversions and would typically eat refined carbohydrates and simple snacks (waffles, pancakes, chips, and crackers). He would not eat foods of mixed texture (applesauce, cereal with milk, etc.) and only ate foods at room temperature. He was able to drink from a sippy cup, open cup, and from a straw. He was not able to blow bubbles, although he enjoyed popping them and would try to blow with a decreased pucker. His parents reported he would tolerate brushing his teeth and they found he actually liked using a vibrating toothbrush. If they tried to introduce a new or different food, he would often cry so much they would concede and give him a familiar food. The speech-language pathologist had his mother use silly faces and noises to encourage Christopher to imitate oral motor movements. Christopher seemed to have adequate oral motor functioning for speech. He did, however, appear to have mild oral motor weakness, which was exhibited by a decreased pucker and decreased ability to sustain oral motor movements for an age-appropriate length of time. On the Rossetti Infant-Toddler Language Scale (Rossetti, 1986) his receptive language skills were at the 18–21-month level and his expressive language skills were at the 15–18-month level. Christopher received a score of 35 on the CARS (Schopler et al., 1986), which placed him in the mildly to moderately autistic range. The team also reviewed the *Diagnostic and Statistical Manual of Mental Disorders* (DSM-IV) (APA, 1994) criteria for autism spectrum disorders (ASD).

The team observed that Christopher had marked impairments in his nonverbal behaviors, ability to form peer relationships, and lack of social and emotional reciprocity. He also had a delay of spoken language and lack of varied make-believe and symbolic play. Further, he displayed a preoccupation with parts of objects. After talking to the team, the parents agreed that Christopher appeared to have characteristics of autism, but asked about the difference between autism and Asperger syndrome. They noted that he appeared to have some higher level skills and said they thought Asperger syndrome was a form of high-functioning autism. The clinic team reviewed the DSM-IV diagnostic criteria for Asperger syndrome.

## Treatment Options Considered

Christopher's clinic team told his family that his language delay and behavior were consistent with the diagnosis of autism. The team explained different treatment options for children with ASD and therapies that would be important for Christopher. The team recommended speech-language therapy in order to increase Christopher's expressive and receptive language and his pragmatic skills. The team also recommended occupational therapy to address Christopher's sensory integration needs and special instruction to address his play skills. The family was given a packet of resources including information about local early childhood centers and their state's early intervention program. The family left the meeting feeling overwhelmed and emotional.

## Course of Treatment

The social worker from the university clinic called the family the next week. The mother worked part time during the day, and the father worked at night. Since the diagnosis was made, the parents had been reading articles they found online. They had contacted the state's early intervention program, and an intervention team was scheduled to visit for the purpose of writing an Individual Family Service Plan (IFSP). The mother indicated she was still feeling overwhelmed and frustrated that Christopher had not been diagnosed sooner, but also more empowered by the information she had found and especially by stories she had read about the benefits of early intervention.

The early intervention case manager, speech-language pathologist, occupational therapist, and special instructor visited the home. They talked about the importance of early intervention and reviewed the university clinic's report. The occupational therapist (OT) and the speech-language pathologist (SLP) described a relationship-based classroom, which used elements of Developmental Individual–Difference Relationship–Based (DIR) and Floortime interventions and included a special instructor (SI), who utilized an Applied Behavior Analysis (ABA) approach to work with children with autism spectrum disorders. Floortime differs from skill-based or behavioral approaches for children with an ASD in many ways. Skill-based interventions attempt to teach a skill by using reinforcers, or by teaching a child to follow a step-by-step picture sequence. These methods target the steps involved in each separate skill sequence. Conversely, Floortime targets underlying problem-solving and cognitive skills.

The team discussed the family's goals for Christopher. The family indicated that they wanted him to communicate more, play with toys more appropriately, and generally engage more with all members of his family. Each team member scheduled a time to work with Christopher. Due to the father's need to work nights and sleep during the day, all team members visited at times when only the mother was able to participate. They explained the importance of the family's role in early intervention and the need for the family to utilize the same techniques throughout Christopher's day.

The next week early intervention services began. Christopher cried the first time the SLP came to see him. He clung to his mother and did not want to look at the toys she brought. She used the time to explain the principles of Floortime to the mother and how she would utilize those in working with Christopher. She provided the mother with an information sheet on the Functional Emotional Developmental Levels (FDLs). These FDLs, described by Dr. Stanley Greenspan and Dr. Serena Wieder (2006), are believed to be necessary for healthy intellectual and emotional growth. These levels are an essential part of the Developmental Individual-Difference Relationship–Based (DIR) theory.

The SLP explained how use of a relationship-based approach would help to increase Christopher's shared attention and engagement. She noted that Christopher had not yet mastered FDL 1 (the ability to remain calm and regulated) and FDL 2 (the ability to sustain shared engagement) and, although he had skills at level 5 (such as the ability to identify letter, shapes, and colors), he was not consistent at any of the levels. The mother confessed that she had read stories about children with an ASD who never learned to talk, and she was worried that Christopher would never use language functionally or would have robotic speech once it was more developed. The SLP shared the hypothesis underlying the theory of DIR, the affect diathesis hypothesis, which also states that children with an ASD have a unique type of biologically based processing deficit involving the connection of affect or intent to processing capacities. These processing capacities include motor planning, sequencing capacities, and symbol formation. Christopher lacked this connection between his intent and his plan or processing capacity. For example, he would have the intent to eat, but often lacked the symbol formation to use words in order to ask for food. This was also the reason that he engaged in some repetitive and aimless behavior. He had the intent to play with toys or books, but not the motor plan or sequencing capacity to reason how to play with toys (Interdisciplinary Council on Developmental and Learning Disorders, 2000). The need to increase back and forth engagement and circles of communication was discussed. By following Christopher's lead, both parents would be able to entice him into opening and closing more circles of communication, thereby increasing his back and forth engagement and shared attention. The mother described Christopher's interests and they made a plan of how to interact when he was engaged in different activities. By the end of the session the mother was using a blanket swing activity to encourage more circles of communication and increasing active waiting time and salient language while keeping Christopher engaged in one activity, sharing meaningful eye contact, vocalizations, and gestures. The SLP discussed the use of the Picture Exchange Communication System (PECS) (Frost & Bondy, 2002), a low-technology augmentative communication system used to help the child understand the function of communication. PECS utilizes a structured behavioral approach to communication and contains six different phases beginning with picture exchange to attain a desired item and moving toward labeling and information gathering. The mother was not comfortable using any method of communication other than speech, but would consider this option. The SLP explained the importance of mirroring back vocalizations to Christopher to show him that he was understood. The mother was encouraged to increase her gestural communication to help Christopher increase his use of gestures to communicate.

When the OT arrived later that week, the mother was excited about things they were trying with Christopher. The OT suggested ways to increase Christopher's sensory integration, motor planning, and sequencing abilities. She followed Christopher's lead and also showed the mother how to challenge him. For example, she demonstrated how to hold on to Christopher's feet when he was swinging and wait for him to vocalize or use eye contact to signal he was ready to swing more. Christopher's mother was surprised at how much Christopher enjoyed play and how engaged he was with the OT during the course of the play.

The SI also visited later that week. She had Christopher sit at a small table with her and talked to the mother about play skills, academic readiness skills, and compliance skills that they could work on with him. She used Discrete Trial Training techniques; for example, when Christopher followed 1-step directions to sit in his chair or imitate gross motor movements, he would receive an edible treat. His mother was excited about his ability to follow directions and imitate, but she did not observe that he was enjoying himself as much as he had with the OT.

During the next 3 months the team continued to work with Christopher. The OT and SLP consulted with one another and co-treated on a monthly basis. The mother looked forward to the relationship-based occupational therapy and speech-language therapy sessions and Christopher would run toward the door when the SLP or OT was coming. During these sessions the adults followed Christopher's interests, ideas, and intentions. The mother was encouraged to interpret all of his behaviors as intentional and meaningful. She was also encouraged to maintain a reciprocal back and forth flow of communication for as long as possible. For example, when Christopher had toys that were similar, such as multiple cars, trucks, or letters, he would want to hold them all. When his mother tried to take them from him, Christopher cried and became dysregulated. The OT and SLP suggested she make a back and forth game out of this activity in order to help him better regulate his body and emotions and maintain shared attention. At first they would sit across from each other and play with their own set of toys, merely sharing the same space. Eventually the mother pretended to take one of his toys, but then tickled him. She was encouraged to expand this play by varying the amount of time between tickling and building the anticipation by using salient language, all the time building back and forth circles of communication with a continuous flow. She learned to use playful obstruction to cover one of his toys with her hand while helping him maintain engagement and self-regulation. The mother was surprised at how much effort she had to put forth when she first started using relationship-based techniques and how it soon transitioned to Christopher doing more of the work.

Although Christopher seemed to be learning from his sessions with the SI, he did not seem as engaged with her and often cried before the sessions. When the team met for the 6-month transition IFSP meeting, they discussed the possibility of enrolling Christopher in a relationship-based early childhood program. The OT and SLP felt he was ready for the classroom program because he was now actively engaged in one-on-one Floortime sessions with them and with the family. He was functioning at FDL level 3, as evidenced by his ability to use and understand gestures and social reciprocity. He also had some skills at level 4, such as engaging in problem-solving activities and imitating gross motor and fine motor actions, and level 5, such as using words in phrases and sentences and also playing symbolically. They also felt he would benefit from Floortime within groups and adult-facilitated dyads. The team agreed to continue services within the home as well as to continue intensive therapy. Although Christopher was making gains with ABA, a skill-based approach, they felt he would make more gains with Floortime, a relationship-based approach. The team, including the parents, decided to place Christopher in the relationship-based program taught by the OT and SLP. He continued to receive occupational and speech-language therapy services in the home and received occupational and speech-language services as well as special instruction in the classroom. The family was invited to observe the classroom program and ask questions about therapy techniques. During the 6-month transition IFSP the family also discussed the need for more intensive feeding services. At the meeting the SLP discussed the use of PECS to increase Christopher's communicative attempts and ability to obtain his wants and needs. The parents felt that although Christopher's speech had increased with the use of Floortime, he needed a more structured approach to communication. The SLP stated that although PECS might increase his requesting skills, it would continue to be important to focus on the meaning and intent of Christopher's communication.

Christopher began attending the relationship-based classroom in the summer of 2004. The transdisciplinary team in the classroom used skill-based approaches to decrease his food aversions and increase his ability to imitate. They also used sensory integration techniques to decrease his tactile defensiveness. They incorporated semistructured problem solving within everyday classroom routines. For instance, they would set out the juice for snacktime but leave the cups in the cabinet and wait for the children to solve the problem of how to get the cups. They also trained the family to use PECS.

Christopher moved quickly from Phase I through Phase III of PECS training. The family was delighted he was requesting more and his frustrations seemed to lessen. The family and classroom staff held up a picture by their face and vocalized for Christopher his request. Soon Christopher would vocalize a request when giving the picture to staff or family. He would comment during circle time by selecting pictures of classmates. Within the home the SLP and OT encouraged the father to engage in at least three 20-minute Floortime sessions daily with Christopher. The transdisciplinary team and the family assessed how to engage Christopher with his sisters and offered suggestions to increase their play together.

At age 3 Christopher transitioned from his early intervention program to his public school district early childhood program. The family and relationship-based team felt Christopher would benefit from enrolling in his community preschool as well as continuing with the relationship-based program. In the 6 months he had been in the program, he had increased his spontaneous initiation and functional language. Using skill-based approaches, he had also increased his ability to imitate and expand his food choices. Through increased sensory motor input at both school and home, he was better regulated and attended to tasks for greater periods of time. Christopher also discontinued his use of PECS. He was now using words to comment and request with meaning and intent. His symbolic play moved from the early concrete stage to more elaborate play involving the sequencing of at least two ideas and adding ideas to play. He continued to need coaxing to remain engaged after a problem was presented during play and to build logical bridges between ideas. The SLP and OT consulted with the community preschool and trained staff to use PECS. They also encouraged the preschool staff to follow Christopher's lead but challenge him at the same time. This collaboration continued for 2 years. His family continued to use the Floortime approach at home, and the father grew increasingly comfortable with the techniques taught to him during speech-language and occupational therapy intervention. His sisters also were encouraged to play with Christopher and were coached by the SLP and OT during intervention time.

## Analysis of Client's Response to Intervention

In August 2007 Christopher began attending his public school regular education kindergarten. Since his diagnosis at the age of 27 months Christopher had made great gains. Utilizing a relationship-based approach the family and his team helped Christopher strengthen his Functional Developmental Emotional Levels (Greenspan & Wieder, 2006). At the age of 5 years, he was still mastering stage 6 of the FDLs (the ability to build logical bridges between ideas) and working on multicausal comparative thinking, FDL stage 7. He used phrases and sentences meaningfully and sustained a reciprocal back and forth flow of communication. Through sensory integration therapy he was better regulated and attended in the classroom setting for longer periods of time. He was able to initiate and sustain interactions with peers, but still needed adult facilitation to terminate play appropriately. When he returned to the university clinic his diagnosis changed from autism spectrum disorder to Asperger syndrome based on his language scores, which were within normal limits. Christopher continued to receive occupational therapy services to address his sensory integration needs. He also received speech-language services within the classroom to strengthen his pragmatic language skills. The family continued to engage Christopher using Floortime techniques.

## Author Note

This case is hypothetical. This case is not based on a real family but on the author's experience with a variety of children.

## References


American Psychiatric Association. (1994). *Diagnostic and statistical manual of mental disorders* (4th ed.). Washington, DC: Author.

Frost, L., & Bondy, A. (2002). *The Picture Exchange Communication System training manual* (2nd ed.). Newark, DE: Pyramid Educational Products.

Greenspan, S., & Wieder, S. (2006). *Engaging autism*. Cambridge, MA: Da Capo Press.

The Interdisciplinary Council of Developmental and Learning Disorders. (2000). *Clinical Practice Guidelines*. Cambridge, MA: Da Capo Press.

Rossetti, L. (1986). *Rossetti Infant Toddler Language Scale*. East Moline, IL: LinguiSystems.

Scholastic Inc. (2001). *The Magic School Bus*. [Video]

Schopler, E., Reichler, R., & Ro, B. (1986). *The Childhood Autism Rating Scale*. Los Angeles, CA: Western Psychological Services.

Sparrow, S., Balla, D., & Cicchetti, D. (1984). *Vineland Adaptive Behavior Scales*. Circle Pines, MN: American Guidance Service, Inc.

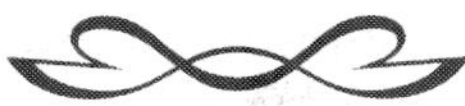

BILINGUAL/LANGUAGE

# CASE 13

# Kana: A Bilingual Preschool Child

*Teri H. Munoz, Noma Anderson, and Shelly S. Chabon*

## Conceptual Knowledge Areas

Children in bilingual environments have different language learning tasks than children in monolingual environments. Being a monolingual speaker means operating with one language in all activities and in all settings. A child who is developing language in a monolingual environment has the task of acquiring, receptively and expressively, the content, forms, and functions of one language. Being bilingual means that an individual exists in settings where two or more languages operate. The extent to which the individual is exposed to and uses both languages can vary as a function of the people with whom and where the person interacts, and with the function of the linguistic task, that is, speaking, comprehending, reading, and writing. A child developing language in a bilingual environment must acquire, receptively and expressively, the content, forms, and functions of two (or more) languages. The nature of the child's linguistic input is a crucial factor. Linguistic input refers to the language models to which the child is exposed. The linguistic goal for many bilingual children is for them to develop proficiency in both languages in all modalities.

There are two processes of bilingual language acquisition. The first, simultaneous language acquisition, refers to acquiring both languages (L1 and L2) at the same time (Roseberry-Mckibbin, 2007). A child 3 years old or younger experiences the benefits of linguistic input from two languages. In the second process, successive, or sequential, language acquisition, a child 3 years old or older acquires a second language (L2) after having developed a first, or primary, language (L1). A typical occurrence of successive language acquisition is a young child who acquires L1 in the home and community settings, enters school as an English language learner (ELL), and subsequently acquires English as his or her L2. A child who is learning English as his or her L2 follows the same sequence of language acquisition as does the monolingual child who is acquiring English.

Irrespective of the child's age or whether the child is displaying simultaneous or successive language acquisition, all of the child's languages should be promoted. Optimum linguistic, cognitive, and academic development occurs when ongoing and continual development of L1 and L2 is facilitated by parents, caregivers, teachers, speech-language pathologists, siblings, peers, and the community. The simultaneous bilingual language learner's growth in linguistic proficiency in both languages should be facilitated. As the successive bilingual language learner progresses through L2 settings, care should be directed to ensure that language skills in L1 are maintained and that the child continues to advance in the acquisition of L1 while acquiring L2.

Competent assessment of the communication development of a bilingual child through the use of standardized tests can be challenging. Competent use of norm-referenced tests is dependent upon many factors, including (1) the standardization methodology employed; (2) the comprehensiveness of the assessment; and (3) the accuracy with which these measurers diagnose the presence, patterns, and severity of a communication disorder. Speech-language pathologists utilizing a battery of diagnostic tests should make every effort to select language tests that are representative of the culture and linguistic systems of the child being tested. Speech-language pathologists also gather case history information by interviewing the child's parents about their perceptions and knowledge of their child's physical, emotional, linguistic, medical, academic, and social development. Not only do parents provide a comprehensive overview of the child's development and medical history, but they have tremendous insight as to whether their child is developing his or her communication in a typical manner. Parents' perceptions are particularly important when assessing ELL children. They have a keen sense of the typical development of L1 as demonstrated by typically developing children of that culture.

An overarching professional responsibility of speech-language pathologists is to become culturally competent and to fully understand second language acquisition. Speech-language pathologists recognize that, as bilingual children are acquiring their language skills, they display language acquisition behaviors that monolingual English speaking children do not. Code switching, which means that the child uses both languages within an utterance, is typical. An example is the sentence: "Mommy, where is *mi muñeca* (my doll)?" Speech-language pathologists appreciate that this is not an example of a communication disorder, but rather two languages learned in a typical, not atypical, manner. Another example is when an ELL child in the early stages of successive language acquisition responds in silence in L2 settings. This is often typical of bilingual language acquisition, although the length of the silent phase depends on the individual. A characteristic of simultaneous bilingual language acquisition is the child who develops dual language systems. For example, the words "water" and "*agua*" initially are not equivalent forms because the child has learned "*agua*" in one context and "water" in a different context. Accordingly, there will be a period of time when the child produces "*agua*" in the settings in which the word was learned and with the initial referents (e.g., the bathtub). Similarly, the child will produce "water" in English language learning contexts and with those referents (e.g., water fountain). Gradually the words become equivalent. This is not a communication disorder, but rather a typical feature of bilingual language acquisition.

Competent assessment includes analyzing language across a variety of settings and interactions. This ecologically valid assessment procedure is essential because bilingual children's communication behaviors are connected to the setting and the people with whom they are interacting. Such a comprehensive process is most effectively conducted when the speech-language pathologist is a member of a multidisciplinary assessment team.

Competent assessment requires that, when assessing bilingual children, the speech-language pathologist determines whether the child is (1) displaying second language learning behaviors (i.e., dialectical differences), not disordered communication; or (2) presenting a communication disorder; or (3) manifesting both dialectical differences related to second language acquisition and a communication disorder. The assessment of bilingual ELL children is best performed by a culturally competent speech-language pathologist who is proficient in the languages spoken by the child and in the appropriate use of assessment instruments. Since the role of a speech-language pathology assessment is to determine the status of the bilingual child's communication development, the child's capability in both languages should be assessed. A monolingual speech-language pathologist may choose to work with a translator to assist with this process.

The American Speech-Language-Hearing Association (ASHA) takes the position that an essential responsibility of speech-language pathologists is to provide clinical services to those who present with communication disorders. It is not appropriate for speech-language pathologists to recommend speech-language pathology services for ELL children who do not present with communication disorders (ASHA Committee on the Status of Racial Minorities, 1983).

There are several approaches speech-language pathologists employ to facilitate the acquisition of English for ELL children who do not exhibit a communication disorder. One approach is to collaborate with parents to guide the linguistic input that children receive in the home. Speech-language pathologists may encourage parents to maintain L1 in the home in conversation, in storytelling, in reading books, in family interaction. The same recommendation may be offered regarding L2, if this is a comfortable language for family interaction in the home. If L2 is not used for family interaction, then L1 must be as rich as possible so that its continued development is ensured. Speech-language pathologists may also collaborate with the child's teacher(s) to guide the linguistic input that the child receives in the classroom to foster the acquisition of L2, emphasizing language content, language forms, and language functions that promote academic success. ASHA acknowledges that parents of a bilingual child may seek the expertise of a speech-language pathologist to teach their child the phonology, semantics, syntax, and pragmatics of English. Though this is elective therapy, it represents a common decision for many parents.

It is the responsibility of the speech-language pathologist to treat the communication disorders that the bilingual child exhibits (American Speech-Language-Hearing Association, 1985). The speech-language pathologist analyzes phonological, syntactic, and pragmatic errors as they are presented in L1 and in L2. A treatment plan is designed that addresses the child's L1 and L2 communication errors.

When a bilingual child is assessed, the child's development in both languages should be captured in order to obtain an appropriate diagnosis. For instance, if speech and language skills in both languages are poor or atypical, this could be indicative of a language disorder. However, if the child's Spanish (L1) skills are commensurate with age level and significantly higher than her or his English (L2) skills, then the speech-language pathologist can consider ruling out a language disorder and implementing appropriate strategies to assist the child with the acquisition of English.

This case describes 4-year-old Kana, a bilingual preschooler. Even though Kana was born in the United States, she exhibited successive bilingual language acquisition.

## Description of the Case

### Background Information

Kana, a 4-year, 6-month-old girl who lived with her mother, her 2-year-old sister, and her maternal grandmother, was a second-generation immigrant from Cuba. The family spoke Spanish at home. Kana was exposed to English at her school and at many social activities. The parents separated when Kana was 6 months old after 7 years of marriage. Kana's family owned a small neighborhood restaurant. Spanish was the language spoken in the restaurant.

Kana was in a prekindergarten class. She had an IQ of 105 and was an ESOL (English Speakers of Other Languages) student. Her school district had ESOL programs with levels ranging from I to V, determined based on a parent questionnaire and oral testing. Level I was for children who had little understanding and expressive English skills. Level V was for children who were able to speak and write English as well as a native speaker (TESOL, March 2006). ESOL assessment conducted at school revealed that Kana was functioning as an ESOL Level IV student, who exhibited occasional syntactic errors and speech sound errors.

### Reason for Referral

Kana's prekindergarten teacher, with 17 years of teaching experience, recommended that she be seen for a complete communication evaluation. She thought that Kana's language difficulties might be the result of her bilingualism and referred the family to a community bilingual speech-language pathologist. Kana's mother provided family history information. She reported that Kana spoke Spanish at home and English at school. She also reported that

Kana's sentences were significantly shorter in both languages than the sentences spoken by her 7-year-old sister when she was Kana's age. The mother described her daughter's speech as "unclear."

## Findings of the Evaluation

Kana was accompanied to the assessment by her mother. She was very sociable and eager to participate. A bilingual speech-language pathologist conducted the evaluation in English and Spanish. Assessment instruments included tests that have bilingual versions, tests that are only in Spanish, and tests that are only in English. The following battery of formal and informal assessments was administered:

- Goldman-Fristoe Test of Articulation-2
- Spanish Articulation Measure (SAM)
- Oral-motor peripheral examination
- Voice screening
- Fluency screening
- Pragmatic checklist
- Informal Language Sample
- Bilingual Expressive One-Word Picture Vocabulary Test (EOWPVT)—Spanish Bilingual Edition
- Bilingual Receptive One-Word Picture Vocabulary Test (ROWPVT)—Spanish Bilingual Edition
- Preschool Language Scale-4 (PLS-4)
- Preschool Language Scale-4, Spanish

### Speech

- ***Goldman-Fristoe Test of Articulation-2:*** The Goldman-Fristoe Test of Articulation assesses the child's production of English consonant speech sounds in single words and in sentences. Kana presented with the following articulation errors in English: /s/ for /θ/, /d/ for/ð/, /ʃ/ for /tʃ/, /s/ for/z/, /t/ for / kl/, /d/ for /b/, /d/ for /p/.
- ***Spanish Articulation Measure (SAM):*** The SAM is an assessment instrument that is used to determine articulation and phonological errors in Spanish of 18 consonants (Mattes, 1995). Kana presented with the following articulation errors in Spanish: /d/ for /b/, /d/ for /p/.

The oral-motor peripheral examination, voice, and fluency were age appropriate.

### Language

Table 13.1 summarizes the evaluation of Kana's oral motor development, voice, fluency, and pragmatic skills.

• ***Pragmatic Checklist:*** Kana was able to take turns appropriately during play activities and social conversations for three-four exchanges. She initiated and maintained topics, made requests, and maintained eye contact with the speaker.

• ***MLU:*** An informal language sample was obtained to determine the mean length of utterance (MLU). Results indicated that Kana had an MLU of 1.7 in both languages. She was at a Stage I of Brown's stages of syntactic development, with an age equivalent of 2–2 years. This was significantly below normal limits for a child her age.

• ***Receptive One-Word Picture Vocabulary Test (ROWPVT)—Spanish-Bilingual Edition:*** This bilingual version of the ROWPVT was administered to assess the level of development of Kana's receptive Spanish and English vocabulary. Children taking the test can respond in both languages; therefore, the scores reflect total acquired vocabulary (Spanish *and* English responses). The test was normed on a national sample of Spanish-bilingual individuals, ages 4 years through 12 years, 11 months (Brownell, 2001b).

TABLE 13.1 Initial Evaluation Results

| Pre-Test | Raw Score | Standard Score | Percentile Rank | Standard Deviation | Age-Equivalence |
|---|---|---|---|---|---|
| ROWPVT—Spanish Bilingual | 20 | 64 | 1 | −2.4 | 3.0 |
| EOWPVT—Spanish Bilingual | 12 | 58 | 1 | −2.8 | 2.0 |
| Preschool Language Scale-4 (Spanish Version) | Auditory Comprehension 34 | 53 | 1 | −3.13 | 2–9 |
| | Expressive Communication 32 | 50 | 1 | −3.13 | 2.6 |
| | Total Language Score 67 | 50 | 1 | −3.3 | 2–9 |
| Preschool Language Scale-4 (English Version) | Auditory Comprehension 34 | 63 | 1 | −2.4 | 2–7 |
| | Expressive Communication 34 | 57 | 1 | −2.8 | 2.4 |
| | Total Language Score 68 | 56 | 1 | −2.9 | 2.5 |

- ***Expressive One-Word Picture Vocabulary Test (EOWPVT)—Spanish-Bilingual Edition:*** This test assesses the expressive vocabulary of individuals who are bilingual in Spanish and English. Like the ROWPVT—Spanish-Bilingual, this version of the EOWPVT permits examinees to respond in both languages and provides the examiner with a total acquired expressive vocabulary (Brownell, 2001a). The EOWPVT—Spanish-Bilingual was normed on a national sample of Spanish-bilingual individuals of ages 4 years through 12 years, 11 months.
- ***The Preschool Language Scale-4—Spanish (PLS-4-Spanish) and the Preschool Language Scale-4 (PLS-4):*** These instruments were administered in both Spanish and English to assess receptive and expressive language skills. The PLS-4 was normed on 1,500 children, birth through 6 years, 11 months of age (Zimmerman, Steiner, & Pond, Spanish ed., 2002). The standardization sample included children with disabilities. Thirty-nine percent of the sample consisted of ethnic minorities. The PLS-4 Spanish edition was normed on 1,188 Spanish-speaking children throughout the United States (Zimmerman et al., 2002).

## Summary

Based on evaluation results, Kana's oral motor development, voice, fluency, and pragmatic skills appeared to be within normal limits for her age and gender. Her spontaneous English language sample included several instances of syntax typical of Spanish. For example, she said, "Car blue" when asked to describe a car. In Spanish, the adjective is placed after the noun, "*Carro azul.*" Kana's total Spanish and English receptive vocabulary development and total Spanish and English expressive vocabulary development appeared to be within normal limits. Scores on the ROWPVT and the EOWPVT suggested that Kana's semantic and concept development, receptively and expressively, were age appropriate. Other language skills, specifically utterance length, overall auditory comprehension, and overall expressive communication, were significantly below age level in both languages, suggestive of a language disorder.

Kana's articulation profile presented with errors that were dialectal (/θ/, /ð/, /tʃ/, and /z/); developmental (/kl/); and delayed (/b/, and /p/). Kana's production of the /θ/, /ð/, /tʃ/, and /z/ was believed to be related to absence of these phonemes in the Spanish phonology system. The /b/ and /p/ phonemes were considered disordered because these two consonants were misarticulated on both the articulation test with Spanish phonemes and on the test with English consonant phonemes. Kana's production of /kl/ was diagnosed as a developmental error, not a misarticulation, because at 4 years of age, a child would not be expected to have acquired correct production of this consonant blend.

## Treatment Options Considered

### Clinical Impressions

This 4-year, 6-month-old girl presented with a severe receptive and expressive language disorder and a mild articulation disorder. Speech and language therapy was recommended. Since she was bilingual, only communication deficiencies that suggested disordered development were addressed in her treatment goals and objectives. Dialectal differences and developmental errors were not incorporated into the treatment plan. Therapy was implemented by two bilingual speech-language pathologists, one working with her in English, the other in Spanish. Kana received therapy 2 times weekly, with one session conducted in Spanish and one in English.

## Course of Treatment

### Therapy

A. *Long-Term Goal:* Improve Receptive Language Skills
   - *Short-Term Objectives*
     1. Follow 1-step directions in 4 out of 6 trials.
     2. Recall 4 of 6 characters and objects in narratives read without prompts with 80% accuracy.

B. *Long-Term Goal:* Improve Expressive Language Skills
   - *Short-Term Objectives*
     1. Combine 2–3 words in spontaneous speech with 80% accuracy.
     2. Name pictures with 80% accuracy.
     3. Produce noun + verb + object utterances with 80% accuracy.

C. *Long-Term Goal:* Improve Articulation Skills
   - *Short-Term Objectives*
     1. Improve articulation of /p/ in the initial position of words with 80% accuracy.
     2. Improve articulation of /b/ in the initial position of words with 80% accuracy.

### Therapy Approach

Therapy sessions included techniques such as modeling, imitation prompts, storytelling, phonemic and verbal cueing for the purpose of eliciting target phonology, and age-appropriate utterances in terms of vocabulary, morphology, and syntax. Age-appropriate materials, such as toys, familiar household and environmental objects, and pictures, were important for language elicitation.

***Outcomes*** After 6 months of therapy, improvement was noted in both Spanish and English.

Kana improved her ability to follow 1-step directions with 28% accuracy in Spanish and with 42% accuracy in English spontaneously and when presented with cues. She was able to recall 4 of 6 characters with 25% accuracy. Kana recalled 4 of 6 characters and objects in narratives read to her (27% in Spanish and 35% in English) spontaneously and when presented with cues.

Kana's expressive language skills improved in Spanish and in English. She combined 2–3 words in connected discourse in Spanish 20% of the time spontaneously and when provided with cues, and she used 2–3 words in connected discourse in English 30% of the time under comparable therapy conditions. Kana named pictures of household objects 20% of the time in

TABLE 13.2 Reevaluation Results

| Post-Test | | Raw Score | Standard Score | Percentile Rank | Standard Deviation | Age-Equivalence |
|---|---|---|---|---|---|---|
| ROWPVT—Spanish Bilingual | | 26 | 66 | 1 | −2.26 | 3–7 |
| EOWPVT—Spanish Bilingual | | 18 | 66 | 1 | −2.26 | 3–0 |
| Preschool Language Scale-4 (Spanish Version) | Auditory Comprehension | 41 | 61 | 1 | −2.6 | 3–5 |
| | Expressive Communication | 39 | 53 | 1 | −3.13 | 3–2 |
| | Total Language Score | 80 | 50 | 1 | −3.3 | 3–3 |
| Preschool Language Scale-4 (English Version) | Auditory Comprehension | 44 | 69 | 2 | −2.0 | 3–8 |
| | Expressive Communication | 45 | 68 | 2 | −2.13 | 3–8 |
| | Total Language Score | 89 | 65 | 1 | −2.3 | 3–7 |

Spanish and in English spontaneously and with cueing. Additionally, at the end of 6 months of therapy, Kana produced noun + verb utterances 20% of the time in Spanish and 23% of the time in English using cues and during spontaneous productions.

Kana's articulation skills also improved. She produced the bilabial speech sounds /p/ and /b/ in the initial position of words in both languages with 80% accuracy

Given the progress that Kana demonstrated in the first 6 months of therapy, a reevaluation of her communication development was conducted. The reevaluation findings are detailed in Table 13.2.

## Analysis of Client's Response to Intervention

With comprehensive assessments in both Spanish and English, Kana's speech and language development was appropriately assessed. There was an understanding of the need for bilingual assessments of her communication development. Kana received bilingual speech-language therapy services from two bilingual speech-language pathologists, one conducting therapy in Spanish on one day and the other conducting therapy in English on another day. With intense and linguistically appropriate therapy services, in 6 months, Kana made favorable progress in both Spanish and English. Kana's therapy continued until her language skills reached age appropriateness. It is very important for children who speak more than one language to have experiences that continuously foster their linguistic, cognitive, and social development in all of their languages across a wide variety of settings—home, school, therapy setting, and community.

## Author Note

This case is fictionalized and was inspired by several children we have worked with.

## References

ASHA Committee on the Status of Racial Minorities. (1983). [Position Statement]. http://www.asha.org/docs/html/PS1983-00115.html

American Speech-Language-Hearing Association. (1985). *Clinical management of communicatively handicapped minority language populations* [Position Statement]. http://www.asha.org/docs/html/PS1985-00219.html

Banks, J. A. (2001). *Cultural diversity and education*. Boston: Allyn & Bacon.

Brownell, R. (2001a). *Expressive One-Word Picture Vocabulary Test* (EOWPVT)—Spanish Bilingual Edition. Novato, CA: Academic Therapy Publications.

Brownell, R. (2001b). *Receptive One-Word Picture Vocabulary Test* (ROWPVT)—Spanish Bilingual Edition. Novato, CA: Academic Therapy Publications.

Mattes, L. (1995). *Spanish Articulation Measures*—Revised Edition. Oceanside, CA: Academic Communication Associates.

Roseberry-McKibbin, C. (2007). Language disorders in children: A multicultural and case perspective. In *The impact of second language acquisition* (pp. 74–75). Boston: Allyn & Bacon.

TESOL, Teachers of English Speakers of Other Languages. (2006, March). *ESL standards for pre-K–12 students*. (March 2006). Retrieved September 10, 2008, from http://www.tesol.org/s_tesol/sec_document.asp?CID=281&DID=6397.

U.S. Census 2000. http://quickfacts.census.gov/main/www/cen2000.html.

Zimmerman, I. L., Steiner, V. G., & Pond, R. E. (2002). *Preschool Language Scale—4th edition*. San Antonio, TX: The Psychological Corporation.


# CASE 14

# Rose: A Preschool Child Who Was Internationally Adopted

*Jenny A. Roberts and Kathleen A. Scott*

## Conceptual Knowledge Areas

Children adopted from abroad constitute a growing population whose communication abilities are of interest to clinicians and other professionals. Internationally adopted (IA) children have high rates of referral for evaluation to speech-language pathologists (SLPs) (Mason & Narrad, 2005), and it is important to understand what puts some IA children at risk for communication disorders.

IA children who are adopted into the United States represent a diverse population. The preadoption experiences of IA children can vary widely in terms of the settings in which they reside, nutrition and health, quality and amount of caregiver interaction, and duration of time spent in institutional or foster care (Johnson, Huang, & Wang, 1998). The social, economic, and political factors related to the country of origin influence the adoption process and the subsequent early development of the internationally adopted child (Mason & Narrad, 2005; Pertman; 2000; Roberts, Krakow, & Pollock, 2003).

For the past 5 years, the majority of children adopted into the United States internationally have come from the countries of China, Russia, and Guatemala (U.S. Department of State, 2007). The reasons why children are made available for adoption may differ from country to country, as well as within regions and settings within individual countries. For example, a large number of children adopted into the United States between 1950 and 1980 came from Korea, due to effects of the Korean War (Simon & Alstein, 1991). In the early 1990s, children from Romania accounted for the largest number of international adoptees. This was due to wide-scale abandonment following the collapse of the Ceausescu regime (Pertman, 2000). For these Romanian adoptees, it was widely reported that many of the children released for adoption were documented to have lived in extremely deprived conditions, were found to be undernourished, and had a variety of cognitive, linguistic, and social delays upon arrival in their new homes (e.g., Rutter et al., 1998).

A different set of social, economic, and political concerns affect the preadoption experiences of children adopted from China. Generally speaking, these children have been abandoned largely due to China's one-child policy, are overwhelmingly girls, and are adopted early in life (i.e., typically prior to 12 months of age) (Cecere, 2001; Rojewski, Shapiro, & Shapiro, 2000). China's institutions are run by a single authority, presumably making care more consistent across the country as a whole. This is important as the vast majority of IA children live in institutional settings prior to their adoption (Johnson & Dole, 1999).

In the past decade, the preadoption care of IA children worldwide has improved, with better institutional living environments and an increased number of children living in foster care (Zeanah et al., 2003). Nevertheless, factors such as the number of caregivers, frequency of caregiver interactions in orphanages, and whether a child receives foster placement varies for individual children (Smyke, Dumitrescu, & Zeanah, 2002), and these variables can have an impact on communication development. For example, a recent study of communication development in children residing in Romanian orphanages documented that both expressive and receptive language abilities were significantly reduced for those children compared to children living in foster care for 1 or more years (Windsor et al., 2007). Thus, although conditions have improved, institutional living environments negatively affect the development of children residing within them, and as a result, IA children are an at-risk group due to their preadoption experiences.

In addition to challenging early life experiences, children who are internationally adopted into the United States are overwhelmingly adopted by monolingual English-speaking families (e.g., Glennen & Masters, 2002), and the children must adjust to an abrupt loss of exposure to their native language. Because of the lack of maintenance of the native language, they are in effect "second first language" learners (De Geer, 1992; Roberts et al., 2005a), in that they are acquiring a second language prior to acquisition of a first language, at a time when their first language is no longer available to them. Thus, they are not precisely like either monolingual or bilingual children. While some IA children develop their second first language rapidly and without apparent difficulty, other children may struggle (e.g., Roberts, Pollock, & Krakow, 2005b). An important question for parents and clinicians alike is whether the trajectory of growth and achievement of language milestones for any individual IA child is within the expected abilities of other IA children. The story of Rose will help illustrate how to determine this.

## Description of the Case

### Background Information

Rose, a 3-year, 3-month-old child, was adopted from China when she was 15 months of age. She was adopted by Tim and Barbara M., who have one biological son, who was 11 years old. The family lived in a suburb of New York City. Tim, age 51, held a Ph.D. in electrical engineering and commuted to New York City daily. Barbara, age 46, held a master's degree in English literature and worked part-time as a proofreader for a major economics magazine. Because of the nature of her work, she worked at home two days a week and commuted to her office, about 40 minutes away, one day a week. Their son attended a nearby public elementary school and was active in after-school sports programs. Tim and Barbara are typical of many parents that adopt internationally in that they are older than parents of preschool-age children, well educated, and financially secure (Fields, 2003; Roberts et al., 2005a; Tan & Marfo, 2006). They had close friends who adopted two girls from China as infants; they wanted another child and felt comfortable with the choice of China as a country from which to adopt.

When Tim and Barbara first met Rose, her Chinese caregivers reported that she was not yet speaking Mandarin Chinese words, the language of the orphanage, although she was making speech sounds. Upon arrival in the United States, Barbara and Tim first took Rose to their son's pediatrician, who had evaluated some IA children before, though was not a specialist in adopted children. Rose's medical records from the orphanage were sparse, but unremarkable. A physical exam at the pediatrician's office revealed an elevated lead level in her blood, which is not unusual for IA children from China (Miller & Hendrie, 2000). She was very small in stature compared to children born in the United States, although within the low average range of children born in China. Her head circumference and weight also fell within these ranges.

Rose soon settled into her new life in the United States and began to gain weight rapidly, though she remained small in stature for her age. Barbara took Rose to many play dates with other children and attended numerous children's events provided by her adoption agency and within her community. Because Tim and Barbara were familiar with the development of the children from China adopted by their friends, they were initially not concerned that Rose spoke very little and seemed to be slow to acquire new English words. She seemed to understand everything that was said to her or asked of her. When she did speak her speech sounded "garbled" to them, and they were not sure at times if she was babbling. Rose loved to be read to and was learning to turn the pages of books. When asked to point to pictures of familiar objects in books, she was easily able to do so. Overall, she appeared to Tim and Barbara to be a happy, bright little girl.

## Reasons for Referral

After Rose had been in the United States for a little over a year, her parents felt that she should be talking more often and articulating more clearly, and their pediatrician advised them to bring Rose to an early intervention clinic affiliated with their local children's hospital. Rose was assessed there at 31 months by several developmental specialists and found, on a general assessment instrument normed on monolingual English-speaking children, to have significantly delayed expressive language, and slightly delayed fine motor skills. She began receiving language stimulation in her home from a developmental educator 3 hours per week. She received services until she turned 3 years of age, 5 months later.

Her Individualized Family Services Plan (IFSP) mandated that she be reevaluated by her local school district when she turned 3 years old. Barbara made an appointment for Rose to be evaluated, but due to a planned month-long family vacation, as well as scheduling difficulties, Rose was not evaluated until she was 3 years, 3 months of age. The following describes her assessment and subsequent treatment plan.

### Assessment Procedure

The SLP assigned to assess Rose's communication skills was familiar with the literature on the language development of IA children. She had learned in her readings of children adopted from China that as a group, by 2 years post-adoption, they were performing within the average or above-average range on a number of standardized tests normed on monolingual English speakers (e.g., Cohen, Lojkasek, Zadeh, Pugliese, & Kiefer, 2008; Roberts et al., 2005a; Tan & Yang, 2005). However, she was not sure if she could use the results of these research studies as a valid type of assessment of Rose. Upon reading further, she learned about the use of "local norms" (Glennen, 2007; Roberts et al., 2005b), and she realized that the best current practice dictated that she interpret Rose's performance on standardized tests in accordance with the norms of IA children established by these research studies, not by the performance of the normative sample of the tests. Thus, she chose a battery of tests that assessed a range of language abilities and whose local norms could be found in the IA literature for children similar to Rose in age and pre-adoption background.

The examiner also collected a careful case history from Barbara, who accompanied Rose to the assessment, and obtained copies of prior assessments and treatment plans. The original assessment by the Early Intervention Clinic included the MacArthur Communicative Development Inventories: Words and Sentences (CDI; Fenson et al., 1993), which is a parent report instrument of expressive vocabulary and early sentence development. The CDI was administered within a few weeks of Rose's first assessment, at 32 months. Barbara, who had completed the CDI, reported that Rose was producing 113 English words.

The examiner obtained permission from Barbara to contact the developmental educator who had worked with Rose in her home. The developmental educator reported that Rose was a "delightful child" with appropriate play and social interaction skills, but whose language skills were only "slowly improving." She also obtained a language sample, during which time Rose and Barbara played with a toy dollhouse and accessories in her office, which the examiner recorded on a small digital audio recorder. She copied the file onto her computer and later transcribed it using a computer program that automates transcription and analysis of language samples (Systematic Analysis of Language Transcripts, SALT; Miller & Chapman, 2000). She also administered several norm-referenced language measures, which included the Peabody Picture Vocabulary Test-III (PPVT-III; Dunn & Dunn, 1997), the Clinical Evaluation of Language Fundamentals-Preschool II (CELF-P II; Semel, Wiig, & Secord, 2004), and the Goldman-Fristoe Test of Articulation-II (GFTA-II; Goldman & Fristoe, 2000).

## Findings of the Evaluation

Table 14.1 shows the results of the standardized tests. From this table it can be seen that, in comparison to monolingual English-speaking norms, Rose's receptive vocabulary on the PPVT-III was in the average range of performance, and her receptive language composite on the CELF-P II was slightly above average. Inspection of individual subtests on the CELF-P II revealed that listening comprehension and understanding of basic concepts was well above average, and that a measure of syntax comprehension (*Sentence Structure*) was in the low average range. In comparison to monolingual English-speaking children, Rose performed significantly more poorly on expressive language measures on the CELF-P II, falling into the clinical range for monolingual English-speaking children on all three expressive language subtests. For example, when asked to repeat sentences said by the examiner in the context of a story (*Recalling Sentences*), Rose frequently omitted whole words of the sentences. On a measure of single word production, however, the GFTA-II, Rose performed within the average range of ability.

In addition to standardized tests, the examiner collected a sample of Rose's spontaneous language while playing with her mother. After transcribing the sample in SALT, she obtained

TABLE 14.1 Standardized Language Assessment Results

| Area Assessed | Measure* | Standard Scores |
|---|---|---|
| Receptive vocabulary | PPVT-III | 111 |
| Single word articulation | GFTA-II | 92 |
| Receptive language index | CELF-P II | 111 |
| Listening Comprehension | | 13 |
| Basic Concepts | | 15 |
| Sentence Structure | | 8 |
| Expressive language index | CELF-P II | 69 |
| Recalling Sentences | | 3 |
| Formulating Labels | | 6 |
| Words and Sentences | | 5 |

Notes: CELF-P II = Clinical Evaluation of Language Fundamentals-Preschool II; GFTA-II = Goldman Fristoe Test of Articulation II; PPVT-III = Peabody Picture Vocabulary Test-III

*"Measure" is not meant to endorse a particular instrument or method of assessment.

scores of mean length of utterance (MLU), number of different root words (NDW), and total number of words used during the session (TNW), along with other basic measures of language that SALT provides. Rose's MLU was 1.98, her NDW was 71, and her TNW was 181. In comparison to English monolingual peers derived from the SALT database, all three of these values fell more than 2 standard deviations below the mean of these children.

The examiner obtained a printout from SALT of the grammatical morphemes that Rose used while playing with Barbara. Using Brown's developmental morphemes as a guide, as provided in SALT, she determined that Rose produced plural –s frequently and had one occurrence of the copula "is." No other free or bound morphemes from Brown's list of 14 grammatical morphemes were observed. She also obtained a printout of all of the utterances that Rose produced. Typical sentences included "draw mommy," "this is fork," and "I want blue." Rose produced many one-word labels of objects in the room and used these single-word utterances to draw her mother's attention to them. This may have contributed to her low MLU. Using a checklist of Brown's morphemes, the examiner quickly probed for the use of morphemes on a subsequent visit, but Rose did not produce any additional morphemes when given the probes.

## Representation of the Problem at the Time of Evaluation

The examiner first compared the assessment results with the published normative data. The normative data indicated that, in comparison to monolingual English-speaking children of the same age, Rose was having primary difficulties with expressive language, which confirmed Tim and Barbara's impressions. Her receptive language appeared to be developing without difficulty. Though syntax comprehension was low average, her other receptive language scores were well within or above the average range on both the CELF-P II and the PPVT-III. In fact, vocabulary understanding was a particular strength. For expressive language, articulation at the single-word level was in the average range according to the results of the GFTA-II, but the CELF-P II expressive language scores were low across the board. The results of the language sample, in comparison to monolingual English-speaking children, also confirmed that in spontaneous use, expressive language appeared below age expectations.

The examiner was not ready to conclude that Rose was performing in the clinical range of ability. In order to do that, she needed to consult the available literature of IA children of similar age, length of exposure to English, and preadoption circumstances to see how Rose compared to them. First, she examined Rose's performance on the CDI when she was 32 months old. Recall that the CDI was administered by specialists at the Early Intervention Clinic where she had received treatment. The examiner consulted several research reports of vocabulary growth of children adopted from China, and determined that 113 words produced on the CDI was a significantly fewer number of words than those produced by other children adopted from China at a similar age and for a similar duration of English language exposure (Krakow & Roberts, 2003; Pollock, 2005, Price, Pollock, & Oller, 2006). For example, for children adopted between 13–18 months of age, Pollock (2005) reported that after 17 months of English language exposure, they were producing on average 340 words on the CDI. Thus, not only was Rose a late talker by monolingual English-speaking norms, more importantly, she was a late talker in comparison to other IA children from China.

Second, the speech-language pathologist examined Rose's performance on the standardized measures with the available normative information on similar standardized measures for children adopted from China. She also examined performance of individual low scoring subjects when it was reported in these papers. She determined that on similar instruments for IA children of a comparable age and duration of English language exposure, Rose was performing below her IA peers in expressive language. For example, Roberts and her colleagues (Roberts et al., 2005a) reported standardized test scores for 55 preschool children adopted from China between 8 and 25 months of age. They reported that the average standard score on the PPVT-III was 117.6, the CELF-P II Receptive language composite score was 120.8, the CELF-P II Expressive language composite score was 118.6, and the GFTA-II standard score was 112.6. Test standard scores across all tests ranged considerably, from a low of 48 to a high of 142. However, only 3 of 55 children performed below 1.25 standard deviations of the mean on two or more composite or test measures. For those 3 children, Roberts et al. (2005a) reported that their standard scores ranged from 76–113 on the PPVT-III, 66–96 on the CELF-P II Receptive language composite, 67–73 on the CELF-P II Expressive language composite, and 48–104 on the GFTA-II. Thus, Rose's standardized expressive language scores were much more comparable to the *low* scoring children in the study than to the group averages.

In addition to reviewing the results of the standardized tests in accordance with the literature on language abilities of IA children, the examiner also consulted the literature with respect to language sample outcomes. Language sample analysis has been used historically by SLPs primarily as a supplement to data obtained from standardized testing (Stockman, 1996), and limitations in the use of language samples as a basis of diagnostic decision making have been noted (Eisenberg, Fersko, & Lundgren, 2001). Little data were available on the spontaneous language abilities of IA children, making data particularly hard to evaluate in diagnostic terms. Only one study of the spontaneous language of IA children from China (Price et al., 2006) was located. In the study, Price and her colleagues reported language sample data on 6 girls adopted from China as infants. At age 3 years, the children's MLUs ranged from 1.9–4.0, NDWs ranged from 72–132, and TNWs from 137–375. Of these 6 girls, the one with the lowest values on all of these measures was performing in the below average range on standardized test measures similar to those used to examine Rose. The researchers also found that parental concern was an important factor in determining the language abilities of the children. The authors of that study concluded that this child was in the delayed range in comparison to other children adopted from China.

Rose's language sample scores were similar to those of the delayed child in Price et al.'s (2006) study. In addition, Tim and Barbara were concerned about Rose's language development. As such, it was felt that the language sample, coupled with parent report, provided crucial information regarding Rose's overall language skills. The examiner recognized that language samples are often used as criterion-referenced measures and are suitable as a source of goal formation (Long & Channell, 2001). It was determined that many appropriate language goals for Rose could be drawn from her initial sample, and with the collection of a second sample, she could use these as baseline and outcome measures in determining progress in therapy. Based upon the careful examination of all of the available testing evidence, along with the established literature on IA children, Rose's prior treatment history, the examiner's clinical experience, and the concern of the family, it was concluded that Rose was performing outside the average range for expressive language in comparison to other girls adopted from China, and she should receive services.

## Treatment Options Considered

From this analysis, long-term treatment goals for Rose were formulated, which were to increase sentence length, use of Brown's grammatical morphemes, and vocabulary diversity. These goals would be simultaneously addressed by targeting infrequently used or unused free and bound grammatical morphemes to lengthen sentences. The specific goals for Rose were to increase her use of three grammatical morphemes that occur early in development (present progressive –ing; irregular past tense, and articles a/the) and that were not present or little used in Rose's language sample. For example, sentences such as "This is fork" would be targeted to be produced with an article ("This is *a* fork").

These findings were discussed with Tim and Barbara, along with the treatment recommendations that Rose be provided with a focused stimulation method for increasing target grammatical morphemes (Weismer & Robertson, 2006). It was explained that focused stimulation provides auditory bombardment of language targets, which would be introduced during play activities, and that the method does not require that children produce the forms they are being exposed to. Conversational recasts (Camarata & Nelson, 2006), in which Rose's phrases and sentences would be expanded, particularly with the morphemes being targeted, would also be used. For example, sentences such as "I want blue" might be recast to Rose as "You want the blue *ball*", which was expected to ultimately help Rose both expand her sentence length and incorporate new vocabulary words. The therapy would occur in the context of play with familiar toys. Finally, shared book reading activities would be incorporated into the treatment sessions to reinforce targeted language goals and provide general emergent literacy support (van Kleeck, 2006).

Barbara and Tim were pleased with these therapy options, because they felt that due to Rose's young age and reduced English language exposure they did not want Rose to be required to produce words and sentences that might be "too difficult for her." They also felt that therapy occurring in a play context was in keeping with their own beliefs of child interaction. They had observed that Rose was "a good listener" and responsive to what was being said around her in her everyday environment. They agreed to begin treatment for 3 months on a weekly basis and for Rose to be reevaluated at the end of that period.

## Course of Treatment

Treatment was conducted as planned. Data were compiled of the number of grammatical morphemes offered in each weekly therapy session (recorded with a silent hand-held "clicker" that added a value each time it was clicked). The therapist pooled the results of morphemes provided in the form of recasts as well as in other contexts. She entered on a simple record sheet the total stimulation offered during each session, which ranged from 32–71 occurrences during each session. She also made notes unobtrusively on a clipboard during the sessions when she heard Rose spontaneously produce any of the target morphemes. Her records showed steady improvement in Rose's production of the target morphemes during their therapy sessions.

To determine whether Rose's use of the target morphemes in therapy had generalized to include the use of other communicative partners, at the end of 3 months, a sample of Rose's language while interacting with her mother was obtained. An audio recording sample was made, copied onto a computer, and transcribed using SALT. Basic measures obtained from SALT revealed that Rose's MLU was now 2.25, her NDW was 108, and her TNW was 231. Although all of these basic measures had increased since the language sample obtained 3 months earlier, Rose's NDW and TNW had particularly improved, with her NDW falling within the range of monolingual English-speaking peers obtained from the SALT database. With respect to Brown's grammatical morphemes, Rose continued to produce plural –s frequently, and several instances of the copula and past tense –ed were observed. For the morphemes targeted during therapy, Rose produced 2 instances of present progressive –ing ("is going" and "he is running"), 1 instance of the irregular past tense (fell), and 4 instances of the article "the." The article "a" was not observed.

## Analysis of Client's Response to Intervention

These results were presented to the mother, who agreed that Rose appeared to be responding to the therapy. The clinician demonstrated how the mother might use both focused stimulation and recast techniques at home and provided her with some parent handouts about increasing language use in preschool-age children. Because Rose was responsive to the therapy, they agreed to continue the therapy for another 3 months and to reevaluate at that time whether additional therapy was needed.

In summary, it was determined that Rose, a 3-year-old child adopted from China as a young toddler, was performing below the range of what is expected for other similar children adopted from China, and she was provided appropriate therapy focused on those language structures that were slow to develop. It was important to Rose's parents that the clinician was well versed in the literature of the language development of IA children, was respectful of their wishes and child-rearing beliefs, and consulted and included them in the therapeutic process. Careful data were maintained of Rose's progress and the clinician was able to demonstrate good improvement in the target structures of language during therapy sessions, as well as in generalization contexts.

## Author Note

This is a fictional case, composed of multiple characteristics drawn from real cases of IA children. It does not represent the characteristics of any individual child and/or family.

## References


Camarata, S. M., & Nelson, K. E. (2006). Conversational recast intervention with preschool and older children. In R. J. McCauley & M. E. Fey (Eds.), *Treatment of language disorders in children* (pp. 237–264). Baltimore, MD: Paul H. Brookes Publishing.

Cecere, L. A. (2001). *The children can't wait: China's emerging model for intercountry adoption*. Cambridge, MA: China Seas.

Cohen, N. J., Lojkasek, M., Zadeh, Z. Y., Pugliese, M., & Kiefer, H. (2008). Children adopted from China: A prospective study of their growth and development. *Journal of Child Psychology and Psychiatry, 49*, 458–468.

DeGeer, B. (1992). Internationally adopted children in communication: A developmental study. Child Language Research Institute, *Working Papers, no. 39*. Lund: Department of Linguistics.

Dunn, L. M., & Dunn, L. M. (1997). *Peabody Picture Vocabulary Test* (3rd ed.). Circle Pines, MN: American Guidance Service.

Eisenberg, S., Fersko, T., & Lundgren, C. (2001). The use of MLU for identifying language impairment in preschool children: A review. *American Journal of Speech-Language Pathology, 10*, 323–342.

Fenson, L., Dale, P. S., Reznick, J. S., Bates, E., Thal, D., Hartung, J., et al. (1993). *Guide and technical manual for the MacArthur Communicative Development Inventories*. San Diego, CA: Singular Press.

Fields, J. (2003). *Children's characteristics and living arrangements: March 2002*. Current Population Reports, P20–547, U.S. Census Bureau, Washington, D.C. (Detailed tables) [http://www.census.gov/prod/www/abs/p20.html; retrieved 8-1-03].

Glennen, S. (2007). Predicting language outcomes for internationally adopted children. *Journal of Speech, Language & Hearing Research, 50*, 529–548.

Glennen, S., & Masters, M. G. (2002). Typical and atypical language development in infants and toddlers adopted from Eastern Europe. *American Journal of Speech-Language Pathology, 11*, 417–433.

Goldman, R., & Fristoe, M. (2000). *Goldman-Fristoe Test of Articulation* (2nd ed.). Circle Pines, MN: American Guidance Service.

Johnson, D. E., & Dole, K. (1999). International adoptions: Implication for early intervention. *Infants and Young Children, 11*, 34–45.

Johnson, K., Huang, B., & Wang, L. (1998). Infant abandonment and adoption in China. *Population and Development Review, 3*, 469–510.

Krakow, R. A., & Roberts, J. (2003). Acquisitions of English vocabulary by young Chinese adoptees. *Journal of Multilingual Communication Disorders, 1*, 169–176.

Long, S. H., & Channell, R. W. (2001). Accuracy of four language analysis procedures performed automatically. *American Journal of Speech-Language Pathology, 10*, 180–188.

Mason, P., & Narad, C. (2005). International adoption: A health and developmental prospective. *Seminars in Speech and Language, 26*, 1–9.

Miller J., & Chapman, R. (2000). *Systematic Analysis of Language Transcripts* [computer software]. *Version 6.1*. Madison, WI: Language Analysis Laboratory, Waismann Center, University of Wisconsin.

Miller, L. C., & Hendrie, N. W.(2000). Health of children adopted from China. *Pediatrics, 105*, 1–6.

Pertman, A. (2000). *Adoption nation*. New York: Basic Books.

Pollock, K. (2005). Early language growth in children adopted from China: Preliminary normative data. *Seminars in Speech and Language, 26*, 22–32.

Price, J. R., Pollock, K., & Oller, D. K. (2006). Speech and language development in six infants adopted from China. *Journal of Multilingual Communication Disorders, 4*, 108–127.

Roberts, J. A., Krakow, R., & Pollock, K. (2003). Three perspectives on language development in children adopted from China. *Journal of Multilingual Communication Disorders, 1*, 162–168.

Roberts, J., Pollock, K. E., Krakow, R., Price, J., Fulmer, K. C., & Wang, P. P. (2005a). Language development in preschool-age children adopted from China. *Journal of Speech, Language and Hearing Research, 48*, 93–107.

Roberts, J., Pollock, K., & Krakow, R. (2005b). Continued catch-up and language delay in children adopted from China. *Seminars in Speech and Language, 26*, 76–85.

Rojewski, J., Shapiro, M., & Shapiro, M. (2000). Parental assessment of behavior in Chinese adoptees during early childhood. *Child Psychiatry and Human Development, 31*, 79–96.

Rutter, M., The English and Romanian Adoptees Study Team. (1998). Developmental catch-up and deficit following adoption after severe global early privation. *Journal of Child Psychology and Psychiatry, 39*, 465–476.

Semel, E. M., Wiig, E. H., & Secord, W. A. (2004). *Clinical Evaluation of Language*

*Fundamentals-Preschool II*. San Antonio, TX: Psychological Corporation, Harcourt Brace Company.

Simon, R., & Alstein, H. (1991). Intercountry adoptions: Experiences of families in the United States. In H. Alstein and R. J. Simon (Eds.), *Intercountry adoption: A multinational perspective*. New York: Praeger.

Smyke, A. T., Dumitrescu, A., & Zeanah, C. H. (2002). Attachment disturbances in young children. I: The continuum of caretaking casualty. *Journal of the American Academy of Child & Adolescent Psychiatry, 41*, 972–982.

Stockman, I. (1996). The promises and pitfalls of language sample analysis as an assessment tool for linguistic minority children. *Language, Speech, and Hearing Services in Schools, 27*, 355–366.

Tan, T. X., & Marfo, K. (2006). Parental ratings of behavioral adjustment in two samples of adopted Chinese girls: Age-related versus socio-emotional correlates and predictors. *Applied Developmental Psychology, 27*, 14–30.

Tan, T. X., & Yang, Y. (2005). Language development of Chinese adoptees 18–35 months old. *Early Childhood Research Quarterly, 20*, 57–68.

U.S. Department of State (2010). Total Adoptions to the United States. Retrieved March 20, 2010, from http://adoption.state.gov/ news/ total_chart.html

van Kleeck, A. (Ed.). (2006). *Sharing books and stories to foster language and literacy*. San Diego: Plural Publishing.

Weismer, S. E., & Robertson, S. (2006). Focused stimulation approach to language intervention. In R. J. McCauley & M. E. Fey (Eds.), *Treatment of language disorders in children* (pp. 175–202). Baltimore, MD: Paul H. Brookes Publishing.

Windsor, J., Glaze, L. E., Koga, S. F., & The Bucharest Early Intervention Project Core Group. (2007). Language acquisition with limited input: Romanian institution and foster care. *Journal of Speech, Language and Hearing Research, 50*, 1365–1381.

Zeanah, C. H., Nelson, C. A., Fox, N. A., Smyke, A. T., Marshall, P., Parker, S. W., et al. (2003). Designing research to study the effects of institutionalization on brain and behavioral development: The Bucharest Early Intervention Project. *Development and Psychopathology, 15*, 885–907.

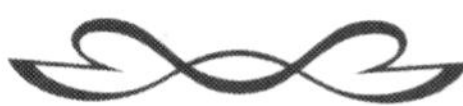

## CLEFT PALATE/SUBMUCOUS

# CASE 15

# Sarah: Submucous Cleft Palate: A Typical Case of Late Diagnosis

*Ann W. Kummer*

## Conceptual Knowledge Areas

### Velopharyngeal Function

The velopharyngeal valve is responsible for closing off the nasal cavity from the oral cavity during speech. Normal velopharyngeal closure is accomplished by the coordinated action of the velum (soft palate) and the pharyngeal walls (the walls of the throat).Velopharyngeal closure is necessary for the production of all speech sounds, with the exception of nasal sounds (m, n, ng). Closure of the velopharyngeal valve is also important for singing, whistling, blowing, sucking, kissing, swallowing, gagging, and vomiting.

During nasal breathing and the production of nasal sounds, the velum rests against the base of the tongue so that the pharyngeal cavity is unobstructed. During the production of oral speech however, the velum raises in a superior and posterior direction and then closes against the posterior pharyngeal wall. As it elevates, the velum has a type of "knee action" where it bends to provide maximum contact with the posterior pharyngeal wall over a large surface. The point where the velum bends is where the paired levator veli palatini muscles interdigitate and pull the velum up and back during contraction. This area can be seen on the oral surface during phonation and is called the *velar dimple*. Examination of the nasal surface of the velum through nasendoscopy reveals a muscular bulge on the top of the "knee" during phonation, the *velar eminence*. It is the result of contraction of the paired musculus uvulae muscles. These muscles provide internal stiffness to the velum and better closure in the midline.

The lateral pharyngeal walls contribute to velopharyngeal closure by moving medially to close against the velum or, in some cases, to meet in midline behind the velum. Both lateral pharyngeal walls move during closure, but there is great variation among normal speakers in the extent of movement. In addition, there is often asymmetry in movement so that one side may move significantly more than the other side.

During velar movement, the posterior pharyngeal wall may move forward to assist in achieving contact, although this forward movement may be slight. Some posterior pharyngeal wall movement is noted in most normal speakers, but its contribution to closure seems to be much less than that of the velum and lateral pharyngeal walls. Some normal as well as abnormal speakers have a defined area on the posterior pharyngeal wall that bulges forward during speech, called the Passavant's ridge. This is a normal variation and is the result of contraction of the superior constrictor muscles.

## Velopharyngeal Dysfunction

Velopharyngeal dysfunction (VPD) refers to a condition in which the velopharyngeal valve does not close consistently and completely during the production of oral sounds. *Velopharyngeal insufficiency (VPI)* is the term usually used to describe an anatomical or structural defect that prevents adequate velopharyngeal closure. Velopharyngeal insufficiency is the most common type of VPD because it includes a short velum, which is common in children with a history of cleft palate after the palate repair. *Velopharyngeal incompetence (VPI)* refers to a neuromotor or physiological disorder that results in poor movement of the velopharyngeal structures. Finally, *velopharyngeal mislearning* refers to inadequate velopharyngeal closure secondary to faulty development of appropriate articulation patterns.

A velopharyngeal opening can cause hypernasality and/or nasal emission with speech. If there is significant nasal emission, consonants will be weak in intensity and pressure, and utterance length will be short due to the need to take frequent breaths to replace the lost air. Compensatory articulation productions may also develop due to inadequate intraoral air pressure for consonant production. Because the air coming from the lungs is perpendicular to the velopharyngeal valve, even a very small velopharyngeal opening will be symptomatic for speech.

## Submucous Cleft Palate (SMCP)

SMCP is a congenital defect that affects the underlying structure of the palate, while the oral surface mucosa is intact. It often involves the muscles and nasal surface of the velum, but can involve the bony structure of the hard palate. Depending on the severity of the SMCP, the defect can range from a slight bifid uvula to a complete submucosal cleft that extends almost to the alveolar ridge.

The characteristics of an SMCP include a bifid or hypoplastic uvula, *zona pellucida* (thin, bluish appearing area) and *diastasis* (separation) of the levator veli palatini muscles, which normally elevate the velum during speech (see Figure 15.1). The diastasis of the muscles can often

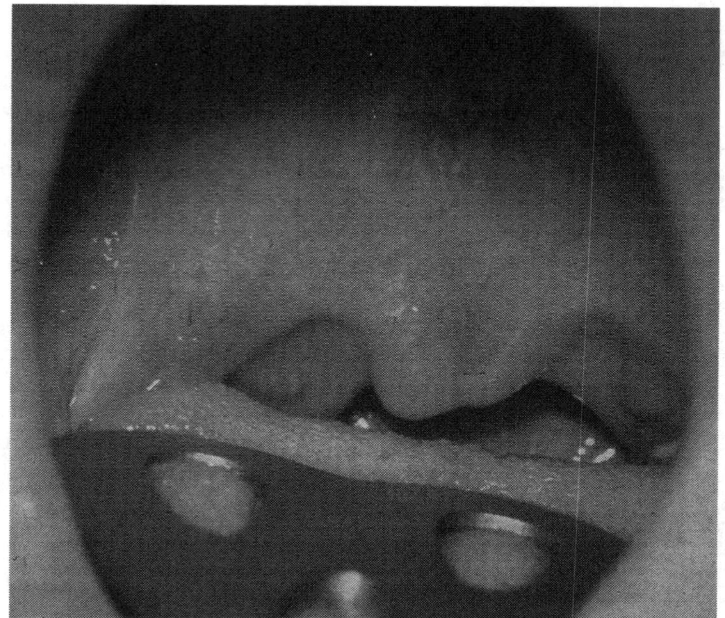

FIGURE 15.1 Submucous Cleft

Note the zona pellucida (thin velum) and wide uvula with a line in midline.

*Source:* From Kummer. *Cleft Palate and Craniofacial Anomalies*, 2E. © 2008 Delmar Learning, a part of Cengage Learning, Inc. Reproduced by permission. www.cengage.com/ permissions

be seen because instead of interdigitating in the middle of the velum, the muscles insert into the posterior border of the hard palate. When they contract during phonation, the velum appears to "tent up" in the shape of an inverted "V"(see Figure 15.2). If the submucous cleft extends through the velum all the way to the hard palate, there may also be a palpable notch in the posterior surface of the hard palate or a groove in the roof of the hard palate.

An *overt submucous cleft palate* is one that can be seen on the oral surface through a simple intraoral examination. An *occult submucous cleft* is a defect in the velum that is not apparent on the oral surface, but can be clearly identified on the nasal surface through nasendoscopy. Because the word "occult" means "hidden" or "not revealed," this malformation is aptly named.

The incidence of SMCP is estimated to be 1 in 1,200 to 2,000 live births, with the true incidence unknown, as many individuals with this condition have few clinical manifestations and often go undiagnosed. SMCP can occur in isolation or as part of a genetic syndrome (such as velocardiofacial syndrome).

The biggest concern with SMCP is that it can cause velopharyngeal insufficiency (VPI). This is because the velum is either too short to reach the posterior pharyngeal wall during speech, or there is a midline defect that interferes with complete closure of the velopharyngeal valve. It has been estimated that one-fourth to one-half of individuals with submucous cleft have associated velopharyngeal dysfunction causing abnormal speech. On the other hand, it is important to recognize that most individuals with a submucous cleft have normal speech.

## Velocardiofacial Syndrome (VCFS)

VCFS is also known as Shprintzen syndrome, De George syndrome, or 22q11.2 syndrome. VCFS is often identified in patients who demonstrate hypernasality with no known cause. In addition to the characteristic hypernasality, affected individuals often have language and learning problems, articulation disorders, and hearing loss. Because communication disorders are common characteristics with VDFS, it is often the speech-language pathologist who first detects the problem and refers the individual for further medical assessment and intervention.

The characteristics of VCFS have been described by many authors (Cable & Mair, 2003; Finkelstein et al., 1993; Ford, Sulprizio, & Rasgon, 2000; Gothelf, 2007; Hay, 2007; Motzkin,

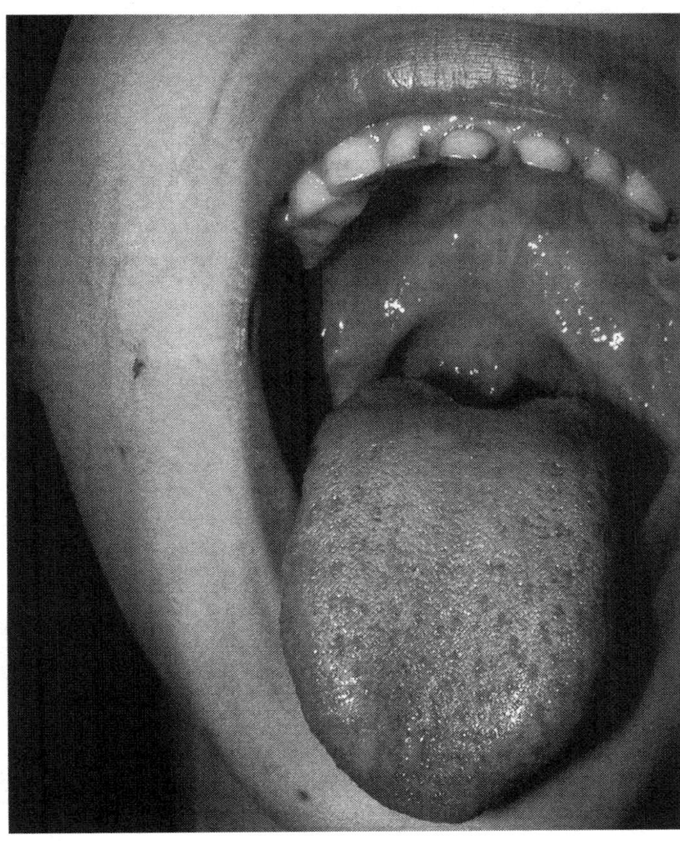

FIGURE 15.2 Submucous Cleft

Note the inverted "V" shape that occurs during phonation. This is the result of abnormal muscle insertion.

*Source:* From Kummer. *Cleft Palate and Craniofacial Anomalies*, 2E. © 2008 Delmar Learning, a part of Cengage Learning, Inc. Reproduced by permission. www.cengage.com/ permissions

Marion, Goldberg, Shprintzen, & Saenger, 1993; Shprintzen, 2000; Stevens, Carey, & Shigeoka, 1990). The basic characteristics are as follows:

- ***Velo:*** There is usually velopharyngeal dysfunction as a result of an overt or submucous cleft or pharyngeal hypotonia. Hypernasality and nasal emission are common findings.
- ***Cardio:*** Minor cardiac and vascular anomalies are common, including ventriculoseptal deviation (VSD); atrial septal defect (ASD); patent ductus arteriosis (PDA); pulmonary stenosis; tetralogy of Fallot; right-sided aortic arch; medially displaced internal carotid arteries; and tortuosity of the retinal arteries. The child may have had a heart murmur at birth.
- ***Facial:*** Facial characteristics include microcephaly, long face with vertical maxillary excess; micrognathia (small jaw) or retruded mandible, often with a Class II malocclusion; nasal anomalies including wide nasal bridge, narrow alar base, and bulbous nasal tip; narrow palpebral fissures (slit-like eyes); malar flatness; thin upper lip; minor auricular anomalies; and others (see Figure 15.3).
- ***Learning and Cognitive Problems:*** Learning disabilities or mild to moderate mental retardation are common. Affected individuals often have difficulty with abstract thinking.
- ***Communication Problems:*** Hypernasality due to velopharyngeal insufficiency and pharyngeal hypotonia is the most common finding. In addition, affected individuals may demonstrate multiple misarticulations, often due to verbal apraxia (Kummer, Lee, Stutz, Maroney, & Brandt, 2007); a high-pitched voice; conductive and/or sensorineural hearing loss; or language disorders with learning problems (D'Antonio, Scherer, Miller, Kalbfleisch, & Bartley, 2001; Kok & Solman, 1995; Scherer, D'Antonio, & Kalbfleisch, 1999; Scherer, D'Antonio, & Rodgers, 2001; Ysunza et al., 2003).
- ***Other Common Physical and Medical Characteristics:*** Other common findings include long slender digits; hyperextensibility of the joints; short stature, usually below

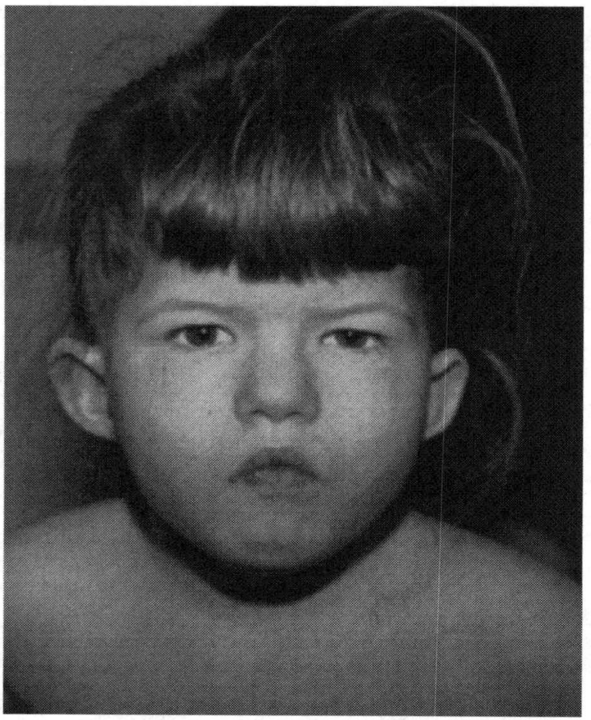

FIGURE 15.3 Velocardiofacial Syndrome

Typical facies of a child with velocardiofacial syndrome. Note the narrow eye openings (palpebral fissures), wide nasal bridge, bulbous nasal tip, thin upper lip, long maxilla (which is why the teeth show), small mandible and low-set ears.

*Source:* From Kummer. *Cleft Palate and Craniofacial Anomalies,* 2E. © 2008 Delmar Learning, a part of Cengage Learning, Inc. Reproduced by permission. www.cengage.com/ permissions

the 10th percentile; Pierre Robin sequence (cleft palate, micrognathia, and glossoptosis with airway obstruction); umbilical and inguinal hernias; and laryngeal web.

- ***Other Common Functional Problems:*** Additional functional problems may include early feeding problems; gross and fine motor delays; social disinhibition; and risk of psychosis in adolescence.

Although there are many common characteristics with velocardiofacial syndrome, the expressivity is widely variable among individuals. Some have only a few characteristics, while others have many. In general, abnormal speech (usually due to velopharyngeal insufficiency and apraxia) is most common.

The cause of velocardiofacial syndrome is a genetic deletion on chromosome 22q11.2 which can occur sporadically in a family that has never had an individual with the syndrome. Once it occurs, it is an autosomal dominant condition, and about 50% of the affected individual's offspring will have the syndrome.

# Description of the Case

## Background Information

The following case report describes a child who was seen in Velopharyngeal Insufficiency/ Incompetence Clinic (VPI Clinic) at Cincinnati Children's Hospital Medical Center. VPI Clinic is conducted by an interdisciplinary team of professionals, consisting of a speech-language pathologist, otolaryngologist/surgeon, and geneticist.

## Reason for Referral

Sarah, age 7 years, 4 months, was referred to VPI Clinic by her pediatrician at the urging of the school speech-language pathologist. Because Sarah had a history of hypernasal speech, the speech-language pathologist wanted an evaluation of velopharyngeal function.

### Pertinent History

Both parents accompanied Sarah to the evaluation. The father was very quiet during the interview, although he occasionally nodded in agreement with the mother's comments. The mother, therefore, was the primary informant and she provided the following information:

***Neonatal History*** Sarah was the product of a full-term pregnancy and normal delivery. She weighed 6 lbs, 10 oz and her Apgar scores were 7 and 9. The only neonatal problem was significant difficulty with breast feeding. The mother reported that after a short period of time, she gave up trying to breastfeed and switched to bottle feeding. Even with the bottle, it took a long time for Sarah to feed. Once she switched to solid foods, Sarah seemed to do fine.

***Medical History*** Sarah had a heart murmur at birth, but this didn't require surgery. However, she was hospitalized at the age of 4 for an inguinal hernia repair. Sarah had chronic ear infections, requiring the insertion of PE tubes on four occasions. When asked where Sarah was on the growth chart, the mother reported that she was at about the 10th percentile for height and close to that for weight. She had been followed by an endocrinologist. Sarah had never been seen by a geneticist or diagnosed with a syndrome.

***Developmental History*** The mother reported that Sarah's developmental milestones were accomplished a little slower than her older sister's, but still within normal limits. Sarah sat alone at 7 months and walked at 14 months. She used single words by 18 months and combined words into short utterances by the age 2 years. Her mother reported that Sarah's speech was initially hard to understand and has always sounded "nasally."

***Treatment History*** Sarah received early intervention services in the home from about 20 months of age until she was 3 years old. When she turned 3, she was enrolled in speech therapy through her school. Sarah continued to receive therapy in school and was currently receiving 2 half-hour sessions per week of individual therapy. The mother noted that although Sarah's articulation and language skills had improved, her speech remained very nasal.

***Social History*** Sarah was the youngest of three children. Her brother and sister had normal speech and no significant medical issues. Her father received speech therapy as a child and reportedly had some learning issues.

***School History*** The mother reported that Sarah was in the second grade. She was generally doing well, but had some difficulties with math.

## Findings of the Evaluation

The following is a summary of the evaluation results:

### Language

Sarah was communicating with complete sentences. An informal screening revealed normal syntax and morphology.

### Speech/Articulation

Articulation placement was characterized by fronting of velars (t/k, d/g); inconsistent nasalization of pressure-sensitive sounds; substitution of ng/l; reduction of blends; and inconsistent voiced/voiceless substitutions. On the sentence level, however, there were many additional inconsistent errors and phoneme omissions. In connected speech, there was a significant increase in omissions and inconsistent errors, apparently due to the increase in utterance length and phonemic complexity.

### Air Pressure/Airflow

There was consistent nasal air emission on all pressure sounds, but this was barely audible. Consonants were very weak in intensity and pressure as a result of the nasal emission.

Utterance length was short due to the loss of air pressure and the need to replenish the supply by taking frequent breaths.

### Resonance

Resonance was severely hypernasal.

### Voice

Voice quality was high in pitch, but otherwise normal.

### Nasometry

Using the Simplified Nasometric Assessment Procedures (SNAP) Test (Kummer, 2005), nasometry revealed a severely high degree of nasalance. The scores were as follows: bilabials-74, lingual-alveolars-69, velars-57, and sibilants-55. A normal score is under about 21 for all four passages. These scores indicated that most acoustic energy during speech was being emitted from the nasal cavity rather than from the oral cavity.

### Intraoral Examination

An intraoral examination revealed evidence of a submucous cleft. The uvula was hypoplastic with a line in the middle. During phonation, the velum formed an inverted "V" shape, which suggested diastasis of the levator veli palatini muscle. The tonsils were not enlarged. Occlusion was in a normal Class I relationship.

### Nasopharyngoscopy

Nasopharyngoscopy showed evidence of a hypoplastic musculus uvulae muscle during phonation. There was also a visible midline notch on the posterior border of the velum. These findings were consistent with a submucous cleft palate. During speech, there was a large velopharyngeal gap due to a short velum and poor lateral pharyngeal wall movement. Observation of the velopharyngeal port during normal nasal breathing showed pulsation of the left carotid artery on the posterior pharyngeal wall. An assessment of the vocal folds revealed a small laryngeal web.

### Additional Observations

Sarah exhibited several dysmorphic facial features, including a wide nasal bridge, bulbous nasal tip, and narrow palpebral fissures (eye slits). She had a long, narrow face and micrognathia (small chin). As the mother reported, Sarah appeared to be very small for her age. Her fingers were long and tapered. On observation the father had several of the same facial features and similarly tapered fingers.

### Examiner Impressions

The preceding results confirmed severe velopharyngeal insufficiency (VPI) as illustrated by a large velopharyngeal opening during speech. The VPI was secondary to a submucous cleft, which had not been previously identified. In addition, poor lateral pharyngeal wall movement (probably due to pharyngeal hypotonia) also contributed to the large opening. The VPI was causing hypernasality, nasalization of consonants, nasal emission, and weak consonants. In addition, there were signs of oral-motor dysfunction in the form of apraxia. These included voicing for voiced phonemes and an increase in inconsistent substitution errors and omissions with an increase in sentence length and phonemic complexity.

There was also very strong physical evidence that the submucous cleft and VPI were secondary to velocardiofacial syndrome. In addition, there were several indications from the history that supported that impression. Finally, there was a suspicion that the father might have had a mild form of VCFS, given his facial features, tapered fingers, and history.

### Parent Counseling

The parents were counseled regarding the results of the evaluation. They had never heard of a submucous cleft and did not understand the mechanics of velopharyngeal function. Therefore, considerable time was spent in explanation, and informational handouts were given to reinforce the learning.

The parents were then told of the suspicion of velocardiofacial syndrome. They had never heard of this syndrome either and the news initially came as a shock. However, as the features were further described, they expressed a degree of relief in knowing that this could explain many of the problems that Sarah was experiencing and that her father had experienced in the past.

## Treatment Options Considered

The team recommendations included the following:

### Genetics Test

The geneticist told the parents that, although the diagnosis of VCFS seemed very likely, this needed to be confirmed with a specific genetic test called a FISH (fluorescent in situ hybridization) test. This test involves taking a sample of blood, then searching for a deletion on chromosome 22q11.2. His recommendation was for both Sarah and her father to have the test.

### Surgical Correction

The team explained to the parents that VPI is a structural problem, and in Sarah's case, it was caused by the submucous cleft and poor lateral wall movement (pharyngeal hypotonia). As such, correction, or at least improvement, of the VPI was necessary before any progress could reasonably be expected in speech therapy. The team also explained that when there is a combination of both VPI and apraxia, correcting the structure defect would give the child the oral air pressure and sound needed to really concentrate on improving articulation skills.

Because of the submucous cleft, the team had discussed two options. One would be to repair the submucous cleft defect and then reevaluate velopharyngeal function to see if a secondary pharyngoplasty was necessary. The second was to do both the cleft repair and a pharyngoplasty at the same time. The team agreed on the second option, given the size of the opening, the pharyngeal hypotonia, and Sarah's age.

Two options for pharyngoplasty were then discussed by the team—a pharyngeal flap, which closes the velopharyngeal port in midline, or a sphincter pharyngoplasty, which narrows the lateral borders of the port. They decided that a pharyngeal flap would be the best procedure in this case because the opening was in midline and very deep. The parents were counseled that with a diagnosis of VCFS, surgery should at least result in improved speech. However, perfect speech may not be likely because there is no way to predict if the flap will result in increased lateral pharyngeal wall movement. In addition to the pharyngeal flap, excision of the laryngeal web was recommended, not only to improve the voice, but also to improve the airway.

### Postoperative Speech Therapy

The parents were told that, although the pharyngeal flap would improve the physical ability to produce sounds, Sarah would require postoperative speech therapy to learn to make the best use of the flap and to improve oral-motor function for speech. In addition to the therapy, the parents would need to work with Sarah every day to practice the skills taught in therapy.

## Course of Treatment

About 6 weeks following her clinic evaluation, Sarah had the palate repair, pharyngeal flap, and laryngeal web excision. The surgeon felt that all went well and the postoperative course was unremarkable. A postoperative VPI Clinic appointment was made for 3 months later.

### Postoperative Evaluation History Update

The parents reported that since the surgery, Sarah's speech was louder and much easier to understand. Even her grandparents could understand her on the phone. Although speech improvement was noted, the mother reported that she still noticed a little nasality.

When asked about the airway, the mother noted that Sarah was not snoring much at night, and that she was sleeping well. She had no signs of sleep apnea.

By this appointment, the genetics test results were available. They revealed that both the father and Sarah had a deletion on chromosome 22q11.2. This confirmed the diagnosis of velocardiofacial syndrome for both, although the father had fewer characteristics and a milder form. Again, the parents indicated that they were relieved to know what caused these problems, what to expect, and what to do about it.

### Postoperative Evaluation Findings

The following is a summary of the postoperative evaluation findings:

***Speech/Articulation*** Articulation was essentially the same as with the preoperative evaluation with one notable exception. Oral consonants were no longer nasalized.

***Air Pressure/Airflow*** There was audible nasal air emission on pressure sounds, and an inconsistent nasal rustle (a loud, friction/bubbling sound, which occurs due to air going through a small opening).

***Resonance*** Resonance was normal and with the increased oral resonance, the volume seemed to be louder.

***Voice*** Voice quality was judged to be essentially normal.

***Nasometry*** Using the SNAP Test, nasometry showed significant improvement in nasalance (bilabials-28, lingual-alveolars-30, velars-27, sibilants-28). Because normal is under about 21, these scores were just a little high.

***Intraoral Examination*** An oral examination showed evidence of the flap donor site. However, the flap could not be seen, which suggested that it was in a good position behind the velum.

***Nasopharyngoscopy*** Nasopharyngoscopy showed the flap to be in good vertical position and in midline. The width of the flap appeared appropriate. Both ports were open wide for normal nasal breathing. During speech, there was lateral pharyngeal wall movement on both sides. The right port closed completely, but a small opening remained in the left port. The vocal folds appeared healthy and moved normally.

## Analysis of Client's Response to Intervention

### Examiner Impressions

The evaluation results revealed significant improvement in velopharyngeal function and thus speech as a result of the pharyngeal flap. However, there was still some nasal emission due to incomplete closure of the left port. The nasal emission was actually more noticeable than before due to the effect of air pressure going through a smaller opening.

## Further Recommendations

Because the problem was with the left port, a left unilateral sphincter procedure was discussed by the team. However, this is the side of the medially displaced carotid artery, making surgery in that area somewhat more difficult. After much discussion, it was decided that the procedure could be done safely and it was recommended to the family.

The family thought about the recommendations for additional surgery, but they were not anxious to put Sarah through another procedure right away. Therefore, they decided to postpone a decision about a touch-up procedure for another year. This seemed reasonable given that the remaining nasal emission was merely "cosmetic." The pharyngeal flap had given Sarah the air pressure and oral resonance to improve speech production skills through speech therapy.

## Author Note

This was based on an actual case. The patient's name was changed to protect her identity.

## References


Cable, B. B., & Mair, E. A. (2003). Avoiding perils and pitfalls in velocardiofacial syndrome: An otolaryngologist's perspective. *Ear, Nose, & Throat Journal, 82*(1), 56–60.

D'Antonio, L. L., Scherer, N. J., Miller, L. L., Kalbfleisch, J. H., & Bartley, J. A. (2001). Analysis of speech characteristics in children with velocardiofacial syndrome (VCFS) and children with phenotypic overlap without VCFS. *Cleft Palate-Craniofacial Journal, 38*(5), 455–467.

Finkelstein, Y., Zohar, Y., Nachmani, A., Talmi, Y. P., Lerner, M. A., Hauben, D. J., et al. (1993). The otolaryngologist and the patient with velocardiofacial syndrome. *Archives of Otolaryngology—Head & Neck Surgery, 119*(5), 563–569.

Ford, L. C., Sulprizio, S. L., & Rasgon, B. M. (2000). Otolaryngological manifestations of velocardiofacial syndrome: A retrospective review of 35 patients. *Laryngoscope, 110*(3 Pt 1), 362–367.

Gothelf, D. (2007). Velocardiofacial syndrome. *Child and Adolescent Psychiatric Clinics of North America, 16*(3), 677–693.

Hay, B. N. (2007). Deletion 22q11: Spectrum of associated disorders. *Seminars Pediatric Neurology, 14*(3), 136–139.

Kok, L. L., & Solman, R. T. (1995). Velocardiofacial syndrome: Learning difficulties and intervention. *Journal of Medical Genetics, 32*(8), 612–618.

Kummer, A. W. (2005). *Simplified Nasometric Assessment Procedures* (SNAP-R): *Nasometer Test and manual.* Pine Brook, NJ: KayPENTAX. The test is included in the equipment manual and is incorporated in the Nasometer software.

Kummer, A. W., Lee, L., Stutz, L. S., Maroney, A., & Brandt, J. W. (2007). The prevalence of apraxia characteristics in patients with velocardiofacial syndrome as compared with other cleft populations. *Cleft Palate-Craniofacial Journal, 44*(2), 175–181.

Motzkin, B., Marion, R., Goldberg, R., Shprintzen, R., & Saenger, P. (1993). Variable phenotypes in velocardiofacial syndrome with chromosomal deletion. *Journal of Pediatrics, 123*(3), 406–410.

Scherer, N. J., D'Antonio, L. L., & Kalbfleisch, J. H. (1999). Early speech and language development in children with velocardiofacial syndrome. *American Journal of Medical Genetics, 88*(6), 714–723.

Scherer, N. J., D'Antonio, L. L., & Rodgers, J. R. (2001). Profiles of communication disorder in children with velocardiofacial syndrome: Comparison to children with Down syndrome. *Genetics in Medicine, 3*(1), 72–78.

Shprintzen, R. J. (2000). Velocardiofacial syndrome. *Otolaryngologic Clinics of North America, 33*(6), 1217–1240.

Stevens, C. A., Carey, J. C., & Shigeoka, A. O. (1990). DiGeorge anomaly and velocardiofacial syndrome. *Pediatrics, 85*(4), 526–530.

Ysunza, A., Pamplona, M. C., Ramirez, E., Canun, S., Sierra, M. C., & Silva-Rojas, A. (2003). Videonasopharyngoscopy in patients with 22q11.2 deletion syndrome (Shprintzen syndrome). *International Journal of Pediatric Otorhinolaryngology, 67*(8), 911–915.

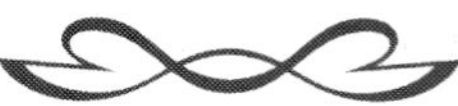

## FLUENCY

# CASE 16

# Oliver: A Preschool Child Who Stutters

*J. Scott Yaruss and Kristin Pelczarski*

## Conceptual Knowledge Areas

Stuttering is a communication disorder that is typically characterized by the production of certain types of disruptions, or *disfluencies*, in the forward flow of speech (Bloodstein & Ratner, 2008). These disfluencies often take the form of part-word repetitions ("li-li-like this"), prolongations ("llllike this"), and blocks ("l—ike this"). Other types of disfluencies, including phrase repetitions ("like this—like this"), interjections ("um," "uh"), and revisions ("I want—I need that"), are also seen, though these are typically judged to reflect normal speech and language development (Conture, 2001).

Fluent and disfluent speech may be accompanied by tension or struggle behaviors as the speaker tries to compensate for the feeling of "loss of control" that accompanies the moment of stuttering (e.g., Perkins, 1990). In older children, adolescents, and adults, stuttering can result in significant negative consequences for the speaker, including negative affective and cognitive reactions, limitations in the ability to perform daily activities involving communication, and restricted participation in social and vocational endeavors (Yaruss & Quesal, 2004). For children, stuttering can result in an adverse educational impact that limits the child's ability to succeed in academic and social settings. These negative consequences may be less common in very young children who stutter, though preschoolers (even typically fluent preschoolers) may experience negative reactions associated with speech disfluencies and stuttering (Ezrati-Vinacour, Platzky, & Yairi, 2001; Vanryckeghem, Brutten, & Hernandez, 2005).

Stuttering typically begins in the preschool years, when a child is between $2\frac{1}{2}$ and 4 years old (Yairi & Ambrose, 1999). It is generally believed to begin gradually and increase in frequency and severity over time, though rapid or sudden onset is also reported (Bloodstein & Ratner, 2008). Most young children who stutter recover within the first 1–2 years postonset (Yairi & Ambrose, 1999). Later recovery is also reported, though recovery after approximately age 7 appears to be significantly less likely (Andrews & Harris, 1964).

Research has demonstrated a strong genetic link for the likelihood of stuttering (Ambrose, Cox, & Yairi, 1997; Ambrose, Yairi, & Cox, 1993; Dworzynski, Remington, Rijsdijk, Howell, & Plomin, 2007; Suresh et al., 2006; Yairi, Ambrose, & Cox, 1996). Boys are more likely to stutter than girls, with an adult male-to-female ratio of approximately 4 or 5 to 1 (Bloodstein & Ratner, 2008). Interestingly, the male-to-female ratio in young children is only approximately 2 to 1, suggesting that young girls may be more likely to recover than young boys (Yairi & Ambrose, 1999). Numerous other factors appear to contribute to the likelihood that young children who stutter will recover from stuttering, including children's language development, their motor abilities, and their temperament (e.g., Bloodstein & Ratner, 2008; Conture, 2001; Yairi, Ambrose, Paden, & Throneburg, 1996). At present, however, there is no way to determine with absolute certainty which children will recover and which children will continue to stutter.

Because of the uncertainty about which children are likely to recover from stuttering, professionals in the field of fluency disorders have engaged in a vigorous debate about whether and when treatment should be recommended for young children who stutter (e.g., Bernstein Ratner, 1997; Curlee & Yairi, 1997). Most practitioners recommend early intervention as the best way to minimize the likelihood that a child will develop chronic stuttering (Conture, 2001). Indeed, numerous studies have shown that the majority of young children who stutter can be helped through treatment (Harris, Onslow, Packman, Harrison, & Menzies, 2002; Millard, Nicholas, & Cook, 2008; Onslow, Costa, Andrews, Harrison, & Packman, 1996; Yaruss, Coleman, & Hammer, 2006). We believe that speech-language pathologists can and should recommend intervention for a young child who stutters if they judge that the child is at risk for developing chronic stuttering.

This case presents a summary that highlights some of the issues clinicians should consider in the diagnosis and treatment of preschool children who stutter. This case history describes the experiences of Oliver, his parents, and his speech-language pathologist from the onset of stuttering through the successful conclusion of treatment. Although some aspects of the scenario are idealized, all reflect the real-life experiences of many of the families that we and our colleagues have evaluated and treated.

## Description of the Case

### Background Information

Oliver was a young boy who lived at home in a rural part of the northeastern United States with his parents and younger sister. He was the product of an unremarkable pregnancy, with no known medical, neurological, behavioral, or social concerns. The family described themselves as being from a middle-class background, and English was the only language spoken in the home. Oliver exhibited normal hearing abilities and had achieved all early speech, language, and motor milestones within normal age expectations. His maternal grandfather had reportedly been a person who stuttered, though there was no other known or reported family history of communication disorders. Oliver was described by his parents, family members, and others as an outgoing child who was "very talkative" and "bright." They added that he "liked to get things right" and sometimes became upset when he made mistakes.

### Reason for the Referral

According to parental reports, Oliver started exhibiting disruptions in his speech when he was approximately 2 years, 10 months old. The parents described these disruptions as including repetitions of parts of words with increasing pitch, stretching of sounds at the beginning of words, and tense pauses when Oliver would move his mouth but no sounds would come out. The parents stated that these disruptions started "overnight" and that Oliver's speech had previously been "quite fluent." In fact, the parents indicated that prior to the onset of stuttering, Oliver had been developing language and speaking skills at an accelerated rate. They stated that he routinely used relatively long and complicated utterances compared to other children his age and that he liked to "tell stories" every night about what he did with his friends during the day.

Oliver's stuttering fluctuated in severity for a period of several months, including some periods when he did not seem to stutter at all and other times when he "could hardly get a word out." The parents believed that he was largely unaware of his speaking difficulties, though he occasionally expressed frustration when he was unable to say what he wanted to say. He continued to talk freely most of the time, though he would occasionally say "never mind" and stop talking when he was having particular difficulty with a word. This behavior in particular caused the parents significant concern for they worried that Oliver might ultimately start talking less because of his speaking difficulties.

After Oliver had stuttered for approximately 3 months, his parents contacted a pediatrician for advice. The pediatrician responded that "most kids outgrow stuttering" and advised them to just "wait and see" whether Oliver would stop stuttering. Further, the pediatrician recommended that the parents not draw attention to Oliver's speech or do anything that might cause him to feel self-conscious about his speaking difficulties. Unfortunately, these recommendations served to increase the parents' fear about the stuttering, for they did not want to do anything that might cause harm to their child. The parents did their best to comply, but often found it difficult to "stand by and watch" when Oliver's stuttering was at its most severe and he was struggling to say even short phrases. On occasion, when Oliver was exhibiting great difficulty speaking, they would tell him to "slow down," and "think about what he was saying." Although this appeared to help him speak more fluently, the parents felt increasingly guilty for talking about Oliver's speaking difficulties in front of him when the pediatrician had told them not to do so.

As the next 3 months passed, the parents' concerns increased dramatically. They began to feel that Oliver was not talking as much as he had when he was younger. They noticed that he was telling fewer stories and giving shorter answers to questions. Episodes of frustration and moments of physical struggle were also more frequent. By this time, Oliver had been stuttering for approximately 6 months and the parents were becoming very worried that he would not recover as easily as the pediatrician had suggested. They were still fearful of drawing attention to stuttering, but they felt that they had to do something to help their son.

## The Search for a Clinician

As a result of their growing fears about Oliver's speech, the parents began to search for information about stuttering. They contacted their pediatrician again but, unfortunately, the pediatrician still expressed doubts about whether action was necessary. This contributed to the parents' apprehension about whether they were "doing the right thing for their child." Still, to be certain about whether Oliver might need help, they searched the Internet. They found websites for organizations such as the Stuttering Foundation of America (SFA; http://www.StutteringHelp.org), the National Stuttering Association (NSA; http://www.WeStutter.org) and Friends: the National Association of Young People Who Stutter (Friends; www.friendswhostutter.org), as well as other sites with suggestions for what to do (e.g., the Stuttering Home Page; http://www.StutteringHomePage.com). At first, they found the volume of information overwhelming. Through careful reading, however, they saw that credible sources recommended that they seek guidance from a licensed and certified speech-language pathologist (SLP). In particular, the SFA, NSA, and Friends provided information about the nature of stuttering in children. Through booklets, pamphlets, and DVDs, the parents learned that although many children do recover from stuttering, it is impossible to tell who will do so without treatment. They also learned that their family history of stuttering placed Oliver at a greater risk for continuing to stutter. This knowledge helped them overcome their reluctance to contact an SLP.

The parents sought to locate a board-recognized specialist via the website of the Specialty Board on Fluency Disorders (http://www.StutteringSpecialists.com), but they were unable to find one in their area. They contacted several specialists by e-mail and found them to be helpful in providing general information about how to help their child. In particular, the specialists confirmed the importance of finding a clinician with expertise in childhood stuttering. Through various sources, the parents obtained the names of several local SLPs whom they interviewed about their experience with children who stutter. They discovered that not all clinicians felt comfortable with fluency disorders (Cooper & Cooper, 1985, 1996; St. Louis & Durrenberger, 1993), and some even echoed the pediatrician's advice to wait to see what would happen. The parents persisted until they found a clinician who was knowledgeable about stuttering. That clinician agreed that based on the length of time since Oliver started stuttering (now more than 8 months), combined with the confirmed family history and the parents' strong concerns, it was appropriate to conduct an evaluation of Oliver's fluency. The goal of the evaluation would be to determine whether treatment would be indicated to help Oliver overcome his stuttering.

## Findings of the Evaluation

Prior to the date of the scheduled evaluation, the parents completed a detailed case history form, in which they provided background information about Oliver's speech and language development, his achievement of developmental milestones, and his early experiences with stuttering and communication. This allowed the clinician to tailor the evaluation to Oliver's individual needs and focus on the specific concerns expressed by Oliver's parents. In particular, the clinician focused her evaluation on trying to determine whether Oliver was at risk for continued stuttering and, as a result, whether he would be in need of treatment to increase his likelihood of developing normally fluent speech.

The evaluation itself consisted of three primary components, each of which was designed to contribute to the clinician's assessment of Oliver's risk for continued stuttering. These components are summarized in the following paragraphs in roughly the same order in which they occurred in the evaluation (Yaruss, LaSalle, & Conture, 1998).

### Parent Interview

While Oliver played with some toys in the therapy room, the clinician conducted a detailed interview with the parents. The interview focused on (a) the onset and development of Oliver's stuttering, (b) the family history of stuttering, (c) Oliver's reactions to his communication difficulties, and (d) the parents' concerns about stuttering. The clinician learned that Oliver had been stuttering for approximately 8 months (two months having elapsed between the parents' decision to seek an evaluation and the scheduling of the evaluation) and that his stuttering had fluctuated somewhat after starting relatively suddenly. The clinician learned about Oliver's grandfather who stuttered and about his sensitivity and occasional negative reactions to stuttering (e.g., the apparent reduction in his willingness to speak freely). In addition, the clinician learned about the parents' concerns about "putting too much pressure" on Oliver while he was young and their fear (based, in part, on what they were told by the pediatrician) about increasing his sensitivity to stuttering. The results of the interview suggested to the clinician that Oliver was at some risk for continuing to stutter and that further evaluation would be prudent (Anderson, Pellowski, Conture, & Kelly, 2003; Conture, 2001; Yairi et al., 1996; Yaruss et al., 1998). At the same time, the clinician would need to gather additional information without increasing the parents' fears about exacerbating Oliver's stuttering.

### Observation of Speech Fluency

Next, the clinician observed while Oliver and his parents engaged in a free play dialogue. In other words, Oliver continued playing with the toys while his parents joined him. The clinician watched from the corner of the room and collected data on the frequency, duration, and type of disfluencies that Oliver exhibited (Yaruss, 1997a, 1998).

Although Oliver was relatively talkative during the evaluation, he exhibited very few speech disfluencies during a 300-word parent-child dialogue. His overall frequency of disfluencies was approximately 7%, and the majority of these disfluencies were phrase repetitions and interjections. Only 4 words out of 100 (2%) were characterized by so-called "stuttered" or "stutter-like" disfluencies (i.e., part-word repetitions, prolongations, and blocks; see Ambrose & Yairi, 1999). The majority of Oliver's disfluencies were brief (less than 1 second) and free of observable physical tension. Still, the clinician observed occasional struggle behaviors during some of Oliver's disfluencies. Overall, however, the surface severity of Oliver's stuttering in the parent-child dialogue was judged by the clinician to be "mild."

The parents immediately expressed their concern that Oliver was so fluent during the evaluation. They explained that he typically stuttered far more than the clinician had observed. In fact, when asked how the speech sample compared to Oliver's speech in other situations, they indicated that it was a "1 or 2" on a 5-point scale, in which a "5" represented Oliver's typical stuttering. The clinician sought to ease the parents' concerns by explaining that it is not uncommon for children to be relatively fluent in clinical settings. The parents added that they observed far more physical tension and struggle in Oliver's speech than he exhibited during the evaluation.

The clinician observed Oliver speaking in other speaking situations to learn more about the variability of Oliver's stuttering (e.g., Yaruss, 1997b). These included a free play dialogue with the clinician in which he described a favorite television show, and a picture description task. Again, Oliver exhibited relatively few stuttered speech disfluencies—far fewer than the parents reported seeing in other situations. Still, the clinician observed occasional tension and struggle behaviors during Oliver's disfluencies, and these were sufficient to cause added concern about Oliver's speech.

Finally, the clinician considered other aspects of Oliver's speech fluency, including his speaking rate and his reactions to stuttering and other difficulties. Oliver was judged by the clinician to use a relatively rapid speaking rate, ranging from approximately 4 to 5 syllables per second. (A typical rate of speech for a preschool child is approximately 3 syllables per second; Pindzola, Jenkins, & Lokken, 1989; Walker, Archibald, Cherniak, & Fish, 1992.) The clinician also observed that Oliver tended to become frustrated easily when playing with a set of building blocks and that he eventually said that he did not want to play anymore because he couldn't get his tower to stand up.

## Speech, Language, and Hearing Testing

The clinician evaluated Oliver's speech, language and hearing abilities. Because Oliver had not previously received a hearing screening, the clinician judged that it was appropriate to conduct a screening and did so using a portable audiometer. Oliver passed the screening bilaterally at 20 dB SPL.

Although the parents had not expressed any concerns about Oliver's speech sound production, receptive and expressive language, or overall communication, the clinician wanted to ensure that latent speech or language difficulties might not be contributing to Oliver's reduced communication. Oliver's scores on the screening portion of the Clinical Evaluation of Language Fundamentals–Preschool 2 (CELF-P2; Wiig, Secord, & Semel, 2004) revealed speech and language abilities within normal limits. In fact, Oliver's language skills were judged to be relatively advanced for his age. (Oliver's standard score was 114, indicating the 82nd percentile.) These results were supported by the clinician's observation that Oliver tended to use long, complex utterances during the free play interaction.

Screening and informal observation suggested that Oliver's speech sound production abilities were probably at the lower ends of normal limits. Oliver exhibited a number of consistent speech error patterns, and his intelligibility was occasionally reduced when the context of communication was unknown to the listener. Thus, the clinician conducted a more specific evaluation of Oliver's speech sound production using the Goldman-Fristoe Test of Articulation-2 (Goldman & Fristoe, 2000). Results indicated that Oliver's articulation abilities were at the 17th percentile (standard score = 88), with consistent error patterns affecting the liquids /l, r/ (which were consistently replaced by the glide /w/ or by a vowel at the ends of words), initial voiceless stops (which were sometimes voiced), and final consonants (which were occasionally deleted). Because most of Oliver's error patterns were inconsistent, they did not cause particular concern. The overall pattern indicated that Oliver's speech sound abilities were still developing.

## Clinical Decision Making

Following the completion of formal testing, the clinician sought to make a decision about whether to recommend speech therapy for Oliver's stuttering. She was aware that there was no way to determine for certain whether Oliver needed therapy; however, she had read that various risk factors might make chronic stuttering more likely (Conture, 2001; Yairi, Ambrose, Paden, & Throneburg, 1996). Based on the results of diagnostic testing, the clinician judged that, even though he did not exhibit very severe observable stuttering during the observation, Oliver was at moderate risk for continuing to stutter. She based this assessment on the positive family history of stuttering; the persistence of stuttering for more than 6 months; speech sound abilities that were still developing in the presence of seemingly advanced expressive language abilities; and the negative reactions he exhibited in response to his stuttering.

## Treatment Options Considered

The clinician shared the results of her evaluation with the parents. In doing so, she emphasized that it was still quite possible that Oliver would recover from stuttering without intervention (e.g., Curlee & Yairi, 1997). Still, she explained that the overall profile indicated that treatment would probably be beneficial to support Oliver's development of normal speech fluency.

The clinician also explained that a number of treatment options were available for children who stutter, including indirect therapy (Gottwald & Starkweather, 1995; Hill, 2003; Starkweather, Gottwald, & Halfond, 1990), direct therapy (Walton & Wallace, 1998), combined direct/indirect approaches (Kelman & Nicholas, 2008; Millard et al., 2008; Rustin, Botterill, & Kelman, 1996; Yaruss et al., 2006), and operant therapy (Harris et al., 2002; Onslow, Andrews, & Lincoln, 1994; Onslow et al., 1996; Onslow, Packman & Harrison, 2003). She added that, based on her reading of the literature, she found both benefits and drawbacks in each of these approaches.

For example, although all treatment for preschool children involves parents, the indirect approach does so without requiring specific corrections of the young child's stuttering as is seen in the operant approach (Onslow et al., 2003). This seemed appropriate for children who might become sensitive to comments about their speech. Still, she explained that the empirical research supporting pure indirect approaches is not fully developed and she would prefer to select a treatment approach that was supported by empirical evidence. On the other hand, although operant therapies are supported by a robust literature, the clinician's own experience suggested to her that these approaches may be better suited for somewhat older children. The clinician expressed her belief that using a purely research-driven approach to selecting a treatment for preschool children who stutter was not straightforward. As a result, it would be necessary for her to combine strategies from a number of data-based approaches to develop an appropriate individualized treatment to address Oliver's stuttering.

The clinician explained that, based on the uncertainty about whether Oliver's stuttering might diminish spontaneously, she would recommend a *staged* treatment approach beginning with methods that were less directly focused on Oliver's fluency and moving toward more direct methods if necessary. This recommendation allowed the clinician to accommodate the parents' ongoing concerns about focusing too specifically on Oliver's stuttering, while still engaging in treatment that would minimize the likelihood of continued stuttering. This recommendation also allowed the clinician to continue monitoring Oliver's speech development to see whether more direct intervention would be required. The parents expressed their agreement with the treatment recommendation, as well as their relief that they would be able to engage in focused activities to help their child without causing him to become too self-conscious about his speech.

The parents ended the evaluation by asking many questions about what they could do to help Oliver's speech at home. The clinician explained that learning such strategies would be a central focus of the early stages of therapy. She recommended that they begin by focusing their attention not only on Oliver's production of speech disfluencies, but also on his overall ability and willingness to communicate. She explained that the most important thing for a young child was his ability to say what he wanted to say, not just whether he could always produce words fluently. She explained that by taking a broader view of the purpose of speaking, the parents would be able to support Oliver's overall communication development. This would promote his ability to communicate successfully regardless of whether he stuttered on a given word or phrase. She explained that therapy would address Oliver's stuttering, and that improvements in fluency would be sought *in the context of good communication skills*.

## Course of Treatment

Although the clinician did not explain all of the details to the parents at the time of the initial evaluation, she had a plan in mind for the course that treatment would likely take, which she would adapt to meet Oliver's needs.

The treatment plan that the clinician adopted was based on the family-focused treatment approach (Yaruss et al., 2006). This treatment seeks to achieve improvements in a young child's fluency by combining parent-focused and child-focused components of treatment while simultaneously working to ensure that both parents and child develop healthy, positive attitudes toward speaking and communication. A schematic depiction of this therapy approach is shown in Figure 16.1.

### Parent-Focused Treatment

The parent-focused components of treatment used in this approach are similar to those described in so-called "indirect" therapies (e.g., Conture, 2001; Gottwald & Starkweather, 1995; Hill, 2003; Kelman & Nicholas, 2008; Millard et al., 2008; Rustin et al., 1996; Starkweather et al., 1990). In general, these aspects of therapy involve helping *parents* learn to modify aspects of the child's communication environment to enhance the likelihood that the child will produce fluent speech. Common parental communication factors that are generally associated with increased fluency include: (a) reduced parental speaking rates (Guitar & Marchinkoski, 2001; Guitar, Schaefer, Donahue-Kilburg, & Bond, 1992; Stephenson-Opsal &

FIGURE 16.1 Schematic Depiction of the Family-Focused Treatment Approach to Treating Preschool Children Who Stutter

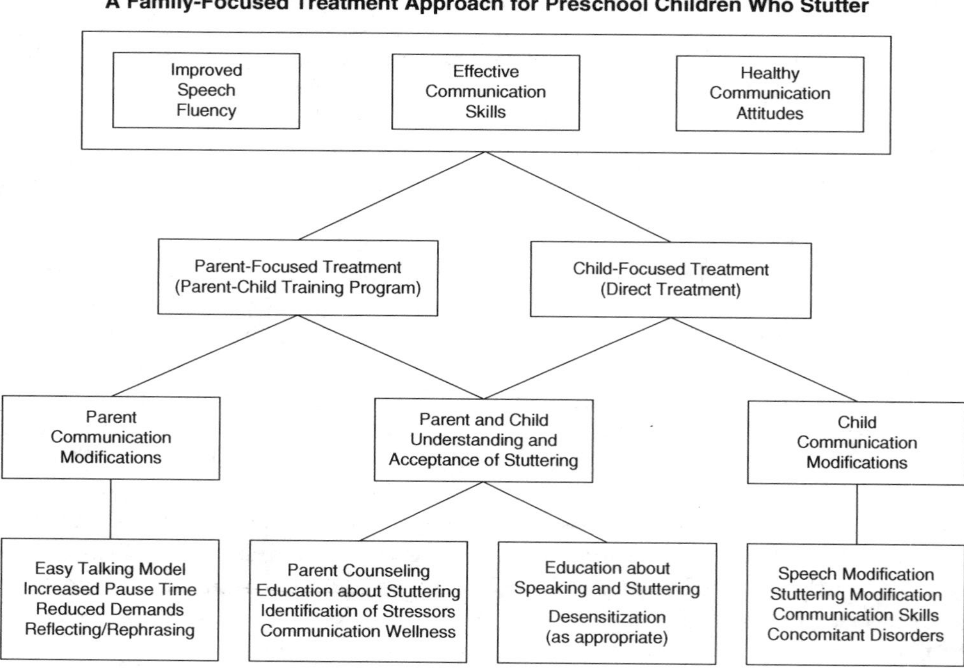


*Source:* Reprinted with permission from Yaruss, J. S., Coleman, C., & Hammer, D. (2006). Treating preschool children who stutter: Description and preliminary evaluation of a family-focused treatment approach. *Language, Speech, and Hearing Services in Schools, 37,* 118–136. Copyright © American Speech-Language-Hearing Association.

Bernstein Ratner, 1988; Zebrowski, Weiss, Savelkoul, & Hammer, 1996), (b) increased pause time following children's utterances (Bernstein Ratner, 1992; Newman & Smit, 1989; Winslow & Guitar, 1994), and (c) reduced parental demands on the child's communication (e.g., minimizing the requirement that the child answer questions or speak in a particular manner) (Conture, 2001; Starkweather et al., 1990). The majority of these changes involve reductions to *time pressure* that the child may experience when trying to communicate. Thus, it is not the specific rate that the parents use that is addressed in therapy; it is the overall sensation of time pressures that the child may perceive. By reducing time pressures, parents can help their child feel that he or she is not rushed to initiate or complete utterances, and this, in turn, can have a positive influence on the child's ability to speak more fluently (Yaruss et al., 2006).

As described by Yaruss et al. (2006), these changes in the parents' communication patterns can be taught during a brief, 6- to 8-session "parent-child training program." The first 2 to 3 of these sessions involve helping parents learn about stuttering and the factors that may contribute to the child's production of disfluent speech. Analogies are introduced that help parents understand that children's speech fluency is more likely to break down under situations of increased time pressure, communication pressure, or general life stress. If these "stressors" can be minimized in a particular situation, then the child is less likely to stutter in that situation. The goal of the early stages of therapy, then, is to try to minimize those pressures as much as is feasible and thereby increase the likelihood that the child will be able to maintain fluency across speaking situations. The next 3 to 4 sessions provide opportunities for the clinician to model, and the parents to practice, specific changes in their communication style that may help to reduce stressors and increase the child's fluency. For example, the clinician may teach the parents to use *slightly* reduced speaking rates to reduce the child's perception of time pressure when speaking. In the context of therapy, the clinician first models the slight reduction in speaking rate while interacting with the child. The parents then have the opportunity to try the modification themselves while receiving feedback from the clinician. This gives the parents the opportunity to directly observe how changes in their own communication style can support the child's production of more fluent speech. These modeling sessions continue until the parents have learned a number of strategies that enhance the child's fluency (e.g., slowing their speaking rates, increasing their use of "pause time," reducing demands on the child's communication). The parent-focused treatment ends with 1 to 2 sessions in which the parents review the strategies that have been helpful for their child and the clinician assesses whether additional treatment (i.e., the child-focused component of treatment) is warranted.

### Child-Focused Treatment

The child-focused components of treatment are similar to those described in so-called "direct" therapies (e.g., Walton & Wallace, 1998). They can be addressed through an open-ended period of treatment in which the child observes, then practices making changes in his or her speaking rate and physical tension to enhance fluency. Specific communication factors that may be associated with increased fluency include: (a) changes in the timing of the child's speech production, and (b) changes in the physical tension the child exhibits during both fluent and stuttered speech (Meyers & Woodford, 1992). Thus, children may be taught to use a slower rate of speech in certain situations in an attempt to enhance their fluency. Or they may be taught to reduce the tightness of their muscles during a moment of stuttering so they are able to move through the disfluency more easily and more smoothly.

Many of these techniques have traditionally been reserved for older children (e.g., Healey & Scott, 1995; Ramig & Bennett, 1995, 1997; Ramig & Dodge, 2005; Reardon-Reeves & Yaruss, 2004; Runyan & Runyan, 1993); however, these approaches can also be used effectively with younger children, (Yaruss et al., 2006). The primary challenge in using more direct treatment strategies with the preschool population is that abstract discussions of speaking rate, pausing, or physical tension are generally too advanced for very young children. These concepts can be made more accessible through analogies that help the child understand the distinction between "too much" (e.g., too much physical tension or too fast speaking rate), "too little" (e.g., too little physical or too slow speaking rate) and "just right" (Yaruss, 2008). For example, when a child is riding a bicycle, he (or she) knows that there are some situations when he can ride as fast as he pleases and other situations when he needs to slow down (e.g., when coming to a curve or when the road is bumpy) or else he will be more likely to fall. When learning to ride a bike, the child rapidly learns that that he will need to change his riding rate depending upon the situation: Sometimes he will ride faster (but not so fast that he will fall down) and other times he will ride more slowly (but not so slowly that he will fall down). He seeks a rate that is somewhere in the middle ("just right"), and the specific rate that is judged to be "just right" will necessarily change from situation to situation. (Note that similar analogies can be constructed for both timing and tension changes using behaviors such as running, shooting baskets, coloring, reading, playing computer games, and, ultimately, talking.)

Of course, treatment cannot rely entirely on analogies. Even if the child understands the importance of using the correct rate when riding a bicycle, this does not mean that he will be able to transfer that understanding to using the correct rate when speaking. Thus, the clinician must explicitly tie the analogy to speech production by pointing out the similarities between riding too fast and talking too fast. For example, the clinician might say, "If we try to go too fast on our bicycle, we will have trouble going where we want to go. The same is true for talking—if we try to go too fast when talking, we will have trouble saying what we want to say." Ultimately, the goal is for children to understand that they may have more difficulty saying what they want to say if they try to go too fast (or use too much tension). At the same time, they may have difficulty saying what they want to say if they try to go too slowly (or use too little physical tension). Thus, they must seek a combination of timing and tension that is "just right" so they can say what they want to say while increasing their speech fluency.

## Parent- and Child-Focused Treatment

One way in which the family-focused treatment approach differs from traditional indirect and direct therapy approaches is that, throughout the therapy process, a significant amount of attention is paid to helping both the parents and child develop and maintain healthy, appropriate *attitudes* toward communication and stuttering (Logan & Yaruss, 1999). The idea that clinicians can talk with preschool children about speaking and stuttering stands in contrast to the advice that has traditionally been given to parents and clinicians about how to treat young children who stutter (Johnson, 1949; Johnson & Associates, 1959). Still, ample research (Harris et al., 2002; Onslow et al., 1994; Onslow et al., 1996; Onslow et al., 2003; Yaruss et al., 2006) has shown that talking to children about their speech does not make stuttering worse. In fact, talking with young children about talking (Logan & Yaruss, 1999; Williams, 1985; Zebrowski & Schum, 1993) can actually help to *reduce* children's concerns about stuttering.

Several strategies can be employed to help parents and children develop healthy attitudes about communication. Most important among these is simply addressing stuttering in an open, honest, and matter-of-fact manner. Thus, rather than avoiding talking about stuttering (Johnson, 1949), parents and children can learn to talk about stuttering openly, acknowledging it as "just something that happens sometimes when children are learning to talk." Parents can learn to treat stuttering just like any other difficulty the child may experience when learning to perform a difficult task. For example, when a child is learning to color, he is likely to color outside the lines. The parent does not avoid talking about this for fear that the child will develop concerns about his coloring abilities! Instead, she simply acknowledges that the child has colored outside the lines and then refocuses the child's attention on the purpose of coloring, that is, creating a picture. Parents respond in a similar fashion when a child trips while learning to walk, falls down while riding a bicycle, reverses letters and numbers, and more.

By acknowledging the child's difficulties with speech production, the parents can help the child understand that there is nothing to fear, and that his message is important, regardless of whether it is produced fluently. The parents' matter-of-fact response helps to maintain a focus on the child's *communication* rather than just his fluency. Of course, improved fluency is an important part of an overall treatment program. That is why these strategies are used as part of a comprehensive treatment approach, including both parent-focused and child-focused components. Before parents can discuss stuttering in an open, matter-of-fact manner, they must first come to terms with their own fears about the child's speech. For this reason, treatment is structured in a staged fashion, with early stages focusing on the parents and later stages addressing the child.

### Structure of Treatment

In an evidence-based approach to treatment, it is important that clinicians be able to adapt the treatment to the individual needs and values of their clients. In the treatment of young children who stutter, this can be seen through the flexible application of various components of the treatment process (parent-focused, child-focused, and both parent- and child-focused) on an as-needed basis. In general, however, the parent-focused components of treatment are typically provided prior to the child-focused treatment. The reason for this is that many children may require *only* the parent-focused components of treatment to achieve normal fluency (Yaruss et al., 2006). Still, both the parent-focused and child-focused components of treatment can be provided simultaneously if the clinician judges that the child is at high risk of continuing to stutter and the clinician is eager to begin work with the child. Combining the parent-focused and child-focused components of treatment allows the clinician to address parental behaviors that may contribute to enhanced fluency while still working directly with the child to enhance fluency. Finally, the child-focused components of treatment can be administered on their own in situations where the parents are unable or unwilling to participate in therapy. Regardless of whether the clinician chooses to start with the parent-focused components or the child-focused components, it is important to incorporate aspects of treatment aimed at helping both the parents and the child develop healthy, appropriate attitudes toward communication.

## Analysis of Client's Response to Treatment

In the present case, the clinician judged that the parents would be active and willing participants in the parent-focused components of treatment. Thus, a plan was developed that started with treatment activities aimed at improving the parents' and child's attitudes toward speaking and stuttering. Child-focused components of treatment were planned for use, as needed, following the initial parent-child training program.

### Parent-Focused Treatment

Both parents attended 6 sessions of the parent-child training program. During the first 2 sessions, they worked with the clinician to identify possible stressors on Oliver's communication, and then they explored ways of minimizing those stressors where possible. For example, they recognized that one factor that probably contributed to Oliver's stuttering was his use of long, complicated sentences, combined with his relatively rapid speaking rate. The parents asked if they should try to get Oliver to use shorter sentences (indicating that they had read this somewhere on the Internet). The clinician responded that she would never want to discourage a child from speaking because of a fear of stuttering. She added that the parents could view Oliver's advanced language skills as a positive aspect of his communication abilities. She underscored this by reiterating the importance of seeking improvements in fluency *in the context of good communication skills*.

Thus, rather than trying to restrict Oliver's speech output, the parents and clinician sought other ways of minimizing the impact that Oliver's long sentences had on his fluency. The clinician highlighted Oliver's speaking rate, suggesting that he might be more fluent if he reduced his speaking rate. She said that although many clinicians discourage parents from telling children to slow down, this advice was largely based on the fear that talking about speech might make the child's stuttering worse. Furthermore, she explained that there were other ways to help Oliver reduce his speaking rate than simply reminding him to slow down. Finally, she explained that the real issue was not really the specific rate that Oliver used but the *time pressure* he might perceive when speaking. The parents stated that they had noticed improvements in Oliver's fluency when they spoke with him in an unhurried manner, so they agreed that this strategy might be helpful.

The clinician then taught the parents that they could help Oliver minimize his sense of time pressure by reducing their own speaking rates. She emphasized that the parents' rate of speech was *not* the cause of Oliver's stuttering—it was Oliver's own rate of speech that was causing the problem. Still, the parents could help Oliver feel that he had more time to say what he wanted to say through changes to their own communication patterns.

During the next 3 sessions, the parents observed the clinician making specific changes in her communication patterns while interacting with Oliver. The parents were given opportunities to try the modifications themselves while the clinician provided feedback. At first, the parents found it quite challenging to reduce their speaking rates and increase their pausing, particularly when engaged in free play. They noticed, however, that Oliver tended to speak more fluently when he had more time to say what he wanted to say. As a result, they were encouraged to continue practicing until their ability to adjust their speaking rates improved. Throughout the process, the clinician emphasized that they were not speaking "too fast" and that they were not to blame for Oliver's stuttering.

During the last session of the parent-child training program, the clinician collected data about Oliver's fluency in the clinical setting, as well as parental reports about Oliver's stuttering in other situations. Results indicated that Oliver's fluency had increased significantly, particularly during situations where the parents were utilizing the strategies they had learned in treatment. Specifically, during a parent-child interaction in the therapy room, Oliver exhibited an average of only 2 stuttered disfluencies per 100 words of conversational speech (1% disfluent), a notable decrease from his stuttering frequency during the evaluation. More importantly, the parents also reported that Oliver's fluency had improved in other situations. They indicated that they rarely saw him struggle with his speech during moments of stuttering, and they reported that tension during fluent speech was practically nonexistent. They stated that he still used a relatively rapid rate of speech most of the time, though they noted that he seemed less concerned when he stuttered. They also reported that he was speaking more and telling stories "like he had before." The parents were pleased with his progress, particularly because Oliver was speaking more freely again. Still, they agreed with the clinician that Oliver's continued stuttering indicated the need for ongoing therapy. Thus, child-focused components of treatment were introduced.

## Parent- and Child-Focused Treatment

Throughout the 6 sessions of the parent-child treatment program, as well as the additional 6 sessions of child-focused treatment described next, the clinician discussed other types of stressors that might affect Oliver's speech. One such stressor that the parents identified during the first 2 sessions was that Oliver became easily frustrated when he experienced difficulty performing any task, not just speaking. As a result, they decided that it would be appropriate to model more appropriate, accepting attitudes toward mistakes of all sorts. For example, the parents tried to react in a matter-of-fact, calm manner when they made minor mistakes like missing the basket when throwing clothes in the laundry, putting a dish in the wrong cupboard, picking the wrong type of snack at the grocery store, and so on. Further, they agreed that they would treat disfluencies in Oliver's speech just like other difficulties he might experience in performing complicated tasks. They worked to overcome their concerns about talking about stuttering. They also learned to pay attention to the *content* of Oliver's messages, not just the fluency with which he produced them. This helped Oliver learn that it was okay to have some disruptions in his speech. In time, this made it easier for him to say what he wanted to say without worrying about whether he was saying it smoothly.

### Child-Focused Treatment

The goal of the child-focused components of treatment was primarily to help Oliver reduce his speaking rate when necessary. Treatment did not specifically address physical tension because of the clinician's observations and the parents' confirmation that his tension had already diminished. The clinician started by introducing the concept of speech disfluencies and explained that some children exhibit disruptions in their speech when they are learning to talk. The clinician further explained that Oliver could learn to change those disruptions by changing certain aspects of how he produced speech.

Various rate analogies were introduced as described above (in particular, bicycle riding, shooting baskets, and coloring), and Oliver quickly saw that he had more difficulty performing various activities when he tried to do them too quickly. For example, he learned that he was more likely to miss a shot when he tried to shoot a basket too quickly. The clinician then tied this to speech production by explaining that missing a basket when he tried to shoot too quickly was similar to producing disfluencies when he tried to speak too quickly. The clinician showed Oliver that shooting more slowly (but not *too* slowly) would increase the chance that he could make the basket—and, similarly, talking more slowly (but not *too* slowly) would increase the chance that he could say what he wanted to say.

Treatment continued for 6 sessions, during which the clinician reinforced lessons about rate modification through additional analogies and focused practice. Oliver's response to this aspect of therapy was rapid and positive. He quickly grasped the analogies and demonstrated his understanding by explaining them to his parents. He showed the parents that he could change his speech and repeated that slowing down "makes it easier" to say what he wanted to say. During this time, the clinician took additional data on Oliver's fluency in the clinical setting and continued to probe Oliver's parents about his fluency at home and in other settings.

After 2 sessions, the parents reported that instances of stuttering had diminished further. They stated that they had directly observed Oliver slowing his speaking rate when he was having difficulty maintaining fluency. Following 4 sessions, the parents indicated that they had not seen any stuttering in Oliver's speech and they asked whether Oliver needed to continue in therapy. The clinician stated that she was reluctant to dismiss Oliver too quickly. She asked that the parents monitor Oliver's speech while he attended 4 additional sessions to ensure that gains in fluency were not simply the result of normal fluctuation. The parents had not seen Oliver maintain his fluency for this long a period since he started stuttering but agreed that attending additional sessions would be worthwhile. After 2 sessions they confirmed that Oliver had continued to speak fluently at home and in other situations and expressed their desire to discontinue therapy. The clinician recommended that they maintain contact through weekly phone conferences until Oliver had maintained his fluency for 3 full months following the end of therapy. They maintained contact through 2 months of weekly phone calls, after which they explained that they no longer had any concerns about Oliver's stuttering and did not see the need for further follow-up. The clinician assured them that they could contact her at any time if they had any other concerns about Oliver's stuttering or overall speech and language development.

## Author Note

This case summarized the evaluation and treatment of a preschool child who stuttered. Although certain aspects of the summary were generalized, the examples represent the types of experiences that the clinicians have seen with numerous preschool children who stutter. As the case summary indicates, early intervention for stuttering can be successful in helping children improve their fluency while simultaneously helping them develop appropriate attitudes toward communication.

## References

Ambrose, N. G., Cox, N., & Yairi, E. (1997). The genetic basis of persistence and recovery in stuttering. *Journal of Speech, Language, and Hearing Research, 40,* 567–580.

Ambrose, N. G., Yairi, E., & Cox, N. (1993). Genetic aspects of early childhood stuttering. *Journal of Speech and Hearing Research, 36,* 701–706.

Ambrose, N. G., & Yairi, E. (1999). Normative disfluency data for early childhood stuttering. *Journal of Speech, Language, and Hearing Research, 42,* 895–909.

Anderson, J., Pellowski, M., Conture, E., & Kelly, E. (2003). Temperamental characteristics of young children who stutter. *Journal of Speech, Language, and Hearing Research, 46,* 1221–1233.

Andrews, G., & Harris, M. (1964). *The syndrome of stuttering. Clinics in developmental medicine, 17.* London: Heinemann Medical Books.

Bernstein Ratner, N. (1997). Leaving Las Vegas: Clinical odds and individual outcomes. *American Journal of Speech-Language Pathology, 6,* 29–33.

Bernstein Ratner, N. (1992). Measurable outcomes of instructions to change maternal speech style to children. *Journal of Speech and Hearing Research, 35,* 14–20.

Bloodstein, O., & Ratner, N. B. (2008). *A handbook on stuttering* (6th ed.). Clifton Park, NY: Thomson/Delmar.

Conture, E. G. (2001). *Stuttering: Its nature, diagnosis and treatment.* Boston: Allyn & Bacon.

Cooper, E. B., & Cooper, C. S. (1985). Clinician attitudes toward stuttering: A decade of change (1973–1983). *Journal of Fluency Disorders, 10,* 19–33.

Cooper, E. B., & Cooper, C. S. (1996). Clinician attitudes towards stuttering: Two decades of change. *Journal of Fluency Disorders, 21,* 119–136.

Curlee, R. F., & Yairi, E. (1997). Early intervention with early childhood stuttering: A critical examination of the data. *American Journal of Speech-Language Pathology, 6,* 8–18.

Dworzynski, K., Remington, A., Rijsdijk, F., Howell, P., & Plomin, R. (2007). Genetic etiology in cases of recovered and persistent stuttering in an unselected, longitudinal sample of young twins. *American Journal of Speech-Language Pathology, 16*(2), 169–178.

Ezrati-Vinacour, R., Platzky, R., & Yairi, E. (2001). The young child's awareness of stuttering-like disfluency. *Journal of Speech, Language, and Hearing Research, 44,* 368–80.

Goldman, R., & Fristoe, M. (2000). *Goldman-Fristoe Test of Articulation–2.* Minneapolis, MN: Pearson Assessments.

Gottwald, S., & Starkweather, C. W. (1995). Fluency intervention for preschoolers and their families in the public schools. *Language, Speech and Hearing Services in Schools, 26,* 117–126.

Guitar, B. & Marchinkoski, L. (2001). Influence of mothers' slower speech on their children's speech rate. *Journal of Speech, Language, and Hearing Research, 44,* 853–861.

Guitar, B., Schaefer, H. K., Donahue-Kilburg, G., & Bond, L. (1992). Parent verbal interactions and speech rate. *Journal of Speech and Hearing Research, 35,* 742–754.

Harris, V., Onslow, M., Packman, A., Harrison, E., & Menzies, R. (2002). An experimental investigation of the impact of the Lidcombe Program on early stuttering. *Journal of Fluency Disorders, 27*(3), 203–214.

Healey, E. C., & Scott, L. A. (1995). Strategies for treating elementary school-age children who stutter: An integrative approach. *Language, Speech, and Hearing Services in Schools, 26,* 151–161.

Hill, D. (2003). Differential treatment of stuttering in the early stages of development. In H. Gregory, *Stuttering therapy: Rationale and procedures* (pp. 142–185). Boston: Allyn & Bacon.

Johnson, W. (1949). An open letter to a mother of a stuttering child. *Journal of Speech and Hearing Disorders, 14,* 3–8.

Johnson & Associates. (1959). *The onset of stuttering.* Minneapolis, MN: University of Minnesota Press.

Kelman, E., & Nicholas, A. (2008). *Practical intervention for early childhood stammering: Palin PCI.* Milton Keynes, England: Speechmark.

Logan, K. J., & Yaruss, J. S. (1999). Helping parents address attitudinal and emotional factors with young children who stutter. *Contemporary Issues in Communication Science and Disorders, 26,* 69–81.

Meyers, S. C., & Woodford, L. L. (1992). *The fluency development system for young children.* Buffalo, NY: United Educational Services.

Millard, S., Nicholas, A., & Cook, F. (2008). Is parent-child interaction therapy effective in reducing stuttering? *Journal of Speech, Language, and Hearing Research, 51*(3), 636–650.

Newman, L. L. & Smit, A. B. (1989). Some effects of variations in response time latency on speech rate, interruptions, and fluency in children's speech. *Journal of Speech and Hearing Research, 32,* 635–644.

Onslow, M., Andrews, C., & Lincoln, M. (1994). A control/experimental trial of an operant treatment for early stuttering. *Journal of Speech and Hearing Research, 37,* 1244–1259.

Onslow, M., Costa, L., Andrews, C., Harrison, E., & Packman, A. (1996). Speech outcomes of a prolonged-speech treatment for stuttering. *Journal of Speech and Hearing Research,* 39(4), 734–49.

Onslow, M., Packman, A., & Harrison, E. (2003). *The Lidcombe Program of early stuttering intervention.* Austin, TX: PRO-ED.

Perkins, W. H. (1990). What is stuttering? *Journal of Speech and Hearing Disorders, 55,* 379–382.

Pindzola, R., Jenkins, M., & Lokken, K. (1989). Speaking rates of young children. *Language, Speech, and Hearing Services in Schools, 20,* 133–138.

Ramig, P. R., & Bennett, E. M. (1995). Working with 7-12 year old children who stutter: Ideas for intervention in the public schools. *Language, Speech and Hearing Services in Schools, 26,* 138–150.

Ramig, P. R., & Bennett, E. M. (1997). Clinical management of children: Direct management strategies. In R. F. Curlee & G. M. Siegel (Eds.), *Nature and treatment of stuttering: New directions* (2nd ed., pp. 292–312). Needham Heights, MA: Allyn & Bacon.

Ramig, P. R., & Dodge, D. M. (2005). *The child and adolescent stuttering treatment and activity resource guide*. Clifton Park, NY: Thompson Delmar Learning.

Reardon-Reeves, N. A., & Yaruss, J. S. (2004). *The source for stuttering: Ages 7–18.* East Moline, IL: LinguiSystems.

Runyan, C. M., & Runyan, S. E. (1993). A Fluency Rules therapy program for school-age stutterers: An update on the Fluency Rules program. In R. Curlee (Ed.), *Stuttering and related disorders of fluency* (pp. 101–114). New York: Thieme Medical Publishers.

Rustin, L., Botterill, W., & Kelman, E. (1996). *Assessment and therapy for young disfluent children: Family interaction.* London: Whurr.

St. Louis, K. O., & Durrenberger, C. H. (1993). What communication disorders do experienced clinicians prefer to manage? *ASHA, 35,* 23–31.

Starkweather, C. W., Gottwald, C., & Halfond, M. (1990). *Stuttering prevention: A clinical method.* Englewood Cliffs, NJ: Prentice-Hall.

Stephenson-Opsal, D. & Bernstein Ratner, N. (1988). Maternal speech rate modification and childhood stuttering. *Journal of Fluency Disorders, 13(1),* 49–56.

Suresh, R., Ambrose, N., Roe, C., Pluzhnikov, A., Wittke-Thompson, J. K., Ng, M. C., et al. (2006). New complexities in the genetics of stuttering: Significant sex-specific linkage signals. *American Journal of Human Genetics, 78*(4), 554–563.

Vanryckeghem, M., Brutten, G., & Hernandez, L. M. (2005). A comparative investigation of the speech-associated attitude of preschool and kindergarten children who do and do not stutter. *Journal of Fluency Disorders, 30,* 307–318.

Walker, J., Archibald, L., Cherniak, S., & Fish, V. (1992). Articulation rate in 3- and 5- year-old children. *Journal of Speech and Hearing Research, 35,* 4–13.

Walton, P., & Wallace, M. (1998). *Fun with fluency: Direct therapy with the young child.* Bisbee, AZ: Imaginart.

Wiig, E., Secord, W., & Semel, E. (2004). *Clinical Evaluation of Language Fundamentals–Preschool* (2nd ed.). San Antonio, TX: The Psychological Corporation.

Williams, D. (1985) Talking with children who stutter. In J. Fraser (Ed.), *Counseling stutterers* (pp. 35–45). Memphis, TN: Stuttering Foundation of America.

Winslow, M., & Guitar, B. (1994). The effects of structured turn-taking on disfluencies: A case study. *Language, Speech, and Hearing Services in Schools, 25,* 251–257.

Yairi, E., & Ambrose, N. (1999). Early childhood stuttering I: Persistency and recovery rates. *Journal of Speech, Language, and Hearing Research, 42,* 1097–1112.

Yairi, E., Ambrose, N., & Cox, N. (1996). Genetics of stuttering: A critical review. *Journal of Speech and Hearing Research, 39,* 771–784.

Yairi, E., Ambrose, N., Paden, E., & Throneburg, R. (1996). Predictive factors of persistence and recovery: Pathways of childhood stuttering. *Journal of Communication Disorders, 29*(1), 51–77.

Yaruss, J. S. (1997a). Clinical implications of situational variability in preschool children who stutter. *Journal of Fluency Disorders, 22,* 187–203.

Yaruss, J. S. (1997b). Clinical measurement of stuttering behaviors. *Contemporary Issues in Communication Science and Disorders, 24,* 33–44.

Yaruss, J. S. (1998). Real-time analysis of speech fluency: Procedures and reliability training. *American Journal of Speech-Language Pathology,* 7(2), 25–37.

Yaruss, J. S. (2008). *Too much, too little, just right.* Eleventh International Stuttering Awareness Day (ISAD) On-line Conference.

Yaruss, J. S., Coleman, C., & Hammer, D. (2006). Treating preschool children who stutter: Description and preliminary evaluation of family-focused treatment approach. *Language, Speech and Hearing Services in the Schools, 37,* 118–136.

Yaruss, J. S., LaSalle, L., & Conture, E. (1998). Evaluating stuttering in young children.

American Journal of Speech-Language Pathology, 7, 62–76.
Yaruss, J. S., & Quesal, R. W. (2004). Stuttering and the International Classification of Functioning, Disability, and Health (ICF): An update. *Journal of Communication Disorders, 37,* 35–52.
Zebrowski, P. M., & Schum, R. L. (1993). Counseling parents of children who stutter. *American Journal of Speech-Language Pathology, 2,* 65–73.
Zebrowski, P. M. , Weiss, A. L., Savelkoul, E. M., & Hammer, C. S. (1996). The effect of maternal rate reduction on the stuttering, speech rates and linguistic productions of children who stutter: Evidence from individual dyads. *Clinical Linguistics & Phonetics, 10(3),* 189–206.

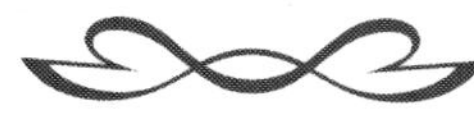

## HEARING

# CASE 17

# Amy: Late Identification of Hearing Loss: A Real-World Story of How a Child Can Fall Through the Cracks

*Paul M. Brueggeman*

## Conceptual Knowledge Areas

According to the U.S. Census Bureau, 5 of the 10 poorest counties in the United States are in South Dakota. The county where this Native American reservation exists is an example. Over 80% of its population is Native American, with over a third of the population living below the poverty level. The population density is quite sparse, with only 6.5 people per square mile. This may seem like a small number, but the average population density for South Dakota in general is 9.9 people per square mile. This county comprises an area that is over 1,000 square miles, so travel to any health care facility can be challenging. Teen pregnancy rates and high school dropout rates are above the national average on this reservation. There is also a well-documented gang problem among teenagers. This is a challenging environment in which to raise children and to find access to appropriate specialty health care in a timely fashion.

The field of audiology is working to lower the age at which permanent hearing loss is identified. Through appropriate universal newborn hearing screening (UNHS) programs, professionals are able to identify most congenital hearing loss early and intervene before hearing loss causes a speech and language delay. Close adherence to recommendations of the Joint Committee on Infant Hearing (JCIH, 2007) by all physicians in the medical community would better ensure that children with hearing loss were not lost in the system. Rural populations, such as those described in this case, are particularly isolated from specialty care related to hearing disorders. Professions other than audiology often have the responsibility for conducting informal "hearing screenings." Unfortunately, these screenings often miss milder forms of hearing loss, and children with hearing loss become lost in the very system of screenings and assessments that is designed to help identify developmentally significant permanent hearing loss.

# Description of the Case

## Background Information

Items that appear in this case study in quotations are direct quotes taken from a recorded interview with the mother, which occurred when Amy was 6 years, 4 months old. This section begins by describing some of Amy's early developmental history and then proceeds to the time when the audiologist first visited with Amy and her mother.

Amy was born full-term at a local hospital weighing 7 lbs, 4 oz. Amy's mother had an uncomplicated pregnancy and received normal prenatal care. At 3 days of age, Amy was rechecked for jaundice due to a concern noted when she was born. The results of this recheck were normal. In South Dakota, newborn hearing screening is not required by law and there is no legal repercussion if a facility does not offer this service. The initial newborn hearing screening performed at the hospital resulted in a "fail" on the screening otoacoustic emission test. Amy's mother was told by the nurse that performed the test that this was because her ear canals were too small. There was no evidence that Amy's ear canals were ever smaller than normal, and no record of a stenosis of the ear canal was provided. Amy was rescheduled for a follow-up newborn hearing screening and failed two subsequent follow-up hearing screenings in her first 2 months of life using transient otoacoustic emissions (TEOAEs). Her mother recalled being told by the physician to "bring her back in a few years and we'll test her again." The JCIH (2007) guidelines for the identification of newborn hearing loss indicate that an immediate referral for an auditory brainstem response (ABR) test to rule out sensorineural hearing loss was in order.

This audiologist first met Amy and her mother at a developmental clinic on a Native American reservation in South Dakota when Amy was 5 years, 3 months old. This is a grant-funded clinic that provides assessments to children age birth through five years on reservation lands. Assessments offered are speech and language, audiology, psychology, nutrition, and others, including quarterly 2-day audiology clinics. The audiologist provides approximately 65 hearing evaluations for children at this one clinic each year. Due to the geography of South Dakota access to specialty health care can be an issue. This is particularly true on reservation lands in western South Dakota. It is not uncommon for families to travel over 40 miles (one way) to have access to health care for their children.

Accompanying the audiologist to this clinic were two doctoral students. One student was in her first year of study for her AuD degree, and the other was in her second year of doctoral study. The University of South Dakota (USD) department has a unique junior/senior clinician model, in which second-year students act as mentors who work alongside faculty in providing supervision and guidance to first-year clinical students. The reservation developmental clinic is housed in a double-wide trailer house converted into clinical space. There are several permanent staff who assist families, provide transportation for families who need specialty care outside of the tribal land area, provide in-home consultations, and perform initial screenings for developmental and other related problems. A wonderful benefit of this clinic is the home-like environment, which includes a cook who is busy throughout the day preparing meals for visiting families.

Services are provided to families who are concerned about their child's development (including hearing concerns) in a relaxed atmosphere where they feel safe and free to share their concerns. It is not uncommon for the staff to wait until the children finish some yogurt or oatmeal before testing begins. Flexibility is the key at these clinics, and that is a learning process in itself for students. Caregivers are asked about the whole family, which is appreciated by most families in this culture. This assists the staff in understanding each family's unique needs and helps to keep in perspective that scheduling an appointment to get cerumen (ear wax) out of a grandson's ear may not be a family's first priority.

It is not unusual for the caregiver accompanying a Native American child to be an aunt, uncle, mother, great-uncle, grandmother, father, or grandfather. It is customary to ask about the relationship between caregiver and child because of how common it is for the network of care to be far-reaching and multigenerational. Before the AuD students travel to these clinics, they receive information regarding Native American culture. This is quite important as the students often do not have the knowledge or experience important to appreciate Native American culture.

## History Information

Amy's mother discussed the instance she first suspected that her daughter had a hearing loss: "She was probably about 4 days old when she had already failed two screening tests, and, well . . . by 6 months, I knew definitely. My mom even pulled me out of the room when we were trying to get her to respond to our clapping and she was, like . . . 'she can't hear, but she can at least see you cry and you don't want her to see that you are scared. . . .' But, yeah . . . I knew early on before all the doctors did." Amy had the normal colds, diaper rashes, runny noses, and coughs and received appropriate medical care when these occurred. She did not have any major medical problems and was generally a very healthy baby.

Amy had her first bilateral ear infection when she was 5 months old and continued to have chronic bilateral middle-ear infections (otitis media) for the next 7 months, which were continuously treated with antibiotics six more times during her first year. A medical examination when Amy was 1 year old included the diagnosis of bilateral otitis media, though the physician noted that "Amy's hearing is grossly intact." During this time, Amy's mother was becoming increasingly worried about Amy's hearing sensitivity, as she noticed that "I would clap my hands and she would just look straight ahead and I would clap over here and she was not getting it. It was scaring me."

By her report, the mother pleaded with her physician on multiple occasions to give her a referral for an ENT or audiologic consult, but was not provided with a "purple card." "Purple cards," as they are referred to by many patients in this area, are referral approval cards for specialty services covered by Medicaid. When asked why she believed she did not get a referral, Amy's mother responded, "I don't think they [physicians] are educated enough about hearing loss to know what to pick up on. . . . They don't have the equipment or the knowledge." Amy's mother went on to say, "Yeah, I mean, it was like . . . I was on a deserted island and the place I needed to go . . . I could see it and knew that it was there, but I just didn't have the bridge to get there. I would ask people and they never knew who I should go to." Amy's mother finally sought specialty care on her own. She had not heard of an "audiologist" before she had her daughter tested as outlined in the following section.

## Previous Audiologic and Related Testing Related to Amy's Case

Amy first had an audiology evaluation when she was 15 months old at the closest audiology clinic to her home, located 100 miles away. On that date Amy had been pulling on her right ear and was not responding to sounds coming from the right side. Tympanometric results were normal, but acoustic reflex testing and otoacoustic emission screening was not completed due to Amy's activity level. The primary recommendation from the audiologist was to follow up with a sedated auditory brainstem response test, with soundfield visual reinforcement audiometry (VRA) testing noted secondarily. Certainly, as pointed out by Thompson (1984), VRA testing could have been attempted on this date of testing.

Amy's second audiologic evaluation was completed at the same clinic when she was 16 months old. It was noted in the case history on test day that Amy was saying "mama, dad, tada, shut up, later, tic-tic, hot." Otoscopy revealed slightly vascular (red) tympanic membranes (eardrums) bilaterally. Tympanometry revealed negative middle-ear pressure at –200 daPa in both ears with normal compliance of the eardrums. Acoustic reflex testing revealed absent reflexes from 500 to 4,000 Hz bilaterally and a "fail" result on the otoactoustic emission (OAE) screening in both ears. No behavioral hearing assessment was attempted. The audiologist did complete a sedated auditory brainstem response (ABR) test, which included the use of 29.3 and 19.3 click rates as well as 500 Hz tone burst stimuli. The evaluation revealed identifiable wave V latencies down to 40 dBnHL for click stimuli and 35 dBnHL for 500 Hz tone-burst stimuli. It was noted that sound-field behavioral testing was not attempted because Amy was too groggy after the sedated ABR to respond in the sound-treated audiologic booth. Amy's mother was told that the test results were consistent with a very mild hearing loss that was suggestive of an upward (more in the low frequencies) sloping hearing loss. The report from this date notes, "While the ABR results would suggest a possible sensorineural component, the bilateral negative middle ear pressure causes me to pause before declaring today's results sensorineural in nature. Certainly, we have absent acoustic reflexes and failed OAEs. However, we can have these with this amount of negative middle ear pressure. It is also possible to have hearing sensitivity affected more in one region than the other due to changes in middle ear pressure." The two recommendations noted on this date included a consultation with an ENT physician regarding Amy's middle ear status and a reevaluation of hearing in 3 months to include repeat tympanometry, OAEs, and sound-field behavioral testing.

A panel of clinical and academic audiologists completed a retrospective review of this case. An overwhelming majority of them found some major discrepancies in how they would interpret the original sedated ABR (and subsequent) sedated ABR test findings. There was considerable artifact error in the low-level stimuli ABR recordings, but the wave V latency found, even at lower intensity levels, is indeed consistent with a sensorineural pathology, not conductive pathology, which was suggested by the audiologist on this date. Conductive pathologies tend to have much longer wave V latencies, versus what is considered to be in the normative range for sensorineural pathologies. The consensus of the review panel was that the test results at the lowest level in which click-ABR results were present was 50 dBnHL in the left ear and 45 dBnHL in the right ear, an indication of the hearing sensitivity in the higher frequency region. Additionally, the lowest 500 Hz tone-burst stimuli level where responses were reliably seen (in retrospect) was at 45 dBnHL in the right ear and 40 dBnHL in the left ear with absent OAEs and absent acoustic reflexes. The interwave latencies, interaural latency differences, morphology, and absolute latencies of the waveforms were interpreted to be consistent with the recommendations published by Hall (2006). At the ENT consultation, held 100 miles from the family's home, the decision was made to place PE (pressure equalization) tubes in both of Amy's ears when she was 18 months old. After Amy received PE tubes, her mother reported that "She got the tubes and . . . I wouldn't have to speak so loudly or look so directly at her so much . . . but I still had to be in close range. So it didn't, like, open them up like I thought it would have, but it did it enough to where the ear infections were coming down to a minimum." Her hearing was not tested, and in fact, over a year went by before Amy returned to the same audiology clinic for follow-up testing. Amy's mother again had difficulty obtaining a referral for specialty (audiologic) evaluation. There also were problems with missed appointments and rescheduling during this period.

Amy was finally reevaluated at the same audiology clinic at 27 months of age. Between 16 and 27 months of age, no speech, language, or hearing evaluations were administered. The decision was made to repeat the sedated ABR. Otoscopy revealed purulent (pus-like) discharge from the right PE tube and an open PE tube in the left eardrum. Tympanometry was performed and results were consistent with an "occluded PE tube with material behind the eardrum" in the right ear and "an open tube that is functioning" in the left ear. There were some issues getting Amy sedated with chlorohydrate on this day, as it was noted it took over 45 minutes for it to "take effect." The results of the sedated ABR for the right ear were described as "no response was obtained at 60 dBnHL suggesting that we have at least a moderate conductive loss in the high frequencies." Amy woke up before 500 Hz tone-burst testing could be performed; however, according to the audiologist, "the last testing revealed responses that would suggest normal hearing in the low frequencies." The results of the sedated ABR for Amy's left ear were described as "able to follow wave V down to 30 dBnHL, which indicated hearing in about the 20–25 dBHL range for mid and high frequencies in the left ear." The audiologist noted that bone conduction testing was not performed because "Amy woke up from the sedation." In the discussion section, the audiologist stated that "we continue to have an incomplete picture of Amy's hearing sensitivity, and because she does not pass on OAE screenings, we feel compelled to arrive at a better picture of her hearing status." No specific recommendations were made for follow-up, except that "we will discuss our experiences with chlorohydrate today with Amy's physician." There was no attempt made to obtain behavioral hearing test information. The American Speech-Language-Hearing Association (ASHA, 2004) points out how important it is to test a child's hearing behaviorally at this age. Amy was over 2 years old and should have been able to respond behaviorally via visual reinforcement audiometry (VRA) or play audiometry.

Amy was reevaluated at the same audiology clinic when she was 30 months of age to repeat the sedated ABR. Amy's mother stated on this date that Amy was saying more words than during the previous assessment. She also reported that Amy was forming short sentences, such as "I said no!" However, Amy's mother and others indicated that many of Amy's words were not understood by others. It was reported that Amy had many articulation errors. Otoscopy revealed that the PE tubes were in place, but appeared occluded. Tympanometric results confirmed that the PE tubes were occluded and that they obtained "normal" middle ear mobility on this measure, evidence that the PE tubes were plugged. The sedated ABR done reportedly showed normal wave V responses to 19.3/sec and 29.3/sec condensation and rarefaction click stimuli down to 20 dBnHL bilaterally. It was noted that the results of the 500 Hz tone-burst ABR test would be consistent with normal hearing sensitivity in the low frequencies. Amy's mother was told that the results suggested or correlated with normal hearing sensitivity. The audiologist noted, "We do know that Amy has struggled with middle ear problems for quite some time. This may have contributed to her speech and language delays. It would be advisable to have her screened for her speech/language development."

These final ABR results were reviewed retrospectively by a panel of academic and clinical audiologists. The results of this retrospective review were quite different from that of the original interpretation from the clinical audiologist who performed the ABR. This panel believed that there were no ABR responses to click stimuli below 40 dBnHL and to tone-burst stimuli below 45 dBnHL in either ear. The panel found that Amy's hearing loss was misdiagnosed as "normal hearing," which seriously delayed the initiation of intervention and treatment. This was the last hearing test performed before this audiologist first saw Amy and her mother 33 months later, when Amy was 5 years, 3 months. It should be noted that no behavioral testing of any kind was attempted up to this point and there had never been a record of present OAEs or acoustic reflexes.

At 42 months of age, Amy's speech and language development was evaluated by a speech-language pathologist in the local school district due to concerns by Amy's mother that "people don't understand Amy at times." The Goldman-Fristoe Test of Articulation-2 was administered and results showed an age-equivalent for single words at 3 years, 2 months (SS ~ 96, RS ~ 25). During conversation, it was noted that Amy used younger speech patterns; however, only single-words were evaluated on this date. Some of the noted errors included /d/ for /g/, /t/ for /k/, /h/ for /t/, /s/ for /th/, final /s/ deletions, and /tl/ for /sl/. Lakota was the primary language spoken in the home, which could have influenced these findings. It was recommended that her progress be monitored.

## Reason for Referral

The audiologist was scheduled to attend a 2-day developmental clinic at the Native American reservation center that was described earlier. Typically he sees children ages birth through 5 years; however, he was told that there was a mother who was concerned that her 5-year old daughter might have a hearing loss. The presenting complaint from Amy's mother was that "Amy says 'huh' a lot, and . . . turns up the TV and headphones way too loud."

## Findings of the Evaluation

The audiologist interviewed Amy's mother about her daughter's hearing, academic, and medical history. Amy spoke quite loudly and seemed not to have the type of normal suprasegmentals (rate, stress, pitch, etc.) expected of a girl her age. She had many articulation errors (particularly high-frequency phonemes) and appeared to be quite hypernasal. These behaviors, combined with her mother's concerns, raised serious "red flags." The audiologist did not yet know anything about the previous testing conducted at other clinics.

A test battery approach, such as that advocated by Diefendorf (1998), was implemented combining both objective and subjective test measures to ensure an accurate measurement of hearing. Results of the audiology testing were as follows:

- Otoscopy: Normal-appearing eardrum landmarks and clear ear canals bilaterally.
- Tympanometry: Testing revealed normal ear canal volumes, middle ear compliance, and tympanometric width bilaterally. Middle ear pressure was recorded at –250 to –265 daPa in both ears.
- Pure Tone Audiometry: Air-conduction testing performed using ER-3A insert earphones revealed a gently sloping (nearly flat) mild to moderate hearing loss bilaterally. Masked bone-conduction testing revealed slight (5–15dB) air-bone gaps at 500 Hz and 1,000 Hz bilaterally. Because of this, the hearing loss was referred to as a mixed type. Amy was able to raise her hand very consistently throughout testing, and as such, test reliability was deemed to be very good. Speech reception thresholds, which were within 5 dB of agreement with Amy's three-frequency pure-tone average (PTA), were recorded at 40 dBHL in the right ear and at 45 dBHL in the left ear.

## Representation of the Problem at the Time of the Evaluation

Following the audiologic evaluation, the results were discussed with Amy and her mother. The audiologist began, "I am sorry, but I have some potentially bad news for you. The results of today's testing are consistent with a hearing loss that has mostly a permanent component." At this point, Amy's mother cried and said, "I knew it, I always knew it. . . . I should have just trusted myself." She was visibly upset about the way her daughter's case had been handled in the past. She said that she had told doctors for years that her daughter could not hear, and that whenever she was tested there always seemed to be something that "clouded" the accuracy of the results.

Amy's mother was interviewed a year after this visit. She recollected,

> I was thinking that day you told me about Amy's hearing, like . . . Did I not take care of myself well enough when I was pregnant? Did I do something while I was pregnant? Like, I ate a lot of hot sauce . . . does that matter? . . . I know it sounds crazy, but you blame yourself for ruining your child, you know. . . . I exercised. . . . I didn't drink or smoke. . . . but you feel so guilty for what happened, you try to find a way to blame yourself. I see other moms drinking while they are pregnant and all this other stuff. You know, what made me so mad is that I did it by the book. Where the **** do other moms get off screwing up their kid's life? You know, it is like I felt I was being punished, like I did something so bad that my kid is being punished too for it. You think of your child of being nothing but perfect . . . then this happens and it's like getting punched in the stomach so hard. I love my kids, so much. . . . I just felt like I'd killed my kid. I was really down . . . I didn't have any help; I didn't know where to go after that day. . . . When they [the field of audiology] says it flips your world upside down, oh . . . it does! There is no way to prepare. But I am glad now that she is taken care of and she is all good now. . . . I remember that day because it was real hard on me and when we sat down at home, Amy asked if hearing aids are going to help and I said "I hope so. . . . " Amy said "Okay," then rubbed my back, gave me a kiss, and said she loved me. . . . I cried for a really long time.

## Treatment Options Considered

### Client Preferences

Four primary recommendations were made after the audiologic evaluation was completed. First, given Amy's articulation errors, an updated speech and language evaluation was requested through her local school district. Second, Amy should be evaluated by an ENT physician due to the small conductive component in her hearing loss and the unknown cause of the permanent sensorineural hearing loss. Third, Amy should have a follow-up hearing evaluation at a regional audiology clinic. Based upon the results of the hearing evaluation and ENT consult, the determination to continue with a hearing aid evaluation at that clinic would be decided. It was felt that Amy would be an appropriate candidate for bilateral BTE hearing aids, but follow-up medical clearance and testing was warranted to better define the nature of her hearing loss. That is, a determination was needed about whether a portion of her loss was medically treatable or whether her hearing loss was stable or going to progress. The fourth recommendation was for Amy and her mother to return to this clinic for (at least) annual hearing evaluations after the hearing aids were ordered and fit to her hearing loss at the other regional audiology clinic.

## Course of Treatment

Nineteen days after this audiologist tested Amy's hearing, she was seen at a local audiology clinic for a follow-up hearing test. The results of this test were consistent with the behavioral findings. Amy's mother was motivated to start the process of acquiring hearing aids for her daughter, so hearing aid options were discussed on this date at this same clinic. It was decided that bilateral mini-BTE hearing aids (pink in color) would be ordered as well as custom earmolds with pink sparkles. The hearing aids that were ordered have direct-audio inputs (DAIs) that can work to link outside inputs (such as a personal FM system) to them. Amy was quite excited about her new hearing aids, as was her mother. The next month, Amy was fit with her new hearing aids. As a standard of care, real-ear verification of the frequency response, gain, and output were performed at the regional audiology clinic. After the optimum gain setting was obtained for soft, moderate, and loud inputs, the volume control was disabled so that it would be held at a constant level.

## Analysis of Client's Response to Intervention

Amy's mother's recollection of the day of the hearing aid fitting, as well as the months that followed, is filled with many successes and a few disappointments. When the audiologist first turned the programmed hearing aids on, Amy said, "Wow, mom, they're kind of loud!" She stood in front of the mirror just looking at them. Amy's mother recalled,

> Every day when she first had them we would tell her how pretty she was with them because some days when she first got them she would say, "I don't want to wear them." . . . I would be like, Amy, you are so pretty with them on, everybody is just jealous of you; they want your hearing aids. Then, she would slap them in!

Following the initial hearing aid fitting, they went to Wal-Mart to get her a gift. There was an elderly woman at the checkout, and Amy said to her, "Look at my new hearing aids, I can hear you now!" Amy's mother reported that their joke on the trip back home was a game of "Can you hear me now?" (like the current cell phone commercials on television). When asked to recall when she noticed Amy's speech and language changing, she stated,

> Oh, it was like a matter of a week, not even a week, and her vocabulary changed. I mean, I am not kidding, just like that! Also, the day she got the hearing aids in, I was talking to her the same I had been for the past 5 years and Amy was like, "Whoa! Mom, I can hear you!" Then, I was like, "Oh, my, I am so sorry!" And then, within like a week we were still seeing more and more "words" from her.

Amy had to teach her dad and grandpa how to care for the hearing aids, because at first they did not know what it meant when they squealed. When asked what her family thinks of the hearing aids, Amy's mother reported,

> We all think it is the greatest thing in the world, except a few of the distant relatives that were initially shocked and were like "oh my gosh," like they had never seen a hearing aid. They just had never seen a child with hearing aids. They have always seen a child with glasses but never a child with hearing aids. Well, now my family is totally on board in helping Amy with her hearing aids.

Amy's mother was asked about her impression of how hearing loss is viewed in the Native American culture. She reported,

> Well, I know how a few people are. One of my really good friends used to act like she loved my kids and thought my kids were great. The day she saw Amy with her hearing aids she said, "Oh, I am so sorry that this happened to you guys and I am so sorry that you had to put those on her head." I was like, "Excuse me? I don't know who the h#@! you think you are, but my kid is beautiful. My kid has hearing aids. There isn't a damn thing wrong with her, she just can't hear well." I said this to Amy later, and she said, "Yep, mom, I know!"

Amy's mother recalled,

> The first day when Amy got her hearing aids, it was like the big talk in grade school because the other kids did not know what Amy was going to get. The teacher told the other children that Amy had something really big that she had to do. So, everybody in her class was all curious. I took her into the classroom and I wanted to stay and make sure that no one was going to make fun of her because she was my kid and I was going to back her up. But she walked in and showed the teachers and said . . . "Look at my hearing aid," and the teacher said "Wow!" and all the little girls came up to her in the classroom and said, "I want them too!" These girls went home and told their mom and dad they wanted hearing aids just like Amy. They thought they were the coolest. So, she never had a problem there [at school], but then, you know, as kids get older they tend to get mean. There are a few kids that bother her about it, but we taught her to tell them, "I am just the same as you are . . . I just can't hear well," and that shuts them up, I guess [laughing]. She has never had a problem. . . . Amy told her teacher how she likes things done with her hearing aids, where she sits and about where the teacher is. So, then . . . after that, Amy got the freedom to sit wherever."
>
> Amy is the only Native American student in her grade, and "even before she got the hearing aids, that was a big step for her to deal with because everybody would look at her [because of her color] everywhere she would go. All the kids now think she is just fine and it's not an issue."

Amy's mother reported,

> After a while, the hearing aids just became routine. I didn't let her mess with them at first because it is an expensive piece of equipment. . . . You know, I got to protect that. I didn't let her mess with them at first a whole lot, but then as she got used to them more and whenever I would clean them or take out the battery she would ask, "Well, mom, what's that, how come you are doing that?" Then, the batteries (size 13) come with cool little sticker things she loved and always wanted to do something with. So, she puts her own batteries in her aids and then she'll turn them on and say "I can hear you, mom!" Now, she gets up in the morning and puts on her robe. This is just so we can have coffee together. Or, she'll be like, "Oh wait, mom, I have to put in my hearing aids" and then she'll come down and give me a hug with them in! I love her.

Almost immediately after Amy was fit with hearing aids, a PLS-4 (Preschool Language Scale) and Battelle Developmental Inventory was administered by the school district, which revealed that her receptive and expressive language fell 1.5 standard deviations below the mean, which qualified her for speech and language therapy services within the school district. Amy was also qualified for services under South Dakota law as a child with hearing impairment. She began language therapy for her receptive and expressive delays, and her teacher performed daily amplification checks. Her speech and language skills continued to develop. Even though her parents separated, they provided a very supportive parenting environment for her. She continued to excel in school and enjoyed playing with her peers.

When asked what she would like to say to future audiology and speech pathology students, Amy's mother reported that audiologists should

> Always listen to a parent. Never force anything really scary on a kid and get to know the kid for what they are. Now that I have said that, please always listen to the parent. A parent spends way more time with that kid than anybody else with the kid. I think if I would have had somebody that would have listened to me early on, we probably could have gotten this [intervention] all done sooner. If they would just have taken an extra 5 minutes and listened to me, they would have definitely gotten to the source of Amy's problem a lot quicker. I mean, it was like Amy was the first Native American kid to ever get hearing aids. Nobody seemed to know that I knew anything.

## Author Note

This material was based on a real case that occurred in South Dakota in 2007 through 2008. The words quoted are the real words of a mother of a child with hearing loss. With permission, the interview of Amy's mother's account of her daughter's case was digitally recorded. Permission was received from the parent as well as the tribal committee where Amy's mother resides. All of the events listed are real, as are the people, test results, and emotions. It is hoped that the depth of feeling associated with this case is communicated to the reader.

## References


American Speech-Language-Hearing Association. (2004). *Guidelines for the audiologic assessment of children from birth to 5 years of age* [Guidelines]. Available from www.asha.org/policy.

Diefendorf, A. O. (1998). The test battery approach in pediatric audiology. In F. H. Bess (Ed.), *Children with hearing impairment* (pp. 71–81). Nashville, TN: Vanderbilt Bill Wilkerson Center Press.

Hall, J. W. (2006). *New handbook of auditory evoked responses*. Boston: Allyn & Bacon.

Joint Committee on Infant Hearing (JCIH). (2007). Year 2007 position statement: Principles and guidelines for early hearing detection and intervention programs. *Pediatrics 120*(4), 898–921.

Thompson, G., & Wilson, W. (1984). Clinical application of visual reinforcement audiometry. *Seminars in Hearing, 5,* 85.


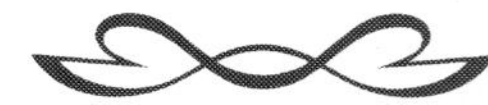

**LANGUAGE/SLI**

# CASE 18

# Tessa: A Preschool Child with a Specific Language Impairment


*Tiffany P. Hogan, Mindy Sittner Bridges, Carole Wymer, and Rebecca Volk*


## Conceptual Knowledge Areas

Everyone loves a good mystery. Children with specific language impairment (SLI) represent an intriguing mystery in the field of speech-language pathology. Children with SLI have a "specific" language deficit despite normal cognitive development and adequate language stimulation. Herein lies the mystery: Why do these children have difficulty learning language when all other key components to language development appear to be present? Moreover, these children are not rare. Approximately 7–10% of children in kindergarten have SLI (e.g., Tomblin et al., 1997). Children are affected across race and socioeconomic boundaries (Tomblin, 1996).

Children with SLI have historically been diagnosed using both inclusionary and exclusionary criteria. The inclusionary criterion is an impairment in language learning. The exclusionary criteria comprise possible reasons for the observed language impairment: cognitive deficits, hearing impairments, adverse environmental factors, neuromuscular disabilities, or severe emotional disorders. Operationally, children are diagnosed with SLI if they have *impaired* language and *normal* nonverbal intelligence.[1] In essence, children with SLI develop normally except in the area of language. In fact, Leonard (1998) noted that the "only thing clearly abnormal about these children is that they don't learn language rapidly and effortlessly" (p. 3).

> **Clinical note:** School-based speech-language pathologists (SLPs) "have never embraced" (Kamhi, 2007, p. 366) the use of nonverbal IQ assessments. In fact, some believe that cognitive testing is not within the scope of practice for SLPs. As such, diagnoses of SLI according to language and nonverbal intelligence scores are common in research but rarely used in clinical settings. Instead, the diagnosis of "language impaired" is applied to describe a broad range of expressive and receptive language impairments in children. If SLI is to be diagnosed, SLPs often obtain a child's nonverbal intelligence scores from a psychologist who has administered an intelligence test.

Although the cause of the language impairment has not been pinpointed, numerous studies have been conducted to characterize children with SLI.

## Family History

SLI tends to run in families. Rice, Haney, and Wexler (1998) reported that the incidence of language disorders among immediate family members is approximately 22%; the incidence of language disorders among family members of a child without SLI is approximately 7%. Further support for a genetic basis of SLI comes from twin studies, in which the risk for SLI is higher for monozygotic twins than dizygotic twins (Bishop, North, & Donlan, 1995).

## Language Impairment

Children with SLI have language learning deficits, likely present at birth. As such, these children typically produce their first words later than children without SLI (Trauner, Wulfeck, Tallal, & Hesselink, 1995). Vocabulary learning continues to be a struggle into early childhood (Gray, 2004). In addition, children with SLI have word retrieval problems (McGregor, Newman, Reilly, & Capone, 2002): They often use nonspecific words such as "stuff" and "thing." When first combining words to make phrases and sentences, children with SLI often omit finite verb markings (Rice, Wexler, & Cleave, 1995). Common errors made by children with SLI include omitting past tense inflections (e.g., "He kick the ball" instead of "He kicked the ball"), omitting present tense inflections (e.g., "She read the book" instead of "She reads the book"), and asking questions without including the verbs "do" or "be" (e.g., "He going?" instead of "Is he going?"). As language skills develop, children with SLI tell stories with fewer specific character references (Finestack, Fey, & Catts, 2006) and fewer story components (McFadden & Gillam, 1996). Moreover, many with SLI develop deficits in pragmatic language skills (i.e., the social use of language) as they become increasingly aware of their language shortcomings in relation to their peers.[2]

It is important to note, however, that children with SLI comprise a heterogeneous group, both in the severity of their language difficulties and in the individual language profiles exhibited. Some show more difficulty expressing themselves, while others have more trouble understanding language. Most often, though, these children have deficits in both expressive and receptive language (Alt, Plante, & Creusere, 2004).

## Comorbidity

Although an SLI diagnosis indicates that a child has a "specific" language deficit, these children are more likely than their typically developing peers to have certain other disorders. In the preschool years, some children with SLI have speech sound disorders in which they have difficulty producing sounds in words (for review a see Leonard, 1998, and see Shriberg, Tomblin, & McSweeny, 1999, for school-age data). Moreover, children with SLI have difficulty acquiring prereading skills such as letter naming and phonological awareness (i.e., the explicit awareness of sound structure of language; Boudreau & Hedberg, 1999). During the school years, approximately half of children with SLI have dyslexia, a word reading impairment (Catts, Adlof, Hogan, & Ellis Weismer, 2005), and many have difficulties understanding what they read (Catts, Fey, Tomblin, & Zhang, 2002). In addition, children with SLI are more likely to have attention deficit disorders compared to age-matched peers (Kovac, Garabedian, Du Souich, & Palmour, 2001).

### Summary of Impairments in Children with SLI

- Acquire first words later than their peers.
- Use less complex sentences with filler words, such as "thing" and "stuff."
- Demonstrate decreased production and comprehension of grammatical markers, most notably verb tense.
- Produce narratives that contain more syntactic errors and fewer essential story grammar components.
- May demonstrate deficient preliteracy skills as preschoolers, including decreased phonological awareness abilities.
- Often exhibit difficulties with word reading and reading comprehension.

## Description of the Case

Tessa, a preschool-age girl (4 years, 6 months), had difficulty communicating with her playmates and family members. As her mother watched her play side by side with cousins and friends, she noticed that Tessa frequently imitated their words and play but had trouble contributing in novel ways to the play or conversation. At home, she was good-natured, playful, and cooperative, but she had difficulty following her parents' instructions and struggled to express her ideas. Tessa's mother described her conversational skills as choppy and noted that she often spoke using "immature" speech with short sentences lacking verb tense markings.

Tessa's preschool teacher also noticed that Tessa had difficulty responding to questions about stories and struggled to stay on topic when describing pictures from books. Based on these concerns, Tessa's mother contacted the university clinic to learn the nature of Tessa's difficulties and what could be done to help her daughter improve her communication.

### Relevant Facts

A full evaluation of Tessa's language and nonverbal skills was conducted for the first time in the spring of 2008. During two evaluation sessions, Tessa's language and cognitive abilities were evaluated using formal speech and language assessments, cognitive assessment, language sampling, parent interview, and informal observation.

In the spring of 2008, Tessa was seen twice a week for 50-minute sessions at the university pediatric clinic by a graduate student clinician. Sessions were supervised by the clinical instructor, and an assistant professor consulted and advised on the case.

Tessa was typically accompanied to therapy by her mother and less frequently by both her mother and father. Initially, Tessa's attendance was intermittent because of her mother's inability to transport her to the clinic due to increased work hours. However, over time, Tessa reliably attended 80% of her scheduled sessions as her mother adjusted her work schedule.

### Background Information

Per parent report, Tessa's birth history was unremarkable following a lengthy, 48-hour labor. Her neonatal reports were normal and she was discharged from the hospital to the care of her parents. She remained healthy and only recently had received hospital care to treat an idiopathic skin disorder.

Gross motor developmental milestones reportedly occurred within normal limits: She sat alone at 6 months and began walking at 12 months of age. Language milestones were delayed: Tessa first babbled at 9 months, produced her first word at 24 months (i.e., "mama"), and began to combine words at 2½ years of age. Per parent report, Tessa had not had an ear infection.

Tessa attended a local preschool. She was planning to attend kindergarten at the public school in her neighborhood in the fall. An only child, Tessa resided with her parents in a single-family home. Her mother reported that she had attended remedial reading and writing classes while in high school and that Tessa's father had repeated the fourth grade. Tessa's mother worked as a card dealer in a local casino. She reported that she did not finish high school and did not like to read. Tessa's mother required a full hour to complete the history and background information documents. Completing the forms and attending to the task appeared to be effortful and fatiguing for her, and she required frequent breaks. Tessa's father worked in a local tire factory. He had earned his high school diploma and completed a few years of technical training.

English was the primary language in their home; however, Tessa's mother speaks both English and Navajo. Per parent report, Tessa heard Navajo spoken infrequently at home and never attempted to speak it.

Tessa's maternal grandparents lived and worked in the Navajo Nation and were employed by the public school system. No information was provided on the paternal grandparents.

## Reasons for Referral

Tessa was referred by her mother for a speech-language evaluation because of her concerns with Tessa's language skills. Although the mother had been concerned for some time, it was Tessa's preschool teacher who encouraged her to contact the university clinic. Tessa's teacher was concerned that the child had difficulty responding to questions about stories and struggled to stay on topic when describing pictures from books.

At the initial meeting, Tessa's mother expressed concerns about frequent communication breakdowns at home. These included her not understanding Tessa's attempts to express herself and her daughter's inability to pay attention and follow directions to complete tasks around the house. She described Tessa's frustration with communication, indicating that Tessa often "checked out" of conversations with her parents and frequently felt left out by her playmates. Tessa's mother expressed a desire to help Tessa before she began kindergarten. She noted that Tessa had many talents that she felt were overlooked by her preschool teacher, such as drawing very detailed pictures and inventing stories that went with the pictures.

## Findings of the Evaluation

Tessa's evaluation consisted of informal observations and interactions, parent interviews, and standardized measures. The following data were obtained. Typical performance is characterized by standard scores above 85 (i.e., the 16th percentile).

### Hearing

A hearing screening (ASHA, 1997) was administered to rule out an undiagnosed hearing impairment. Tessa passed the screening at 20 dB for 1,000, 2,000, and 4,000 Hz in both ears.

### Speech Skills

The Goldman Fristoe Test of Articulation-2 (GFTA-2; Goldman & Fristoe, 2000) was administered to assess Tessa's speech sound system, and the results are summarized in Table 18.1. Her scores for the GFTA-2 were: 0 errors, 119 standard score, and >92 percentile rank. Based on

TABLE 18.1 Goldman Fristoe Test of Articulation–2 Summary

| Raw Score | Standard Score* | Confidence Interval (95%) | Percentile Rank | Concern? |
|---|---|---|---|---|
| 0 | 119 | 113–125 | > 92 | No |

*The standard scores are based on a mean of 100 and a standard deviation (SD) of 15.

TABLE 18.2 Preschool Language Score–Fourth Edition Summary

| | Raw Score | Standard Score (SS)* | SS Confidence Band (95% level) | Percentile Rank (PR) | PRs for SS Confidence Band Values | Concern? |
|---|---|---|---|---|---|---|
| Auditory Comprehension | 35 | 65 | 56–74 | 1 | 1–4 | Yes |
| Expressive Communication | 38 | 65 | 58–72 | 1 | 1–3 | Yes |
| Total Language Score | 130 | 61 | 53–69 | 1 | 1–2 | Yes |

*The standard scores are based on a mean of 100 and a standard deviation of 15.

these scores and conversational analyses of speech, Tessa's speech sound system was considered to be within normal limits for her chronological age.

## Basic Pragmatic Skills

Tessa's pragmatic skills were assessed to be within normal limits based on observations of her interactions with others. Tessa's mother did not report any concerns regarding social function at her daughter's preschool or home. During interactions with the clinician, Tessa engaged in appropriate turn-taking, eye contact, joint attention, and intonation and prosody. Because there were no concerns in this area, no standardized tests were administered.

## Expressive and Receptive Language Skills

The Preschool Language Scale–Fourth Edition (PLS-4; Zimmerman, Steiner, & Pond, 2002) (Table 18.2) was administered as a standardized measure of Tessa's expressive and receptive language skills. It was chosen because it displays acceptable sensitivity (.80) and specificity (.88) for diagnosing specific language impairment using a cut-point of $z$ score $>-1.5$ (Spaulding, Plante, & Farinella, 2006). That is, based on the psychometric properties of the PLS-4 a clinician has confidence that a child scoring below $-1.5$ $z$ score (77.5 standard score) is truly language impaired. Tessa's scores on the PLS-4 are listed in Table 18.2 followed by an interpretative summary.

***Auditory Comprehension Summary*** The auditory comprehension subscale of the PLS-4 is designed to assess comprehension of basic vocabulary, concepts, and grammatical markers. Tessa was able to identify colors, understand negatives in sentences, and demonstrate appropriate use of objects in play. For example, she was correctly able to identify a picture when given the prompt, "Look at all the babies. Show me the baby who is *not* crying" from a field of four pictures. However, she had difficulty with inferences, identifying categories, following directions with cues, and qualitative concepts (e.g., long, tall, short, and shapes). Tessa had particular difficulty following verbal instructions such as, "Get the cup and give the bear a drink." Tessa's performance on this subtest indicated that her receptive language abilities were markedly impaired, as she scored more than 2 standard deviations below the mean for her chronological age.

***Expressive Communication Summary*** The expressive communication subscale of the PLS-4 examined verbal development and social communication. Tasks include naming common objects, describing objects, and expressing quantity. Tessa was able to use basic word combinations (e.g., noun + verb, noun + verb + adjective) and quantity concepts (e.g., "How many chicks are here?"), and answer logical questions (e.g., "She is sleepy. What would you do if you were sleepy?"). She had difficulty using possessives, naming objects, completing analogies, and describing how objects are used. Tessa's performance on this subtest indicated that her expressive language abilities were markedly impaired as she scored more than 2 standard deviations below the mean for her chronological age.

***Total Language Score Summary*** Tessa's overall performance on the PLS-4 indicated that her core language abilities were more than 2 standard deviations below the mean. To this end, Tessa's overall language score was below the first percentile, indicating a significant impairment in both receptive and expressive language abilities.

## Language Sample Analysis

A conversational sample of 50 utterances was collected during the evaluation. Tessa was friendly and talkative; therefore the sample was obtained easily. An analysis of the language sample showed that Tessa had difficulty formulating grammatically and semantically correct sentences. She had particular difficulty with pronouns and often interchanged he/she within sentences. In addition, Tessa had some word finding problems as evident by many pauses and false starts. Moreover, she often used a circumlocutory sentence pattern including vacuous words such as "thing" and "stuff."

## Emerging Literacy Skills

Tessa's emergent literacy skills were assessed because children with language impairments are at significant risk for literacy impairments. The Test of Preschool Early Literacy (TOPEL; Lonigan, Wagner, & Torgesen, 2007) was administered to assess Tessa's emerging literacy skills. A summary of Tessa's results follows in Table 18.3.

***Print Knowledge Summary*** The Print Knowledge subtest of the TOPEL measures a child's familiarity with print materials, such as holding books appropriately, turning pages, and pointing to pictures. Tessa's score on this subtest indicated that she was developing print knowledge skills in line with her chronologically age-matched peers.

***Definitional Vocabulary Summary*** The Definitional Vocabulary subtest of the TOPEL measures a child's use of spoken vocabulary. Tessa was able to identify simple objects and their uses (e.g., "What do you put on pancakes?"). Tessa's scores on this portion were within the normal range for her chronological age.

***Phonological Awareness Summary*** The Phonological Awareness subtest of the TOPEL measures a child's ability to manipulate sounds in words. Tessa was able to delete initial syllables and sounds from words and blend sounds to form words. Tessa's scores on this portion were within the normal range for her chronological age.

***Early Literacy Index Summary*** The Early Literacy Index is an average score based on Print Knowledge, Definitional Vocabulary, and Phonological Awareness subtest scores. Tessa's prereading skills were age-appropriate on this index.

## Nonverbal Intelligence

The Kaufman Assessment Battery for Children–Second Edition (KABC-II; Kaufman & Kaufman, 2004) was administered to measure Tessa's nonverbal intelligence. Tessa was able to accurately recognize faces, create matching patterns, and imitate hand movements. The

TABLE 18.3 Test of Preschool Early Literacy Summary

| | Raw Score | Standard Score* | Percentile | Concern? |
|---|---|---|---|---|
| Print Knowledge | 12 | 92 | 30 | No |
| Definitional Vocabulary | 40 | 90 | 25 | No |
| Phonological Awareness | 14 | 93 | 32 | No |
| Early Literacy Index | 275 | 90 | 25 | No |

*The standard scores are based on a mean of 100 and a standard deviation of 15.

TABLE 18.4 Kaufman Assessment Battery for Children–Second Edition Summary

| | Raw Score | Standard Score (SS)* | SS Confidence Band (95% level) | Percentile Rank | Concern? |
|---|---|---|---|---|---|
| Nonverbal Index | 33 | 89 | 82–98 | 23 | No |

*The standard scores are based on a mean of 100 and SD of 15.

results of the KABC-II indicated that Tessa's nonverbal intelligence scores were within normal limits compared to her age-matched peers (see Table 18.4).

### Overall Summary

Tessa presented with impaired expressive and receptive language abilities. She struggled to express her thoughts and ideas, as characterized by word finding problems, vacuous circumlocutions, and immature morphology and syntactic structure (e.g., omitted verb tense and agreement and gender reversal). In addition, Tessa's discourse patterns were marked with broad and empty speech and cognitive inflexibility. She had problems following verbal instructions. Tessa's pragmatic skills were normal and age appropriate. Her speech sound system was age appropriate. Her nonverbal intelligence was within normal limits. These observations were confirmed by Tessa's mother. In sum, Tessa presented with specific language impairment.

## Treatment Options Considered

Treatment decisions were made using an evidence-based practice, three-pronged approach (Sackett, Straus, Richardson, Rosenberg, & Haynes, 2000) in which scientific evidence, clinical experience, and client preferences were considered.

### Client Preferences

The ultimate goal of language treatment is to improve the client's language functioning in daily living. To better understand Tessa's functional language needs, the clinicians had a discussion with her parents. Both parents indicated that they wanted Tessa to communicate her ideas more clearly with precise words and age-appropriate grammar. Additionally, they expressed their desire for Tessa to be able to tell stories about her day and also to share stories, both real and make-believe, with her friends. They wanted Tessa to "develop friendships." Finally, they noted that they were concerned that Tessa would struggle with the kindergarten curriculum that she would encounter the following year. They wanted Tessa to "feel good" about her artistic strengths and to overcome her language weaknesses. Logistically speaking, they also said that transporting Tessa to therapy at the university clinic might be a struggle because of her mother's variable work schedule.

### Clinical Experience

The clinical team met to determine Tessa's language goals in light of their discussions with Tessa's parents. Based on parent concern and observed language weaknesses, the clinicians decided that treatment goals should focus on strengthening receptive and expressive vocabulary and morphosyntax skills, as well as narrative production. It was noted that Tessa's parents would be informed of the Individuals with Disabilities Education Improvement Act (IDEA, 2004) and then be provided with contact information for Tessa's public school special education services office. According to IDEA, children are eligible for free school-based services from birth to 21 years if they meet school-based criteria for treatment.

Before consulting the research literature, clinical experiences surrounding the treatment of language were discussed. The team considered the implementation of a therapy program that trains parents to stimulate language skills in the home environment (Girolametto & Weitzman, 2006). It was noted that this approach would accommodate Tessa's parents' concern that they might have difficulty transporting her to the university clinic due to work- and preschool-based scheduling conflicts. A treatment approach that targets grammar and vocabulary using focused stimulation revolving around play activities (Ellis Weismer & Robertson, 2006) was also considered. Finally, it was noted that recent treatment research focused on improving expressive grammatical targets and vocabulary as well as narrative structure (Finestack, Fey, Sokol, Ambrose, & Swanson, 2006). The team felt that a narrative-based treatment approach would meet Tessa's parents' desire to see their daughter's story-telling abilities improve. Moreover, they thought that Tessa's pictures could be incorporated into treatment, and, as such, the treatment would provide a nice format for utilizing (and showcasing) Tessa's artistic abilities. However, it was noted that the narrative intervention had been developed for older children with SLI (Swanson, Fey, Mills, & Hood, 2006) and, as such, modifications to the intervention would likely need to be in place for Tessa, a preschool child. With these three treatment approaches in mind for Tessa, the clinicians evaluated the external scientific evidence.

## Scientific Evidence

To focus the search for scientific evidence, a foreground question was developed that included four components: (P) patient/problem, (I) intervention, (C) comparison/contrast, and (O) outcome. These questions have been termed PICO questions, an acronym for the four components (Sackett et al., 2000). The foreground question was:

1. For a preschool child with SLI (P), does a focused stimulation treatment program (I) increase vocabulary and morphosyntax skills in narrative language (O) better than a parent training program aimed at stimulating language in the home environment (C)?

First, to learn about each technique and its supporting evidence, the clinicians read book chapters devoted to outlining each treatment approach. The focused stimulation method is outlined in a chapter by Ellis Weismer & Robertson (2006). The parent-focused model for stimulating language in the home environment is outlined in a chapter by Girolametto & Weitzman (2006). Both chapters are located in a book edited by McCauley & Fey (2006). In addition, the narrative-based language intervention approach was reviewed by the clinicians. This approach is overviewed in a research article by Swanson et al. (2005) and a book chapter by Finestack et al. (2006). The literature on this approach confirmed that the narrative-based program was created for older children with SLI, while the focused stimulation and parent training approaches were geared toward younger children.

Next, a database search was conducted using the ASHA website online journals search page, a members-only electronic search engine of ASHA journal articles. The book chapters and search of external evidence allowed the clinicians to determine that focused stimulation and parent training yielded similar vocabulary and morphosyntax improvements in children with language impairments (Fey, Cleave, Long, & Hughes, 1993; Girolametto, Pearce, & Weitzman, 1996).

## Treatment Decision and Language Goals

After reading and reviewing the external evidence, the clinicians decided on a treatment approach for Tessa, pending approval by her parents. The intervention would include focused stimulation within a modified narrative-based language intervention approach administered during bi-weekly university clinic therapy sessions. Moreover, Tessa's drawings would be used to generate stories for treatment. To supplement the clinic intervention plan, Tessa's parents would watch and discuss the therapy sessions with the clinicians to learn language stimulation techniques for use in the home environment. The proposed intervention was presented to the parents, who agreed that the approach targeted Tessa's language needs and was a reasonable plan for both home and clinic-based instruction. They especially liked the idea of using Tessa's drawings in each session to promote her strength as an artist. They were also hopeful that including narratives in the therapy sessions would directly improve Tessa's ability to tell stories at home and at school. Tessa's mother did not like the idea of including only a home-based program, as she did not feel comfortable serving as the sole stimulation for Tessa's language. Instead, she wanted intervention to be provided at the clinic, where she could watch the sessions and learn techniques to supplement therapy at home. Thus, she was comfortable with learning from the clinicians and completing home-based assignments. In sum, the intervention for Tessa was chosen based on scientific evidence, clinical experience, and client preferences. It was determined that Tessa's prognosis for success was good because she was motivated to produce language through narrative productions, Tessa's parents were supportive of the intervention plan, and Tessa's language sample indicated the presence of grammatical structures indicative of potential to learn more complex structures (Pawlowska, Leonard, Camarata, Brown, & Camarata, 2008).

Basic, intermediate, and specific treatment goals (Fey, 1986) were set for Tessa. These goals address vocabulary, grammatical forms, and oral narratives.

### Tessa T.'s Basic Goal

To improve Tessa's ability to orally produce complete, sequential, meaningful narratives to increase her ability to communicate in her everyday environments such as home and preschool.

### Tessa T.'s Intermediate Goals

#### *Vocabulary*

Tessa will show expressive knowledge of previously unknown words encountered in narratives.

#### *Grammatical Forms*

Tessa will spontaneously produce finite verb markings in oral narratives.
Tessa will spontaneously produce correct subject-verb agreement in oral narratives.

#### *Narratives*

Tessa will produce sequential, meaningful oral narratives that include key story elements.

### Tessa T.'s Specific Goals

#### *Vocabulary*

Tessa will correctly label 4 pictures representing previously unknown words (2 nouns and 2 verbs) at 90% accuracy each week.
Tessa will retell one narrative in the therapy room each week including 3 of the 4 newly learned words.

#### *Grammatical Forms*

Tessa will correctly produce regular past tense verbs at 90% accuracy while generating and retelling oral narratives in the therapy room.
Tessa will use a personal pronoun (i.e., he, she) when referencing characters at 90% accuracy while generating and retelling oral narratives in the therapy room.

#### *Narratives*

Tessa will include all essential story elements (i.e., characters, setting, problem/goal, actions, and resolution/ending) while generating and retelling oral narratives in the therapy room.

## Course of Treatment

The language intervention chosen for Tessa was a hybrid approach that included focused stimulation on specific vocabulary and grammatical forms (Ellis Weismer & Robertson, 2006) in the context of narrative-based language instruction (Finestack et al., 2006). A horizontal goal attack strategy was implemented in which all specific treatment goals were targeted each session. In addition to the clinician-directed intervention, Tessa's parents watched therapy sessions and were explicitly instructed on ways to mimic the graduate student clinician's language stimulation techniques in the home environment. These techniques included recasting Tessa's productions and expanding them to include verb tense marking and targeted vocabulary.

## Treatment Sessions

Each treatment session followed a similar sequence. One clinician-driven narrative was used per week (i.e., two sessions). Tessa generated one narrative each session. Each of the five language goals were targeted each session.

***Vocabulary and Grammatical Forms Probes*** At the beginning of each session, Tessa was presented with pictures of two nouns and two verbs from the clinician-generated oral narrative previously presented in the treatment session. To elicit spontaneous productions of these newly learned words, the student clinician used the following prompts: "These are new words you heard in the story you heard last session. What did we call this?" and "In our story, one of your characters did this—he ______." Tessa was prompted to name the verb, including a past tense verb marking. Finally, the clinician probed for pronouns by showing Tessa a picture of two characters, one male and one female, from previous narratives. Tessa was then prompted to say a sentence about the character after a clinician-model. For example, "He likes to play. Who likes to play?" at which time Tessa would be required to say, "He likes to play." Each probe, verb and personal pronoun, included 10 test words. Corrective feedback was provided after each probe.

***Clinician-Generated Narrative*** Each week the graduate student clinician generated a narrative in consultation with Tessa's mother to include events from Tessa's home and school. The narratives included two main characters, one male and one female. Noun and verb targets were chosen based on frequency counts (Dale & Fenson, 1996). Each story contained two high-frequency verbs that were not targeted for treatment (i.e., known verbs) and two mid- to low-frequency verbs that were targeted for treatment (i.e., unknown verbs). The same procedure was followed for the selection of nouns for each story. To visually represent the story elements crucial for a narrative, color-coded elements were presented to Tessa. This procedure was adapted from the narrative-based language intervention discussed in Finestack et al. (2006). First, Tessa was presented with the two story characters pasted on purple construction paper. Next, she was shown the story setting on blue construction paper. Third, the clinician presented the picture of the story's problem pasted on green construction paper. Fourth, Tessa was shown the story's action (i.e., resolution to the problem). The picture of the action was pasted on red construction paper. Finally, a picture of the story's ending/resolution was shown pasted on an orange piece of construction paper. The clinician explained to Tessa that stories have to include these colors of the rainbow. Each story element was explained as it was shown to Tessa. For example, the clinician told Tessa that characters are people in a story. Tessa was given a rainbow to represent the colors of the elements in the story. As the clinician told the prescripted story, she picked up each color-coded element and placed it on a storyboard, a large whiteboard, which was on the therapy table. The title of the story was written on the board and read to Tessa. When introducing each story element, the clinician emphasized the targeted vocabulary words and the grammatical forms (i.e., personal pronouns and regular past tense) that she wanted to teach. Tessa was given a colored sticker to place on the rainbow for each story element. The sticker was a smiley face that was the same color as the story element. Tessa was prompted to repeat each sentence of the story as it was given. If errors were present in the sentence repetition, the clinician modeled the sentence again without requiring another repetition. An example story follows with targeted words and forms underlined for emphasis.

EXAMPLE CLINICIAN-GENERATED STORY
Title: The Fall

- Bob and Sue are friends. (characters on purple paper)
- They go to school every day. (setting on blue paper)
- One day Bob was playing outside. He tripped over a rock on the sidewalk. He scraped his knee! (problem on green paper)
- Sue helped him. She pulled his hand. Bob stood up again. (action on red paper)
- Bob was happy that Sue helped him. He started to play on the merry-go-round. She played on the merry-go-round too. (resolution/ending on orange paper)

The vocabulary words targeted in this story were *sidewalk, merry-go-round, tripped,* and *scraped*. The familiar verbs were *helped, pulled, started,* and *played*. The clinician emphasized personal pronouns and past tense verb markings through increased loudness, raised pitch, and word elongation.

***Client-Generated Narrative*** After Tessa repeated each sentence of the clinician-generated story, she was asked to retell the story. During the retelling, Tessa's use of the newly learned vocabulary and grammatical forms, personal pronouns, and past tense verb marking was tallied. The clinician then told the story to Tessa again while highlighting the story elements using the rainbow visual prompts. Tessa was then presented with more color-coded character, setting, problem, action, and resolutions/ending pictures. She was instructed to create another story using "the rainbow" as a cue for including all story elements. Sequencing was not a focus, thus, she could choose story elements at random. Tessa was then instructed to tell her story one rainbow color at a time in a sequence, starting with the characters. Tessa's use of story elements, specific vocabulary words, and grammatical forms was tallied. If an error was present, the clinician recasted Tessa's sentence including all relevant information with correct productions and, at times, expanded content.

***Homework*** At the end of the session Tessa's mother was given the clinician-derived story. She was asked to read it to Tessa as Tessa drew a picture of the story. Tessa's mother was also provided the vocabulary that she was to emphasize while reading the story and while interacting with Tessa throughout the week. A rainbow and stickers were provided to Tessa's mother to assist Tessa, as she used her drawing to retell the story while including all of the story elements. Tessa's mother was encouraged to remind Tessa to "use the rainbow" when she told stories.

***Narrative Probe*** For each session, Tessa brought a picture she had drawn representing the clinician-driven story that was presented in the previous therapy session. She was given a rainbow to represent story elements and asked to tell the story using the same words that Rebecca and her mother used as they told the story. Tessa was given a smiley face sticker color-matched to each of the story elements she successfully included in her narrative. The clinician tallied Tessa's use of targeted vocabulary and grammatical forms (i.e., personal pronouns and past tense) as Tessa retold the story. This probe was administered each session after the vocabulary and grammatical forms probe. Note that the amount of opportunities to determine correct use of grammatical structures and new vocabulary learning varied across probes depending on the richness of Tessa's story retelling. Thus, the narrative probe served two purposes: (a) to assess the use of story elements in narrative retell, and (b) to determine the generalization of vocabulary and grammatical targets to functional language use (i.e., narrative production).

## Analysis of the Client's Response to Intervention

Tessa attended bi-weekly therapy sessions for 8 weeks. She made the most progress learning new vocabulary words and using personal pronouns, while her production of past tense verb markings showed less improvement. Figure 18.1 displays data for each target across the twice weekly sessions. Likewise, her narratives often continued to lack focus, and she struggled to learn the concepts associated with the story elements (e.g., characters). Nonetheless, her enthusiasm for learning showed each session, and she expressed how much she liked including

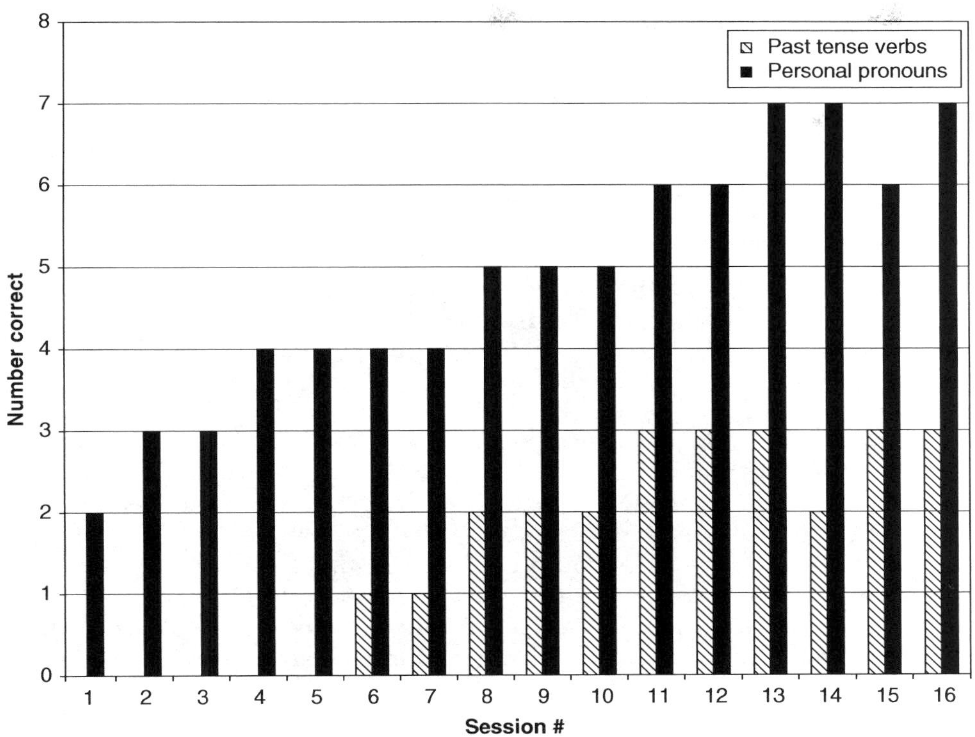


FIGURE 18.1 Treatment Probe Data Across 8 weeks for Grammatical Forms: Past Tense Verbs and Personal Pronouns (10 Total Points Possible per Probe)

her drawing in the story retell. Tessa's mother reported that she was more confident when telling stories at home, and Tessa asked her often, "Did I use the rainbow?" Tessa's parents reported that they felt better able to stimulate her language at home by explicitly pointing out new vocabulary words, by expanding upon her sentences emphasizing correct grammatical forms, and by "telling stories" each evening, a ritual they expressly enjoyed. Tessa's preschool teacher noticed an increase in her confidence, but she noted that Tessa continued to struggle when communicating in the classroom compared to her peers.

The graduate student clinician, in consultation with her supervisors, implemented several adaptations to Tessa's language intervention to respond to Tessa's difficulty producing past tense verb markings and narrative story elements. First, she strived to use more concrete, direct language when explaining the story elements. It was hypothesized that Tessa's receptive language problems impeded her ability to understand complex concepts. This adaptation seemed to work, as Tessa began to show increased use of narrative elements. Of course, this improvement could have been due to time in therapy as well. Swanson et al. (2005) showed limited success using a narrative-based language intervention after 6 weeks. They predicted that more treatment could have led to more gains. This may be especially relevant when working with a preschool child with more immature language than a school-age child. Another adaptation made in treatment was the use of forced choice when probing past tense verb acquisition. Tessa was asked to determine whether a sentence with or without past tense verb marking was grammatically correct. As such, receptive language goals have been added to supplement the original expressive language targets. She showed progress in this area and, in turn, her production of past tense verb markings increased. When Tessa generated her own narratives, she often lost sight of the narrative story elements and began to stray from the story. The graduate student clinician then touched Tessa's rainbow to cue her to include the story elements and stay on topic. This adaptation seemed to work; Tessa's attention was often redirected to the rainbow, and she started to include more story elements.

## Further Recommendations

At the time of this study, Tessa was making progress in treatment; however, she had much to learn. Additionally, generalization to the attainment of goals outside of the therapy room needed to be explicitly addressed to ensure functional improvement in Tessa's language abilities. For example, parent and teacher rating forms (cf. Newman & McGregor, 2006) may be included to determine generalization of treatment targets.

### Other Considerations

- Tessa's parents were directly instructed on ways to improve Tessa's language skills in the home environment. Per parent request, goals were not set to quantify Tessa's parents' learning of language stimulation techniques. Goals directly targeting parent training have been used by the clinical team in other cases.
- Narrative story elements were taught to Tessa to explicitly increase her narrative abilities. However, because Tessa is a preschool child, expectations for learning these elements were lower than they would have been if she were older and in grade school. Research shows that narrative development is a protracted process that spans from early childhood through the school years (Gillam & Pearson, 2004).
- Tessa's narrative abilities were not formally assessed. A formal assessment (e.g., Gillam & Pearson, 2004; Hughes, McGillivray, & Schmidek, 1997) would have more thoroughly quantified Tessa's narrative skills to gain a better overall picture of her abilities and to determine the effect of treatment on targeted structures as well as untargeted structures.

## Author Note

The authors would like to thank their clients and their clients' parents for serving as inspiration for the hypothetical case study. We also thank Mary Alt, Lizbeth Finestack, Jill Hoover, and Cameron Kliner for helpful comments on earlier drafts of this case. Hogan's Fall 2008 Preschool Language Disorders course members provided valuable feedback from the student perspective.

## Endnotes

1. Normal nonverbal abilities in children with SLI are defined as the attainment of a standard score greater than 70 on a nonverbal intelligence test (see Plante, 1998), although some studies require that children with SLI exhibit a standard score of 85 or greater (e.g., Stark & Tallal, 1981; Tomblin et al., 1997). It should be noted that even though children with SLI exhibit *normal* nonverbal skills, on average, they score in the lower end of the normal range on nonverbal intelligence tests (e.g., 87–95 mean standard score).
2. See Leonard (1998, pp. 77–85) for a comprehensive summary of studies related to social language use in children with SLI.

## References

Alt, M., Plante, E., & Creusere, M. (2004). Semantic features in fast-mapping: Performance of preschoolers with specific language impairment versus preschoolers with normal language. *Journal of Speech, Language, and Hearing Research, 47*, 407–420.

ASHA. (1997). Audiologic screening guidelines—Pediatric section. *ASHA*, IV–74gi.

Bishop, D. V. M., North, T., & Donlan, C. (1995). Nonword repetition as a behaviour marker for inherited language impairment: Evidence from a twin study. *Journal of Child Psychology and Psychiatry, 37*, 391–403.

Boudreau, D. M., & Hedberg, N. L. (1999). A comparison of early literacy skills in children with specific language impairment and their typically developing peers. *American Journal of Speech-Language Pathology, 8*, 249–260.

Catts, H. W., Adlof, S. M., Hogan, T. P., & Ellis Weismer, S. (2005). Dyslexia and specific language impairment: Same or different developmental disorder? *Journal of Speech, Language, and Hearing Research, 48*, 1378–1396.

Catts, H. W., Fey, M. E., Tomblin, J. B., & Zhang, X. (2002). A longitudinal investigation of reading outcomes in children with language impairments. *Journal of Speech, Language, and Hearing Research, 45,* 1142–1157.

Dale, P. S., & Fenson, L. (1996). Lexical development norms for young children. *Behavior Research Methods, Instruments, & Computers, 28,* 125–127.

Ellis Weismer, S. & Robertson, S. (2006). Focused stimulation approach to language intervention. In R. J. McCauley & M. E. Fey (Eds.), *Treatment of language disorders in children* (pp. 77–103). Baltimore, MD: Paul H. Brooks Publishing.

Fey, M. E. (1986). *Language intervention with young children*. San Diego, CA: College-Hill Press.

Fey, M. E., Cleave, P. L., Long, S. H., & Hughes, D. L. (1993). Two approaches to the facilitation of grammar in children with language impairment: An experimental evaluation. *Journal of Speech and Hearing Research, 36,* 141–157.

Finestack, L. H., Fey, M. E., & Catts, H. W. (2006). Pronominal reference skills of second and fourth grade children with language impairment. *Journal of Communication Disorders, 39,* 232–248.

Finestack, L. H., Fey, M. E., Sokol, S. B., Ambrose, S., & Swanson, L.A. (2006). Fostering narrative and grammatical skills with "syntax stories." In A. van Kleeck (Ed.), *Sharing books and stories to promote language literacy* (pp. 319–346). San Diego, CA: Plural Publishing.

Gillam, R. B., & Pearson, N. A. (2004). *Test of narrative language.* East Moline, IL: LinguiSystems.

Girolametto, L., Pearce, P. S., & Weitzman, E. (1996). Interactive focused stimulation for toddlers with expressive vocabulary delays. *Journal of Speech and Hearing Research, 39,* 1274–1283.

Girolametto, L., & Weitzman, E. (2006). It takes two to talk—The Hanen program for parents: Early language intervention through caregiver training. In R. J. McCauley & M. E. Fey (Eds.), *Treatment of language disorders in children* (pp. 77–103). Baltimore, MD: Paul H. Brooks Publishing.

Goldman, R., & Fristoe, M. (2000). *Goldman-Fristoe Test of Articulation–Second Edition.* Bloomington, MN: Pearson Assessments.

Gray, S. (2004). Word learning by preschoolers with specific language impairment: Predictors and poor learners. *Journal of Speech, Language, and Hearing Research, 47,* 1117–1132.

Hughes, D. L., McGillivray, L., & Schmidek, M. (1997). *Guide to narrative language: Procedures for assessment.* Greenville, SC: Super Duper Publications.

Individuals with Disabilities Education Improvement Act. 20 U.S.C. § 126–16 *et seq.* (2004).

Kamhi, A. G. (2007). Thoughts and reflections on developmental language disorders. In A. G. Kamhi, J. J. Masterson, & K. Apel (Eds.), *Clinical decision making in developmental language disorders.* Baltimore, MD: Paul H. Brookes Publishing.

Kaufman, A. S., & Kaufman, N. L. (2004). *KABC-II: Kaufman Assessment Battery for Children–Second Edition.* Bloomington, MN: Pearson Assessments.

Kovac, I., Garabedian, B., Du Souich, C. & Palmour. (2001). Attention deficit/ hyperactivity in SLI children increases risk of speech/language disorders in first-degree relatives: A preliminary report. *Journal of Communication Disorders, 34,* 339–354.

Leonard, L. B. (1998). Children with specific language impairment. Cambridge, MA: MIT Press.

Lonigan, C. J., Wagner, R. K., & Torgesen, J. K. (2007). *Test of Preschool Early Literacy.* Austin, TX: PRO-ED.

McCauley, R., & Fey, M. ( Eds.). (2006). Treatment of language disorders in children. Baltimore: Brookes.

McFadden, T. U., & Gillam, R. B. (1996). An examination of the quality of narratives produced by children with language disorders. *Language, Speech, and Hearing Services in Schools, 27,* 48–56.

McGregor, K. K., Newman, R. M., Reilly, R. M., & Capone, N. C. (2002). Semantic representations and naming in children with specific language impairment. *Journal of Speech, Language, and Hearing Research, 45,* 998–1014.

Newman, R. M., & McGregor, K. K. (2006). Teachers and laypersons discern quality differences between narratives produced by children with and without SLI. *Journal of Speech, Language, and Hearing Research, 49,* 1022–1036.

Pawlowska, M., Leonard, L. B., Camarata, S. M., Brown, B., & Camarata, M. N. (2008). Factors accounting for the ability of children with SLI to learn agreement morphemes in intervention. *Journal of Child Language, 35,* 25–53.

Rice, M. L., Haney, K. R., & Wexler, K. (1998). Family histories of children with SLI who show extended optional infinitives. *Journal of Speech, Language, and Hearing Research, 41,* 419–432.

Rice, M., Wexler, K., & Cleave, P. (1995). Specific language impairment as a period of extended optional infinitive. *Journal of Speech and Hearing Research, 38,* 850–863.

Sackett, D. L., Straus, S. E., Richardson, W. S., Rosenberg, W., & Haynes, R. B. (2000).

*Evidence-based medicine: How to practice and teach EBM.* Edinburgh, Scotland: Churchill Livingston.

Shriberg, L. D., Tomblin, J. B., & McSweeny, J. L. (1999). Prevalence of speech delay in 6-year-old children and comorbidity with language impairment. *Journal of Speech, Language, and Hearing Research, 46,* 1461–1481.

Spaulding, T. J., Plante, E., & Farinella, K. (2006). Eligibility criteria for language impairment: Is the low end of normal always appropriate? *Language, Speech, and Hearing Services in the Schools, 37,* 61–72.

Stark, R. E., & Tallal, P. (1981). Selection of children with specific language deficits. *Journal of Speech and Hearing Research, 46,* 114–122.

Swanson, L. A., Fey, M. E., Mills, C. E., & Hood, L. S. (2006). Use of narrative-based language intervention with children who have specific language impairment. *American Journal of Speech-Language Pathology, 14,* 131–143.

Tomblin, J. B. (1996). Genetic and environmental contributions to the risk of specific language impairment. In M. L. Rice (Ed.), *Toward a genetics of language* (pp. 191–210). Mahwah, NJ: Lawrence Erlbaum.

Tomblin, J. B., Records, N., Buckwalter, P., Zhang, X., Smith, E., & O'Brien, M. (1997). Prevalence of specific language impairment in kindergarten children. *Journal of Speech, Language, and Hearing Research, 40,* 1245–1260.

Trauner, D., Wulfeck, B., Tallal, P., & Hesselink, J. (1995). Neurologic and MRI profiles of impaired children. Technical report CND-9513, Center for Research in Language, University of California at San Diego.

Zimmerman, I. L., Steiner, V. G., & Pond, R. E. (2002). *Preschool Language Scales–Fourth Edition.* San Antonio, TX: The Psychological Corporation.

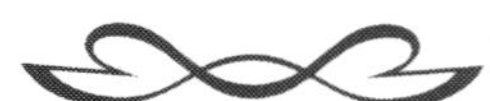

## PHONOLOGY/ARTICULATION

# CASE 19

# Tom: Complex Disorder Traits in a Three-Year-Old Boy with a Severe Speech Sound Disorder

*Beate Peter*

## Conceptual Knowledge Areas

### Speech Sound Disorder: Single Clinical Entity or Discrete Subtypes?

Many children have difficulty with speech production in the absence of known causes and other communication deficits, a condition commonly called speech sound disorder (SSD). Compared to their peers, these children have more trouble being understood by their listeners.

How can children with SSD be grouped into distinct disorder subtypes? Clinicians and researchers differ in the way they answer this question. For instance, Bauman-Waengler

(2000) proposes a phonetic-phonemic continuum, where the phonetic pole of the disorder continuum captures articulatory errors that are produced consistently, while the phonemic pole represents systematic speech sound errors based on phoneme class. An example of a phonetic error would be a laterally distorted /s/ sound in all attempts at the sound, and a phonemic error would be [tʌp]/cup, [do]/go, and [wɪn]/wing—in other words, all velar sounds are produced in an alveolar place of articulation. The continuum allows for pure phonetic or phonemic error patterns as well as for mixed forms. Dodd's taxonomy of childhood speech disorders is based on a psycholinguistic model of the speech processing chain (Dodd, 1995). Speech disorder subtypes are classified by error types, e.g., articulation disorder versus delayed phonological development; deviant-consistent versus deviant-inconsistent phonological errors. Shriberg and colleagues (e.g., Shriberg et al., 2005) base their disorder classification on suspected etiology, giving rise to subtypes related to genetic factors, otitis media, motor involvement, psychosocial involvement, and speech errors. Several other taxonomies coexist in the literature. It is unknown which of them describes speech sound disorder subtypes with the greatest clinical and statistical relevance. In a recent study, Peter and Stoel-Gammon (2008) found that some children with SSD also show evidence of global timing inaccuracy during speech-related as well as during hand tasks. The same children also had difficulty with expressive language. We hypothesized that this disorder profile may represent a separate subtype related to central difficulties with timing accuracy and associated effects on speech and language skills. In what follows, two proposed SSD disorder subtypes, childhood apraxia of speech (CAS) and phonological processes, are outlined.

## Childhood Apraxia of Speech

Childhood apraxia of speech (CAS) is conceptualized as a motor planning disorder. It is one of the subtypes in Shriberg et al.'s (2005) taxonomy. In a recent position statement issued by the American Speech-Language-Hearing Association (ASHA) (2007), CAS is described as "a neurological childhood (pediatric) speech sound disorder in which the precision and consistency of movements underlying speech are impaired in the absence of neuromuscular deficits." As thoughts are converted into speech sounds, motor planning is viewed as one of the steps preceding the actual muscle activity in the articulators. During this phase, which only takes fractions of a second, a blueprint of the sequence and basic parameters of speech movements is constructed. Evidence for this preparatory step comes from research in adults with, and without, motor speech disorders and includes the observation that it takes longer to respond to a complex utterance prompt than to a more basic one. This "sequence length effect" has been observed in speech as well as other motor activities (e.g., Canic & Franks, 1989). Numerous and only partially compatible CAS feature lists coexist in the literature, for instance, Davis, Jakielski, and Marquardt (1998), Hall (2000a, b), and Hickman (1997). Shriberg et al. (2003) name those features deemed most plausible in the context of motor planning deficits. Their list is organized into segmental and suprasegmental speech errors and includes the following features: articulatory struggle (groping), particularly on word onsets, transpositional (metathetic) substitution errors reflecting sequencing constraints on adjacent sounds, marked inconsistencies on repeated tokens of the same word type, proportionally increased sound and syllable deletions relative to overall severity of involvement, proportionally increased vowel/diphthong errors relative to overall severity of involvement, inconsistent realization of stress (i.e., prominence on syllables or words), inconsistent realization of temporal constraints on both speech and pause events, and inconsistent oral-nasal gestures underlying the percept of nasopharyngeal resonance.

While there is widespread agreement that CAS is a severe form of SSD requiring intense intervention, no rigorously derived therapy efficacy data are currently available (American Speech-Language-Hearing Association, 2007). In addition to standard speech therapy, options include augmentative and alternative communication strategies, oral motor exercises, gestural cueing, melodic intonation therapy, and linguistic approaches.

## Phonological Processes

During the early years of clinical practice, speech sound errors were addressed individually. As alluded to in the description of Bauman-Waengler's (2000) taxonomy of SSD, a phonemic view of speech sound errors is based on the idea that sounds can be grouped into classes, for instance, by place of articulation such as alveolar or velar; by manner of articulation such as stops, fricatives, or glides; or by voicing. Speech sound errors can affect several sounds within the same class. For instance, a child who has trouble with the /s/ sound, replacing it with [t], may also have difficulty with /f, θ/, substituting [p] and [t], respectively, a pattern called "stopping" because stops are produced instead of fricatives. Systematic sound substitutions are often referred to as phonological processes, and in therapy, they are addressed by sound class rather than as individual sounds.

Phonological processes can be observed in different linguistic structures including segments, syllables, and words. Table 19.1 lists selected phonological processes and some examples from clinical practice. Because many children with severe SSD show several error patterns at once, some examples contain multiple errors.

Multiple processes can affect the same word production. For instance, [wi]/tree shows evidence of both gliding and cluster reduction. Three phonological processes are evident in [daʊn]/clown: cluster reduction, velar fronting, and prevocalic voicing. In some cases, it may not be clear at first which phonological process is at play. [gɔg]/dog could be an example of assimilation or backing. A close look at other productions will resolve the ambiguity. Care must be taken to distinguish between phonological processes and expressive language deficits. Final consonant deletion and unmarked plurals or missing third person singular verb endings may result in the same word production. Probing for other syntactic markers will shed light on the underlying disorder. For more detailed information on phonological processes, consult Edwards and Shriberg (1983), Hodson and Paden (1991), and Williams (2003).

Errors in speech production can be explained through multiple models. For instance, a clinician working from a phonological process perspective might classify [bu]/blue as the phonological process of cluster reduction, while a clinician more comfortable in a motor planning framework may view this error type as a planning error triggered by a complex phonetic environment. The former is a linguistic perspective, while the latter emphasizes motoric elements of speech production.

TABLE 19.1 Examples of Selected Phonological Processes, by Linguistic Level and Underlying Mechanism

| Affected Structure | Mechanism | Phonological Process | Example |
|---|---|---|---|
| Segment | Place of articulation | Fronting | [ti]/key<br>[so]/show |
| | | Backing | [sʌm]/thumb |
| | Manner of articulation | Stopping | [ti]/see |
| | | Gliding | [wɛd]/red |
| | | Affrication | [haʊts]/house |
| | Voicing | Prevocalic voicing | [bədʒæmaz]/pajamas |
| | | Final devoicing | [slaɪt]/slide |
| Syllable | Quantity of syllable constituents | Cluster reduction | [bu]/blue |
| | | Final consonant deletion | [haʊ]/house |
| | Quality of syllable constituents | Assimilation | [lɛ́lo]/yellow |
| Word | Quantity of word constituents | Syllable deletion | [bun]/balloon |
| | | Syllable insertion | [θəlaɪd]/slide |

## Description of the Case

### Background Information

Tom had just celebrated his third birthday when he was referred for a clinical evaluation of his speech skills. Tom's father, Mike, was a pediatrician and his mother, Andrea, was a health insurance professional with expertise in early childhood education. They had been concerned about Tom's communication skills for some time, and as soon as Tom became eligible for an evaluation through the public school system, they contacted the district.

### Reason for Referral

During the phone interview prior to the evaluation, Andrea stated that Tom was generally in excellent health and that he was outgoing and curious, adding that he did not show interest in joint book reading, preferring other, more gross-motor–based activities. Tom's speech development was his parents' main concern. Andrea reported that she and Mike could only understand approximately 50% of Tom's utterances; that he produced sentences of 3 to 4 words in length, such as "help me, please" and "put it on, Mom"; and that they had no concerns regarding other aspects of his communication skills, e.g., voice, fluency, receptive and expressive language. She declined the school district's offer to conduct a full evaluation including language and cognitive functioning, suggesting that this could be scheduled later if concerns arose.

During the intake interview, Andrea reported that there were no birth complications, and Tom appeared to be in perfect health during his early weeks and months. He reached all typical developmental milestones, with the exception that he did not start walking until age 15 months. Between the ages of 4 and 16 months, he spent time in day care, but after 16 months of age stayed home full-time with his mother. His main social contacts were his immediate family, including an older brother and his cousins.

Tom's parents began to notice that he did not start to talk as they expected.

"He wasn't speaking," his mother said. "He showed no signs of verbal communication."

One of Mike's nephews, a boy five years older than Tom, had received speech therapy because of severe speech delays, and Andrea recalled that her sister had been in speech therapy as a young child. Mike's brother had undergone therapy as a child to remediate stuttering. Mike and Andrea were keenly aware of the difference between Tom's speech development and that of his older brother, and they continued to watch him closely.

When Tom was 2 years old, his vocabulary consisted of 5 words that could be understood and an untold number of words he attempted to say, unsuccessfully. To determine what Tom was trying to say, Andrea and Mike used various strategies. Often, they told him to "slow down and try again." When they thought he was requesting something, they guessed at what it might be and asked him to verify. Although they never questioned his ability to understand them, they requested a formal hearing evaluation at a local children's hospital when Tom was 2 years, 7 months. Findings were consistent with normal hearing.

By now, Tom was showing signs of frustration as his parents and older brother could not understand much of what he said. He expressed his frustration by growling, crying, or lashing out, which seemed particularly out of character. Perhaps worst of all, sometimes he gave up trying to talk when he was asked to repeat what he had just said.

In all other areas, Tom appeared to be developing within or above age expectations. His giftedness in spatial reasoning became apparent as he worked complicated puzzles, completed crafts projects, and drew pictures with a level of sophistication typical of much older children. As he approached his third birthday, Tom's parents decided to seek professional intervention.

"It seemed to us that he was not nearly as independent as he should be for his age," his mother concluded. "He was not able to advocate for himself sufficiently."

### Findings of the Evaluation

Tom arrived for his evaluation accompanied by his mother. The evaluation consisted of a conversational speech sample, an oral structural/functional examination, and standardized articulation testing.

Approximately 20% of Tom's utterances were judged as intelligible. He was unwilling to interact with the clinician directly, clinging to his mother. When his mother tried to engage him in a conversation, he responded with single words or simply shouted, "No!" He seemed restless, jumping up from his chair frequently to explore materials in the room.

The oral structural/functional and articulation examinations were influenced by Tom's young age, his substantial frustration levels related to communication tasks, and his refusal to interact with unfamiliar adults. Although the oral/functional examination could not be completed, it revealed extremely large faucial tonsils, a fairly large tongue, and a forward tongue carriage. A medical follow-up was suggested to rule out sleep apnea due to the size of the tonsils. Andrea was receptive to this advice. She reported that Tom never had any difficulty with chewing and swallowing food.

Articulation testing began with the Goldman-Fristoe Test of Articulation-2 (GFTA-2; Goldman & Fristoe, 2000). When Tom became uncooperative, the Structured Photographic Articulation Test Featuring Dudsberry (SPAT-D; Kresheck & Tattersall, 1993) was used. Both tests sample all consonants of English in initial, medial, and final positions. Tom complied for the first few test items and was then unwilling to continue, shouting, "No!" and leaving his chair despite many efforts to redirect him. Andrea was able to elicit several more test words by asking him to imitate her model. She prompted additional speech samples by asking questions like, "What is your favorite breakfast food?" Table 19.2 lists Tom's single word productions from the two attempts to administer standardized testing, as well as single-word responses to questions posed by his mother.

An estimate of Tom's relational phoneme inventory was constructed from his single-word productions while naming pictures, imitating his mother's models, answering questions, and engaging in conversational productions. Using the SPAT protocol, at least 30 errors were noted, which translated to a percentile ranking of 5. If the clinician had been able to sample all phonemes in all tested word positions, the error score would likely have increased. Based on this estimate, Tom easily qualified for 30 minutes of weekly therapy services, using a cutoff rule of 7th percentile ranking or lower, compared to same-age children.

TABLE 19.2 Word Productions During the Initial Evaluation

| **Items from Articulation Testing** | | **Words Elicited in Conversation** | |
|---|---|---|---|
| ***Word Transcription*** | ***Gloss*** | ***Word Transcription*** | ***Gloss*** |
| haɵ | house | to | toy |
| ðíðʊ | scissors | bókəno | vulcano |
| kέgɪ | carrot | piɵ | please |
| naf | knife | gámɑ, dámɑ | grandma |
| ʤέwo | jello | nópaʊ | snow-plough |
| ʃawáf | shovel | ʃɔ́ʃɔʧ | sausage |
| wun | spoon | pébʌkəʔ | play bucket |
| vɔʧ | watch | bɔɵ | blocks |
| túba | toothbrush | ða | yeah |
| bǽʔtʌb | bathtub | ðέɵ | yes |
| ʤǽmɑð | pajamas | | |
| ɵek | snake | | |
| vímlŋ | swimming | | |
| bun | balloon | | |
| kέɵ | skates | | |
| ɵíblŋ | sleeping | | |
| pέðɛn, pέnɛ | present | | |
| fi | three | | |
| gáwað | glasses | | |
| Kɔʔ | clock | | |
| ápen | airplane | | |

It was concluded that Tom had a severe SSD with components of multiple disorder subtypes. For instance, he had a frontal lisp, as evidenced by consistently placing his tongue too far forward during production of /s, z/, and he consistently substituted [ð] for /j/, even in high-frequency words like "yeah" and "yes." This aspect of his speech would be classified as a phonetic error in taxonomies such as Bauman-Waengler's (2000), and his tongue size and carriage may have been a physical contributor to these sound errors. Tom also showed evidence of several phonological processes. For instance, he exhibited gliding as in [ʤέwo]/jello, cluster reduction as in [nópaʊ]/snowplough, syllable deletion as in [bun]/balloon, and assimilation errors such as [kέgɪ]/carrot and [ʃóʃɔʧ]/sausage. Tom's speech sound inventory was additionally characterized by a kind of "musical chair" game for /ɵ, f, s/ and their voiced cognates. Tom was capable of producing interdental fricatives, because he substituted them for /s, z, j/. In words requiring /ɵ/, however, Tom produced [f] instead. This aspect of his speech was clearly not a phonetic error; rather, it represented a phonologic system shift. Finally, several aspects of his speech were consistent with childhood apraxia of speech, for instance, vowel errors as in [to]/toy and [naf]/knife; sequencing errors such as those in [ʃawáf]/shovel and [gáwað]/glasses; a lexical stress error, [bókənо] /volcano; and variable productions of several words, for instance, [gámɑ, dámɑ ]/grandma and [pέðέn, pέnɛ]/present.

The information gathered during the intake activities led to the conclusion that Tom was a young child with a severe SSD of mixed type (phonetic, phonemic, and apraxic). The barriers he experienced in trying to express his thoughts had begun to cause him a significant level of frustration. His frequent use of the word "no" was seen as a desperate strategy to have at least some level of control using speech. Because of his lack of interest in joint book reading, he did not receive systematic exposure to hearing objects labeled with speech sounds.

## Treatment Options Considered

- *Traditional therapy, which includes auditory activities ("ear training") and structured speech production tasks*. The target speech sounds are produced in increasingly complex contexts, beginning with the individual sound and progressing to syllables, words, phrases, and so on, until they have generalized to conversational speech. Targets are usually, but not always, selected starting with the most developmentally appropriate and most stimulable ones. This approach has been widely used and would be most appropriate for Tom's /s, z, j/ errors. See Williams (2003) for published efficacy data on specific aspects of traditional therapy.
- *Pattern-based therapy to address* Tom's *phonological processes, for instance, minimal opposition therapy, in which target word pairs differ only in one aspect of articulation (manner, place, or voicing), or maximal opposition therapy, in which target word pairs differ in more than one aspect of articulation*. Efficacy of minimal pair therapy in general is unclear as reports have been contradictive (Saben & Ingham, 1991; Weiner, 1981). In a study of three children, Gierut (1990) showed that maximal opposition therapy was more effective than minimal opposition therapy.
- *Cycles (Hodson & Paden, 1991), a programmed approach tailored to children with multiple phonological processes*. Each session begins and ends with auditory exposure, preferably using amplified speech. Therapy focuses on one phonological process at a time, switching to another one after a short course of therapy, for instance, 6 to 18 therapy hours, regardless of whether the child mastered the pattern. Once all processes are addressed in therapy, the next therapy cycle begins. Although this approach is widely used, no published efficacy data are available.
- *Phonotactic therapy, working on syllable and word shapes first and focusing on segment accuracy later.* Velleman (2002) showed that this approach facilitates the phonetic accuracy of segments.

## Course of Treatment

A therapy program was designed for Tom that considered the different elements of his SSD, his need to focus attention on auditory representations of words, his young age, and his frustration with communication activities. A modified course of Hodson and Paden's (1991) Cycles approach was adopted because it provided focused listening activities and a systematic way to work on Tom's phonological processes. Goals related to phonetic, phonotactic, and apraxic errors were also incorporated into the overall framework. Therapy targets for the first cycle were switched every other month and included the following:

- Consonant clusters, regardless of accuracy of cluster constituents such as /s, l/ to build Tom's syllable shapes first, then refine the accuracy of the segments
- CVCV words with different consonants to address the apraxic-like sequencing errors and work on Tom's ability to sequence consonants across a bisyllabic word
- Vowels and diphthongs
- / θ, f/ contrasts, which were an area of confusion in Tom's phoneme inventory

The second cycle expanded on the scope of the first to additionally include /j/. The [ð] substitution for /j/ was treated from an articulatory perspective. Gliding was not addressed during the first and second cycles because of Tom's young age. Articulatory work on /s, z/ was interspersed to reinforce the work on /θ, f/ contrasts, using an orthodontic model, a rubber tongue, and a mirror as visual aids. Because /s, z/ frequently do not emerge until later, they were not treated with the same intensity as the other sound errors.

Therapy was greatly enhanced by daily homework. Tom's parents were extremely supportive and made sure that Tom completed his assignments. They took turns reading word lists to him every night before bedtime, which became a comfortable ritual for him. Games and crafts were used to reinforce the relevant sound contrasts at home.

An additional goal of therapy was to address Tom's frustration with verbal communication. Therapy was designed to give him many opportunities to control his environment and to empower him as a stakeholder in his own therapy. One way to accomplish this was to create a speech folder for which he had responsibility. He was expected to carry his speech folder into the therapy room to show his homework. Another strategy was to give him choices about his weekly therapy schedule. In a plastic pocket holder, pictures of all the activities for the therapy sessions were waiting for Tom. He decided on the order ("What should we do first today, Tom?") and checked them off when completed. Because he was reluctant initially to participate in the listening activities using a tape recorder, Tom chose who would push the "Start" button, and which stuffed animal was going to join him while listening.

## Analysis of Client's Response to Intervention

### Progress in Therapy

When Tom started therapy, he had not been in a structured school setting, and separating from his mother was difficult. Andrea's presence during the first few sessions was helpful because she observed the activities and was able to continue them at home. Summer break came after the first two months of therapy, and during that time, Tom started preschool. When he returned for therapy in September, he had acquired new interaction skills and more independence. He was able to participate in therapy without his mother present, and his outbursts completely ceased.

The combined elements of therapy and the consistent home practice soon paid off. At the end of the first year of therapy, vowel accuracy was 100% in conversational speech, cluster reductions had been eliminated in words with prompts, CVCV words were 100% accurate in words with prompts, and /r/ had fully emerged without therapy. The Individual Education Plan (IEP) for Year 2 was modified accordingly. The residual consonant sequence errors and cluster reduction errors were combined into one goal ("Produce all consonants in multisyllabic words in the correct sequence"). Tom's speech was still characterized by a consistent frontal lisp and consistent substitutions of [ð] for /j/ and [f] for /θ/. According to parent report, Tom's overall communication behaviors had improved dramatically. In preschool, he interacted with his teachers and peers, and his speech was understood by others most of the time.

During Year 2, Tom was served by a different speech-language pathologist while his first therapist was on academic leave. Tom focused mainly on correct production of /s, z, j/ and progressed to the word level. At the end of Year 2, he began working on the [f] for /θ/ substitution again. All of his phonologic errors were fully resolved in conversational speech.

During the initial evaluation, Tom's parents had been made aware of his large tonsils and advised to rule out any medical sequelae such as inadequate oxygenation during sleep. Almost exactly two years later, Tom underwent tonsillectomy because of medical concerns. Andrea reported that the surgery had immediate and dramatic benefits, in that his breathing during the day had become much quieter, and he slept now without "snoring like a train."

Overall, Tom responded well to therapy. He started kindergarten, continuing to receive speech therapy to address the residual issues related to his more phonetic-based errors and the [f] for /θ/ substitution. His speech therapist reported that he appeared to have an extensive vocabulary and a good command of expressive syntax. With his new set of interaction skills, he had a great prognosis for a successful school experience socially and academically.

## Author Note

This case study is based on an actual client. The names of the child and his family members have been changed to protect their identity. The child's parents and the school district where he was served gave their explicit consent to publish this case study. The parents reviewed and approved this case prior to publication.

## References


American Speech-Language-Hearing Association (2007). *Childhood apraxia of speech* [Position Statement]. Available from http://www.asha.org/docs/html/PS2007-00277.html.

Bauman-Waengler, J. (2000). *Articulatory and phonological impairments: A clinical focus.* Boston: Allyn & Bacon.

Canic, M. J., & Franks, I. M. (1989). Response preparation and latency in patterns of tapping movements. *Human Movement Science, 8*, 123–139.

Davis, B. L., Jakielski, K. J., & Marquardt, T. P. (1998). Developmental apraxia of speech: Determiners of differential diagnosis. *Clinical Linguistics and Phonetics, 12*, 25–45.

Edwards, M. L. & Shribery, L. D. (1983). *Phonology Applications in Communication Disorders*. San Diego, CA: College Hill.

Gierut, J. A. (1990). Differential learning of phonological oppositions. *Journal of Speech and Hearing Research, 35*, 1049–1063.

Goldman, R., & Fristoe, M. (2000). *Goldman-Fristoe Test of Articulation 2*. Circle Pines, MN: American Guidance Service.

Hall, P. K. (2000a). A letter to the parent(s) of a child with developmental apraxia of speech: Part I: Speech characteristics of the disorder. *Language, Speech, and Hearing Services in Schools, 31*, 169–172.

Hall, P. K. (2000b). A letter to the parent(s) of a child with developmental apraxia of speech: Part III: Treatment of DAS. *Language, Speech, and Hearing Services in Schools, 31*, 179–181.

Hickman, L. A. (1997). *The apraxia profile: A descriptive assessment tool for children.* San Antonio, TX: Communication Skill Builders.

Hodson, B. W., & Paden, E. P. (1991). *Targeting intelligible speech. A phonological approach to remediation* (2nd ed.). Austin: PRO-ED.

Kresheck, J., & Tattersall, P. (1993). *Structured Photographic Articulation Test Featuring Dudsberry*. De Kalb, IL: Janelle Publications.

Peter, B., & Stoel-Gammon, C. (2008). Central timing deficits in children with primary speech disorders. *Clinical Linguistics & Phonetics, 22*, 171–198.

Saben, C. B., & Ingham, J. C. (1991). The effects of minimal pairs treatment on the speech-sound production of two children with phonologic disorders. *Journal of Speech and Hearing Research, 34,*1023–1040.

Shriberg, L. D., Campbell, T. F., Karlsson, H. B., Brown, R. L., McSweeny, J. L., & Nadler, C. J. (2003). A diagnostic marker for childhood apraxia of speech: The lexical stress ratio. *Clinical Linguistics and Phonetics, 17*, 549–574.

Shriberg, L. D., Lewis, B. L., Tomblin, J. B., McSweeny, J. L., Karlsson, H. B., & Scheer, A. R. (2005). Toward diagnostic and phenotype markers for genetically transmitted speech delay. *Journal of Speech, Language, and Hearing Research, 48*, 834–852.

Velleman, S. L. (2002). Phonotactic therapy. *Seminars in Speech and Language, 23*, 43–56.

Weiner, F. (1981). Treatment of phonological disability using the methods of meaningful minimal contrast: Two case studies. *Journal of Speech and Hearing Disorders, 46*, 97–103.

Williams, A. L. (2003). *Speech disorders. Resource guide for preschool children.* Clifton Park, NJ: Thomson Delmar Learning.

# CASE 20

# Molly: Cognitive-Linguistic Intervention with a Preschool Child Who Has a Visual Impairment

*Jean Pedigo*

## Conceptual Knowledge Areas

Children with normal vision are exposed, by direct instruction and through incidental learning, to a wide variety of experiences, beginning at birth. At least 80% of the information they take in from the world around them is taken in through vision (Hill & Blasch, 1980).

Since an infant begins acquiring language with early prelinguistic interactions with her parents, it is evident what a crucial role vision plays in the learning of language. Baby seeks to make eye contact, Mother smiles and talks to her, Baby coos back. Later on, Mother does funny things with her tongue as Baby gazes at her intently, and then Baby tries to imitate that tongue movement. Soon Mother gains Baby's attention and points to the object in her hand and says, "Bottle!" After she's done that numerous times, Baby says, "baba" because she now realizes that thing is called a bottle. And so it goes. This routine is repeated thousands and thousands of times over the course of Baby's first year, as Mom and Dad and all other persons in Baby's life teach her the names of all the objects she encounters every day. They also demonstrate actions for her. One day she realizes that running looks different from walking, and they both are far stranger than crawling. Thus Baby starts to learn verbs. Before she's mastered verbs, she starts hearing about size and color and location. Will she ever learn it all? Of course she will, and she'll do it in a relatively short period of time and without even thinking about it, because she can *see*.

To gain an appreciation for the role that vision plays in language and cognitive and social development, an examination of commonly used developmental checklists is recommended. For example, the Rossetti Infant-Toddler Language Scale (Rossetti, 1990) assesses many behaviors that are partially or completely reliant on vision, ranging from seeking to maintaining eye contact with an adult (0–3 months) and searching for the speaker (0–3 months), to looking at familiar people and objects when they are named (9–12 months), to pointing to pictures on request (18–24 months). Among the visual behaviors assessed on the Hawaii Early Learning Profile (HELP; Furuno et al., 1998) are localizing sound with eyes (3–5 months), reaching purposefully for an object (5–6 months), responding to facial expressions (6–7 months), and identifying self in a mirror (15–16 months). By contrast, far fewer behaviors involving vision are listed in the cognitive, social, and language sections of the Oregon Project for Preschool Children Who Are Blind or Visually Impaired (Anderson, Boigon, Davis, & deWaard, 2007).

Language acquisition without the benefit of vision, or with severely impaired vision, may be daunting for children and their parents. Educators and professionals often fail to appreciate the fundamental differences between the way sighted and visually impaired children learn.

Sighted children organize their perceptions of objects and living beings from *whole to part.* First, the entire object is seen, and then the components are evaluated one by one. A house may be a big cube with a pointed top, but on closer examination, a roof and windows and doors are noted, and perhaps there are shutters and a porch, too. A dog is a furry animal with four legs, two ears, and a tail. The child who is blind or visually impaired learns about that dog by tactual exploration, first feeling one leg, and the second, then the third and fourth, and then examining its tail, its ears, and eventually piecing those separate components into a whole animal. She will use other senses, too. She may smell the dog and listen to him bark and growl, and feel his tail move. That child is learning about her world from *part to whole,* and unlike her sighted peers, she likely will need repetitive exposures to new concepts before mastery is assured.

Obviously, not every person with a visual impairment learns in this manner, but those who are totally blind and those with severely impaired vision do. One needs to be mindful of the amount of time and effort needed to learn without the benefit of sight. Ferrell (1997) describes this process of receiving information in bits and pieces from several sources (e.g., multiple senses) as similar to putting a jigsaw puzzle together without knowing what it is supposed to look like.

Besides approaching things from a *part to whole* perspective, children who are blind or visually impaired also must learn additional information that their sighted peers do not need to think about in order to navigate their way through the sighted world, such as knowing where they are in space, learning how to move safely through their environment, understanding how to use low-vision devices and environmental cues, and learning visual efficiency training in order to improve residual vision. These and many other compensatory skills fall under the broad title of the Expanded Core Curriculum, and students with visual impairments should receive instruction addressing all of the specific skills needed to ensure their academic success. As students get older, the Expanded Core Curriculum also addresses independent living skills, recreation and leisure skills, prevocational education and career planning, and self-advocacy (LaVenture, 2007).

Experiential learning opportunities should be arranged for children with visual impairments so they have a chance to learn through tactile exploration what other children learn through seeing. Activities involving auditory, olfactory, and gustatory experiences in addition to tactile input are especially meaningful. It is important to allow enough time to explore and integrate information, to provide clear explanations and descriptions, and for repetitive practice and review in order to achieve mastery of new learning.

## Description of the Case

### Background Information

Molly is a 22-month-old-girl who was diagnosed with Leber's congenital amaurosis (LCA) as an infant. She was seen in her home by a certified Teacher of the Visually Impaired (TVI) starting at age 6 months. Initially, her parents were primarily concerned with her visual skill development, but in recent months both her parents and her vision teacher observed that she was not meeting developmental milestones in several domains. She was referred for an interdisciplinary team evaluation by her vision teacher. The results of the communication portion of the evaluation are described in the following paragraphs.

### Reason for Referral

Molly was the second child of Jane and David. She was delivered without incident and was a healthy 6-pound baby. No hearing difficulties were identified on a screening done in the hospital, and her early weeks at home were typical and uneventful. In her first few months, however, her parents began to suspect there was something wrong with her vision. She did not regard their faces or make eye contact the way her older brother had when he was her age, and other visual behaviors did not seem quite right. She failed to follow objects or people moving across her field of sight, search for faces or colorful toys, and exhibited limited head movement except when reacting to auditory stimuli. At 4 months, the parents took her to a pediatric ophthalmologist, who examined her and then ordered an electroretinogram (ERG). This test revealed a marked reduction in retinal function, and soon thereafter Leber's congenital amaurosis was diagnosed. LCA is believed to be caused by abnormal development of the photoreceptor cells in the retina. It is genetically passed and can result in progressive central field loss, peripheral field loss, loss of color vision and detail, nystagmus (rapid involuntary movement of the eyes), and eccentric viewing (viewing peripherally to compensate for a central field loss). Excessive poking or rubbing of the eyes is also characteristic.

An early childhood special education teacher who was also a certified Teacher of the Visually Impaired (TVI) initiated services to Molly and her parents in the home. She worked directly with Molly and also educated her parents regarding routines and games they could play that would encourage Molly to use her vision as she played with toys, and helped them adapt the surroundings to include high contrast and good lighting and minimize visual and auditory clutter. She provided the parents with resources related to LCA and parent support groups. Over time, the TVI taught Molly to approximate signs for *more* and *all done*, and they engaged in early reciprocal turn-taking activities. Her parents indicated on Molly's first Individual Family Service Plan (IFSP) that their goal for their daughter was for her to meet developmental milestones age appropriately. In terms of communication development, they wanted her to proceed through cooing and babbling stages on to single words and by 18–24 months to start putting two words together, similar to the sequence they had experienced with her older brother.

According to her parents, at 6 months Molly's prelinguistic development seemed to be on schedule. She cooed, she responded to her parents' voices, she calmed to music and to their voices. By 18 months, she had a vocabulary of 10 words; she followed a few simple directions and was beginning to walk with assistance. She demonstrated a beginning understanding of cause-effect, she showed preferences for certain toys, and the concepts of *in* and *out* were emerging as she played with shape sorters and other container-type toys. However, she rarely engaged in solitary vocal play, and she did not initiate communication with her brother or parents by using signs, vocalizations, or word approximations. When encouraged, she would sometimes wave *bye-bye* or imitate words. Although she loved movement and jumped on the bed with her hands held, she did not move on her own to explore her surroundings as her brother had done.

## Findings of the Evaluation

Molly was brought to the arena assessment by her mother. In this type of assessment, professionals from several disciplines (e.g., occupational therapist [OT], physical therapist [PT], speech-language pathologist [SLP], TVI, Certified Orientation and Mobility Specialist [COMS]) evaluate the child together in a play-based setting. Molly did not exhibit significant apprehension in the presence of strangers but seemed to keep track of where her mother was by turning her head when she heard her mother's voice, or smiling when she understood something her mother said about her. Although initially tentative and reserved, Molly was easily engaged in play with the PT, OT, SLP, COMS, and TVI throughout the session.

### Expressive Language

Molly did not use any words or word approximations during this evaluation but did spontaneously sign *more* on a few occasions to continue activities she was enjoying, and she spontaneously signed *all done* when she heard the examiner say, "We're all done with that drum now." The mother answered questions regarding her daughter's expressive communication from the Rossetti Infant-Toddler Language Scale, which placed Molly in the 9–12 month range with a few scattered skills above that. Her chronological age at the time of this evaluation was 22 months. She used *mama* and *dada* meaningfully; she vocalized a variety of syllables in a variety of situations; she indicated a desire for a change in activities by signing *all done*; she was able to imitate the sounds a cat, a dog and a truck make; and she enjoyed singing and engaging in finger plays. She did not name a variety of toys and functional objects on request, did not shake her head to indicate *no*, did not combine vocalization and gesture to obtain desired objects, did not ask "what's that?" and did not use action words.

### Receptive Language

Molly followed several simple directions such as *sit down* and *give me the ball* with minimal assistance. She did not visually search for toys in the area, but when they were within her reach, she was able to find familiar objects (bear, ball, baby) by tactile exploration. The mother again provided information for the Rossetti Infant-Toddler Language Scale, and Molly's receptive skills were also found to be in the 9–12 month range, again with some skills above that. She was able to identify 4 body parts on herself on request, understand a few prepositions, follow simple commands, and participate in playing patty cake with some assistance. She did not attend to pictures or look at people when they were named; she did not identify objects by category, point to action words in pictures, or choose one object from a group on request.

### Pragmatics

Most of the early skills in this area involve visual behaviors such as seeking to make eye contact with the caregiver (0–3 months), imitating facial expressions (3–6 months), and pointing to objects (15–18 months), and Molly did not exhibit these behaviors. She did, however, imitate some of her brother's vocalizations and she engaged in a few turn-taking activities with him and her parents. Her mother reported that Molly rarely interacted with other children, even though there were several children in the family and in the neighborhood who were close in age to her and her brother, and there were frequent opportunities for playing together. She said Molly enjoyed being near the other children but rarely participated in activities with them, despite adult encouragement.

### Gestures

Few of the skills on this portion of the Rossetti Infant-Toddler Language Scale were reported. Molly did not cover and uncover her face when she was playing peek-a-boo, did not reach upward to indicate she wanted to be picked up, and did not point to an object to indicate awareness of it—all skills typically seen in sighted children at 9–12 months. She did not shake her head to indicate *no* (12–15 months) and did not lead her caregiver to a desired object or toy, pretend to dance to music or pour from a container (18–21 months). She did learn to blow kisses and wave *bye-bye* on request but did not initiate those gestures at 22 months.

## Summary and Recommendations

The evaluation revealed mild to moderate delays in fine motor, gross motor, social, communication, and adaptive skills. Based on informal assessment, behavioral observations, and parent report, her expressive language, receptive language, and pragmatic behaviors reflected delays of 33–50%. Standardized testing could not be done because Molly was unable to see stimulus pictures used in these instruments. In addition to the Rossetti Infant-Toddler Language Scale, portions of the Oregon Project for Preschool Children Who Are Blind or Visually Impaired and the Hawaii Early Learning Profile (HELP) were also used, and the results were similar to the Rossetti scale findings.

## Treatment Options Considered

### Natural Environment

Although Molly had been seen by a TVI since she was 6 months old, the assessment confirmed that she needed to receive services from an OT, an SLP, and a COMS. These services could be provided in her home once a week. The advantage to receiving services in the natural environment was that Molly would learn functional skills and routines where she would be using them most often. Concern about her having to generalize skills learned elsewhere would be minimal.

### Center-Based Intervention

Near Molly's home there was a specialized preschool for children who are blind and visually impaired. Its focus was on a multisensory approach to early education that addressed the sensory needs of this population while giving children opportunities to learn through practice. It was based on principles that have been developed to facilitate meaningful learning experiences for children who are blind and visually impaired and included skills addressed by the Expanded Core Curriculum. It utilized specialized equipment and assistive technology that enhance learning opportunities and offered socialization activities with sighted peers in each classroom.

## Course of Treatment

The assessment team recommended that Molly attend preschool two half-days per week to provide her with intensive exposure to a setting rich in experiential learning opportunities and conducive to optimizing functional vision skills. At that time, she would receive speech therapy, occupational therapy, and orientation and mobility training in the classroom provided by a certified TVI. In the interim she continued to be seen by her TVI in the home.

Molly started preschool shortly after her second birthday. She adjusted to her new surroundings reasonably quickly and was able to separate from her mother without serious difficulty. Her schedule included 30-minute therapy sessions twice weekly with an occupational therapist and speech-language pathologist and two 15-minute sessions weekly with the orientation and mobility specialist (COMS). Some of the therapy sessions were conducted in quiet rooms; others were integrated into classroom activities. Vision services were provided in the classroom, which was staffed by a TVI and two teaching assistants for 7 students, including 2 sighted peers. Although the classroom looked similar to most preschool classrooms, it was organized with the needs of the visually impaired in mind. Visual clutter was kept to a minimum, good contrast and lighting were provided throughout the room, and closed circuit TV (CCTV), a computer, a braillewriter, and age-level books in print and braille were provided. Adjacent to the classroom was an observation room where parents and others could watch the activities in the classroom.

### Treatment Goals

Molly's Individual Family Service Plan (IFSP), which had been developed when she first began receiving services in the home, indicated that the parents' goals for her were:

1. Continue to learn names of objects
2. Feed herself with utensils
3. Walk independently and safely around the home
4. Use at least 50 words to get her needs met

At preschool, goals 2 and 3 were addressed by the OT and COMS, respectively; goals 1 and 4 remained priorities in her speech therapy sessions at preschool but were revised slightly with the parents' concurrence; and a social-communication goal was added:

#### Goal 1: Molly will use 2-word phrases to express her wants and needs and respond to simple questions

- ***Baseline:*** Molly occasionally used single words to get what she wanted and sometimes signed *more* to indicate that she wanted to continue an activity or that she wanted more of something to eat or drink. She occasionally signed *all done* when she wanted to stop an activity. She did not respond to questions either with gestures or words.

- ***Response to Treatment:*** Molly's vocabulary increased fairly rapidly once therapy began at school, and she began using 2-word combinations occasionally after the first month. She was consistently using 2- and 3-word utterances by the end of the year, but progress with answering questions was slow. She was able to spontaneously respond with *yes* or *no* about half the time by the end of the year.

### Goal 2: Molly will learn 20 new object labels and 10 new action words and use them in functional communication with her teachers and parents

- ***Baseline:*** Molly used approximately 10 object labels.
- ***Response to Treatment:*** Naming familiar objects and toys was a focus of individual therapy, and she learned the meaning of several action words through carefully planned experiential learning opportunities to establish the conceptual basis for the new labels and actions. These labels and actions were then reinforced in her other therapies (e.g., running and jumping in orientation and mobility sessions) and on the playground as well as in her routine classroom activities. Molly consistently used well over 75 new object labels and 25 new action words at the time of her discharge from therapy.

### Goal 3: Molly will respond to an adult's greeting or departure spontaneously by waving or saying hi or bye while looking toward the person's face

- ***Baseline:*** Molly rarely responded to greetings or waved unless cued when therapy commenced.
- ***Response to Treatment:*** Molly only needed occasional cues to face the speaker and respond with *hi* or *bye* appropriately by the end of the school year. It should be noted that this was only with adult speakers. She infrequently responded to greetings initiated by classmates and other children.

## Treatment Planning/Considerations

***Cognitive-Linguistic*** Many category names are abstract—food, clothes, songs—and are especially puzzling to children with visual impairments who do not have mental images of category members (e.g., cake, bananas, carrots) to reference in attaching meaning to the category name (food, for example). Functional activities can help in teaching abstract category names by tactually referencing concrete category members.

The child with a visual impairment typically learns in the *part to whole* sequence, so a dog, a pig, and a sheep may all seem the same because they have four legs. Teaching is often focused on tactual experience of the features that distinguish them; for example, the dog has a long hairy tail, the sheep is woolly, and the pig has very short legs and a curly tail.

Because blind children do not see personal referents, pronouns are frequently confused. A tactile cue such as taking the child's hand and helping her to pat her chest while modeling "*I* want a drink of juice," and practicing it while engaging in turn-taking routines that focus on I/you references is often effective.

Experiential learning is suggested for early action words such as *sit, run, touch* and *jump*, and it is strongly recommended for verbs like *come/go* and *give/take* for the child to differentiate the directionality of their meaning. This is also recommended for other expressions such as *here/there* and *this/that.*

***Social Skills*** Because many of the social aspects of communication are reliant on nonverbal visual signals such as eye contact, facial expressions, gestures, and body language, it is not surprising that children who are blind or visually impaired predictably have difficulty with these skills. For some children, the very earliest communication between mother and child—shared gaze—does not occur, and this has a profound effect on subsequent forms of early social communication. Babies who do not see do not automatically turn toward a person speaking to them and attempt to establish eye contact. Toddlers must be cued to face the speaker even though they may not be able to see that person at all. This skill may need to be taught and reinforced, sometimes for several years, before it is habituated in young children. Molly could see people near her but was not able to establish eye contact or perceive facial expressions, so she sometimes did not know whether the person was talking to her or to another child nearby. Giving a tactile cue (e.g., a tap on her shoulder) is one way to indicate intent, but addressing the child by name is the most efficient way. For children who do have some functional vision and are able to make eye contact but do not automatically do it, verbal cues should be given whenever it is appropriate.

Most children are taught social gestures such as waving, clapping, blowing kisses, and shaking hands, but when the child does not see well, it takes considerably more time and practice to master these gestures. Young children with visual impairments need to be made aware when they are in situations that call for one or more of these social gestures, since they may not see the child a few inches away, for example, who has reached out to hand them something.

Turn-taking in conversation requires special attention for the child with a visual impairment because she is not able to "read" the body language and facial expressions of her conversation partners. Therapy groups that focus specifically on social communication and conversational rules can be useful in teaching successful interactions with both sighted individuals and those with visual impairments.

## Conclusion

Heightened awareness of the different ways sighted and nonsighted children learn is the key to successful cognitive-linguistic intervention. Providing meaningful experiential opportunities for learning is imperative and requires diligent planning and collaboration among the various professionals in order to utilize any functional vision the children may have and facilitate the use of compensatory skills to ensure successful learning.

## Author Note

Molly is a composite character based on children with Leber's congenital amaurosis who were on the author's caseload at the Children's Center for the Visually Impaired. Permission to use information related to these children was given by the children's parents prior to the writing of this case.

## References


Anderson, S., Boigon, S., Davis, K., & deWaard, C. (2007). *The Oregon Project for Preschool Children Who Are Blind or Visually Impaired* (6th ed.). Medford, OR: Southern Oregon Education Service District.

Ferrell, K. A. (1997). What is it that is different about a child with blindness or visual impairment? In P. Crane, D. Cuthbertson, K. A. Ferrell, & H. Scherb (Eds.), *Equals in partnership: Basic rights for families of children with blindness or visual impairment.* Watertown, MA: Hilton/Perkins Program of Perkins School for the Blind and the National Association for Parents of the Visually Impaired.

Furuno, S., O'Reilly, K., Hosaka, C., Inatsuka, T., Zeisiloft-Falbey, B., & Allman, T. (1998). *Hawaii Early Learning Profile: Ages birth to three years*. Palo Alto, CA: VORT.

Hill, E. W., & Blasch, B. B. (1980). Concept development. In R. L. Welsh & B. B. Blasch (Eds.), *Foundations of orientation and mobility*. New York: American Foundation for the Blind Press.

LaVenture, S. with Allman, C. B. (2007). Special education services: What parents need to know. In S. LaVenture (Ed.), A parent's guide to special education for children with visual impairments. New York: American Foundation for the Blind Press.

Rossetti, L. (1990). *The Rossetti Infant-Toddler Language Scale*. East Moline, IL: LinguiSystems.

PART III

# School-Age Child Cases

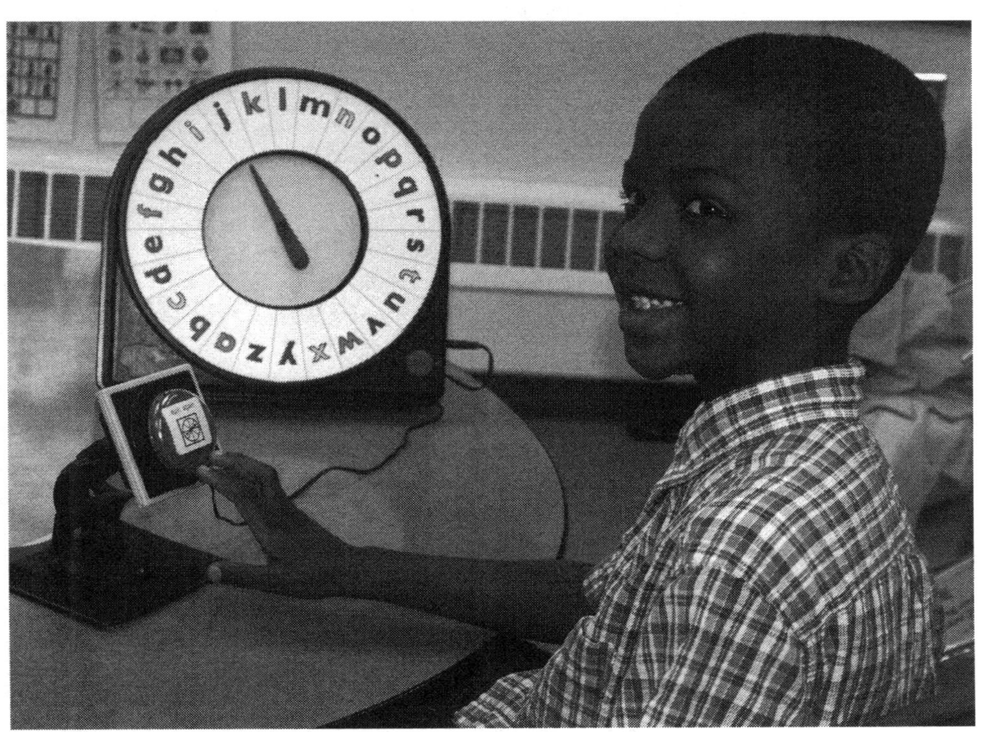

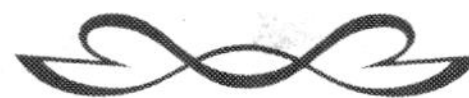



# CASE 21

# Sarah: Childhood Apraxia of Speech: Differential Diagnosis and Evidence-Based Intervention

*Kathy J. Jakielski*

## Conceptual Knowledge Areas

An understanding of this case requires the reader to have a strong knowledge base in phonetics and phonology. The reader also will benefit from having knowledge of the acquisition of speech in typically developing children, from canonical babbling through mastery, including an understanding of both segmental and suprasegmental components. Several textbooks contain overviews of these skills (e.g., Bauman-Waengler, 2008; Bernthal, Bankson, & Flipsen, 2009; Bleile, 2004; Vihman, 1996).

Childhood apraxia of speech (CAS) is a pediatric motor speech disorder that shares some common characteristics with non-CAS speech impairment; however, CAS is a distinct disorder that is differentially diagnosed using a complex of symptoms. It is important to be able to discern if a child with disordered speech exhibits CAS or nonapraxic speech impairment based on the child's specific symptoms. The best single source currently available to increase the reader's general understanding of CAS is the Technical Report published by the American Speech-Language-Hearing Association (ASHA, 2007). It is also important for the reader to be familiar with the principles of cognitive motor learning, as well as with how specific principles relate to speech production. One recent summary of motor learning theory can be found in an article published by Maas et al. (2008).

## Description of the Case

### Background Information

At age 6 years, 3 months, Sarah was brought to the College Center for Speech, Language, and Hearing (College Center) by her mother for a speech evaluation with concerns regarding the nature of Sarah's speech disorder. Sarah first was diagnosed with speech delay at age 2 years, 5 months and she had received ongoing speech intervention since that time. Sarah and her mother recently had moved to the area from another state, and the speech-language pathologist (SLP) at Sarah's new public grade school had referred Sarah to the local craniofacial clinic with concerns regarding fluctuating hypernasal speech quality. Findings from the craniofacial team were negative for structural abnormalities; however, members of the team raised concerns regarding apraxic-like speech symptoms. The team then referred the family to the College Center for a differential assessment of Sarah's speech impairment.

## Client History

The following information was secured from a parent questionnaire, a review of medical records, and parent conferencing that specifically explained and probed early and later vocal and verbal behaviors.

Sarah was the only child in a family that consisted of her biological mother and herself. Sarah's parents separated when she was 2-½ years old; they divorced when she was 4 years old. Sarah and her mother moved from another state to a lower-middle-class neighborhood that was close to the College Center when Sarah turned 6 years old, just prior to entering first grade, so that the mother could secure employment. Sarah's mother had a high school diploma and worked in sales for a furniture company. Sarah's home life was reported to be stable, with an attentive mother and an environment in which Sarah's needs were met.

Sarah's birth followed a full-term, unremarkable pregnancy. She weighed 7 pounds, 11 ounces and was 20 inches long at birth. Her Apgar score one minute after birth was 7, and five minutes after birth was 9. She produced a healthy birth cry. Sarah was breast-fed until she was approximately 6 months old; she demonstrated no difficulty sucking or swallowing. Early weight and height gains were normal for her age and sex. Throughout infancy, Sarah exhibited normal sleeping patterns and her overall health was excellent. Hearing was normal, with no history of middle ear infections.

Sarah was described as a quiet infant, producing only a limited number of sounds and engaging in minimal sound play. Canonical babbling emerged at approximately 14 months of age; babbling volubility was low. Early vocalizations were characterized by reduplicated strings of stops and nasals combined with a limited number of vowels. Sarah's mother did not remember hearing Sarah produce jargon or long, variegated strings of babble. Sarah's early communication consisted of gestures, home signs, and vocalizations. Her first intelligible word, /du/ for juice, was produced at 20 months of age; first words consisted of juice, me, no, mama, dada, doggie, and more. The mother reported that Sarah always appeared to comprehend what was said to her, including single words, short sentences, and multistep commands. At age 2-½ years, Sarah began to demonstrate some behavior problems, such as throwing her toys, squealing/yelling in anger, and hitting others. Sarah's mother reported that those behaviors appeared to be linked to Sarah's frustration at not being able to communicate well enough to express her needs. Once Sarah began to receive early intervention services, her expressive language increased and the negative behavior problems decreased.

Sarah's motor development was unremarkable except for delays in some fine motor hand skills, including stacking small blocks, placing pieces into shape sorters, and manipulating small toys; later Sarah exhibited difficulty correctly holding crayons/pencils and buttoning and zippering. No excessive drooling, eating problems, or food sensitivities were reported.

Shortly after Sarah's second birthday, her pediatrician referred her to the local early intervention program for motor and communication assessments. The physical therapist's assessment revealed normal gross motor development. The occupational therapist (OT) assessed Sarah's visual, sensory, and physical capabilities; results revealed mild delays in fine motor development, specifically in eye-hand coordination and in-hand manipulation. The SLP's assessment revealed normal play skills, normal receptive language development, moderate delays in expressive language, and mild delays in speech production. At age 2 years, 6 months, Sarah began receiving 60-minute sessions of combined, in-home OT and SLP services once every other week. Early speech goals targeted building a communication system comprised of gestures and signs paired with verbalizations. CAS initially was suspected; however, it was ruled out based on Sarah's "age appropriate oral-motor skills, including adequate tongue and jaw strength and movement, absence of excessive drooling, and good ability to chew and swallow food."

Sarah was enrolled in her public school's preschool speech and language program at age 3 years. She remained in the preschool program until she entered kindergarten at age 5 years. While in the preschool program, Sarah received direct speech and language services throughout the 9-month school year; however, OT services were decreased to monthly consultations for the first year that she was in the program, after which OT services were discontinued based on goal attainment. Speech and language goals consisted of increasing Sarah's expressive language and eliminating the phonological process of final consonant deletion using stops /p, b, t, d, k, g/ and nasals /m, n/ in single words. Sarah continued to make progress on the goals throughout her enrollment in the preschool program, although her progress remained slower than was predicted. These same goals were continued once Sarah reached kindergarten, with the addition of another goal—eliminating the phonological process of stopping of fricatives in words.

At the beginning of first grade, in her new school, Sarah had comprehensive language and cognitive testing. She also underwent an articulation screening; articulation testing was deferred pending the findings of the craniofacial clinic. Language testing was conducted by administering the Clinical Evaluation of Language Fundamentals, Fourth Edition (CELF-4; Semel, Wiig, & Secord, 2003) and by analyzing a 30-utterance spontaneous language sample. Testing revealed receptive language skills consistently in the average range of performance; expressive language performance in the areas of word structure, recalling sentences, formulated sentences, and morphosyntax was below average. Cognitive testing was conducted using the Wechsler Preschool and Primary Scale of Intelligence-III (WPPSI-III; Wechsler, 2002). Findings revealed a low-average Verbal IQ score of 86 and an average Performance IQ score of 102—a 16-point difference between quotients. Results from the informal speech screening indicated a severe speech impairment characterized by highly unintelligible speech.

Sarah's mother described Sarah as easygoing, happy, shy, socially immature, and a child who preferred to play alone. She stated that Sarah was willing to repeat herself several times in an attempt to be understood.

## Reasons for Referral

The family came to the College Center seeking a better understanding of the nature of Sarah's speech disorder. Sarah's school-based SLP also expressed the need for a differential diagnosis of Sarah's speech disorder. Sarah recently had language and cognitive testing upon transferring to her new school; therefore, the family and the SLP sought a speech-only evaluation at the College Center.

## Findings of the Evaluation

Sarah separated easily from her mother at the start of testing. Sarah interacted appropriately with the examiner and completed all tasks cooperatively and with good effort. She remained compliant throughout the 50-minute assessment session.

Sarah was tested using a variety of articulation measures, which included the Goldman-Fristoe Test of Articulation-2 (GFTA-2; Goldman & Fristoe, 2000), the Kaufman Speech Praxis Test for Children (KSPT; Kaufman, 1995), and the Fletcher Time-by-Count Test of Diadochokinetic Syllable Rate (DSR; Fletcher, 1973; see also Fletcher, 1972). During testing, informal attempts were made in conversation to elicit multiple tokens of words, as well as to elicit a variety of multisyllabic words. Informal observations focused on the suprasegmental aspects of Sarah's speech. A record review was completed to obtain information regarding Sarah's hearing ability and oral structures and functioning.

Following the completion of testing, standardized and informal analyses of the speech data were completed. Test scores were derived when possible; informal analyses yielded phonetic and error inventories for consonants, vowels, and word shapes; and observations were noted regarding suprasegmental production.

### GFTA-2

The Sounds-in-Words subtest of the GFTA-2 was administered to assess Sarah's production of speech sounds in spontaneous single words. She exhibited a total of 40 errors on this subtest, resulting in a raw score of 40. This raw score equated to a standard score of 47 and placed her below the first percentile for her age and sex.

## KSPT

The KSPT was designed to provide information regarding a child's motor speech proficiency. The KSPT consists of 4 levels—Oral Movement, Simple Phonemic and Syllabic, Complex Phonemic and Syllabic, and Spontaneous Length and Complexity levels—and contains a variety of tasks that increase in motor speech complexity within and across levels. The KSPT was normed on children up to 72 months of age (i.e., 6 years); therefore, Sarah's age of 6 years, 3 months exceeded the test's normative data, necessitating descriptive-only reporting of findings.

On the first, most basic level, the Oral Movement Level, Sarah exhibited 1 error on the 11 tasks, demonstrating difficulty rounding her lips to produce a lip pucker. All other oral-motor movements were completed easily, smoothly, and without difficulty. Sarah exhibited 2 errors on the 63 tasks on the Simple Phonemic and Syllabic Level. She exhibited no difficulty producing isolated vowel (monophthong and diphthong) imitations, singleton consonant productions, CV productions, reduplicative CVCV productions, and CVC homorganic productions (i.e., same place of articulation, as in the word /tod/, which has two alveolar consonants). She did exhibit 1 error out of 4 possible errors on tasks requiring $V_1CV_1$ or $V_1CV_2$ imitations and 1 error out of 6 possible errors on tasks requiring $CV_1CV_2$ imitations; in both of these instances, Sarah misarticulated a target vowel (as in, omə/umə, babo/bəbo). She also exhibited 2 out of 13 possible errors on simple consonant synthesis tasks requiring word-final /b/ and /d/ productions.

Tasks on the third level, the Complex Phonemic and Syllabic Level, can be used to evaluate speech movements in 6 different contexts. Some tasks can be used to test complex consonant production (designated as C) in C, CVC, and CVC productions. Other complex tasks include CCVC, $C_{front}VC_{back}$ and $C_{back}VC_{front}$, CVCVC, CVCVCV, and CVC to CVCV(C) to CVCV(C)CVC productions. Of the 91 productions elicited, Sarah misarticulated 39. Errors included difficulty producing affricates and some of the fricatives in isolation and in words. Sarah misarticulated 6 of the 15 clusters tested. She also exhibited difficulty imitating 5 of the 7 multisyllabic stimuli (i.e., cantaloupe, television, invitation, Cinderella, and puhtuhkuh); she assimilated sounds and omitted syllables. Sarah also demonstrated difficulty producing the medial syllable in the polysyllabic words tested; all of her productions were reduced to 2 syllables from 3 (e.g., wɪndo/wɪndosɪl).

Sarah's performance on the Spontaneous Length and Complexity Level was based on her spontaneous speech sample that was collected in play. Analysis revealed an increase in consonant, vowel, and word shape errors in conversational speech. Suprasegmental errors also were noted in rhythm (irregular syllable timing noted) and lexical stress (overstressing all syllables in multisyllabic words). There were numerous vowel errors exhibited in multisyllabic words and in spontaneous speech, and speech variability was noted on multiple productions of the same words. Overall, Sarah's conversational speech was rated as being partially intelligible (i.e., a score of 3–4, indicating "decodable speech").

## DSR

The DSR was administered to assess Sarah's ability to rapidly and accurately sequence reduplicated CV strings (i.e., pə, tə, kə, fə, lə, pətə, pəkə, təkə, pətəkə). Sarah's performance on all of the diadochokinetic (DDK) tasks indicated production rates that ranged from 2 to 4 times slower than the normative data provided for other 6-year-old children. Sarah especially exhibited difficulty on the multisyllabic repetition tasks. In addition, results revealed numerous misarticulations that were characterized by consonant substitutions and omissions, frequent vowel substitutions (i.e., a/ə substitutions), and poor rhythmicity, in addition to the slower rates.

## Record Review

A review of current (i.e., findings from the craniofacial team assessment) and past (i.e., early intervention and kindergarten) records revealed that Sarah's bilateral hearing was normal; she had no history of middle ear infections. Oral structures and functions also were normal for speech production.

## Phonetic Inventory

The phonetic inventory is a list of all of the consonants, vowels, and word shapes a child produces, regardless of target accuracy. For example, the word "truck" consists of 4 speech sounds, /t/, /r/, /ə/, and /k/, and the word shape is consonant-consonant-vowel-consonant (i.e., CCVC). If a child articulates the word correctly, then the child's phonetic inventory contains word-initial cluster /tr/, word-final singleton /k/, vowel /ə/, and word shape CCVC. On the other hand, for example, if a child produces the word as "tut," then the child's phonetic inventory would contain word-initial /t/, word-final /t/, vowel /ə/, and word shape CVC. The phonetic inventory provides important information regarding what sounds and sound combinations a child is capable of producing.

Sarah's consonant, vowel, and word shape phonetic inventories derived from the words she produced during testing are displayed in Table 21.1. It is important to note that every singleton consonant and vowel had the opportunity to be produced at least three times; almost all of the consonants had the opportunity to occur in every permissible word position at least one time.

## Error Inventory

The error inventory is a description of errors and error patterns exhibited by a child. Sarah's consonant, vowel, and word shape error inventories derived from the words she produced during testing are displayed in Table 21.2.

TABLE 21.1 Sarah's Phonetic Inventory at the Time of Testing

| Consonants | | Vowels | Word Shapes |
|---|---|---|---|
| **Initial Position** | | **Monophthongs** | |
| stops: | p b t d k g | i ɪ e ɛ æ | CV |
| nasals: | m n | ə a | CVCV(CV) |
| glides: | w j | u ʊ o ɔ | CVC |
| fricatives: | f v s h | | CCVC |
| affricates: | | **Diphthongs** | CVCCV |
| liquids: | l r | aɪ aʊ ɔɪ | VCVC |
| clusters: | pl bl kw gr fr | **Rhotics** | |
| **Medial Position** | | ɚ ɪɚ ɛ́ɚ uɚ | |
| stops: | p b t d k g | ɔɚ aɪɚ aʊɚ | |
| nasals: | n | | |
| glides: | | | |
| fricatives: | s | | |
| affricates: | | | |
| liquids: | l r | | |
| clusters: | mp nd | | |
| **Final Position** | | | |
| stops: | p t g | | |
| nasals: | m n | | |
| glides: | | | |
| fricatives: | s | | |
| affricates: | | | |
| liquids: | l | | |
| clusters: | | | |

TABLE 21.2 Sarah's Error Inventory at the Time of Testing

| Consonants | Vowels | Word Shapes |
|---|---|---|
| **Initial Position**<br>71% accuracy<br>2 most frequent types of errors:<br>• substitution of /d/ for consonants not in repertoire<br>• consistent substitution of /d/ for /s/ | **Monophthongs**<br>85% accuracy<br><br>Majority of errors were random substitutions of one monophthong for another monophthong | 45% accuracy<br><br>95% accuracy matching number of syllables in words |
| **Medial Position**<br>45% accuracy<br>2 error patterns:<br>• substitution of /d/ for medial consonants 64% of the time<br>• reduplication of initial-position consonant 36% of the time | **Diphthongs**<br>85% accuracy<br><br>Consistent error pattern of reducing a diphthong to a monophthong (for example, a/aɪ) | Word shape errors were result of:<br>• omissions of cluster segments<br>• omissions of final consonants |
| **Final Position**<br>42% accuracy<br>3 observations:<br>• omitted final consonant in 58% of monosyllabic and multisyllabic words ending in a consonant<br>• omitted final consonant in 39% of words ending in a stop or fricative<br>• substitution of random consonant in 42% of words ending in a consonant | **Rhotics**<br>90% accuracy<br><br>Consistent error pattern of reducing a rhotic to a monophthong (for example, ə/ɚ) | |
| **Consonant Clusters**<br>31% accuracy<br>2 error patterns:<br>• reduced clusters to a single cluster segment in 65% of misarticulated clusters<br>• substitution of /d/ or another singleton consonant in 35% of misarticulated clusters | | |

## Suprasegmental Observations

The suprasegmental aspects of Sarah's speech that were noted included rate of speech, vocal pitch, vocal quality, loudness, and lexical stress. Sarah's rate of speech was judged to be normal for her age. Her pitch was normal for her sex and age; however, she exhibited difficulty lowering her pitch to "sound like a daddy" during play. The quality of her voice was good, with the exception of intermittent hyponasal and hypernasal resonance that primarily was noted on words comprised of nasal phonemes. Sarah produced speech with appropriate loudness and demonstrated the ability to switch from whispered speech to normal speech to loud speech. She exhibited lexical stress errors on approximately 15% of the multisyllabic words she produced; she tended to produce equal-excessive stress on all syllables.

## Assessment Summary

Speech testing at the College Center when Sarah was age 6 years, 3 months revealed a severe speech impairment. The characteristics exhibited are as follows:

- An incomplete phonetic inventory for consonants /ŋ, θ, ð, z, ʃ, ʒ, ʧ, ʤ/
- An incomplete phonetic inventory for word shapes containing consonant clusters and final consonants
- Many more consonants and vowels in her phonetic inventory than she produced correctly in words
- Atypical consonant and vowel substitutions
- A high percentage of consonant omission errors
- A nondevelopmental nature to her sound development (e.g., mastery of /l/ and /r/, but omission of word-final stop consonants)
- Poor vowel accuracy in words
- An increased number of errors as stimuli increased in length and/or phonetic complexity
- An inaccurate production of lexical stress in multisyllabic words
- A reduced number of syllable productions on DDK tasks
- Arrhythmicity in syllable productions on DDK tasks
- Fluctuating nasal resonance in the absence of structural abnormalities or muscle weakness

A review of speech and language, medical, and parent reports revealed that Sarah also had a positive history of speech concerns that included the following:

- Delayed emergence of canonical babbling
- Decreased volubility of canonical babble
- A limited number of speech sounds in babble
- Decreased volubility of vocal play
- An absence of jargon
- Gestures substituted for words
- Delayed onset of first words
- An early diagnosis of speech and expressive language impairment
- Good language comprehension
- Behavior problems prior to increased expressive language output
- Highly unintelligible speech
- Slow progress in speech intervention
- Fine motor delays and history of occupational therapy
- Verbal IQ lower than performance IQ

## Differential Diagnosis

There is no single marker that can be used to diagnose CAS; rather, a complex of characteristics must be considered. Speech characteristics that were considered when differentially diagnosing the nature of Sarah's speech impairment included the observed and reported symptoms in Table 21.3.

For additional evidence of motor speech impairment, a qualitative analysis of Sarah's specific speech errors was completed. Several findings revealed motor-based errors. Sarah's preference for a single stop phoneme (i.e., /d/), numerous assimilation errors, numerous sound and syllable omissions, and reduction of clusters to singleton consonants all can be considered simplification of the motor speech plan. There was no evidence that Sarah omitted final consonants because she did not understand the concept of word-final consonants. In fact, she produced a limited but diverse variety of word-final consonants. Sarah's preference for open syllables was similar to the pattern found in infant canonical babbling in which open-syllable productions predominate. It has been argued that syllables ending in vowels are motorically less complex than syllables ending in closants (i.e., consonant-like sounds; for an overview, see Davis & MacNeilage, 1995). Based on the complex of symptoms discussed and a

TABLE 21.3 CAS Differential Symptoms

| Characteristic | Observed/Reported Characteristic | Indicators* |
|---|---|---|
| vocal development | delayed onset; limited output | characteristic of CAS |
| oral structures | no structural abnormalities | speech impairment cannot be attributed to a structural deficit |
| nonspeech oral-motor functioning | normal nonspeech oral-motor functioning | speech impairment cannot be attributed to an oral-motor deficit |
| hearing status | normal hearing | speech impairment cannot be attributed to an auditory deficit |
| sensory-motor status | history of fine motor disorder | characteristic of CAS |
| diadochokinesis | reduced number of productions<br>arrhythmic productions | characteristic of CAS |
| linguistic status | average receptive language<br>below-average expressive language | commonly reported finding in children with CAS |
| cognitive status | low-average verbal IQ<br>average performance IQ | speech impairment cannot be attributed to a cognitive deficit |
| speech intelligibility | highly unintelligible for age | characteristic of CAS |
| speech assessment findings | numerous consonant errors<br>vowel errors<br>unusual consonant and vowel errors<br>nondevelopmental errors<br>increased complexity = increased number of errors<br>lexical stress errors | when all of these symptoms are combined, highly characteristic of CAS |
| speech intervention | history of slow progress over 3-½ years of speech intervention | characteristic of CAS |
| environmental factors | attentive mother<br>enriched preschool/school environments<br>history of medical care | speech impairment cannot be attributed to an environmental deficit |

* Note: CAS is considered a symptom complex; a single marker for CAS does not exist.

preponderance of evidence suggesting a motor speech planning deficit, a diagnosis of CAS was confirmed.

## Treatment Options Considered

Numerous approaches to remediating speech impairment are available; these approaches historically have been described as being either articulatory or phonological in nature. Articulatory approaches also are referred to as phonetic- or motor-based approaches. Examples of articulatory approaches include traditional sound production training (Van Riper & Erickson, 1996), postural restructuring of motor planning therapy (PROMPT; Chumpelik, 1984), sensory-motor–based intervention (McDonald, 1964), and integral stimulation (Rosenbek, Hansen, Baughman, & Lemme, 1974; Strand & Skinder, 1999). Phonological approaches also are referred to as linguistic- or language-based. Examples of phonological approaches include the cycles approach (Hodson & Paden, 1991), Metaphon therapy (Howell & Dean, 1991), and minimal pair contrast therapy (Weiner, 1981).

CAS is a disorder that disrupts motor planning and/or programming for speech, thus a motor-based intervention approach would be congruent with the inherent motor-planning difficulty experienced by children with CAS. Integral stimulation was selected for working with Sarah because it is a cognitive- and motor-based approach for remediating speech impairment (for an overview, see Maas et al., 2008). In addition, while very few treatment efficacy studies on children with CAS have been published, three such studies have been published on integral stimulation that provide evidence of its effectiveness in treating children with CAS (Rosenbek et al., 1974; Strand & Debertine, 2000; Strand, Stoeckel, & Baas, 2006). To date no other intervention approach has been demonstrated to be more effective for treating children with CAS. Also, the College Center SLP had approximately10 years of experience successfully employing this approach with several children with CAS, and Sarah's school SLP was willing to learn the techniques.

All of the motor-based approaches, including integral stimulation, contain three similar components. These consist of an establishment phase (when a new movement pattern is learned), a stabilization phase (when the new movement pattern is produced automatically in practiced contexts), and a generalization phase (when the new movement pattern is produced automatically in novel contexts). Integral stimulation is a drill-intensive, cognitive-motor approach to speech intervention that is used to focus on decreasing the frequency and types of feedback cues provided to the child. Maximal cueing is the initial technique used to establish a new sound movement pattern, followed by (in decreasing order of support) simultaneous production, mimed production, immediate repetition, successive repetition, delayed repetition, question response, reading, and so on. Simultaneous production is when the SLP and child say the target utterance at the same time. Mimed production is when the SLP mouths the target while the child watches the SLP and says the target aloud. Immediate repetition is when the SLP models the target and the child repeats the target directly following the model. Successive repetition is when the child imitates the SLP's initial model several times successively without being provided an additional model. Delayed repetition is when the child imitates the SLP's model after waiting for several seconds after the model is provided. Question response is when the child spontaneously produces the target utterance after being asked a question by the SLP. Cueing begins with the SLP providing maximal multisensory input and a slowed speech rate. The SLP then slowly fades temporal and tactile cues as the child demonstrates the ability to take increasing responsibility for the assembly, retrieval, and execution of the motor speech plan at a normal speech rate.

## Course of Treatment

Following the assessment, Sarah's mother enrolled her in twice-weekly 20-minute individual speech intervention sessions at the College Center. The center's schedule consisted of fall and spring 14-week semesters, separated by a 6-week winter vacation. Sarah's school SLP agreed to follow the speech goals developed at the College Center. Sarah's school speech intervention schedule consisted of two 20-minute individual sessions weekly; school speech intervention was scheduled on alternate days when Sarah was not seen at the College Center. Between both sites, Sarah received 20 minutes of speech intervention 4 days a week. The school SLP also saw Sarah for two 20-minute group language intervention sessions per week.

The integral stimulation cueing hierarchy used with Sarah consisted of six levels, including (from most to least support) simultaneous production, mimed production, immediate repetition, successive repetition, delayed repetition, and question response. Productions were scored using Strand and Debertine's (2000) 0–2 point scale. A score of 2 indicated that the utterance was produced with no articulation errors. A score of 1 indicated that the utterance was intelligible and contained only 1–2 articulation errors. A score of 0 indicated that the utterance did not meet the criteria for a score of 1 or 2. Sarah's school SLP learned integral stimulation methods and used the same cues and cueing hierarchy that were used at the College Center. Sarah's articulation goals for the dual-site, 9-month intervention period follow.

### Goal 1

*In response to cognitive-motor learning principles incorporated into integral stimulation intervention, Sarah will increase her phonetic inventory to include the fricatives /θ, ð, z, ʃ/.*

***Related Subgoal 1*** To decrease Sarah's preference for open word shapes.

***Related Subgoal 2*** To increase Sarah's vowel accuracy in monosyllabic words.

- ***Objective 1:*** Sarah will correctly produce /θ/ and /ʃ/ in word-final position in functional monosyllabic words and short sentences.
- ***Objective 2:*** Sarah will correctly produce /ð/ and /z/ in word-initial position in functional monosyllabic words and short sentences.
- ***Objective 3:*** Once Sarah demonstrates approximately 50% accuracy on objectives 1 and 2 at the level of successive repetition, vowel production accuracy also will be targeted.

***Rationale*** Increasing Sarah's phonetic repertoire to include the four target fricatives would increase her overall speech intelligibility. Learning how to produce these sounds in words would add an increased level of complexity to her motor speech skill repertoire. In typically developing children, voiceless fricatives emerge first in word-final position, so teaching word-final production of /θ/ and /ʃ/ was selected to simulate the developmental context. In addition, teaching /θ/ and /ʃ/ in word-final position would help to eliminate Sarah's preference for open word shapes. Working on /ð/ and /z/ in word-initial position would increase intelligibility of Sarah's speech by eliminating her preference for /d/ in word-initial position. Last, addressing vowel accuracy once the consonant targets were emerging would lead to increased speech intelligibility. Stimuli initially consisted of monosyllabic words in an attempt to minimize the articulatory demands on Sarah as she learned how to produce the four later-mastered fricatives.

## Goal 2

*In response to cognitive-motor learning principles incorporated into integral stimulation intervention, Sarah will increase correct production of a variety of speech sounds in functional multisyllabic words that are comprised of sounds already in her phonetic repertoire.*

- ***Objective 1:*** Sarah correctly will produce all phonemes in 10 functional multisyllabic words selected by Sarah and her mother.
- ***Objective 2:*** Sarah correctly will produce all phonemes in up to 20 multisyllabic words selected from the Grade 1 National Reading Vocabulary List. (TampaREADS, n.d.).

***Rationale*** Multisyllabic word production is similar to connected speech production, so Sarah's ability to correctly produce multisyllabic words would lead to increased overall articulatory proficiency and intelligibility. Sarah's ability to produce multisyllabic words should help her communicate more independently and help her to express her needs and wants more effectively at home and school, and in other social situations. Using words that Sarah selects should help to increase her interest in intervention and should increase her practice time, as those words should have a high frequency of occurrence for Sarah. Using words from the Grade 1 National Reading Vocabulary List (e.g., before, after, today, tomorrow, cannot, etc.) should increase Sarah's speech intelligibility, as well as help to avert potential reading problems.

## Goal 3

*In response to cognitive-motor learning principles incorporated into integral stimulation intervention, Sarah will correctly produce all of the speech sounds in 6 functional sentences.*

***Rationale*** Sarah's ability to correctly produce the sounds in the target sentences would increase her overall speech intelligibility and help her to communicate more independently. Sentences targeted contained personal information that was important for Sarah to be able to convey to unfamiliar listeners. Examples of target sentences included: "My name is Sarah xxx," "My phone number is 794-xxxx," "I live in Rock Island, Illinois," and "My address is xx Pine Road."

## Analysis of Client's Response to Intervention

Sarah's overall response to speech intervention was slow but steady throughout the academic year. She remained positive and enthusiastic about attending therapy and worked hard during her sessions at the College Center and at school. Sarah attended a total of 110 20-minute speech sessions over the 9-month period, totaling approximately 37 hours of speech intervention between both sites. Typically, all three goals were addressed in each session. The number of target utterances practiced varied, depending on her success on a goal within and across sessions. Smaller target sets tended to be used as Sarah established new sounds and word shapes, with stimuli increasing in number as she became more successful.

### Goal 1

Sarah initially exhibited the slowest overall progress on this goal. Sarah began intervention able to produce the target phonemes only when provided a very slow speech model and tactile cues. Sarah initially made the most rapid progress on /θ/ and /ʃ/ in word-final position; after approximately 16 sessions, she could produce these sounds in target words in immediate repetition with scores of 1 and 2. She made slower progress on /ð/ and /z/ in word-initial position; after approximately 16 sessions, Sarah could produce these sounds in words in mimed productions with scores of 1. After the first 50 sessions, she was able to produce all four fricatives in target words and contexts with scores of 1 on successive repetition tasks. Sarah demonstrated the most regression on this goal after she returned to the College Center from winter break, even though she had received some school-based intervention for 3 of the 6 weeks. By the end of the school year, Sarah was able to correctly produce the target fricatives in target utterances with scores of 1 and 2 on delayed repetition tasks.

### Goal 2

Sarah demonstrated the most rapid progress on and pleasure with this goal. She began intervention producing target multisyllabic words with scores of 0 and 1 in simultaneous production with moderate cues (e.g., slowed model, exaggerated movements, etc.). Her most frequent error was omitting syllables. To initiate work on this goal, therapy began by having Sarah produce strings of 3–5 CV words containing sounds in her phonetic repertoire. For example, Sarah simultaneously produced baa-baa-baa-baa with the SLP, and once able to do this in successive repetition, the string would be changed (for example, to baa-bee-bee-baa). Toward the latter part of the first month of intervention, Sarah had learned to produce repetitive word strings containing sounds from her phonetic inventory intelligibly and with decreased cues; a list of 10 multisyllabic words then was developed by Sarah, her mother, and the SLPs. After approximately 2-½ months of intervention (i.e., ~40 sessions), Sarah consistently produced the 10 target words with scores of 2 in response to questions. Multisyllabic word targets then were selected from the Grade 1 National Reading Vocabulary List. (TampaREADS, n.d.).

By the end of another 40 intervention sessions, Sarah was consistently producing those words with scores of 2 in response to questions. In addition, Sarah demonstrated the ability to read over half of the target words by sight.

### Goal 3

Sarah exhibited good progress on this goal, demonstrating functional mastery after receiving the equivalent of 5 months of intervention (i.e., ~80 20-minute sessions). Sarah began intervention on this goal needing maximal cues (e.g., slowed model, exaggerated movements, simultaneous production, etc.) to achieve scores of 0 and 1. After approximately 2 months of intervention, she consistently produced target utterances with scores of 1 and 2 in immediate repetition of a model. After 5 months of intervention, she consistently produced all of the target utterances with scores of 2 in delayed repetition, and with scores of 1 and 2 in question response. This goal was discontinued in the middle of the spring semester (i.e., after the equivalent of approximately 5 months of intervention); however, Sarah's teacher periodically asked Sarah questions to elicit the target utterances. Her teacher reported that Sarah maintained intelligibility and largely correct articulation of all 6 sentences until the end of the school year.

In summary, Sarah demonstrated success on all three speech goals. Based on her progress in response to integral stimulation intervention at the end of first grade, the College Center SLP predicted that Sarah's speech likely would resolve to normal if she continued to receive frequent speech intervention sessions over the next several years. Sarah's speech gains were also apparent to Sarah herself. She clearly expressed her excitement over "learning to talk better" and by the spring of first grade, Sarah more frequently initiated conversation with her peers, volunteered to answer in class, and talked on the telephone.

## Author Note

The case described is not based on an actual client.

## References


American Speech-Language-Hearing Association. (2007). *Childhood apraxia of speech* (Technical Report). Retrieved from www.asha.org/policy.

Bauman-Waengler, J. (2008). *Articulatory and phonological impairments: A clinical focus* (3rd ed.). Boston, MA: Allyn & Bacon.

Bernthal, J. E., Bankson, N. W., & Flipsen, P. (2009). *Articulation and phonological disorders: Speech sound disorders in children* (6th ed.). Boston, MA: Allyn & Bacon.

Bleile, K. (2004). *The manual of articulation and phonological disorders: Infancy through adulthood* (2nd ed.). Clifton Park, NY: Thomson Delmar Learning.

Chumpelik, D. (1984). The PROMPT system of therapy: Theoretical framework and applications for developmental apraxia of speech. *Seminars in Speech and Language, 5*, 139–156.

Davis, B. L., & MacNeilage, P. F. (1995). The articulatory basis of babbling. *Journal of Speech and Hearing Research, 38*, 1199–1211.

Fletcher, S. G. (1972). Time-by-count measurement of diadochokinetic syllable rate. *Journal of Speech and Hearing Research, 15*, 763–70.

Fletcher, S. G. (1973). *Fletcher time-by-count test of diadochokinetic syllable rate.* Tigard, OR: C.C. Publications.

Goldman, R., & Fristoe, M. (2000). *Goldman-Fristoe test of articulation* (2nd ed.). Circle Pines, MN: American Guidance Service.

Hodson, B. W., & Paden, E. P. (1991). *Targeting intelligible speech: A phonological approach to remediation* (2nd ed.). Austin, TX: PRO-ED.

Howell, J., & Dean, E. (1991). *Treating phonological disorders in children: Metaphon—theory to practice.* San Diego, CA: Singular Publishing.

Kaufman, N. R. (1995). *Kaufman speech praxis test for children.* Detroit, MI: Wayne State University Press.

Maas, E., Robin, D.A., Austermann Hula, S.N., Freedman, S.E., Wulf, G., Ballard, K.J., et al. (2008). Principles of motor learning in treatment of motor speech disorders. *American Journal of Speech-Language Pathology, 17*, 277–298.

McDonald, E.T. (1964). *Articulation testing and treatment: A sensory motor approach.* Pittsburgh, PA: Stanwix House.

Rosenbek, J. C., Hansen, R., Baughman, C. H., & Lemme, M. (1974). Treatment of developmental apraxia of speech: A case study. *Language, Speech, and Hearing Services in Schools, 1*, 13–22.

Semel, E., Wiig, E. H., & Secord, W. A. (2003). *Clinical evaluation of language fundamentals* (4th ed.). San Antonio, TX: Harcourt Assessment.

Strand, E. A., & Debertine, P. (2000). The efficacy of integral stimulation intervention with developmental apraxia of speech. *Journal of Medical Speech-Language Pathology, 8*, 295–300.

Strand, E. A., & Skinder, A. (1999). Treatment of developmental apraxia of speech: Integral stimulation methods. In Caruso, A. & Strand, E. A. (Eds.), *Clinical management of motor speech disorders in children* (pp. 109–148). New York: Thieme.

Strand, E. A., Stoeckel, R., & Baas, B. (2006). Treatment of severe childhood apraxia of speech: A treatment efficacy study. *Journal of Medical Speech-Language Pathology, 14*, 297–307.

TampaREADS. (n.d.). *Reading key.* Retrieved March 26, 2010, from http://tampareads.com.

Van Riper, C., & Erickson, R. (1996). *Speech correction: An introduction to speech pathology and audiology* (9th ed.). Englewood Cliffs, NJ: Prentice-Hall.

Vihman, M. M. (1996). *Phonological development: The origins of language in the child.* Cambridge, MA: Blackwell.

Wechsler, D. (2002). *Wechsler preschool and primary scale of intelligence* (3rd ed.). San Antonio, TX: Psychological Corporation.

Weiner, F. (1981). Treatment of phonological disability using the method of meaningful minimal contrast: Two case studies. *Journal of Speech and Hearing Disorders, 46*, 29–34.

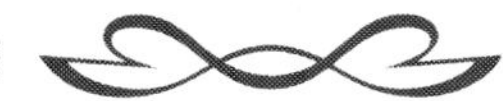

## ARTICULATION/PHONOLOGY

CASE **22**

# David: Of Mouth and Mind: An Articulation and Phonological Disorder in a Young School-Age Child

*Susan T. Hale and Lea Helen Evans*

## Conceptual Knowledge Areas

### Referral Questions and Assessment Decisions

When parents or school personnel report that a child has speech that is "delayed" or "difficult to understand" or even "unintelligible," the speech-language pathologist must make some important initial decisions about whether and how to assess the child. A referring statement, whether oral or written, brings immediate questions to mind.

- Is the child experiencing speech differences that are within the range of normal performance expected for children of the same age?
- Are the speech sound differences misarticulations or phonological error patterns, or is there evidence of both?
- Is it possible that there are other concomitant problems such as receptive or expressive language delays/disorders, hearing loss, oral motor or structural differences, developmental delays, or behavioral issues?
- How consistent are the errors across speech contexts, and can the child improve the errored productions with instruction?
- What is the likelihood that the speech pattern will have an effect on academic achievement in the areas of reading, spelling, or writing?

Initial impressions about the possible answers to these questions will come from a thorough case history. However, each question must also be answered through direct observation and interaction with the child. An accurate assessment of a disorder of articulation/phonology rests not only on the information obtained from the case history and the direct observations but also on the clinician's sound conceptual and experiential framework for addressing articulation and phonological disorders. Specifically, the clinician must have the following knowledge and skills:

- Theoretical knowledge of normal aspects of development for articulation and phonology, which may affect both assessment and remediation decisions
- Clinical knowledge and skill using appropriate articulation/phonology assessment protocols
- Clinical knowledge and skill using evidence-based remediation approaches for articulation/phonological disorders

## Developmental Articulation/Phonology Models

To appropriately evaluate and remediate a phonological disorder, the clinician must have a working knowledge of the theories of developmental phonology. Many strategies have been suggested as possible models of phonological development. Vihman (2004) cites original authors and includes reasonably comprehensive descriptions of the following models: the behaviorist model, the natural phonology model, the generative phonology model, the prosodic model, the cognitive model, the biological model, the self-organizing model, and the nonlinear model.

Whereas the behavioral and structural models, based more on deductive rather than empirical thinking, have largely fallen out of favor, the remaining models address more currently accepted ideas regarding the presence or absence of universals, systematization, and the accuracy or inaccuracy of the child's speech perception from the beginning (Vihman, 2004). Maturation and practice clearly influence phonological development. Models that suggest the child engages in problem solving and also brings nonlinear learning related to prosody and segmental knowledge to the task complement most commonly used approaches for remediation (Vihman, 2004). As with any aspect of communication development, the model or models that the clinician accepts affect the clinical decision-making process. However, Vihman (2004) cites Macken and Ferguson, who stated that one point on which "virtually all theoretical persuasions can agree is the *systematic* nature of the child's simplifications and restructuring of adult words."

## Assessment Rationale

In order to evaluate the presence or absence of a disorder of articulation or phonology, the well-prepared clinician should have a reasonably standardized protocol for assessment. Certain aspects of the child's history, physical makeup, and sensory and oral motor abilities must be assessed. Physical causes (hearing loss, problems with oral structures or their functioning) for the disorder must be ruled out with accepted measurement protocols.

Objective, reliable, and valid assessment of the child's current speech and language status is essential. Receptive and expressive language must be evaluated to assure that the problems in articulation are not compounded by problems in the language system. Additionally, the objective measures of speech sound production, which often occur in word-only contexts, must be supplemented with subjective observations in naturalistic and interactive environments.

Although the discussion of the current case focuses on thorough assessment illustrative of a clinical "ideal," Tyler et al. (2002) remind us that there is a need for balance between the ideals of thoroughness and efficiency. Evaluation appointments typically must progress from history to the final step of informing and counseling parents within a time span that is reasonable in the clinical setting and within the attention span of the child being evaluated. The current case is presented with the assumption that those measures not completed in the initial assessment were conducted during the first clinical session. Specific measures and their results are provided.

## Intervention Models

In addition to a basic understanding of the theories of developmental phonology, the clinician must also have a working knowledge of the theoretical approaches to clinical remediation. Kahmi (2006) explored the fundamental similarities and differences in current clinical approaches. Accordingly, he delineates the following five models: (1) normative, (2) bottom-up, discrete skill, (3) language-based, (4) broad-based, and (5) complexity-based.

According to the normative view, decisions regarding the presence or absence of a speech sound disorder, as well as decisions regarding the nature or severity of the disorder, are based on comparison of the client's speech to that of other children who are developing speech sounds typically. With this clinical approach, the clinician would begin treatment with targets no smaller than the syllable but would focus primarily on treatment beginning at the word level. Kamhi (2006) cautions that comparing the phonological learning of a child with a disorder to the normative sequence may lead to erroneous conclusions. Additionally, Kamhi (2006) suggests that most effective interventions for phonological disorders rely, at some point, on teaching the production of the target sound in isolation, a phenomenon that does not occur in normal development.

A bottom-up, discrete skill approach is the basis for two different treatment models. The traditional motor approach (Van Riper & Emerick, 1984) rests on the initial teaching of auditory discrimination for errored phonemes and moves to a stepwise progression of production in isolation, words, phrases, sentences, and finally, conversation. The second branch of the bottom-up, discrete skill approach assumes that physical practice of the oral musculature outside the context of communication increases the accuracy of speech sound production in communication. Therefore, clinicians adhering to this approach incorporate oral motor exercises into a treatment protocol. Both models are widely used. Kamhi (2006) reports a lack of evidence that the oral motor approach improves speech production. He further indicates that while the traditional motor approach is supported by efficacy data, it has notable limitations (Kamhi, 2006).

Language-based approaches consider speech to be inexorably entwined with language. Taking into account the synergistic nature of phonology and language, clinicians who adhere to this approach focus therapy within the context of naturally occurring interactions and do not decontextualize the communication with direct instruction or practice. This protocol indirectly addresses speech sound errors. Kamhi (2006) cites prevailing findings that indicate that direct treatment is necessary for children with significant speech delays.

A broad-based approach to therapy combines parts from many different treatment approaches including the normative approach and the bottom-up discrete skill approach. The broad-based paradigm is probably most widely applied in the form of Hodson's cycles approach (Hodson & Paden, 1991). This model considers movement in a stepwise progression as well as in teaching speech sound motor movements. Like the normative approach, this broad-based approach bases target selection on typical speech sound development. Finally, this model gives the clinician the flexibility to use any form of evidence-based treatment that is effective for a particular child. Kamhi (2006) cites limited studies supporting a cycles approach as being more efficacious than other approaches.

Finally, the complexity approach addresses more complex targets first, which, when corrected, create the greatest positive change in overall speech-sound production with a resulting generalization to non-targeted (less complex) sounds. Kamhi (2006) notes that despite numerous studies supporting the efficacy of this model of treatment, clinicians do not typically select goals in regard to complexity principles.

Regardless of the approach chosen, current research has indicated that all of the models detailed above are effective (Kahmi, 2006). Gierut (2005) indicated that the treatment target chosen for therapy was more important than the way in which it was taught. Kamhi (2006) summarizes this viewpoint by stating that "one treatment approach has not proved to be better than another."

## Description of the Case

### Background Information

David D., a 6-year, 4-month-old male, was seen for a speech-language evaluation in the Pediatric Speech-Language Clinic of the Vanderbilt Bill Wilkerson Center (the Center), Nashville, TN. A certified and state licensed SLP saw David for his evaluation. David was accompanied to the evaluation by his mother, his two younger sisters, and his maternal grandmother. The clinician briefly observed David interacting with his sisters. Then, his sisters left the examination room with the grandmother to play on the playground. David's mother provided case history information and then observed the testing session from the observation room. She returned to the examining room at the conclusion of the session in order to receive the results of the assessment. David separated from his sisters and mother easily and was readily engaged with the toys in the testing room. He then transitioned smoothly to the activities of the evaluation. He was cooperative and communicative throughout the session. When the clinician had difficulty understanding him, he repeated his messages up to three times before showing signs of frustration. When asked why he thought he was at the Center, David responded, "Because my friends don't understand me sometimes."

#### History

David was from an upper-middle-class family who had just moved to the area. His father was an attorney, and his mother did not work outside the home. She indicated that "my children are my focus" at this particular stage in life. She held a degree in elementary education. David was the oldest of three siblings. He had two younger sisters, one age 3 years and one who was 15 months old. The parent reported that the two younger children had speech and language development commensurate with other children their ages. Other familial communication disorders were not reported.

Pregnancy and birth history for David were unremarkable. Medical history was significant for recurrent otitis media (three to four episodes per year) treated with antibiotics. After placement of pressure equalization (PE) tubes when David was 3 years old, further ear infections were not noted. David achieved all developmental milestones at the expected ages.

At the time of the evaluation David had just completed kindergarten. He had not attended a day care, preschool or prekindergarten program, in his previous home town. Teacher checklists indicated that while he was very reticent in groups of his peers and in volunteering to answer questions aloud in class, David excelled in kindergarten and surpassed all of the state-determined benchmarks including phonetic awareness and identification and conceptual knowledge of numbers and colors. He had a sight-word vocabulary of 50 words. Additional teacher report revealed that David exhibited some aggressive interactions on the playground that typically occurred when he attempted to verbally engage his peers.

David's mother brought him to the Center due to his poor intelligibility. She expressed concern about the discrepancy between his level of intelligence and his speech intelligibility and his growing frustration level. Additionally, his mother reported that David's sisters were more intelligible even though they were younger than he and that unfamiliar adults in unfamiliar contexts were not able to understand David much of the time. On the day of the speech/language evaluation, the clinician, as an unfamiliar listener, noted that David's intelligibility in connected speech was less than 50%. Intelligibility improved when the clinician could relate David's word production to a limited and known context or when he was producing single words. David's sisters did not seem to be concerned about his speech. They did not respond verbally when David said something that they did not understand; however, they were attentive to his words and actions and seemed to gain an understanding of his intended messages through the gestalt of the situation. David had no prior history of evaluation or therapy for speech or language issues.

## Reasons for Referral

The concern of the parents, which was supported by observations from David's kindergarten teacher, caused the mother to seek a speech-language consultation. She was most anxious to proactively address any barriers to academic achievement that his speech and language might present and to reduce the presence of social frustration.

## Findings of the Evaluation

### Oral Mechanism Examination

An examination of the oral mechanism revealed normal and intact oral structures. General symmetry of the face at rest and while making specific movements was observed to be within normal limits. Off-target groping, uncoordinated movements, or signs of weakness were not noted. Structural and functional integrity of the lips and tongue were intact. Structural and functional integrity of the hard and soft palates appeared to be intact. Velopharyngeal incompetence or insufficiency was not noted; however, there was a slight inflammation of the faucial tonsils (located between the anterior and posterior faucial pillars). When asked about it, the mother indicated that David was just getting over a sore throat. The integrity of the teeth and dental arches were intact with normal occlusal relationships. However, the upper right central incisor was noted to be loose, which was judged to be normal at David's age for a deciduous tooth. Repetitive tongue and lip movements and palatal elevation for the sustained /ah/ vowel were judged to be within normal limits.

### Standardized Assessment Measures

***Goldman-Fristoe Test of Articulation-2 (GFTA-2; 2000)***—This assessment instrument, initially published in 1969, is appropriate for clients 2 years of age through 21 years, 11 months of age, measures speech sound production in the word initial, medial, and final positions as well as in consonant blends. Using 34 pictures and 53 words, this evaluation of sound production uses indications of substitutions, distortions, and omissions to describe speech sounds at the word level. In addition to assessing speech sound production in individual words, the assessment also evaluates connected speech in a somewhat restricted manner by eliciting sentences/conversational speech from the client through story retelling. A third component of the GFTA-2 is a stimulability assessment of individual phonemes at the syllable, word, and sentence levels. David's raw score on the GFTA-2 was 24. This raw score converted to a standard score of 70, a percentile rank of 7, and an approximate age equivalent of less than 2 years. Errors included the data in Table 22.1.

***Khan-Lewis Phonological Analysis-2 (KLPA-2; 2002)***—Originally published in 1986, this assessment instrument uses the information obtained by the GFTA-2 to identify phonological processes that could be active in the child's speech sound system. This assessment evaluates

TABLE 22.1 The Goldman-Fristoe Test of Articulation-2—Errors

| **Initial Position** | **Medial Position** | **Final Position** |
|---|---|---|
| w/r, t/ th (voiceless), b/v, t/s, d/z, d/th (voiced), bw/br, dw/dr, fw/fr, gw/gr, kw/kr, t/sl. t/st, tw/tr | t/sh, w/r, -/th (voiceless), b/v, t/w, and d/th (voiced) | w/r, t/ th (voiceless), b/v, and t/s |

* Note: In the notations, errors are listed by position with slash marks; that is, if a child produced "dog" as "gog," the substitution would be indicated as being in the initial position as g/d. If the consonant was omitted, the omission would be indicated as a "-". For example, if the child produced "dog" as "do," the error would be indicated in the final position as -/g/. Results of stimulability testing indicated that David was stimulable for all phonemes in at least one context with the exception of /r/, which was not stimulable at any level.

the GFTA-2 information for 12 developmental and 3 nondevelopmental processes. David's raw score on the KLPA-2 was 31. This raw score converted to a standard score of 68, a percentile rank of 6, and an approximate age equivalent of 3 years, 2 months. Developmental processes and percentage of occurrence noted included deletion of final consonants (2% occurrence), stopping of fricatives and affricates (42% occurrence), cluster simplification (11%), and liquid simplification (45%).

***Preschool Language Scale-4 (PLS-4; 2002)***—Originally published in 1969, this assessment instrument for children birth to age 6 years, 11 months evaluates the child's ability to understand language directed toward him or her (auditory comprehension subtest) as well as to use language to communicate with others and to effect change in the environment (expressive communication subtest). David's raw score on the auditory comprehension subtest of the PLS-4 was 61. This raw score converted to a standard score of 103, a percentile rank of 58, and an approximate age equivalent of 6 years, 6 months. David's raw score on the expressive communication subtest of the PLS-4 was 65. This raw score converted to a standard score of 99, a percentile rank of 47, and an approximate age equivalent of 6 years, 3 months. Combined, these raw scores were 126. The combined standard scores converted to a total language standard score of 101, a percentile rank of 53, and an approximate age equivalent of 6 years, 7 months.

### Informal Descriptive Measures

An analysis of a connected speech sample was used to augment the information obtained from the standardized assessment measures, since the standardized measures focused primarily on production of speech sounds at the single word level. Assessment of the speech sample was accomplished with both an independent analysis (assessment of speech sound productions without reference to the adult targets of the word) and a relational analysis (assessment of the child's speech sound production as those productions relate to the adult targets). Results of independent and relational analyses performed on a connected speech sample taken while David engaged in free play with his sisters and later his mother yielded speech sound inventories as well as phonological process usage similar in nature to those found with the standardized assessments.

### Audiological Screening and Screening Tympanometry

Normal results were obtained from a hearing screening at 20 dB SPL for the frequencies 500–8,000 Hz. Otoscopic evaluation of the external ear and middle ear was unremarkable. It was noted that the PE tubes were no longer in place. Screening tympanometry revealed Type A tympanograms bilaterally, suggesting normal mobility of the middle ear structures. Results suggested the presence of normal hearing for speech purposes as well as middle ear functioning within normal limits.

### Speech Sound Discrimination Testing

Informal testing indicated that David was able to appropriately discriminate between speech sounds in a variety of contexts.

### Voice

Voice quality and pitch were normal for David's age and gender.

### Fluency

David had normal speech fluency in connected speech.

## Representation of the Problem at the Time of Evaluation

David exhibited age-appropriate receptive and expressive language skills, normal fluency, and normal voice production. However, his production of the sounds of language did not appear to be age-appropriate at the time of the evaluation. Standardized and informal assessments indicated that he exhibited both an articulation disorder (inability to produce /r/) and immature phonological processes (stopping of fricatives and affricates and cluster reduction). Although analysis indicated the presence of the process of gliding of liquids, it was judged that this finding was due to David's inability to produce /r/ rather than to a phonological process affecting all of the liquids. This observation was supported by David's ability to produce /l/ in a variety of contexts.

In summary, David exhibited delayed articulatory/phonological development. He substituted w/r in word initial and medial positions and in all consonant blends containing /r/, and this pattern was judged to be a motor error for the production of /r/. In addition, he exhibited the phonological processes of stopping of fricatives and affricates, and cluster reduction. The process of cluster reduction did not occur at a level of consistency to warrant remediation. However, the process of stopping of fricatives and affricates was strongly present and had a significant impact on David's intelligibility. Individual therapy was recommended at a frequency of 2 times per week for 1-hour sessions to address /r/ errors and the phonological process of stopping of fricatives/affricates.

## Treatment Options Considered

In accordance with the preceding hypothesis, David had both phonological process usage as well as motoric articulation errors. The two types of errors warranted different remediation approaches. In view of the treatment models presented and the conclusions regarding efficacy by Kamhi (2006), a hybrid approach to speech sound remediation was chosen. This approach included elements of the traditional model (to address his articulation error in the production of /r/) and the broad-based approach (to address those speech sound errors that occurred due to inappropriate phonological process usage, notably, stopping of fricatives and affricates).

## Course of Treatment

Therapy was designed to work briefly on the traditional, motoric production of /r/ before moving to a more cycles-based approach for remediation of the phonological process of stopping of fricatives and affricates. After a short traditional production activity designed to teach the placement of the /r/ phoneme, each therapy session was divided into the following sequence: (1) review of previous session's production targets, (2) listening activity for the identified phonological process, (3) target word review to incorporate new exemplars for the process being addressed, (4) production practice in play-based activities, (5) stimulability probing, (6) return to listening activity for the day's exemplars, and (7) discussion of home programming.

A vertically structured articulation treatment approach was employed. At the initiation of therapy, activities were planned to coincide with David's current level of functioning. Comprised of drill play, these activities consisted of turn-taking games in which turns focused on the imitation and then spontaneous production of the /r/ phoneme initially in isolation, syllables, monosyllabic CVC words, and sentences. David had to reach criterion of mastery at each level before moving to the next.

Although a more broad-based phonological approach was chosen, only one phonological process was deemed to be severely affecting David's intelligibility—the stopping of fricatives and affricates. The percentage of occurrence of the phonological process of gliding of liquids was directly attributed to the absence of the /r/ phoneme. The percentage of occurrence of the phonological process of cluster reduction was fairly small and was not felt to affect intelligibility to a great extent. Since the clinician and client were only focused on one phonological process, the treatment approach was more vertical in nature though the sequence of therapy activities from a cycles-based approach was incorporated. For each session, the first activity incorporated review of the previous week's practice words with the client. The client was not required to make any judgments of the words or to produce any of the previous week's targets.

The second activity consisted of a listening activity in which the child did not actively participate but rather listened to the clinician's production of the week's target words. For the listening activity, there were typically between 10 and 12 words that contained the target sound. (Although it was not used with David, this activity may be done with the use of an amplification device. Additionally, during this activity the clinician may contrast the correct production of the target with the misarticulation.)

The third activity consisted of creation of target word cards. Within the context of this activity, the clinician and the client chose between 3 and 5 of the target words, which were represented by created pictures. These representations took different forms including line drawings, photocopied pictures, stickers, and appropriate representations from magazines. The name of the picture represented was written on each of the cards.

The fourth activity comprised the majority of each therapy session and consisted of production practice, which is similar to production practice in many other therapy approaches. The client and the clinician engaged in experiential play that focused on the target words and required production of the target in order to continue with or take a turn in the activity. By incorporating experiential play, all aspects of environmental stimuli can be utilized to aid in production.

The fifth activity, stimulability probing, is used to plan for the target words for the following week. During this activity, the clinician attempted to discover what words the client possessed the ability to imitate. After the stimulability probing, the listening activity implemented earlier in the therapy session was repeated using the same word list.

The final activity, the home program, was discussed with the client's parent at the end of the therapy session. With this activity, the parent was given a word list of 10 to 12 target words similar in nature but different from the target words used in therapy. The parent was instructed to read the list to the child at least once a day in a manner similar to the listening activities used in therapy. Additionally, the picture cards that were created by the clinician and child at the beginning of the therapy session were sent home for daily practice.

## Analysis of the Client's Response to Intervention

Following 1 month of therapy, David was able to produce /r/ imitatively following direct clinician model and was suppressing the phonological process of stopping of fricatives to 37% in words. Following 3 months of therapy, David was still mispronouncing the /r/ in words when he produced them spontaneously; however, he was beginning to self-correct at the word level. Additionally, he was suppressing the phonological process of stopping of fricatives to 20% or less in words. Following 6 months of the previously described therapy, David was able to spontaneously produce /r/ in words and had decreased the use of the phonological process of stopping of fricatives to 20% occurrence in connected speech.

## Further Recommendations

The treatment regimen recommended after the evaluation was effective in improving David's speech. After 6 months of intervention, he was observed to be 90% intelligible in connected speech. His production of /r/ was correct in all contexts with the exception of highly complex consonant blends; that is, he still produced a w/r in the words *mushroom* and *shrub* in single-word contexts. Additionally, his production of /r/ in conversational contexts continued to be inconsistent, but it was accurate in at least 80% of the conversational contexts. Also after 6 months of remediation, he no longer used a stop for fricatives, but stops were observed occasionally for the affricates in phrases and in conversation. Following the reevaluation at the 6-month juncture, it was recommended that David continue with the current course of therapy until spontaneous production of /r/ was noted consistently in conversational speech and until the use of the phonological process of stopping of affricates was extinguished.

David's mother was pleased with his progress after 6 months of treatment. A conference with David's first-grade teacher resulted in the report that David was eager to participate in class discussions and to answer questions or read words from the board. She also stated that the other children understood David readily and that there were few instances when he was requested to repeat what he had said in conversation. David's mother wanted him to continue in therapy until his speech was error-free and asked frequently if it was reasonable to expect that he would no longer need therapy once this school year was completed.

## Author Note

David is a fictional school-age client who was used to represent common articulation and phonological error patterns as well as an expected course of treatment and recovery.

## References


Gierut, J. (2005). Phonological intervention: The how or the what? In A. Kamhi & K. Pollock (Eds.), *Phonological disorders in children: Clinical decision making in assessment and intervention* (pp. 201–210). Baltimore: Brookes.

Goldman, R., & Fristoe, M. (2000). *Goldman-Fristoe Test of Articulation-2.* Minneapolis, MN: Pearson Assessments.

Hodson, B., & Paden, E. (1991). *Targeting intelligible speech: A phonological approach to remediation* (2nd ed.). Austin, TX: PRO-ED.

Kamhi, A. G. (2006). Treatment decisions for children with speech-sound disorders. *Language, Speech, and Hearing Services in Schools, 37,* 271–279.

Khan, L., & Lewis, N. (2002). *Khan-Lewis Phonological Analysis-2.* Circle Pines, MN: American Guidance Service.

Tyler, A. A., Tolbert, L. C., Miccio, A. W., Hoffman, P. R., Norris, J. A., Hodson, B., et al. (2002). Five views of the elephant: Perspectives on the assessment of articulation and phonology in preschoolers. *American Journal of Speech-Language Pathology, 11,* 213–214.

Van Riper, C., & Emerick, L. (1984). *Speech correction: An introduction to speech pathology and audiology* (7th ed.). Englewood Cliffs, NJ: Prentice Hall.

Vihman, M. M. (2004). Early phonological development. In J. E. Bernthal & N. W. Bankson (Eds.), *Articulation and phonological disorders* (5th ed). Boston: Allyn & Bacon.

Zimmerman, I. L., Steiner, V. G., & Pond, R. E. (2002). *Preschool Language Scale* (4th ed.). Minneapolis, MN: Pearson Assessments.


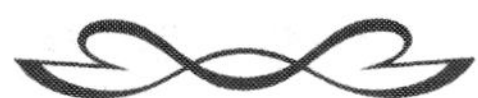

**AUDITORY PROCESSING**

# CASE 23

# Emily and Jeff: School-Age Children with Auditory Processing Disorder


*Deborah Moncrieff*


## Conceptual Knowledge Areas

In the past, filtered words and speech-in-noise have been used to assess monaural low-redundancy skills in children suspected of having auditory processing disorder (APD). Dichotic listening tests have also been used to assess binaural integration (repeat what is heard in both ears) and binaural separation (ignore one ear and repeat what is heard in the other ear) in these same children. Temporal processing skills have been evaluated with time-compressed speech, masking level difference, and gap detection tests. In these cases, the focus will be on the use of dichotic listening tests to identify children with a specific deficit in binaural integration, an important auditory processing skill that has been linked to language, reading, and learning disorders.

## Description of Case 1

This case contrasts assessment procedures that have been historically used to diagnose an APD with new procedures that can specifically characterize a binaural integration type of APD. In addition to highlighting a new diagnostic approach, this and the second case also demonstrate the failure of traditional remediation techniques such as FM systems and computerized auditory training programs to facilitate auditory processing skills. The resistance of binaural integration deficits to improve under traditional therapies has led to the development of an auditory training therapy that is specifically targeted to remediate these deficits in schoolchildren. The new auditory training therapy will be discussed in Case 2.

### Background Information

For more than 30 years, children have been diagnosed with APD on the basis of poor performance across a variety of sensitized speech and nonspeech listening tests. Commonly used clinical tests cover a variety of auditory processing skills with little effort to demonstrate weakness across two or more tests that assess the same skills. This has led to criticism that the construct of APD is poorly defined and that without valid constructs of the types of weaknesses the child is experiencing, there can be no practical approach to treat the deficits and reasonably measure outcomes. This case illustrates the benefits of repeated evaluations with tests that assess the same basic auditory skills and the additional benefits of follow-up assessments to determine whether there have been any gains in auditory processing ability as a result of development or remediation.

### Reason for Referral

Emily was brought to the clinic by her mother to be evaluated for APD. At the time of the first appointment, Emily was 8 years, 11 months old and in the third grade at a local elementary school. She was receiving special education services under a 504 Plan that had been initiated when she was 6 years old, shortly after she had been diagnosed with an APD. Under the 504 Plan, Emily was given an FM listener to use in school, but her mother reported that Emily was still having difficulty with auditory information.

#### History

Emily was born following a protracted labor of 44 hours. During her toddler years, she experienced multiple chronic ear infections and was once hospitalized for an ear infection and allergic reaction to medication. She wore glasses for reading, but was in good health and developing normally. She lived with her parents and a younger sister and was generally cheerful, enthusiastic, and cooperative both at home and school.

The initial diagnosis of APD at age 6 years was based upon an overall performance level of 81% on one-half of the Staggered Spondaic Words Test (SSW; Katz, 1986); 26% in the right ear and 20% in the left ear on the Binaural Separation of Competing Sentences (Willeford, 1977); 20% in the right ear and 28% in the left ear on Filtered Speech (Willeford, 1977); and 90% in both ears on Rapid Alternating Sentences Perception (Willeford & Bilger, 1978). The SSW result was interpreted as a moderate deficit and the results from the Filtered Speech and Binaural Separation of Competing Sentences subtests were reported to be 3 and 2 standard deviations below normal, respectively. It was recommended that in addition to the use of an FM listener, Emily would benefit from simplified instructions, preferential seating, additional visual cues for teaching, and verbal rehearsal.

Over the next 2 years, Emily continued to have significant academic difficulties in school and was assessed for intelligence, attention, psychosocial, emotional, and speech and language abilities. Results from those evaluations are detailed in Table 23.1. Of particular note was the discrepancy between a high-average nonverbal intelligence score of 135 on the Test of Nonverbal Intelligence (TONI; Brown, Sherbenou, & Johnsen, 1997) and a low-average verbal

TABLE 23.1 Evaluation Results

| Test | Age | Test/Subtest | Score | Interpretation |
|---|---|---|---|---|
| **TOLD-P** | 6–9 | | SS = 85 | Low-average verbal |
| **TONI** | 6–9 | | SS = 135 | High-average nonverbal |
| **WJ Cog** | 8–2 | Short-Term Memory | SS = 85 | Low-average |
| | | Memory for Sentences | SS = 88 | Low-average |
| | | Memory for Words | SS = 86 | Low-average |
| | | Comprehension Knowledge | SS = 94 | Average |
| | | Picture Vocabulary | SS = 92 | Low-average |
| | | Oral Vocabulary | SS = 96 | Average |
| | | Auditory Processing | SS = 92 | Low-average |
| **WISC-III** | 8–2 | Verbal | 97 | Average |
| | | Performance | 100 | Average |
| | | Full Scale | 98 | Average |
| **CELF-3** | 8–2 | Receptive Language | 88 | |
| | | Expressive Language | 84 | |
| | | Total Language | 85 | Age equivalent 7–3 |
| **(After FastForWord)** | 8–6 | Receptive Language | 114 | |
| | | Expressive Language | 98 | |
| | | Total Language | 106 | Age equivalent 8–7 |
| **GORT** | 8–2 | **Form A**: Reading Rate | GE = 2.5 | |
| | | Reading Accuracy | GE = <1.9 | |
| | | Reading Passage | GE = < 1.9 | |
| | | Reading Comprehension | GE = 3.7 | |
| | | Oral Reading Quotient | 97, Rank 42% | Average |
| | | **Form B**: Reading Rate | GE = 2.2 | |
| | | Reading Accuracy | GE = < 1.9 | |
| | | Passage Score | GE = < 1.9 | |
| | | Comprehension Oral Reading | GE =1.9 | |
| | | Oral Reading Quotient | 85, Rank 16% | Low-average, Below cognitive |
| **WIAT** | 8–2 | Reading | SS = 94, 34% | Low-average |
| | | Basic Reading | SS = 93, 32% | Low-average |
| | | Reading Comp | SS = 98, 45% | Average |
| | | Mathematics | SS = 112, 79% | High-average |
| | | Numerical Operations | SS = 107, 68% | Upper-average |
| | | Spelling | SS = 101, 53% | Average |
| **Child Behavior Checklist** | 8–2 | Behavior Problems | WNL | |
| **Copeland Symptom Checklist for ADD** | 8–2 | Inattention/Distractability | WNL | |
| | | Impulsivity | WNL | |
| | | Overactivity/Hyperactivity | WNL | |
| | | Underactivity | WNL | |
| | | Noncompliance | WNL | |
| | | Attention-Getting Behavior | WNL | |
| | | Immaturity | WNL | |
| | | Emotional Difficulties | WNL | |
| | | Poor Peer Relations | WNL | |
| | | Family Interaction Problems | WNL | |
| | | Poor Achievement | Mild to moderate | |
| | | Cognitive & Visual-Motor Problems | Mild to moderate | |

score of 85 on the Test of Oral Language Development-Preschool (TOLD-P; Hammill & Newcomer, 1996). Further testing revealed low-average performance on several language and reading measures. At the age of 8 years, 3 months, Emily completed the FastForWord™ (Scientific Learning Corporation, 1997) training program and achieved excellent performance scores across all of the program subtests. A post training speech and language evaluation with the Clinical Evaluation of Language Fundamentals-3 (CELF-3; Semel, Wiig, & Secord, 1995) reflected language gains of 1 year, 4 months within a period of 5 months.

Despite these successes, Emily continued to have difficulty attending to and understanding auditory information. She was getting A's and B's in school, but was struggling with reading. Knowing the importance of good reading skills, Emily's mother wondered whether auditory processing weaknesses might be interfering with Emily's ability to learn to read.

## Findings of the Evaluation

At age 8 years, 11 months, Emily was reassessed for APD. Emily's pure tone air conduction thresholds and speech recognition thresholds were within normal limits for both ears (PTA < 20 dB HL; SRT = 5–10 dB HL). There was no evidence of middle ear disorder and ipsilateral acoustic reflexes were present in both ears. Word recognition scores were 100% in both ears, suggesting an excellent ability to repeat words one ear at a time in quiet.

Two auditory processing tests were used to evaluate Emily's performance, the Test for Auditory Processing Disorders in Children (SCAN-C; Keith, 2000) and the Staggered Spondaic Words Test (SSW; Katz, 1986). The results from those tests are detailed in Table 23.2. Based on standard scores alone, the results obtained by Emily on the SCAN-C would have indicated normal performance, but her right ear significantly outperformed her left ear on the two subtests in which her ears were placed in competition. A comparison of the individual results obtained for each ear demonstrated that for both dichotic listening subtests of the SCAN-C (Competing Words and Competing Sentences) and for the SSW (also a dichotic listening test), Emily had significant difficulties identifying words presented to her left ear at the same time that words were being presented to her right ear.

### Interpretation

Emily had a binaural integration type of APD that interfered with her ability to successfully integrate competing information arriving simultaneously at the two ears. Binaural integration during dichotic listening tests depends upon structural integrity within the ascending auditory nervous system and appropriate allocation of attentional resources during challenging listening experiences. There is strong evidence of binaural integration deficits among children with reading disorders who are assessed with dichotic listening tests (Lamm & Epstein, 1994; Moncrieff & Black, 2008; Morton & Siegel, 1991).

TABLE 23.2 Results from the SCAN-C and SSW Tests

| Test | Age | Test/Subtest | Score | Interpretation |
|---|---|---|---|---|
| **SCAN-C** | 8–11 | Filtered Words | SS = 14 | WNL |
| | | Auditory Figure | SS = 10 | WNL |
| | | Ground | SS = 10 | WNL |
| | | Competing Words | R 83%, L 47% | Significant interaural asymmetry |
| | | | SS = 8 | WNL |
| | | Competing Sentences | R 100%, L 10% | Significant interaural asymmetry |
| **SSW** | 8–11 | Right Non-Competing | 100% | WNL |
| | | Right Competing | 95% | WNL |
| | | Left Competing | 73% | Abnormal |
| | | Left Non-Competing | 93% | WNL |

The structural model of dichotic listening states that (1) information ascends via contralateral auditory pathways to the opposite side of the brain, and (2) ipsilateral auditory pathways are suppressed when both ears are simultaneously activated by differing input (Kimura, 1967). As a result, information presented to the right ear ascends directly to the language-dominant left hemisphere of the brain (typical in 80% of right-handed and 50% of left-handed individuals). Information presented to the left ear ascends indirectly, arriving first in the right hemisphere and then transferring via the corpus callosum to the language-dominant left hemisphere. This indirect routing of the auditory signal from the left ear can account for some loss of information, but in most individuals, the loss leads to only a small decrement in performance for material presented toward the left ear. A significant decrement has been attributed to poor interhemispheric transfer via the corpus callosum, but it is also possible that auditory neural pathways ascending from the left ear may be disordered.

The attention model of dichotic listening states that once linguistic material is presented, there is a priming of the language-dominant left hemisphere, which then leads to an advantageous allocation of attention to material being presented toward the right ear (Kinsbourne, 1970). Under this hypothesis, a listener who performs normally in the right ear and poorly in the left ear may be experiencing difficulties with appropriate allocation of attentional resources. This would result in a decreased ability to overcome the natural bias toward the right ear and to attend more to the information presented toward the left ear.

Because there had been no evidence that Emily had an attention deficit disorder (see results in Table 23.1), it seemed unlikely that her difficulty with processing the words presented toward her left ear was the result of poor attentional resources during the dichotic listening tests. Her strong performance for information presented toward the right ear was consistent with the most recent language results that indicated no significant disorder of language. It seemed plausible that Emily's difficulty with binaural integration stemmed from poor transmission of auditory information arriving at the left ear. Whether this was due to poor interhemispheric transfer via the corpus callosum or the result of poor transmission through ascending auditory pathways from the left ear was not known from these results.

## Treatment Options Considered

Emily's mother had considered the Earobics™ program (Cognitive Concepts, 2000) and it was recommended that Emily complete Earobics™ and continue in ongoing language exercises (Wiig, 1992) as recommended by her speech-language pathologist. To explore potential physiologic weaknesses that might be underlying her binaural integration deficit, it was recommended that she be evaluated with a middle latency response (MLR).

## Course of Treatment

### Findings from the MLR Evaluation

The MLR was recorded in response to biphasic click stimuli presented at the rate of 12 per second to the right and left ears. The early components of the MLR, the Na response and the Pa response, were present for input to both ears at latencies of approximately 19 msec and 35 msec, respectively. As shown in Figure 23.1, the peak-to-peak amplitude of the MLR (from maximum negativity of the Na response to maximum positivity of the Pa) was greater for input to the left ear (shown in black, 0.514μV) than for input to the right ear (shown in gray, 0.378μV). This pattern of greater amplitude for the response from the left ear had been observed in other children with binaural integration deficits (Moncrieff, Byrd, & Bedenbaugh, 2002). With similar latencies for responses from the right and left ears, there was no evidence of any delay in the interhemispheric transfer of neural activation. Instead, it appeared that the asymmetry was occurring in the ascending pathways for auditory information, with greater activation for input to the left ear than for input to the right ear.

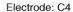


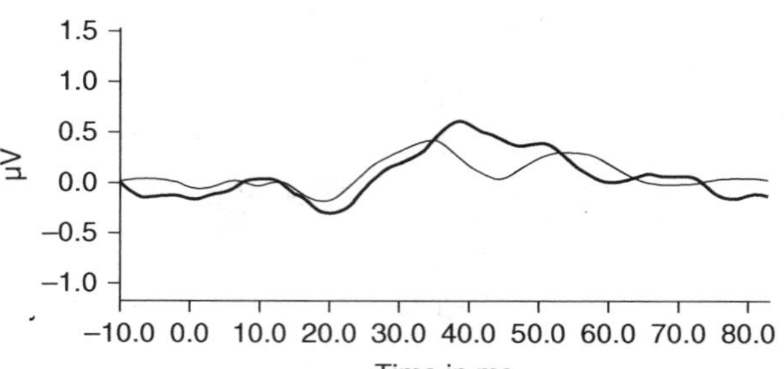


FIGURE 23.1 Findings from the MLR Evaluation

### Follow-Up Evaluation

Despite earning A's in conduct, Emily had even greater difficulty in the fourth grade, and her performance was inconsistent throughout the school year. Her mother was concerned that despite the language exercises and participation in Earobics™ training, Emily's difficulties were not diminishing. Emily was reevaluated by the student services department of her public school district near the end of the fourth-grade year. Evaluation results are detailed in Table 23.3.

### Findings from the Follow-Up Evaluation

Emily's mother asked the school district to provide an independent educational evaluation for Emily, including a language evaluation. Her request was denied and the matter was referred for a due process hearing. In the meantime, Emily returned to the clinic for a follow-up evaluation for APD to see if any of the binaural integration difficulties had resolved. The goal was to use different dichotic listening tests to determine if the same pattern of a left-ear weakness would emerge with new stimuli. Emily was 10 years, 2 months of age. She was assessed with three dichotic listening tests, Competing NU-6 Words (Moncrieff, 2004), Dichotic CVs Test (Hugdahl & Andersson, 1987), and the Randomized Dichotic Digits Test (Moncrieff & Wilson, 2008). She was also assessed with the Pitch Pattern Sequence Test (Pinheiro & Musiek, 1985). Results from those tests are detailed in Table 23.4.

## Analysis of Client's Response to Intervention

The significant interaural asymmetry observed in the initial APD evaluation a little more than a year previously was still present in this evaluation. Across all 3 tests, Emily performed significantly better with information presented toward her right ear than with information

TABLE 23.3 Evaluation Results Near the End of the 4th-Grade Year

| Test | Age | Test/Subtest | Score | Interpretation |
|---|---|---|---|---|
| **WISC-III** | 9–8 | Verbal | 95 | Average |
| | | Performance | 99 | Average |
| | | Full Scale | 97 | Average |
| **WJ-R** | 9–8 | Letter-Word Identification | 103 | Average |
| | | Passage Comprehension | 97 | Average |
| | | Calculation | 118 | Average |
| | | Applied Problems | 105 | Average |
| | | Dictation | 98 | Average |
| | | Broad Reading | 99 | Average |
| | | Broad Math | 112 | Average |
| | | Skills (E Dev) | 101 | Average |
| | | Proofing | 122 | Average |
| | | Basic Writing Skills | 111 | Average |

TABLE 23.4 Results from the Competing NU-6 Test, Randomized Dichotic Digits Test, and Pitch Pattern Sequence Test

| Test | Age | Test/Subtest | Score | Interpretation |
|---|---|---|---|---|
| **Competing NU-6 Words Test** | 10–2 | Right Ear | 66% | Significant interaural asymmetry |
| | | Left Ear | 40% | |
| **Dichotic CV Test** | 10–2 | Nonforced condition | | |
| | | Right Ear | 53% | Large right-ear advantage |
| | | Left Ear | 20% | |
| | | Forced Right condition | | |
| | | Right Ear | 50% | |
| | | Left Ear | 23% | |
| | | Forced Left condition | | Demonstrates ability to attend preferentially toward left ear |
| | | Right Ear | 33% | |
| | | Left Ear | 33% | |
| **Randomized Dichotic Digits Test** | 10–2 | Single Digits | | |
| | | Right Ear | 100% | WNL |
| | | Left Ear | 89% | Abnormal |
| | | Double Digits | | |
| | | Right Ear | 94% | WNL |
| | | Left Ear | 83% | WNL |
| | | Triple Digits | | |
| | | Right Ear | 93% | WNL |
| | | Left Ear | 57% | Abnormal |
| | | | | Significant interaural asymmetries during single and triple digit conditions |
| **Pitch Pattern Sequence** | 10–2 | Right Ear | 67% | Below normal |
| | | Left Ear | 77% | Borderline |

presented toward her left ear. Despite efforts to remediate her auditory processing difficulties with Earobics™ and language intervention programs, Emily still demonstrated a significant binaural integration deficit during dichotic listening tasks.

## Further Recommendations

A novel therapy approach that would involve training the weaker ear to perform at more normal levels during dichotic listening tasks was proposed. To conduct the therapy, a variety of dichotic materials were created so that each participant could receive different stimuli during 30-minute sessions. Participants were to participate in training 3 times per week for 4–6 weeks. Emily was encouraged to enroll in therapy, but she was unable to participate. Both of her parents worked and the driving time between home and the training site was 1.5 hours each way. Therapy was developed and several children were enrolled in Phase I and Phase II clinical trials (Moncrieff & Wertz, 2008). Results from this approach with another child with a similar binaural integration deficit type of APD are presented as Case 2.

# Description of Case 2

This case highlights the benefits that may be obtained when a child with a binaural integration deficit type of APD receives auditory training targeted specifically at that deficit.

## Background Information

Following enrollment in Auditory Rehabilitation for Interaural Asymmetry (ARIA), children have been shown to perform at more normal levels in both ears during dichotic listening tests. In some instances, children have also demonstrated significant improvements in listening skills after the training experience (Moncrieff & Wertz, 2008). In this case, a binaural integration deficit was remediated following enrollment in ARIA shortly after the initial diagnosis of APD. A point of interest is that the child continued to demonstrate difficulties with short-term memory for some complex stimuli following the training. This led to a recommendation for additional training beyond ARIA. It is plausible that this need for additional therapy beyond ARIA may occur in children with APD.

## Reason for Referral

Jeff was brought to the clinic by his father for an evaluation for APD when he was 7 years, 11 months of age. He was in the second grade at a local elementary school where he was receiving special education resources. He was referred to the laboratory by his speech-language pathologist who had been working with him on difficulties with articulation, syntax, and pragmatic language skills.

## History

Jeff was born prematurely and was diagnosed immediately after birth with jaundice. In the newborn nursery, he was given oxygen treatment. He began to speak at 1 year of age but was slow to put words together. By age 3 years, he had had 8 ear infections in either the left ear (5) or in both ears (3). At age 6 years, Jeff's hearing was evaluated because of his parents' concerns that he frequently misunderstood words. At that time, his hearing results were normal, but the audiologist recommended that he use an FM system at school. Jeff used the FM system for several months, but his parents asked that it be discontinued when he began the next school year. At that time, Jeff was 7 years old and was using Earobics™ at home and working on language skills at a university speech and language clinic. The clinician noted concerns that Jeff might have an auditory processing disorder and recommended an evaluation.

## Findings of the Evaluation

Jeff's father provided responses to the Children's Auditory Processing Performance Scale (CHAPS; Smoski, Brunt, & Tanahill, 1998). It was noted that Jeff had the greatest difficulty when listening with background noise. He also had mild difficulties when listening with multiple inputs, with skills involving memory, and with skills involving attention. His score on the CHAPS placed him in the at-risk category. On an unpublished Auditory Processing Difficulties Checklist developed by the author for intake purposes in the clinic, Jeff's father noted the greatest difficulties in the types of skills related to the integration type of APD with some mild difficulties in the types of skills related to the auditory decoding type of APD (Bellis & Ferre, 1999).

Jeff's pure tone air conduction thresholds and speech recognition thresholds were within normal limits for both ears (PTA < 20 dB HL; SRT = 0–5 dB HL). There was no evidence of middle ear disorder and ipsilateral acoustic reflexes were present in both ears. Word recognition scores were 100% in both ears, suggesting an excellent ability to repeat words one ear at a time in quiet.

Jeff was evaluated with the Test for Auditory Processing Disorders in Children (SCAN-C; Keith, 2000), Digits in Multi-talker Babble (Wilson, Burks, & Weakley, 2005), Words in Multi-talker Babble (Wilson, Abrams, & Pillion, 2003), and the Dichotic Words Test (Moncrieff, 2004). Results from all tests are detailed in Table 23.5. The SCAN-C was used as an initial evaluation tool to identify areas of auditory processing weaknesses. Based on standard scoring, Jeff had difficulties with listening in background noise, with binaural integration, and with binaural separation. Any standard score of 5–7 represents borderline performance and any score of 4 or lower represents disordered performance on the SCAN-C.

In Jeff's case, performance on the Competing Words subtest was below normal for both ears (43% in the right ear and 7% in the left ear), but there was a significant interaural

TABLE 23.5 Results for the Test for Auditory Processing Disorders in Children, Digits in Multi-talker Babble, Words in Multi-talker Babble, and the Dichotic Words Tests

| Test | Age | Test/Subtest | Score | Interpretation |
|---|---|---|---|---|
| **SCAN-C** | 7–11 | Filtered Words | SS = 10 | WNL |
| | | Auditory Figure Ground | SS = 5 | Borderline |
| | | | SS = 4 | Disordered |
| | | Competing Words | R 43%, L 7% | Significant interaural asymmetry |
| | | | SS = 9 | WNL |
| | | Competing Sentences | R 100%, L 0% | Significant interaural asymmetry |
| **Digits in Babble** | 7–11 | Right Ear | –3.33 dB SBR | Borderline |
| | | Left Ear | 0.67 dB SBR | Abnormal |
| | | | | Normal for age 7 is approximately –6 to –9 dB SBR |
| **NU-6 Words in Babble** | 7–11 | Binaural | 14.4 dB SBR | Abnormal |
| | | | | Normal for age 7 is approximately 7–10 dB SBR |
| **Dichotic Words Test** | 7–11 | Right Ear | 58% | Abnormal |
| | | Left Ear | 14% | Abnormal |
| | | | | Poorer than normal in both ears with a significant interaural asymmetry |

asymmetry of 36%. This suggested that in addition to the problems with binaural integration, Jeff may have had a fundamental problem with language since even in his dominant ear with direct access to the language-dominant left hemisphere, his performance was not at a normal level. This same pattern can be seen in the results from the Dichotic Words Test on which he demonstrated weaknesses in both ears and an interaural asymmetry of 44%.

The two speech-in-babble tests were used as follow-up measures to assess Jeff's ability to handle speech presented in background noise because of his borderline score on the Auditory Figure Ground subtest of the SCAN-C. With digits-in-babble, 7-year-old children can usually identify 50% of the presentations at a level that is approximately 6 to 9 dB below the level of the background noise. Jeff's performance started to decline below 50% at only 3 dB below the level of the background noise in his right ear and at a level slightly above the level of the background noise in his left ear. With words-in-babble, 7-year-old children need presentations to be approximately 7 to 10 dB above the background noise in order to identify 50% of them. This is because a closed set of highly familiar digits (the numbers 1 through 10) are more easily identified in background noise than an open set of single-syllable words. Jeff's ability to identify the words began to decline below 50% at 14.4 dB above the background noise. Both of these results confirm that Jeff had difficulty listening in background noise as suggested by his father in response to the two initial questionnaires.

## Interpretation

Results from the APD evaluation supported a diagnosis of an auditory decoding type of APD based on poor results in both ears during speech-in-noise and dichotic listening tests. Significantly poorer results in his left ear supported a diagnosis of the integration type of APD. Both of these were further supported by results from the two listening questionnaires filled out by Jeff's father.

## Recommendation

Jeff was advised to return to the clinic in 3 months to be further evaluated and to then enroll in the ARIA training program. The purpose of the reevaluation was to measure the stability of the results obtained at this first appointment and to establish pretraining measures prior to enrolling Jeff in ARIA. In the meantime, the speech-language pathologist at Jeff's school tested him with the Test of Auditory Processing Skills (TAPS-3; Martin & Brownell, 2005).

TABLE 23.6 Results from the TAPS-3 and Two Additional Dichotic Listening Tests at the Clinic Reevaluation

| Test | Age | Test/Subtest | Score | Interpretation |
|---|---|---|---|---|
| **Test of Auditory Processing Skills** | 8–1 | Word Memory | SS = 5 | Abnormal |
| | | Sentence Memory | SS = 4 | Abnormal |
| | | Auditory Comprehension | SS = 6 | Abnormal |
| **Dichotic Words Test** | 8–2 | Free Recall Conditions | | |
| | | Right Ear | 78% | WNL |
| | | Left Ear | 38% | Abnormal<br>Significant interaural asymmetry of 40% |
| | | Directed Response Conditions | | |
| | | Right Ear | 72% | WNL |
| | | Left Ear | 28% | Abnormal<br>Significant interaural asymmetry of 44% |
| **Randomized Dichotic Digits Test** | 8–2 | Single Digits | | |
| | | Right Ear | 100% | Norms not yet available for 8-year-olds on this test (right ear cut-off for 10-year-olds is 97.6% for single digits, 89.7% for double digits, and 82.4% for triple digits). Results demonstrate a significant interaural asymmetry across listening conditions; potentially normal performance in right ear. |
| | | Left Ear | 78% | |
| | | Double Digits | | |
| | | Right Ear | 78% | |
| | | Left Ear | 50% | |
| | | Triple Digits | | |
| | | Right Ear | 80% | |
| | | Left Ear | 43% | |

## Follow-Up Evaluation

Results from the TAPS-3 at school and the two additional dichotic listening tests at the clinic reevaluation supported the diagnosis of a binaural integration type of APD. As shown in Table 23.6, Jeff performed at or near normal levels for input to his right ear, but he continued to demonstrate significant weaknesses for input to the left ear across both tests.

## Interpretation

The improved performance seen in his right ear across the two tests suggested that Jeff might have been more comfortable with the testing situation at the second appointment. The weaknesses attributed to a possible language disorder at the first appointment might have been due to discomfort and anxiety. Jeff was a very conscientious child who always wanted to do his best and was concerned that he might displease someone by his behavior. He often asked how he was doing throughout the testing session and needed lots of encouragement, so it is plausible that as he became more relaxed, performance in his right ear improved to more normal levels.

## Treatment Options Considered

It was recommended that Jeff enroll in the ARIA training for a 4–6 week period. The training would take place 3 times per week for 30 minutes per session. It involved listening to a variety of dichotic material presented so that the intensity of information delivered to the right ear was reduced until performance in the left ear improved to more appropriate levels. Once the left ear's performance was stable at a normal level, the intensity of input to the right ear could then be systematically increased across training sessions. Depending upon the dichotic material being presented, fine adjustments of as little as 1 dB HL would be made to the intensity of information going into the right ear so that left ear performance could be maintained. At any time that left ear performance dropped, the intensity of input to the right ear was again reduced until left ear performance improved.

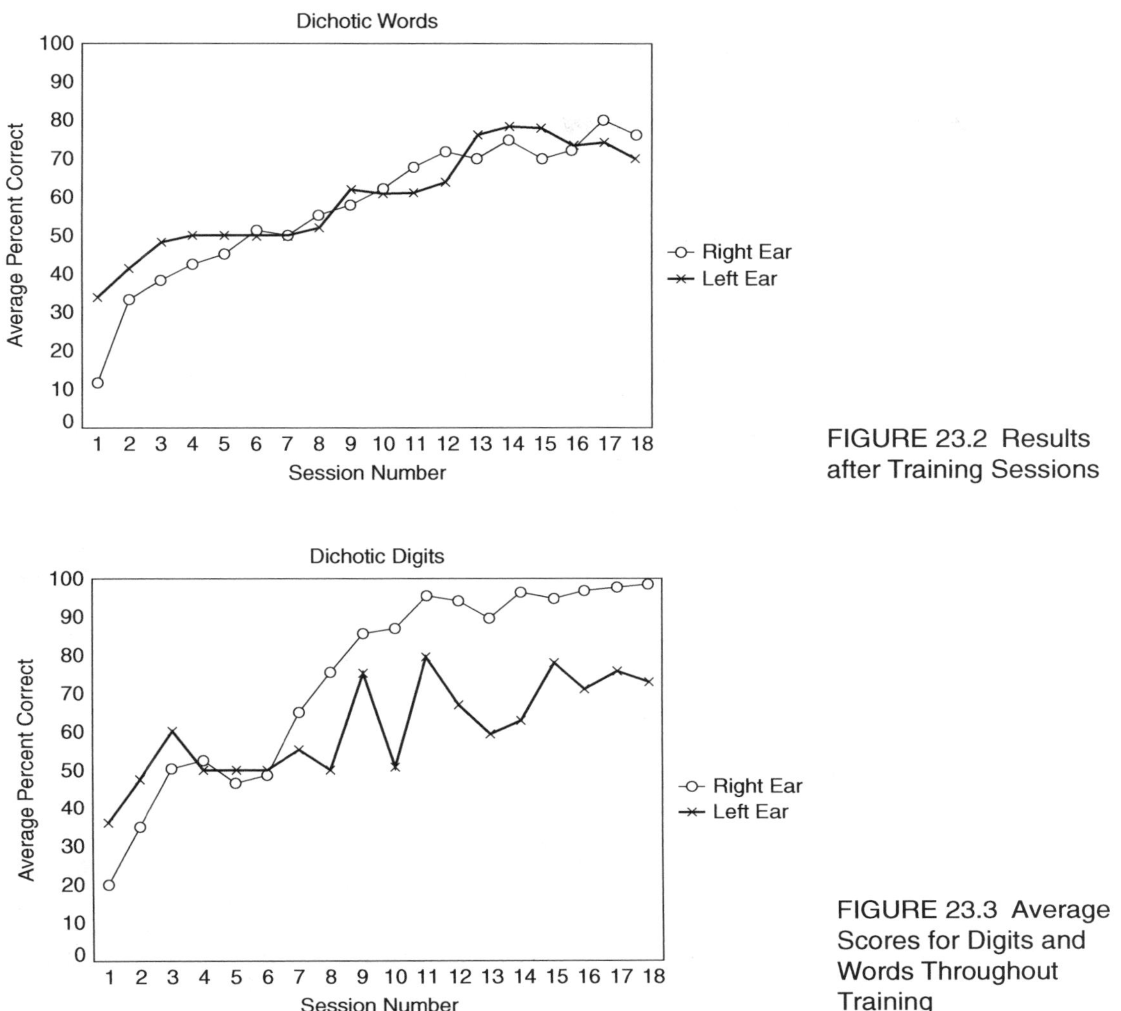


FIGURE 23.2 Results after Training Sessions

FIGURE 23.3 Average Scores for Digits and Words Throughout Training

## Course of Treatment

### Results from the ARIA Training

Jeff participated in a total of 18 training sessions. As shown in Figures 23.2 and 23.3, his left ear showed steady improvement for both words and digits across the ARIA training. As shown in Figure 23.2, performance in the two ears for words was essentially normal at the end of training. As shown in Figure 23.3, performance in the left ear for digits showed some improvement, but compared to words, the left ear continued to significantly lag behind the right ear. The digits results shown in Figure 23.3 are averages for all types of stimuli, so it includes average results for single, double, and triple digit pairs. Jeff did very well in his left ear for single and double presentations of digits throughout training, but whenever he needed to identify digits presented in triple pairs, performance in his left ear would drop off significantly. This drop in performance was most evident during sessions 10, 12, 13, and 14.

## Analysis of Client's Response to Intervention

### Posttraining Evaluation

Following training, binaural integration was again tested with the same dichotic listening tests that were used before training. Jeff was also reassessed with the TAPS-3 by his speech language pathologist. Results of the posttraining evaluation are detailed in Table 23.7.

TABLE 23.7 Results of the Posttraining Evaluation

| Test | Age | Test/Subtest | Score | Interpretation |
|---|---|---|---|---|
| **Test of Auditory Processing Skills** | 8–9 | Word Memory | SS = 8 | WNL |
| | | Sentence Memory | SS = 7 | WNL |
| | | Auditory Comprehension | SS = 8 | WNL |
| **SCAN-C Competing Words Subtest** | 8–9 | Overall | SS = 10 | WNL |
| | | Right Ear | 67% | WNL |
| | | Left Ear | 60% | WNL |
| **Dichotic Words Test** | 8–9 | Right Ear | 74% | WNL |
| | | Left Ear | 72% | WNL |
| **Randomized Dichotic Digits Test** | 8–9 | Single Digits | | Norms not yet available for 8-year-olds on this test (right ear cut-off for 10-year-olds is 97.6% for single digits, 89.7% for double digits, and 82.4% for triple digits). Results demonstrate a significant interaural asymmetry **only in the triple pairs condition.** |
| | | Right Ear | 100% | |
| | | Left Ear | 94% | |
| | | Double Digits | | |
| | | Right Ear | 97% | |
| | | Left Ear | 82% | |
| | | Triple Digits | | |
| | | Right Ear | 100% | |
| | | Left Ear | 50% | |

### Interpretation

Left ear performance with Competing Words, Dichotic Words, and with single and double digits with Randomized Dichotic Digits improved following ARIA training. The degree of asymmetry observed between the two ears following the ARIA training was appropriate for a child Jeff's age for all measures except triple digit pairs on which he demonstrated a 50% interaural asymmetry. In addition, Jeff's scores from the 3 subtests of the TAPS were all within the normal range following the ARIA training. Since Jeff's left ear weaknesses were only evident with triple digit pairs, it seemed plausible that Jeff did not have sufficient resources in verbal working memory to hold and process information that involved 6 critical elements. When asked to hold and process 2 to 4 critical elements in single or double digit pairs, Jeff had no problem with identifying information from either the right or the left ear.

## Further Recommendations

Jeff's parents reported that he was engaging more actively in peer-related conversations at home and at school and that he appeared to be significantly better able to follow auditory instructions. They noted that it was much easier for Jeff to stay focused on auditory messages in general, especially when there were no other distractions. They were still concerned, however, that his attention could be distracted by multiple inputs and that under those circumstances, he seemed to do more poorly. It was suggested that Jeff might benefit from participation in a newly developed program (Klingberg, Forssberg & Westerberg, 2002) for enhancing working memory in children with a variety of attention-based difficulties. The training is given for 5 weeks and can be conducted at home with appropriate coaching support. It was recommended that Jeff consider this or another training program that would facilitate his ability to hold and process multiple critical elements that he hears.

## Author Note

These two cases are largely based on real clients who gave permission for use of data related to their diagnosis and training.

## References


Bellis, T. J., & Ferre, J. M. (1999). Multidimensional approach to the differential diagnosis of central auditory processing disorders in children. *Journal of the American Academy of Audiology, 10,* 319–328.

Brown, L., Sherbenou, R. J., & Johnsen, S. K. (1997). *Test of Nonverbal Intelligence* (3rd ed.). Upper Saddle River, NJ: Pearson Education.

Cognitive Concepts. (2000). Earobics [Computer software]. Boston, MA: Houghton Mifflin Harcourt.

Hammill, D. D., & Newcomer, P. L. (1996). *Test of Language Development-Primary* (3rd ed.). Upper Saddle River, NJ: Pearson Education.

Hugdahl, K., & Andersson, B. (1987). Dichotic listening and reading acquisition in children: A one-year follow-up. *Journal of Clinical and Experimental Neuropsychology, 9*, 631–649.

Katz, J. (1986). *SSW test user's manual.* Vancouver, WA: Precision Acoustics.

Keith, R. (2000). Development and standardization of SCAN-C Test for Auditory Processing Disorders in Children. *Journal of the American Academy of Audiology, 11*, 438–445.

Kimura, D. (1967). Functional asymmetry of the brain in dichotic listening. *Cortex, 3,* 163–168.

Kinsbourne, M. (1970). The cerebral basis of lateral asymmetries in attention. *Acta Psychologica Amsterdam, 33,* 193–201.

Klingberg, T., Forssberg, H., & Westerberg, H. (2002). Training of working memory in children with ADHD. 781–791.

Lamm, O., & Epstein, R. (1994). Dichotic listening performance under high and low lexical work load in subtypes of developmental dyslexia. *Neuropsychologia, 32*, 757–785.

Martin, N. A., & Brownell, R. (2005). *Test of Auditory Processing Skills* (3rd ed.). Greenville, SC: Super Duper Publications.

Moncrieff, D. (2004). *New tests of auditory processing.* Presentation at the Annual Convention of the American Speech-Language-Hearing Association, Philadelphia.

Moncrieff, D. W., & Black, J. R. (2008). Dichotic listening deficits in children with dyslexia. *Dyslexia, 41*, 54–75.

Moncrieff, D. W., Byrd, D. L., & Bedenbaugh, P. H. (2002, March). *MLR in children with a dichotic left-ear deficit.* Presentation at American Auditory Society Annual Meeting, Scottsdale, AZ.

Moncrieff, D. W., & Wertz, D. (2008). Auditory rehabilitation for interaural asymmetry: Preliminary evidence of improved dichotic listening performance following intensive training. *International Journal of Audiology, 47,* 84–97.

Moncrieff, D. W., & Wilson, R. H. (2008, accepted for publication). Recognition of randomly presented 1-, 2-, and 3-pair dichotic digits by children and young adults. *Journal of the American Academy of Audiology.*

Morton, L. L., & Siegel, L. S. (1991). Left ear dichotic listening performance on consonant-vowel combinations and digits in subtypes of reading-disabled children. *Brain and Language, 40*, 162–180.

Pinheiro, M. L., & Musiek, F. E. (1985). Sequencing and temporal ordering in the auditory system. In M. L. Pinheiro & F. E. Musiek (Eds.), *Assessment of Central Auditory Dysfunction: Foundations and Clinical Correlates* (pp. 219–238). Baltimore: Williams & Wilkins.

Scientific Learning Corporation. (1997). Fast ForWord Language [Computer software]. Berkeley, CA: Author.

Semel, E., Wiig, E. H., & Secord, W. A. (1995). *Clinical Evaluation of Language Fundamentals* (3rd ed.). San Antonio, TX: Psychological Corporation.

Smoski, W. J., Brunt, M. A., & Tannahill, J. C. (1998). Listening characteristics of children with central auditory processing disorders. *Language, Speech, and Hearing in Schools, 23,* 145–149.

Wiig, E. H. (1992). *Language intervention for school-age children: Models and procedures that work.* Buffalo, NY: Educom.

Willeford, J. (1977). Assessing central auditory behavior in children: A test battery approach. In R. W. Keith (Ed.), *Central Auditory Dysfunction* (pp. 43–72). New York: Grune & Stratton.

Willeford, J. A., & Bilger, J. M. (1978). Auditory perception in children with learning disabilities. In J. Katz (Ed.), *Handbook of clinical audiology* (2nd ed., pp. 410–425). Baltimore: Williams & Wilkins.

Wilson, R. H., Abrams, H. B., & Pillion, A. L. (2003). A word-recognition task in multitalker babble using a descending presentation mode from 24 dB to 0 dB signal to babble. *Journal of Rehabilitation Research and Development, 40*, 321–327.

Wilson, R. H., Burks, C. A., & Weakley, D. G. (2005). A comparison of word-recognition abilities assessed with digit pairs and digit triplets in multitalker babble. *Journal of Rehabilitation Research and Development, 42*, 499–510.

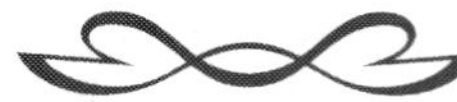



CASE **24**

# Sam: Assessment and Intervention for a School-Age Child with Complex Communication Needs and Physical Impairments

*Pam Hart and Suzie Wiley*

## Conceptual Knowledge Areas

### Overview of AAC

Assistive technology involves the use of tools to achieve tasks that would otherwise be difficult or impossible to achieve through traditional means alone. Within the general field of assistive technology, augmentative and alternative communication (AAC) is an area of research and clinical focus that involves finding ways to compensate for severe difficulties with spoken and written modes of communication (ASHA, 2005). The field of AAC has been shaped by the recognition that all persons, regardless of type or severity of disability, have the basic right to communicate.

Individuals with complex communication needs and severe physical impairments, such as the case presented here, may require a system of strategies to achieve communicative competence across a variety of environments and communication partners. For example, in a school setting with familiar communication partners, a child may use a vocalization such as "aaaah" to indicate "I have something to say, please come here," and then once having the attention of the listener, use a high-tech dynamic display system with switch input to communicate a message, followed by a facial expression or gesture to indicate agreement or disagreement of the listener's interpretation and response to the message. This same child in the home environment may be able to communicate mostly by gestures and facial expressions and may not require the aided communication strategies as frequently when communicating with his or her parents. The authors advocate for a multimodal communication approach that uses all of the individual's natural skills along with any necessary electronic and non-electronic aids. Person-centered planning is critical when assessing an individual for an AAC system. Additionally, different strategies may work better with more or less familiar communication partners. Clinicians must understand and consider the communication needs of the individual across environments with more and less familiar communication partners (Blackstone & Hunt-Berg, 2003).

### Assessment and Intervention Considerations

Assessment and intervention for individuals who use AAC includes considerations across (a) the general and specific vocabulary needs of the individual, (b) how symbols will be used to represent vocabulary, (c) selection of a device and/or system of strategies to transmit the messages, (d) the method of access that will be used by the individual, and (e) meaningful learning and communication opportunities that will be developed and implemented to promote the communicative competence of the individual using AAC (Beukelman & Mirenda, 2005). Although it is beyond the scope of this case to provide comprehensive coverage of all of these issues, components related to the case presented here are discussed in the following sections.

Traditionally, AAC strategies are divided along a continuum from low-tech to high-tech, differentiated by those with computer chips and integrated circuits vs. those without (Lloyd, Fuller, & Arvidson, 1997). Specific voice output communication aids vary from those that transmit only one message to those with text to speech capabilities and storage for hundreds of messages. Messages within AAC systems are represented by symbols. Unaided symbols include things that individuals can do with their bodies to augment communication such as gestures, signs, vocalizations, and facial expressions. Aided symbols require a device or aide external to the user's body for transmission and may include tangible items such as real, miniature, or partial objects; photographs; pictures; various symbol sets; and traditional or modified orthography (Beukelman & Mirenda, 2005). Selection of a symbol set depends partly on an individual's ability to understand concrete vs. abstract representations of vocabulary along with the general developmental level and physical skills for input.

In the process of considering overall vocabulary needs and how vocabulary will be represented in an AAC system, it is important to determine the cognitive, linguistic, sensory, perceptual, and physical abilities of the individual (McEwen, 1997) and how these can be accommodated within an AAC system. Principles of human factors represent ways in which individuals interact with technology and have been applied to individuals with disabilities to better understand the difficulties encountered when assistive technology strategies are implemented. Baker's (1987) basic ergonomic equation, later adapted by King (1999), is a model useful to understanding the ways that various human factors affect the successful use of an AAC device. The model posits that the motivation of the AAC user must exceed the sum of physical effort (the actual physical exertion required to complete the task), cognitive effort (the overall level of cognition necessary to operate the system), linguistic effort (the level of linguistic knowledge required to understand the symbol system), and time load (the amount of time it takes the AAC user to communicate a message) to result in a successful outcome.

Another issue for young children who require AAC is how to balance the need for immediate communication with allowances for developmental vocabulary and future language and literacy stimulation via AAC. It has been found that children with complex needs receive fewer early language and literacy experiences at home, possibly due to the increased physical demands of caring for a young child with severe impairments (Light & Smith, 1993). Additionally, the attempt to reduce linguistic, physical and cognitive effort, and time load of using AAC systems has resulted in systems based on iconic, rather than alphabetic representations of language (King, 1999). Increased knowledge and understanding of the language-literacy connection in typical populations has raised questions about the influence of various AAC icon-based symbol sets on later literacy development in children with complex communication needs. This asymmetry requires children who use AAC to understand the language of the AAC system and the alphabetic orthography of English to develop functional literacy and communication skills (Bishop, Rankin, & Mirenda, 1994; Koppenhaver & Pierce, 1994; McNaughton, 1993). While much remains uncertain as to the influence of language representation in AAC on overall language and literacy development, there is general agreement regarding the importance of regularly occurring early literacy experiences that allow for language-literacy connections to emerge in meaningful contexts.

## Alternative Access

Children with complex communication needs related to severe physical impairments may require alternative access to AAC systems. A familiar method of device access is direct selection. Direct selection on an AAC device is when an individual is able to use his or her body or a tool such as a pointer to directly touch the device to make choices. Anyone who has pressed the keys of a keyboard has used direct selection. However, if an individual's motor skills limit his or her ability to use direct selection, alternate methods of input may need to be considered. One example is switch scanning. There are many options when designing the scanning setup of an AAC device. In general terms, the individual activates the switch using a reliable movement that does not increase tone, affect posture/positioning, or overfatigue muscles. The activation of the switch begins a scanning (also referred to as highlighting) process on the screen of the device. Options are highlighted as they become available and the individual activates the switch again when the desired choice is highlighted. Critical considerations in successful switch access include (a) determining a movement that can be initiated, consistently released, and repeated without negatively influencing normal tone, (b) determining the motor and cognitive demands of timing the switch activation to make a selection, and (c) isolating the ability to visually process the scanned items as the highlight moves across the device options in a way that allows the brain to "make sense of" and "react to" the visual information it receives.

For some individuals with physical impairments, scanning may be the best option for access to a communication device. For individuals with cognitive impairment and physical impairment, however, methods to decrease the cognitive demands of scanning may need to be explored. For example, researchers have explored the learning demands of scanning in typical populations and found that they exceed the capabilities of typically developing 2-year-olds. Subsequently, a redesigned approach to scanning that reduced the cognitive load was developed. Rather than only highlighting the scanned icons, the size of the icon increased as it was scanned. This approach showed promise with typical populations but more research is needed to explore applications to populations with physical and cognitive impairments (McCarthy et al., 2006).

New developments in high-tech AAC systems with eye gaze access have recently emerged in the market. These systems show promise for individuals unable to use direct selection or scanning due to severe physical limitations. For these individuals, the use of eye gaze may be preferable to scanning as a more direct, efficient method of access. Other technologies that may assist with AAC access in the future include components of systems such as the Cyberlink. The Cyberlink is a computer interface that reads voltage at the user's forehead from brain waves, minute facial movements, and eye movements. Researchers have reported favorable outcomes from trials with the Cyberlink in which two children with cerebral palsy were taught to "click" and control a mouse cursor for games and communication purposes. In this study, both participants acquired some skill with the system, and one participant met higher-level skills, indicating this system was a good match for the participant's skills (Redstone, 2006). Additional research and development is needed in the area of alternative access for individuals with severe physical impairments.

## AAC in Educational Settings

In educational settings, speech-language pathologists work as part of a team to implement AAC strategies for students with complex communication needs (ASHA, 2005). Other primary team members include occupational therapists, physical therapists, educators, administrators, parents and other caregivers, and, of course, the person who will be using the AAC system. Legislation requires the consideration and acquisition of necessary pieces of assistive technology, including AAC strategies, to be included in Individualized Education Programs (IEPs) of students who require such tools to meet their potential (PL 101-476, 1990). Through this mandate, school-based IEP teams attempt to evaluate the need for assistive technology, determine funding, and coordinate services and programs to integrate assistive technology across the curriculum. Children with complex communication needs due to severe physical impairments such as cerebral palsy are among those who could most benefit from AAC strategies. Sadly, because of the level of physical impairment, children in this population often struggle for many years before successful access methods to the AAC devices are determined and implemented (Redstone, 2006).

For students who use AAC as a primary means of communication, successful educational inclusion requires careful planning and implementation. Challenges may be encountered due to factors such as a lack of familiarity with assistive technology and AAC by team members and the extensive need for time to program and update vocabulary contained within an AAC device to increase its educational relevance. Additionally, educators and parents may be concerned that use of AAC will decrease or inhibit any natural speech produced by the child. In response to this general concern, researchers analyzed data from cases of AAC intervention for individuals with developmental disabilities and found no evidence that use of AAC decreased or inhibited speech production. Most often, introduction of AAC co-occurred with a modest increase in speech production (Millar, Light, & Schlosser, 2006).

Another aspect of successful educational inclusion is acceptance of the individual who uses AAC by his or her peer group. Individuals who use AAC have been found to have decreased social interaction opportunities (Light, 1988) with most communication generated via AAC directed toward adult communication partners (Sack & McLean, 1997). The range of communicative functions of school-age children who use AAC has been reported to primarily consist of requesting, rejecting, and greeting (Seigel & Cress, 2002). This is far less diverse than communicative functions observed in school-age children with typical abilities. Naturalistic interventions in which the AAC system is incorporated into regularly occurring social activities with groups of children should be provided to increase peer acceptance and as a means to model a variety of communicative functions. Outcomes across 16 students from a special needs program indicated that with adequate planning, commitment, and collaboration, it was possible to achieve successful inclusion and socialization for children who used AAC (Hunt-Berg, 2005).

## Description of the Case

### Background Information

Sam was a 10-year-old male who attended Elmwood Elementary School where he spent most of his day in a self-contained program for children with severe multiple impairments. Sam was born with a form of spastic cerebral palsy and, as a result, was unable to walk or speak and had severely limited use of his hands. He used a manual wheelchair for mobility. Sam's parents reported that his vision was satisfactory with a recent examination indicating 20/20 acuity. At the time of the first meeting, Sam used unaided symbols for communication including turning his head to the right to indicate "yes" and pointing his head downward with his chin against his chest to indicate "no." Sam's communication participation consisted mainly of responding to yes/no questions to try to indicate his basic wants and needs and to participate in the modified curriculum he received in the self-contained room. In addition to his yes/no response, Sam used a few vocalizations that his family and close caregivers were able to interpret as indications that he wanted to change activities, was in pain and needed to be adjusted in his wheelchair, or was tired and needed to lie down.

Recently, Sam's IEP team met to discuss Sam's goals and progress. During this meeting, Sam's mother expressed concerns about Sam's limited system of communication. Sam's physical therapist, occupational therapist, speech-language pathologist, and classroom teacher were also concerned about his lack of expressive communication but disagreed as to whether he had the cognitive skills to operate an AAC system. After much discussion, all team members eventually agreed to contact an assistive technology center for consultation. The following assessment and intervention information represents the team evaluation by the occupational therapist and speech-language pathologist at an assistive technology program with input and participation from the client's school-based team.

#### Client History

Sam's mother had a normal pregnancy with a difficult delivery via forceps during which Sam suffered oxygen deprivation. During the first several months of Sam's development several motor abnormalities were noted, and eventually he was diagnosed with spastic cerebral palsy. Sam received early intervention services that included speech-language therapy, occupational therapy, physical therapy, and early childhood special education. Sam's early intervention speech-language pathologist (SLP) initially focused on feeding and swallowing strategies. Once feeding and swallowing needs had been effectively addressed, the SLP shifted focus to stimulation and development of Sam's receptive and expressive language skills. Progress in all areas was difficult due to the severity of his physical impairments.

Sam lived at home with his mother, father, and younger sister. Sam's mother did not work outside the home and his father was an electrical engineer. The severity of Sam's needs placed a strain on the relationship between Sam's mother and father. Sam's father felt that the mother "babied" Sam too much and wanted Sam to go to college, find employment, and live as independently as possible following high school.

Sam attended elementary school and spent most of his day in a self-contained class for children with severe physical and cognitive impairments. He interacted with his typical peers during physical education, art, and music. Sam's physical impairments required considerable time and care. Subsequently, the amount of direct instruction related to the curriculum that Sam received was greatly reduced compared to his same-age peers. A paraprofessional assisted with Sam's care but had little training in communicating with Sam and felt that Sam probably did not understand what she said to him. Most of Sam's needs were anticipated rather than elicited and there was little opportunity for reciprocal interaction in this setting.

## Reasons for Referral

Sam was referred to the assistive technology center for evaluation to determine AAC strategies that would maximize his ability to communicate in educational, home, and community settings while allowing for growth in overall language and literacy skills.

### Evaluation Summary

***Language Skills*** This area was informally assessed via observation and interaction with Sam along with reports from Sam's parents, his school SLP, and other educational team members. Sam's expressive language skills were judged to be profoundly impaired. He was nonverbal but able to vocalize a few sounds when excited or frustrated. During this evaluation, vocal behavior was observed in response to highly preferred activities. Sam was able to say "eee" when he became excited about these activities. No other vocal behaviors were observed. Attempts to elicit additional vocal behaviors through imitation and prompting were not successful. Parents and his SLP reported that Sam was able to produce a few other vocalizations that were not observed during this evaluation. Based on Sam's lack of progress in verbal skills over the previous years and the nature/type of his physical impairment, it was not anticipated that his verbal skills would be a primary means of communication in the future.

Sam's receptive language skills were judged to be an area of relative strength. He showed some understanding of speech at the conversational level as noted by appropriate "yes" and "no" responses to questions during the evaluation. His facial expressions appeared to indicate understanding of humor, as he would smile appropriately at the examiners in response to something he thought was funny. From a field of four pictures, Sam was able to identify the picture named by the examiner 80% of the time. Sam's educational team concluded that Sam understood basic directions and conversation in the classroom such as, "no," "wait," and "are you ready to go?"

Sam's written language skills in reading and spelling were difficult to assess, but it appeared that he continued to be in the early stages of literacy development. Using eye gaze with letters placed in the four quadrants of a piece of paper, Sam was able to look toward the requested letter approximately 50% of the time. He was not able to demonstrate other word reading or basic spelling skills at the time of this evaluation.

***Cognitive Ability*** Sam's educational team was uncertain of his overall level of cognitive ability. During this evaluation, Sam exhibited good ability for new learning with the use of speech-generating devices. He also demonstrated good attention to all assessment tasks during this evaluation.

***Vision Status*** Although recent testing indicated Sam had 20/20 acuity, other visual skills needed to be assessed for visual perception of a potential communication system, including how the eyes work together. Contrast sensitivity (the ability to perceive varying intensities) and visual field perception (the visual surround that can be viewed as the eye stares straight ahead) appeared intact. Sam was expected to be able to perceive varying degrees of color contrast on the display images and recognize the need to look at all areas of the device for possible communication buttons. Extraocular muscle imbalance was observed, as Sam did not maintain his gaze on a target with both eyes simultaneously. Additionally, it was noted that with visual tracking activities, Sam presented with extraocular muscle weakness demonstrating difficulty coordinating movements of both eyes together. Sam denied double vision; however, he tried to alternate between the use of each eye to compensate for the limited ability to use the eyes together. Enlarging the icons and font on devices was likely to increase visual perception as he alternated his view between each eye.

***Hearing Status*** Although not formally assessed during this evaluation, previous assessments of hearing were within normal limits per report of Sam's mother. Additionally, Sam was able to respond appropriately to the voice output of several communication devices presented during the evaluation.

***Physical Status*** Sam was dependent for all activities of daily living. He used a wheelchair for mobility and had a lap tray in place when seated in the wheelchair. Functional movement patterns were significantly limited due to spasticity. He was dependent for wheelchair mobility and transfers. During this assessment, he was unable to accurately use direct selection to access a dynamic or static communication display. Use of a keyguard was helpful for increasing accuracy, but range of motion continued to limit access to the entire display. When reaching toward the device, spasticity increased causing him to flex forward in his wheelchair. Use of switch scanning was introduced and Sam showed some good responses to this activity. The switch was placed at the outer aspect of Sam's knee and he was able to accurately activate the switch by pressing slightly outward to start the scanning process upon request. He exhibited difficulty attending to the scanning pattern on the screen of the speech-generating device, but with cues, was able to activate the switch again to play the recorded message upon request. Icons were enlarged to 1" square in size to maximize visual perception of the options being scanned. The device was placed upright on his lap tray to provide better posture while viewing the display.

## Specific Daily Functional Communication Needs

Sam's primary communication environments included his home, school, and church. He needed to effectively communicate messages that provided identifying/ biographical information, express physical status/needs, make choices during daily activities, enhance social closeness with peers and caregivers, offer information about past and present experiences, participate in curriculum activities at school, and express feelings and opinions with familiar and unfamiliar communication partners across multiple environments.

## Current Communication Strategies

Sam used some limited head movements to indicate "yes" and "no." He used a few vocalizations that were understood by caregivers to indicate comfort/discomfort or happiness/sadness. Sam also used eye gaze to indicate preferred places in the room and some limited expression of preferred activities when his communication partner held two items in front of him and asked him, "Which one do you want?" Clearly, Sam's receptive language skills surpassed what he was able to convey expressively. Attempts to teach Sam to use sign language had not been successful due to his severe motor impairment. Sam's current expressive language system of mostly unaided strategies significantly limited the quantity and quality of expressive language opportunities for him.

## Representation of the Problem at the Time of Evaluation

Sam's communication needs far exceeded what he was able to achieve with unaided strategies. Sam needed access to high-tech AAC tools that would allow for the extensive vocabulary and literacy tools required to participate more fully in the general education curriculum and socially with his peers.

### Assessment with Speech-Generating Devices

Several speech-generating devices were presented to Sam during this evaluation. Sam demonstrated the ability to use switch scanning to find requested icons and was able to navigate between multiple page sets after brief instruction. Using the onscreen keyboard with the device, Sam was able to identify the letters of his first name. Based on these results, with consideration of Sam's current and future needs, a high-tech device with dynamic display and large storage capacities was recommended. Additional considerations included specific capabilities of the device to meet current needs while allowing for continued language and literacy development. The required features of a device for Sam included:

- A durable device that could be placed on his lap tray or mounted to his wheelchair and accessed via switch input
- Text-to-speech capabilities to support and stimulate Sam's continued literacy development
- Rate enhancement strategies including prestored messages, abbreviation expansion, word prediction, and communication partner reader capability
- High-quality screen that would be clearly visible in outdoor and indoor environments
- Picture symbols and/or digital photo capabilities based on concrete representations of items, ideas, wants/needs
- Capability to change the number, size, and spacing of icons
- High-quality voice output that could be heard in situations with background noise
- Adequate battery life to be used throughout the day

## Course of Treatment

Sam's educational team obtained a device on loan from their state assistive technology program that fulfilled the above requirements. The team had the device for 6 weeks to evaluate Sam's response and progress. Interventions included naturalistic, game-oriented sessions to build his desire to communicate and enhance motivation for overcoming the physical effort, time load, and cognitive and linguistic load factors (Wood & Hart, 2007). Initially, games were designed to build Sam's knowledge of semantics and pragmatics. Using books and simple guessing games such as "I Spy" and "Go Fish," the members of Sam's team provided many opportunities during the day, across multiple environments, for Sam to use the device. Additionally, Sam's peers were included and in some instances, provided the voicing for unique phrases recorded into the device such as a "whining" message that would allow Sam to express his dismay at an undesirable situation with appropriate inflection for his age.

To demonstrate the use of the device, the educational team implemented an augmented input strategy in which the communication partner used the device to communicate back and forth with Sam. This provided a scaffolding effect that is often not possible with augmented communicators. In many instances, the augmented communicator is the only person communicating via AAC in his or her environment. Children with typical abilities are provided consistent verbal models of their production, whereas children who use AAC rarely receive this type of model. Augmented input helps to provide this model while building reciprocity in communication exchanges (Beukelman & Mirenda, 1995). Sam was also taught how to use unaided strategies to support efficiency of communication with the AAC device. For instance, Sam learned to vocalize to first gain the attention of a communication partner prior to creating a message with the AAC device.

## Analysis of the Client's Response to Intervention

Sam's response to the device trial period was positive. By the end of the 6 weeks, Sam was able to use his device to:

- Navigate to the correct page within the device using switch input to find and activate specific messages upon request.
- Adjust basic settings on the device such as volume and on/off controls.
- Interact with peers during games in which preprogrammed pages within the device allowed Sam to ask and answer appropriate questions related to the game.
- Initiate basic greetings and farewells with peers and caregivers.
- Extend turn-taking during a conversation with caregivers and/or peers to 3 comments on the same topic.
- Use the onscreen keyboard and switch input to find a target letter.

## Further Recommendations

After reviewing Sam's response to the trial period, it was recommended to purchase a similar device that could travel between home and school. Future language and literacy goals with continued progress in using the device could include (a) working with the onscreen keyboard and word prediction to spell basic vocabulary skills and advance these skills as appropriate across a multiple linguistic perspective (see Hart, Scherz, Apel, & Hodson, 2007), (b) development of narrative language skills via AAC to tell stories and describe events, (c) increasing Sam's access to the general education curriculum across subject areas via AAC, and (d) helping Sam to develop a more active role in communication by learning how to express helpfulness and elicit opinions and ideas from others.

As evident from this case, the authors believe that successful implementation of AAC requires participation from a multidisciplinary team of professionals who are willing to think beyond traditional models of assessment and intervention. With clients such as Sam, initial determination of cognitive and linguistic skills is often difficult due to the complexity of physical impairments. In such cases, caution should be exercised when making general assumptions about overall potential and ability. Until proven otherwise, each individual should be considered as having unlimited potential but perhaps lacking an effective means of expression. As clinicians, our task is to identify appropriate resources and tools that will allow individuals like Sam to participate meaningfully and achieve their highest potential.

## Author Note

The presented case was fictional.

## References


American Speech-Language-Hearing Association. (2005). *Roles and responsibilities of speech-language pathologists with respect to augmentative and alternative communication: Position statement* [Position Statement]. Retrieved from www.asha.org/policy.

Baker, B. (1986, November). Systematic approaches to vocabulary selections for communication aid users. Short course, American Speech-Language Hearing Association (ASHA), Annual Conference, Detroit, Michigan.

Beukelman, D., & Mirenda, P. (2005). *Augmentative and alternative communication, supporting children and adults with complex communication needs.* Baltimore, MD: Paul H. Brookes Publishing.

Bishop, K., Rankin, J., & Mirenda, P. (1994). Impact of graphic symbol use on reading acquisition. *Augmentative and Alternative Communication, 10*, 113–125.

Blackstone, S., & Hunt-Berg, M. (2003). *Social networks: A communication inventory for individuals with complex communication needs and their communication partners.* Monterey, CA: Augmentative Communication.

Hart, P., Scherz, J., Apel, K., & Hodson, B. (2007). Analysis of spelling error patterns of individuals with complex communication needs and physical impairments. *Augmentative and Alternative Communication, 23,* 16–29.

Hunt-Berg, M. (2005). The bridge school: Educational inclusion outcomes over 15 years. *Augmentative and Alternative Communication, 21*, 116–131.

King, T. W. (1999). *Assistive technology: Essential human factors.* Needham Heights, MA: Allyn & Bacon.

Koppenhaver, D. A., & Pierce, P.L. (1994). *Written language development research in AAC.* Paper for the International Society for Augmentative and Alternative Communication Research Symposium.

Light, J. (1988). Interaction involving individuals using augmentative and alternative communication systems: State of the art and future directions. *Augmentative and Alternative Communication, 4*, 66–82.

Light, J., & Smith, A. (1993). Home literacy experiences of preschoolers who use AAC systems and of their nondisabled peers. *Augmentative and Alternative Communication, 9*, 10–25.

Lloyd, L., Fuller, D., & Arvidson, H. (1997). Introduction and overview. In L. Lloyd, D. Fuller, & H. Arvidson (Eds.), *Augmentative and alternative communication: A handbook of principles and practices* (pp. 1–17). Needham Heights, MA: Allyn & Bacon.

McCarthy, J., Light, J., Drager, K., McNaughton, D., Grodzicki, L., Jones, J., et al. (2006). Re-designing scanning to reduce learning demands: The performance of typically developing 2-year-olds. *Augmentative and Alternative Communication, 22*, 269–283.

McEwen, I. R. (1997). Seating, other positioning, and motor control. In L. Lloyd, D. Fuller, & H. Arvidson (Eds.), *Augmentative and alternative communication: A handbook of principles* (pp. 280–298). Needham Heights, MA: Allyn & Bacon.

McNaughton, S. (1993). Graphic representational systems and literacy learning. *Topics in Language Disorders, 13*, 58–75.

Millar, D., Light, J. C., & Schlosser, R. W. (2006). The impact of augmentative and alternative communication intervention on the speech production of individuals with developmental disabilities: A research review. *Journal of Speech, Language, and Hearing Research, 49*, 248–264.

Redstone, F. (2006). A training program for the use of the cyberlink control system for young children with cerebral palsy. *Technology and Disability, 18*, 107–115.

Sack, S. H., & McLean, L. K. (1997). Training communication partners: The new challenge for communication disorders professionals supporting persons with severe disabilities. *Focus on Autism and other Developmental Disabilities, 12*, 151–158.

Siegel, E. B., & Cress, C. J. (2002). Overview of the emergence of early AAC behaviors: Progression from communicative to symbolic skills. In J. Reichle, D. R. Beukelman, & J. C. Light (Eds.), *Exemplary practices for beginning communicators: Implications for AAC* (pp. 25–57). Baltimore, MD: Paul H. Brookes Publishing.

Wood, L., & Hart, P. (2007). Language facilitation in augmentative and alternative communication. In A. Kamhi, J. Masterson, & K. Apel (Eds.), *Clinical decision making in developmental language disorders* (pp. 323–336). Baltimore: Paul H. Brookes Publishing.

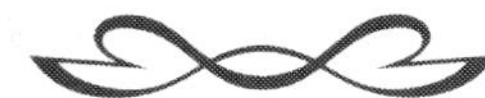

# Autism

# CASE 25

# Diego: A School-Age Child with an Autism Spectrum Disorder

*Erin Brooker Lozott and Jamie B. Schwartz*

## Conceptual Knowledge Areas

The term *autism spectrum disorders (ASDs)* is often used synonymously with the term *pervasive developmental disorders (PDD)*. Pervasive developmental disorder is an umbrella term that includes the following five diagnoses: childhood disintegrative disorder, Rett syndrome, autism disorder, pervasive developmental disorder-not otherwise specified (PDD-NOS), and Asperger's disorder. Diagnostic criteria for each of these pervasive developmental disorders can be found in the *Diagnostic and Statistical Manual of Mental Disorders-IV* (DSM-IV; APA, 1999).

Autism spectrum disorders (ASDs) are present from birth or early in life and are characterized by impairments in social interaction and communication, and by repetitive and stereotyped patterns of behavior, interests, and activities. There are currently no medical tests for detecting ASDs. There are, however, a variety of hypotheses related to causes. Current biologic research suggests a genetic basis, although additional causal hypotheses include a teratogenic agent (prenatal, neonatal, or cumulative), a metabolic error, or mutations/natural errors of brain organization (see Volker & Lopata, 2008 for a review). Consequently, ASDs are lifelong disorders that require ongoing intervention.

The prevalence rates for autism spectrum disorders are now believed to be 1:150 (Centers for Disease Control, 2007) and affect all cultures and economic groups. ASDs vary in age of onset, severity of symptoms, and comorbidity with other disorders (e.g., cognitive impairment, seizure disorder, attention-deficit/hyperactivity disorder) and are often more common in boys than in girls. Impairments in social communication, language and behavior differ across individuals as well as within the individual over time (National Research Council, 2001).

Individuals with ASD typically present with a documented language disorder prior to the age of 3. Language disorders can vary in degree of severity ranging from mild to profound expressive, receptive, and pragmatic disorders. Current evidence suggests that at least 71% of individuals with ASD may develop verbal language in some capacity (Chakrabarti & Fombonne, 2001). Language is typically used for a limited range of functions and is often repetitive and inflexible in nature. Language difficulties also frequently include pronoun reversal, echolalia, limited understanding of multiple meaning words or phrases, limited understanding of nonliteral language, difficulties in comprehending discourse, and deficits in producing oral narratives. Language impairments have a direct impact on an individual's ability to acquire many necessary social skills (e.g., greetings, friendships, social exchanges, maintaining social interactions, understanding nonverbal communication). Deficits in social skills influence the ability to develop meaningful relationships and negatively affect academics (Bellini, Peters, Benner, & Hopf, 2007).

Current research suggests that the literacy development of children with ASDs parallels their oral language development. Additionally, it has been shown that individuals with ASDs can learn to read and write meaningfully (Mirenda, 2003). Since spoken and written language development are interconnected and mutually enhance each other, it is not surprising that instruction in reading has been found to enhance the oral language skills of some individuals with ASDs (Colasent & Griffith, 1998; Craig & Sexton Telfer, 2005; Koppenhaver & Erickson, 2003). Current scope of practice guidelines for speech-language pathologists indicate that interventions targeted toward individuals with ASDs include both a language and literacy focus (ASHA, 2006). Therefore, it is imperative that speech-language pathologists understand the nature of literacy and the typical development of reading and writing as well as disorders of language and literacy and their relationships to each other. Furthermore, speech-language pathologists should have training to administer and interpret literacy-based assessments and obtain the knowledge and skills needed to target areas that lead to spoken and written language growth. Targeting both language and literacy skills in individuals with ASD supports literacy instruction in the classroom environment, enhances the ability to achieve academic success, and ultimately affords an individual with ASD access to gain increased success in a variety of life skills.

## Description of the Case

Diego is a six-and-a-half-year-old male diagnosed with PPD-NOS. He was initially diagnosed with classic autism at 3 years of age. Three months after the initial diagnosis the same neurologist revised the diagnosis to PDD-NOS after administering the widely used screening instrument, Autism Behavior Checklist (ABC) (Krug, Arick, & Almond, 1993).

### Background Information

#### Developmental, Medical, Family, and Educational History

Diego was a product of a 33.5-week dyzogotic twin gestation delivered via cesarean section. He was in a neonatal intensive care unit (NICU) for approximately 1 week following birth. Past medical history included inguinal hernia repairs and surgical removal of a cyst under his tongue. No major illnesses, head injuries, or seizures were reported. Neurological examinations were unremarkable. Audiological evaluations revealed hearing within normal limits bilaterally. At 3 years of age, Diego was evaluated by an alternative medicine physician who prescribed a variety of supplements (e.g., proactive enzyme plus, biomega 3, citrus seed extract, B-complex plus) which Diego took for approximately 6 months to control chronic diarrhea. Since then his family has had him on a gluten- and casein-free diet. He has been followed medically by a pediatric neurologist, a general practice pediatrician, and a developmental pediatrician. Recently he was placed on Strattera (10 mg, once a day), a drug used to treat attention-deficit/hyperactivity disorder (ADHD) in an attempt to control inappropriate behavior.

Diego's early motor milestones were within normal limits. As a toddler he was reported to climb on everything and would try to escape through doors and windows. However, early speech and language milestones were globally delayed. In the first 2 years of his life, Diego would not respond to his name when called; was nonverbal; would not wave hello or goodbye; was not pointing; and was not participating in reciprocal interactions. Despite continuing significant speech and communication delays, speech and language therapy was not initiated until Diego was 3 years of age. Following 6 months of therapy he began imitating words; however, his speech was highly unintelligible. He used a limited repertoire of gestures spontaneously to communicate his wants and needs. Maladaptive behaviors (e.g., hitting, kicking biting, screaming) frequently were used for communication when frustrated. Also at age 3, Diego began attending a full-day preschool program, 5 days a week, in a varying exceptionalities classroom.

Over time, with continued speech-language intervention and placement in a full-time preschool program, Diego's speech, language, and communication skills markedly improved. At the time of the evaluation, he communicated via verbal language and his speech was primarily intelligible. He was able to combine 3 to 4 sentences in response to questions on familiar topics. However, when engaged in spontaneous conversation, he typically reverted to 1- to 3-word utterances and tended to intersperse utterances he had previously heard (i.e., delayed echolalia). He frequently had difficulty adding new information to a topic and/or demonstrating fluent conversational volley and reciprocity while communicating. During conversations and social interactions, he inconsistently used eye gaze shift to socially reference his communication partner or referent. In addition to Diego's growth in speech, language, and communication, he had made significant gains in his activities of daily living (ADLs). Diego was fully bowel and bladder toilet trained, and he dressed himself independently.

Diego resided at home with his mother, father, twin sister, and younger brother. Although Diego's twin sister did not exhibit characteristics of ASD, it was suspected that she might have a learning disability. The family resided in a rural community and considered themselves to be middle class. English was the only language spoken in the home. Diego's mother did not work outside the home and was the primary caregiver. His father was a firefighter/paramedic. Other caregivers included maternal and paternal grandparents. The family's primary goals for Diego were to increase his social interactions with peers and improve his behavior in all settings. They believed that for Diego to reach his potential, inclusion was the only educational option for him.

Diego attended a public school where he was placed full-time in a regular education kindergarten classroom. He was taught by a regular education classroom teacher and assisted 1 to 2 hours a day by a paraprofessional. He received "pull-out" speech and language therapy in a small group, twice a week for 30-minute sessions, by a school-based, licensed and certified speech-language pathologist. Diego began taking Straterra, 7 months into the school year, to help regulate his ability to attend and control inappropriate classroom behaviors.

## Reason for Referral

Diego was referred for speech-language pathology services because of his globally delayed speech, language, and communication skills.

## Findings of the Evaluation

When Diego entered kindergarten, the school-based speech-language pathologist administered both a receptive language measure, Peabody Picture Vocabulary Test-4 (Dunn, 2006), and an expressive language measure, Expressive One-Word Picture Vocabulary Test (Brownell, 2000). Standard scores for both tests fell within the average range, 102 and 105 respectively, based on his chronological age. A language sample was obtained while the clinician and Diego engaged in play with a variety of age-appropriate materials. Due to time constraints the clinician conducted a cursory analysis of the language sample. Her analysis indicated that Diego used both simple and complex sentences when responding during conversations but only used short, simple sentences when initiating conversation. Occasionally, phrase repetitions were embedded within his utterances and instances of delayed echolalia were noted. Although his speech was primarily intelligible, Diego consistently substituted /f/ for unvoiced "th," /v/ for voiced "th," and /t/ for /k/. During the play activities, he engaged in reciprocal interactions and used all materials appropriately.

Early in the second half of kindergarten, the Stanford Achievement Test Series (10th ed.) was administered in the classroom setting. Based on test results, Diego's overall achievement score indicated functioning at the K.1 (beginning kindergarten) level. He exhibited strengths and weaknesses across the areas assessed (i.e., reading, listening comprehension, mathematics, social studies, science). His strengths were in isolated single word reading and sentence reading (scores falling within the end of kindergarten to beginning of first grade range). His areas of difficulty centered on letter and sound correspondences, listening comprehension, mathematics, social studies, and science (scores falling within the prekindergarten to beginning of kindergarten range). The speech-language pathologist noted that Diego appeared to be acquiring a sight word vocabulary but was having difficulty with letter and sound correspondences, suggesting difficulties in phonemic awareness. Although his single word vocabulary knowledge was age appropriate, he appeared to have difficulty understanding connected speech and written language.

After obtaining results of the Stanford Achievement Test Series (10th ed.), the speech-language pathologist administered several subtests from the Woodcock Reading Mastery Test-Revised (Form G) (Woodcock, 1987). Since Diego was taking the medication Straterra to improve his attending skills, it was hypothesized that he might perform better on selected early literacy measures. However, results were consistent in the areas of word identification (single word reading), word attack (decoding pseudo-words), and passage comprehension (reading comprehension). His relative strength was in single word reading (beginning first grade level), while decoding and reading comprehension scores were at the beginning kindergarten level. These results revealed that although medication may have improved his attending skills, he appeared to present with difficulties in phonemic awareness and listening and reading comprehension.

The speech-language pathologist asked Diego's classroom teacher and family to complete the Autism Social Skills Profile (ASSP) (Bellini, unpublished manuscript) to obtain additional information about social skills functioning since Diego continued to exhibit intermittent difficulties in the classroom even with medication. Based on teacher and parent report, Diego exhibited difficulties in two primary social skill areas: social reciprocity (i.e., asking questions to request information about a topic or a person; maintaining the "give and take" of conversations; joining a conversation without interrupting; considering multiple viewpoints; speaking with an inappropriate volume); and detrimental social behaviors (i.e., maintaining an appropriate distance when interacting with peers; making inappropriate comments; engaging in socially inappropriate behavior; misinterpreting the intentions of others). On the other hand, Diego was reported to exhibit strengths in social participation (i.e., inviting peers to join in activities; joining in activities with peers during structured and unstructured activities; engaging in one-on-one peer interactions as well as group interactions; and occasionally engaging in solitary activities in the presence of peers).

### Problem

Diego presented with social communication, language, and literacy deficits that negatively influenced his social interactions, academic achievement, and ability to function independently in a regular education classroom setting with same-age non-disabled peers.

### Hypothesis

If Diego received intervention with a focus on pragmatic language and social skills training with positive behavioral supports, in both small group and classroom settings, and he received an integrated approach to language and literacy instruction in the classroom, with individual instruction as needed, then he would be successful in a regular education classroom independent of direct adult support.

## Treatment Options Considered

A number of treatment options were considered and discussed with the family based on Diego's strengths and current needs. Three primary treatment areas were decided upon following review of scientific evidenced-based research, review of records (including formal and informal assessments and observations) and the family's desire to increase appropriate social interactions and behavior. These treatment areas included social skills training (e.g., initiating and maintaining social interactions; discourse skills; self awareness; understanding nonverbal communication; adhering to classroom rules and routines); integrated language and literacy instruction (e.g., oral language including narrative development and story retelling; phonemic awareness; vocabulary and concept development; listening and reading comprehension; and writing); and behavior modification intervention (e.g., speaking with appropriate volume; maintaining an appropriate distance when interacting with peers; making appropriate comments; engaging in socially appropriate behaviors). Although these three broad treatment areas are consistent with current best practices for individuals with ASDs, advantages and disadvantages of any treatment approach should continue to be reviewed and understood prior to implementation. (See Ali & Frederickson, 2006; Bellini et al., 2007; Buettel, 2008; Lee, Simpson, & Shogren, 2007; Tutt, Powell & Thornton, 2006; Wheeler, Baggett, Fox, & Blevins, 2006 for reviews.)

## Course of Treatment

An integrated approach to treatment was initiated during the second half of Diego's kindergarten year following a review of records and evaluation information. This integrated treatment approach was implemented across settings (i.e., collaboration within the regular education classroom and during pull-out group speech and language intervention). Parent and peer training were interspersed throughout the intervention programming. The social skills training occurred primarily within the classroom setting as well as during nonacademic activities (e.g., recess, lunch). This occurred multiple times each day, incorporating a number of strategies that have been found to be effective in teaching social skills to individuals with ASDs. Strategies utilized included social stories, visual supports, targeted scripts, and role playing with same aged, nondisabled peers (Delano & Snell, 2006; Sansosti, 2006).

The integrated language and literacy instruction focused on oral language, phonemic awareness, vocabulary and concept development, listening comprehension, and writing. Language and literacy goals were primed during pull-out group speech and language therapy sessions (twice a week for 30-minute sessions) and then maintained and generalized within a variety of academic lessons and activities in the regular education classroom in collaboration with the classroom teacher. A number of strategies were incorporated to facilitate and enhance Diego's language and literacy skills. Interactive read-alouds, story retelling and dramatizing books, and shared and interactive writing activities were used to enhance comprehension and extend vocabulary, develop narrative story schema, and draw attention to letters and sounds. Both narrative and expository texts were used in activities (Bellon, Ogletree, & Harn, 2003; McCormick, 2003). Phonemic awareness instruction was embedded in shared reading of books and poems with alliteration and rhyme and taught explicitly through letter-sound matching, blending, and segmenting activities. Although there is a paucity of empirical research focusing on teaching literacy skills to individuals with ASDs, the speech-language pathologist selected intervention strategies that had some documented support to promote literacy development (Bellon et al., 2003; Colasent & Griffith, 1998; Koppenhaver & Erickson, 2003; Lanter & Watson, 2008) and met Diego's language and literacy needs.

A functional behavior assessment (FBA) was conducted to determine the need for a behavior intervention plan (BIP). A behavior intervention plan was then developed and implemented across the school day targeting the following areas: keeping hands and feet to self (i.e., inappropriate touching of others), keeping an appropriate distance between self and others during social interactions (i.e., personal space), using an "inside voice" versus yelling within the classroom, and using socially "acceptable" language within the school environment (Buschbacher & Fox, 2003). Visual supports and social stories were incorporated to enhance Diego's comprehension of new behavioral expectations. Family members and professionals were encouraged to implement the plan on a daily basis to ensure consistency, rate of success, and continuity across people and settings.

## Analysis of the Client's Response to Intervention

The integrated intervention approach was begun 3 months prior to the end of the school year. Overall clinical impressions of Diego's response to intervention were positive. In the area of social skills, he made gains in his ability to maintain social exchanges by engaging in brief conversations with peers that related to his preferred topics or familiar experiences. The ability to adhere to classroom rules and routines appeared to be emerging. In the area of language and literacy, improvements were seen in phonemic awareness. Diego advanced in his ability to detect and produce rhymes and his invented spellings reflected emerging knowledge of letter and sound correspondences. Diego's story retelling ability improved, but oral narrative production continued to be difficult for him. Listening comprehension (and hence reading comprehension) continued to require a great deal of support. Behaviorally, Diego demonstrated continued improvement. His ability to keep his hands and feet to himself, stay within his own personal space, and keep his volume to a level appropriate for an "inside voice" improved dramatically. Intermittently, Diego continued to need reminders as to which language is or is not "socially acceptable" at school and when socially interacting with peers. The initiation of medication may have played a considerable role in enhancing the rate of Diego's success in responding positively to the intervention plan.

Diego's classroom teacher submitted a narrative report on Diego's progress. She noted that he was "extremely strong in most academic areas." She related that although Diego had difficulty staying on task and following rules at the beginning of the school year, his behavior was clearly improving. She attributed this improvement to the medication Diego was taking. The teacher also commented that the collaboration with the speech-language pathologist to improve Diego's social, language, and academic skills was a positive experience. She stated that Diego would be promoted to first grade, but indicated that he would continue to need support with observing rules and regulations, following directions promptly, staying on task for longer periods of time, and demonstrating "good" listening skills.

The clinician expressed concern that without explicit, ongoing, integrated intervention in language and literacy, and social skills training, Diego would struggle socially as well as academically the next school year. She noted that full-time inclusion in a regular education classroom might need to be reevaluated as the continued least restrictive and best placement option if the proper supports were not in place to support Diego's continued success.

## Further Recommendations

The clinicians recommend that Diego receive ongoing social skills training, integrated instruction in language and literacy, and positive behavioral support on a daily basis, across setting. This would prepare him for success in a regular education classroom as well as for social interaction with nondisabled peers during nonacademic activities, independent of direct adult support.

## Author Note

The authors wish to acknowledge and thank all of the children and their families with whom we have worked over the years. Our case study is a compilation of multiple cases of school-age children with autism spectrum disorders. The Institutional Review Board (IRB) at the University of Central Florida (UCF) was contacted prior to writing this case study. Since this is a fictionalized case study based on multiple true cases, IRB approval was not necessary.

## References

Ali, S., & Frederickson, N. (2006). Investigating the evidence base of social stories. *Educational Psychology in Practice, 22*(4), 355–377.

American Psychological Association. (1999). *Diagnostic and statistical manual of mental disorders* (4th ed.). Washington, DC: Author.

American Speech-Language-Hearing Association. (2006). *Guidelines for speech-language pathologists in diagnosis, assessment, and treatment of autism spectrum disorders across the life span.* Available from http://www.asha.org/docs/html/GL2006-00049.html

Bellini, S. (in press). *The autism social skills profile.* Shawnee Mission, KS: Autism Asperger Publishing.

Bellini, S., Peters, J. K., Benner, L., & Hopf, A. (2007). A meta-analysis of school-based social skills interventions for children with autism spectrum disorders. *Remedial and Special Education, 3,* 153–162.

Bellon, M., Ogletree, B., & Harn, W. (2003). Repeated storybook reading as a language intervention for children with autism: A case study on the application of scaffolding.

*Focus on Autism and Other Developmental Disabilities, 15*(1), 52–58.

Brownell, R. (2000). *Expressive One-Word Picture Vocabulary Test.* Novato, CA: Academic Therapy Publications.

Buettel, M. P. (2008). Research-based social-emotional interventions for Asperger syndrome: A meta-analysis. *Dissertation Abstracts International Section A: Humanities and Social Sciences, 68*(7-A), 2823.

Buschbacher, P. W., & Fox, L. (2003). Understanding and intervening with the challenging behavior of young children with autism spectrum disorder. *Language, Speech, and Hearing Services in Schools, 34,* 217–227.

Centers for Disease Control and Prevention. (2007). Prevalence of autism spectrum disorders. *Autism and Developmental Disabilities Monitoring Network,* 14 Sites, United States, 2002. MMWR SS 2007; 56 (No. SS-1).

Chakrabarti, S., & Fombonne, E. (2001). Pervasive developmental disorders in preschool children. *Journal of the American Medical Association, 285*(24), 3039–3099.

Colasent, R., & Griffith, P. (1998). Autism and literacy: Looking into the classroom with rabbit stories. *The Reading Teacher, 51*(5), 414–420.

Craig, H. K., & Sexton Telfer, A. (2005). Hyperlexia and autism spectrum disorder: A case study of scaffolding language growth over time. *Topics in Language Disorders, 25*(4), 364–374.

Delano, M., & Snell, M. E. (2006). The effects of social stories on the social engagement of children with autism. *Journal of Positive Behavior Interventions, 8*(1), 29–42.

Dunn, L. M. (2006). *Peabody Picture Vocabulary Test-4.* Circle Pines, MN: American Guidance Service.

Koppenhaver, D., & Erickson, K. (2003). Natural emergent literacy supports for preschoolers with autism and severe communication impairments. *Topics in Language Disorders, 23*(4), 283–292.

Krug, D. A., Arick, J. R., & Almond, P. J. (1993). *Autism behavior checklist (ABC).* In *Autism Screening Instrument for Educational Planning (ASIEP-2).* Austin, TX: PRO-ED.

Lanter, E., & Watson, L. R. (2008). Promoting literacy in students with ASD; The basics for the SLP. *Language, Speech, and Hearing Services in Schools, 39,* 33–43.

Lee, S.H., Simpson, R. L., & Shogren, K. A. (2007). Effects and implications of self-management for students with autism: A meta-analysis. *Focus on Autism and Other Developmental Disabilities, 22*(1), 2–13.

Mirenda, P. (2003). He's not really a reader . . . : Perspectives on supporting literacy development in individuals with autism. *Topics in Language Disorders, 23*(4), 271–282.

McCormick, S. (2003). *Instructing students who have literacy problems.* Upper Saddle River, NJ: Merrill/Prentice Hall.

National Research Council. (2001). *Educating children with autism.* Committee on Educational Interventions for Children with Autism. Washington D.C.: National Academy Press.

Sansosti, F. J. (2006). Using video modeled social stories to increase the social communication skills of children with high functioning autism/Asperger's syndrome. *Dissertation Abstracts International: Section B: The Sciences and Engineering, 66*(9-B), 5104.

*Stanford Achievement Test Series* (10th ed.). (2003). San Antonio, TX: Harcourt Educational Measurement.

Tutt, R., Powell, S., & Thornton, M. (2006). Educational approaches in autism: What we know about what we do. *Educational Psychology in Practice, 22*(1), 69–81.

Volker, M. A., & Lopata, C. (2008). Autism: A review of biological bases, assessment, and intervention. *School Psychology Quarterly, 23*(2), 258–270.

Wheeler, J. J., Baggett, B. A., Fox, J., & Blevins, L. (2006). A review of intervention studies conducted with children with autism. *Focus on Autism and Other Developmental Disabilities, 21*(1), 45–54.

Woodcock, R. N. (1987). *Woodcock Reading Mastery Test-Revised* (Form G). Circle Pines, MN: American Guidance Service.

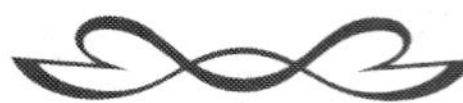



# CASE 26

# Manuela: Cultural and Linguistic Diversity: A Bilingual Child with a Speech and Language Disorder

*Brian Goldstein*

## Conceptual Knowledge Areas

Providing clinical services to bilingual children is not the same as providing them to monolingual children. Having input in and using more than one language complicates the process of assessment and subsequent treatment. Thus, speech-language pathologists (SLPs) must be prepared to alter their "standard of care" with bilingual children. The purpose of this case is to show how assessment and treatment differ for bilingual children in comparison to monolingual peers. To that end, three aspects of the clinical process will be the focus of this case: (1) assess speech and language skills in both languages; (2) take into account sociolinguistic variables; and (3) provide treatment in both languages (Goldstein, 2006).

### Assess in Both Languages

Research on the speech and language development (and disorders) of bilingual children indicates that it is similar, although *not* identical, to monolingual development (e.g., Marchman, Martínez-Sussman, & Price, 2000). This finding holds for bilingual children with language disorders as well. For example, Paradis, Crago, Genesee, and Rice (2003) found that the morphological skills of bilingual children with specific language impairment (SLI) were commensurate with those of age-matched monolingual English and monolingual French speakers with SLI. Thus, as bilingual children gain more linguistic experience over time, their speech and language skills become more like those of monolinguals. However, it is also likely that the language skills of bilinguals will be asymmetrically distributed across the two languages such that knowledge in one language is not necessarily replicated in the other. For example, Peña, Bedore, and Rappazzo (2003) found that bilingual children showed better performance in English than in Spanish on some tasks (e.g., receptive similarities and differences) but also better performance in Spanish on other tasks (e.g., expressive functions). Findings from these types of studies show the necessity of completing an assessment in both of the bilingual child's languages.

### Consider Sociolinguistic Variables

Although the speech and language skills of bilingual children are similar to monolingual peers, those skills might be tempered differentially by the sociolinguistic environment (Hammer, Miccio, & Rodriguez, 2004). Historically, sociolinguistic variables have been related to language dominance (i.e., which is the "stronger" language?) and type of bilingual (e.g., simultaneous or sequential). However, these descriptors do not allow the clinician to delve deeply into the child's bilingual background. Thus, in assessing bilingual children, SLPs should obtain information on language history (age at which the child hears and uses each language), language environment (environments in which the child hears and uses each language), language input/output (frequency with which the child hears and uses each language), and language proficiency (how well the child uses each language). Consideration of how the bilingual child develops and uses both languages will result in a more reliable and valid assessment and subsequently will link to treatment.

### Provide Treatment in Both Languages

Because bilingual children show distributed skills in each of their two languages and bilingual speech and language development is not equivalent to that of monolingual speakers, it is almost certain that treatment will need to occur in both languages at some point during the treatment process. Kohnert and Derr (2004) and Kohnert, Yim, Nett, Fong Kan, and Duran (2005) proposed two approaches to treating speech and language disorders in bilingual children. First, the bilingual approach maintains that SLPs should improve language skills common to both languages. Along those same lines, Yavaş and Goldstein (1998) recommended initially treating errors/error patterns exhibited with relatively equal frequency, in both languages. Second, the cross-linguistic approach maintains that the linguistic skills unique to each language should be targeted. Kohnert and colleagues emphasize that SLPs likely will utilize both approaches during treatment with bilingual children.

Analyzing the speech and language skills of bilingual children is a complicated task. Analysis is aided by assessing in both languages, considering the sociolinguistic variables, and providing intervention in both languages. These three parameters set the backdrop for the following learning objectives and case study.

## Description of the Case

Manuela Torres is a 5-year, 8-month-old bilingual (Spanish-English) female who attends first grade at the Marín School. She was referred to the speech-language pathologist (SLP) by her classroom teacher as she tends to be "quiet" in class and is not making expected academic progress. Her mother, Sra. Ana Torres, was interviewed by phone in Spanish, her language of preference. During the evaluation, which occurred in both Spanish and English, case history information was obtained, formal testing was performed, and a language sample was recorded. The results of the evaluation are summarized in the following paragraphs.

### Background Information

Manuela's birth history was normal. Her mother reported that she reached all developmental motor milestones at the appropriate times, but she had difficulty with toilet training; Manuela was completely trained at age 4 years, 6 months. Regarding her medical history, Manuela's mother stated that she has had multiple cases of whooping cough, which have not reoccurred for over 2 years. Mrs. Torres reported that results from an in-school hearing screening were normal, and she has no concerns about Manuela's hearing. According to school records, Manuela's hearing (pure tone and impedance) was screened at school approximately 3 months prior to the assessment and found to be within normal limits.

Manuela lived at home with her mother, father, and two brothers (age 4 years and age 8 months). Sra. Torres did not work outside the home, and Sr. Torres worked in the maintenance department for the school district. Manuela also spent time with her grandmother. Manuela attended preschool for 1 year at a community Head Start 5 times a week and was instructed in both Spanish and English. Manuela's 4-year-old brother attended the same Head Start program.

## Reason for Referral

Manuela's language environment consisted of both English and Spanish since birth. However, until the time she entered preschool, she heard and used more Spanish than English. Sra. Torres estimated the frequency with which Manuela heard and used each language was 75% Spanish and 25% English. Manuela spent the majority of her day hearing and using English (approximately 80% of the time) at home and in school. The rest of the day (about 20% of the time) she heard and used the Puerto Rican dialect of Spanish. At the Marín School, Manuela heard English almost exclusively in her classroom from the classroom teacher, although the aide in the classroom used Spanish to reinforce instructions and information from the classroom teacher. In school, nearly 100% of Manuela's productions were in English, according to Manuela's teacher. Manuela's teacher reported her English proficiency as a 3 (speaks the language with some errors) on a 0–4 point scale (Restrepo, 1998). Sra. Torres rated Manuela's Spanish proficiency (how well she uses the language) as a 2 (speaks the language with a relatively large number of errors) on the same 0–4 point scale.

Sra. Torres reported that at age 2 years Manuela spoke her first words, which were in Spanish (e.g., *dáme* [give me] and *mío* [mine]), and that at age 3 years she began combining 2 and 3 words in Spanish and English (e.g., *mi perro* [my dog]; *dáme manzana* [give me apple]; *uh-oh mommy*). Sra. Torres started showing concern about Manuela's speech and language skills 1 year prior to this evaluation as she noticed Manuela was not "speaking as well as the other children" in her preschool class. She did not express her concern to the school as she thought they would let her know, "if something was wrong." Her main concern was Manuela's articulation, especially in Spanish. However, she understood less than half of Manuela's utterances in Spanish. At the time of this study intelligibility had increased to about 75%. Manuela's teacher was concerned not only about her articulation in English but also about her expressive language skills, especially her grammar in English.

## Findings of the Evaluation

Manuela's speech and language skills were assessed in both Spanish and English. To assess those skills, the phonology subtest of the Bilingual English-Spanish Assessment (BESA) (Peña, Gutiérrez-Clellen, Iglesias, Goldstein, & Bedore, in development) and the Wiig Assessment of Basic Concepts-English (Wiig, 2004) and Spanish (WABC) (Wiig & Langdon, 2006) were administered. An oral-peripheral mechanism screening was conducted, and language samples in both Spanish and English were collected.

### Behavior

Manuela behaved well and appeared to have an attention span typical for her age. She interacted well with the clinician during play and was engaged in the testing activities, but was initially reluctant to talk.

### Oral Peripheral Examination

An informal oral-peripheral assessment was completed during the evaluation. Her facial symmetry and oral musculature appeared to be within normal limits. Her mouth appeared to be symmetrical during speech and at rest. Diadochokinetic rate was within normal limits (Shipley & McAfee, 2004).

### Phonology

Manuela's phonology was assessed in Spanish and English using the BESA (Bilingual English-Spanish Assessment) phonology subtest. Scoring was completed taking dialect features into account such that those features were not scored as errors (Goldstein & Iglesias, 2001).

Manuela exhibited a severe phonological disorder based on consonant accuracy less < 50% in both languages (Gruber, 1999). Scores for the Spanish and English phonology subtests are displayed in Figure 26.1.

| | |
|---|---|
| Consonant Accuracy: Spanish | 48.78% |
| Vowel Accuracy: Spanish | 87.14% |
| Consonant Accuracy: English | 48.5% |
| Vowel Accuracy: English | 84.91% |

FIGURE 26.1 Scores for BESA Phonology Subtest—Spanish and English

Phoneme accuracy is listed in Table 26.1. These results provide further evidence of a phonological disorder given the expectation of near 100% accuracy on the majority of phonemes at this age in English (Smit, Hand, Freilinger, Bernthal, & Bird, 1990) and in Spanish (Jimenez, 1987).

Manuela demonstrated a high frequency of occurrence (> 10%) for phonological patterns in Spanish and English (Table 26.2): cluster reduction, initial cluster reduction, final consonant deletion, stopping, and backing. These patterns are ones that are typically suppressed by the time a child reaches Manuela's age. It also should be noted that the frequencies of occurrence were largely similar in both languages, although there were two exceptions: initial consonant deletion occurred in Spanish but not in English, and gliding occurred in English but not in Spanish.

## Language

Receptive and expressive language skills were assessed in both English and Spanish using the WABC-Level 2 (English and Spanish).

TABLE 26.1 BESA Phonology Subtest—Phoneme Accuracy

| Phoneme | Percent Correct: Spanish | Percent Correct: English |
|---|---|---|
| p | 100% | 89% |
| b | 86% | 100% |
| t | 85% | 80% |
| d | 70% | 65% |
| k | 67% | 89% |
| g | 75% | 75% |
| m | 100% | 100% |
| n | 80% | 55% |
| ɲ | 90% | n/a |
| ŋ | n/a | 100% |
| f | 67% | 50% |
| v | n/a | 50% |
| θ | n/a | 15% |
| ð | 50% | 22% |
| s | 14% | 17% |
| z | n/a | 50% |
| ʃ | n/a | 12% |
| ʒ | n/a | n/a |
| ʧ | 66% | 50% |
| ʤ | n/a | 42% |
| l | 33% | 20% |
| ɹ (as in *red*) | n/a | 9% |
| ɾ (flap) | 11% | n/a |
| r (trill) | 6% | n/a |
| w | n/a | 95% |
| j | 85% | 90% |

TABLE 26.2 Phonological Patterns Displayed

| Phonological Pattern | Percentage of Occurrence | | Example | |
|---|---|---|---|---|
| | ***Spanish*** | ***English*** | ***Spanish*** | ***English*** |
| Cluster Reduction | 71% | 69% | "nego" for "negro" | "toe" for "toast" |
| Initial Cluster Reduction | 87% | 83% | "tabo" for "clavo" | "dop" for "stop" |
| Final Consonant Deletion | 15% | 33% | "ku" for "cruz" | "bri" for "bridge" |
| Initial Consonant Deletion | 20% | 0% | "ama" for "cama" | n/a |
| Stopping | 30% | 24% | "keño" for "señor" | "tum" for "thumb" |
| Consonant Backing | 15% | 13% | "ke" for "tren" | "come" for "thumb" |
| Gliding | 0% | 22% | n/a | "wing" for "ring" |

***Receptive Language*** Results from the receptive portion of the WABC indicated receptive skills that were within normal limits. Manuela achieved a standard score of 88 on the WABC-English and a standard score of 90 on the WABC-Spanish, which placed her scores slightly below the mean, but still within normal limits. She could follow one- and two-step commands. In both Spanish and English, she accurately identified many objects, parts of objects, and objects within a category (body parts, food items, animals, and clothing). She pointed to the correct use of objects, recognized actions in pictures and in play, and made inferences. Manuela demonstrated comprehension of quantitative concepts, part/whole relationships, and descriptive concepts such as *heaviest*, *slowest*, and *dark* in English and *débil* (weak), *menos* (less), and *tarde* (late). She also appeared to understand pronouns and accurately identified the colors of objects (in English only). Although Manuela had difficulty with spatial concepts in both languages during testing (e.g., *inside*), she was able to demonstrate this skill during play. Concepts that were not answered correctly on the test tended to be condition concepts in Spanish (e.g., *oscuro* [dark]) and quantity concepts in English (e.g., *half*). During play, Manuela appeared to understand all wh- questions with the exception of *when*.

***Expressive Language*** Results from the expressive portion of the WABC (English and Spanish) found Manuela's skills to be moderately delayed. She achieved the following scores:

| | *English* | *Spanish* |
|---|---|---|
| Standard score | 80 | 73 |
| Confidence interval (90%) | 72–89 | 64–82 |
| Percentile rank | 9th | 1st |

Manuela showed similarities and differences on the WABC by language. In both languages, she knew concepts of weight/volume (e.g., *thin*, *heavy* in English and *bajo* [under], *delgada* [thin] in Spanish) and distance/speed/time (e.g., *slow*, *late* in English and *lejos* [far], *viejo* [old] in Spanish). She exhibited differences across languages as well. In English, she showed difficulty with concepts of condition/quality (e.g., *neat*, *quiet*, *straight*). In Spanish, she showed difficulty with concepts of location/direction (e.g., *izquierdo* [left], *tercera* [third], *al frente* [in front]).

A conversational language sample of 75 utterances in English and 62 utterances in Spanish was collected. In the sample, Manuela mainly used 3- and 4-word utterances in both languages, although she did show that she is capable of producing longer utterances (e.g., *My mom come in the car over here*). By this age, children typically should be able to produce complex utterances of at least 5 to 6 words. Mean length of utterance-words (MLUw) was calculated in both languages as a measure of grammatical complexity. MLUw was calculated rather than MLUm (morphemes) to provide comparable measures across languages (Anderson, 1999). Manuela's MLUw from the conversational sample was 3.74 in Spanish and 3.85 in English. An MLUw under 4 places her language complexity at the level of a child age 3 years 6 months to 4 years.

In the sample, Manuela used more nouns than verbs in both languages. To answer questions, she also produced a relatively large number of unconjugated verbs (infinitives such as *comer* [to eat] in Spanish and "to sleep" in English). When producing verbs, she used many general all-purpose verbs such as *tengo* [I have] and *quiero* [I want] in Spanish and *like, got, put, want* in English, as well as action verbs in Spanish (*ven* [come], *salta* [jump]) and in English (kick, crash, jump), and modal auxiliaries and concatenatives in English (wanna, gonna). She used possessive (*mío* [mine], *tuyo* [yours], his, my) and personal pronouns in Spanish (*yo* [I], *tú* [you]) and in English (he, you, I, it, me). Manuela inconsistently used the following constructions (*denotes omission of required element):

- ***Articles:*** *put* ***the*** *car* vs. *my mom crashed in front of * police*
- ***Irregular past tense* (in English only):** *My mom bought it* vs. *I can* ***broke*** *it*
- ***Plurals:*** *uvas* (grapes) vs. *two ball**
- ***Possessive nouns:*** *my, his* vs. *you see my ma* car right there?*
- ***Auxiliaries and copulas:*** *I * tired, what * this?, then he * leaving, I wish my mother * buy me that*

To measure lexical diversity, number of different words (NDW) was calculated. NDW was .31 (23 different words) in English and a slightly higher .42 (26 different words) in Spanish. In both languages, NDW was less than expected for her age (Miller, 1987). By age 7 years, English-speaking children produced, on average, 173 different words in a 100-utterance sample (Leadholm & Miller, 1992). In Spanish, children of approximately the same age as Manuela produced 70 different words (Muñoz, Gillam, Peña, & Gulley-Faehnle, 2003).

Manuela did not always demonstrate the ability to communicate her wants and needs in an age-appropriate fashion. At times, she relied on action verbs to make requests. For example, when a toy did not function, she brought it to a clinician and said, "Do this." When asked, "Do what?" she replied, "Jumping" to refer to the balls that moved up and down inside the toy. When asked what she was doing while playing with the hula hoop, she responded, "*Trata* (try)." There were instances, however, when she demonstrated the ability to construct appropriate requests but did not do so. For example, to ask the clinician to tie her shoe she said, "My tie it" and "Make it." Afterward, however, she said, "My dad can tie it" and "I can tie my shoes."

By 5 to 6 years old a child typically uses adult-like grammar most of the time. Manuela's inconsistent omission of articles, verbal morphology, auxiliaries, and copulas are not typical for a child her age. By this age she should be able to put 5–6 word sentences together consistently. Although the sample shows that she is capable of producing longer utterances (e.g., *I gonna throw hard over there* and *Tengo un gato en mi casa* [I have a cat at my house]), she typically used short utterances that did not adequately communicate her thoughts or requests.

***Pragmatics*** Manuela's pragmatic skills were demonstrated in informal (play) testing situations. She engaged in play with the clinician and warmed up quickly. She showed appropriate levels of eye contact, turn-taking, and joint attention. She demonstrated an excellent ability to request information and actions from the clinician (e.g., *¿qué es esto?* [what is this?]). With puppets, Manuela created characters and told the clinician which one was the daddy, the mommy, and the baby (based on sizes of the dolls). Manuela was very outgoing and playful with any task asked of her.

***Voice and Fluency*** Voice and fluency were examined informally and found to be within normal limits.

## Treatment Options Considered

Manuela was evaluated formally and informally in both English and Spanish. Based on the results of testing, she exhibited a moderate expressive language disorder and a severe articulation disorder in both languages that was impacting her ability to be understood. Both areas of weakness should be addressed in therapy twice per week.

## Course of Treatment

Results of Manuela's comprehensive assessment revealed that she exhibited a moderate expressive language disorder and a severe articulation disorder in both languages. Manuela received 2 1-hour treatment sessions per week, and this phase of treatment lasted 8 weeks.

Three initial treatment goals were implemented. For Goals 1 and 2, a bilingual treatment approach was utilized initially, given that both languages were affected, although not identically. The selection of this approach was based on the work of Kohnert and colleagues (Kohnert & Derr, 2004; Kohnert et al., 2005) and Yavaş and Goldstein (1998), who suggested initially treating errors/error patterns exhibited with relatively equal frequency in both languages. For Goal 3, a cross-linguistic approach was utilized as all errors were in only one language. The following description states the goal, rationale, implementation procedure, and results of treatment.

### Goal 1

*Manuela will suppress the use of the phonological patterns: stopping and cluster reduction.*

- ***Rationale:*** Both patterns were frequently occurring in both languages. By Manuela's age, both patterns should be suppressed entirely or infrequently occur in English (Bernthal & Bankson, 2004) and Spanish (Goldstein, Fabiano, & Washington, 2005). Moreover, these goals represented two types of patterns: syllabic (cluster reduction) and substitution (stopping).
- ***Implementation:*** Treatment occured in both languages, with equal time in English and Spanish. One session per week was conducted in English, and 1 session per week was conducted in Spanish. Both types of patterns (syllabic and substitution) were addressed in each session.
- ***Results of Treatment:*** As noted in Table 26.3, percentages of occurrence decreased for both patterns. However, the frequency of occurrence decreased more for cluster reduction in Spanish than in English. This result was most likely due to differences in clusters in the two languages. Spanish has only 2-member clusters in onset position (e.g., *plato* [plate]) versus 3 for English (e.g., *string*) (Hammond, 2001).

### Goal 2

*Manuela will increase her mean length of utterance to 4.5 words in conversation in both Spanish and English.*

- ***Rationale:*** MLUw was below age expectations in both languages (Bedore, 2004 for Spanish and Shipley & McAfee, 2004 for English). In conversation, Manuela produced mainly utterances of 3 and 4 words.
- ***Implementation:*** Treatment occurred equally in both languages. One session per week was conducted in English, and 1 session per week was conducted in Spanish.
- ***Results of Treatment:*** After 8 weeks of treatment, MLU increased in both languages, although slightly more so in English. The slight English advantage is likely the result of two factors. First, Manuela was exposed to more English during the day than to Spanish. In the classroom setting, instruction was almost exclusively in English. Second, Spanish is a pro-drop language, meaning that subject nouns and pronouns are

TABLE 26.3 Results of Treatment for Phonological Patterns

| | Spanish | | English | |
|---|---|---|---|---|
| **Pattern** | ***Pretreatment*** | ***Posttreatment*** | ***Pretreatment*** | ***Posttreatment*** |
| Cluster Reduction | 71% | 33% | 69% | 50% |
| Stopping | 30% | 18% | 24% | 15% |

TABLE 26.4 Results of Treatment for MLU

| MLUw | Spanish | | English | |
|---|---|---|---|---|
| | *Pretreatment* | *Posttreatment* | *Pretreatment* | *Posttreatment* |
| | 3.74 | 4.10 | 3.85 | 4.25 |

largely optional (Bedore, 2004). Thus, utterance length may be less than that of English, which is not a pro-drop language. Results are displayed in Table 26.4.

### Goal 3

*To produce irregular past tense verbs in English in 80% of obligatory contexts.*

- ***Rationale:*** Manuela produced irregular past tense verbs only in English. Accuracy for these verbs was approximately 30%. At her age, she should be producing these verbs accurately (Shipley & McAfee, 2004).
- ***Implementation:*** Treatment occurred in English only. However, cross-linguistic generalization was monitored in Spanish through the use of a probe list of sentences containing irregular past tense verbs and via elicitation in conversation.
- ***Results of Treatment:*** After a course of treatment, accuracy on irregular past tense verbs in English increased from 30% to almost 50%. In Spanish, Manuela accurately produced 1 of 10 irregular verbs in the elicited sentences. In conversational speech, 6 irregular verbs were attempted and 1 was produced correctly. Thus, even though irregular verbs in Spanish were not targeted, some cross-linguistic generalization might have been occurring.

## Further Recommendations

Assessing and treating bilingual children with speech and language disorders is a complicated task given the increasing but general lack of developmental research studies, paucity of valid and reliable assessment tools, and few treatment studies with this group of children. Evidence-based practice, however, also dictates considering clinical judgment and the client's goals in the provision of clinical services (Dollaghan, 2007). The interaction of these three components suggests that SLPs need to assess in both languages, consider sociolinguistic variables, and treat in both languages as a means to provide reliable and valid services to bilingual children.

## Author Note

The case study presented is hypothetical.

## References


Anderson, R. (1999). Loss of gender agreement in L1 attrition: Preliminary results. *Bilingual Research Journal, 23*, 319–338.

Bedore, L. (2004). Morpho-syntactic development. In B. Goldstein (Ed.), *Bilingual language development and disorders in Spanish-English speakers* (pp. 163–185). Baltimore: Brookes.

Bernthal, J., & Bankson, N. (Eds., 2004). *Articulation and phonological disorders* (5th ed.). Boston, MA: Allyn & Bacon.

Dollaghan, C. (2007). *The handbook for evidence-based practice in communication disorders.* Baltimore, MD: Paul H. Brookes Publishing.

Goldstein, B. (2006). Clinical implications of research on language development and disorders in bilingual children. *Topics in Language Disorders, 26*, 318–334.

Goldstein, B., Fabiano, L., & Washington, P. (2005). Phonological skills in predominantly English, predominantly Spanish, and Spanish-English bilingual children. *Language, Speech, and Hearing Services in Schools, 36*, 201–218.

Goldstein, B., & Iglesias, A. (2001). The effect of dialect on phonological analysis: Evidence from Spanish-speaking children. *American*

*Journal of Speech-Language Pathology, 10,* 394–406.

Gruber, F. (1999). Probability estimates and paths to consonant normalization in children with speech delay. *Journal of Speech, Language, and Hearing Research, 42,* 448–459.

Hammer, C. S., Miccio, A. W., & Rodriguez, B. L. (2004). Bilingual language acquisition and the child socialization process. In B. Goldstein (Ed.), *Bilingual language development and disorders in Spanish-English speakers* (pp. 21–50). Baltimore: Paul H. Brookes Publishing.

Hammond, R. (2001). *The sounds of Spanish: Analysis and application (with special reference to American English).* Somerville, MA: Cascadilla Press.

Jimenez, B. C. (1987). Acquisition of Spanish consonants in children aged 3–5 years, 7 months. *Language Speech and Hearing Services in the Schools, 18*(4), 357–363.

Kohnert, K., & Derr, A. (2004). Language intervention with bilingual children. In B. Goldstein (Ed.), *Bilingual language development and disorders in Spanish-English speakers* (pp. 311–342). Baltimore, MD: Paul H. Brookes Publishing.

Kohnert, K., Yim, D., Nett, K., Fong Kan, P., & Duran, L. (2005). Intervention with linguistically diverse preschool children: A focus on developing home language(s). *Language, Speech, & Hearing Services in Schools, 32,* 153–164.

Leadholm, B., & Miller, J. (1992). *Language sample analysis: The Wisconsin guide.* Madison, WI: Wisconsin Department of Public Instruction.

Marchman, V., Martínez-Sussman, C. & Price, P. (2000, June). *Individual differences in early learning contexts for Spanish- and English-speaking children.* Paper presented at Head Start's 5th National Research Conference, Washington, DC.

Miller, J. F. (1987). *A grammatical characterization of a language disorder.* Proceedings of the First International Symposium on Specific Speech and Language Disorders in Children, London, England.

Muñoz, M., Gillam, R., Peña, E., & Gulley-Faehnle, A. (2003). Measures of language development in fictional narratives of Latino children. *Language, Speech & Hearing Services in Schools, 34,* 332–342.

Paradis, J., Crago, M., Genesee, F., and Rice, M. (2003). French-English bilingual children with SLI: How do they compare with their monolingual peers? *Journal of Speech, Language, and Hearing Research, 46,* 113–127.

Peña, E., Bedore, L. M., & Rappazzo, C. (2003). Comparison of Spanish, English, and bilingual children's performance across semantic tasks. *Language, Speech & Hearing Services in Schools, 34,* 5–16.

Restrepo, M. A. (1998). Identifiers of predominantly Spanish-speaking children with language impairment. *Journal of Speech, Language, and Hearing Research, 41,* 1398–1411.

Shipley, K., and McAfee, J. (2004). *Assessment in speech-language pathology: A resource manual* (3rd ed.). San Diego, CA: Singular Publishing Group.

Smit, A., Hand, L., Freilinger, J., Bernthal, J., & Bird, A. (1990). The Iowa articulation norms project and its Nebraska replication. *Journal of Speech and Hearing Disorders, 55,* 779–798.

Wiig, E. (2004). *Wiig Assessment of Basic Concepts-English.* Greenville, SC: Super Duper Publications.

Wiig, E., & Langdon, H. (2006). *Wiig Assessment of Basic Concepts-Spanish.* Greenville, SC: Super Duper Publications.

Yavaş, M., & Goldstein, B. (1998). Phonological assessment and treatment of bilingual speakers. *American Journal of Speech-Language Pathology, 7,* 49–60.

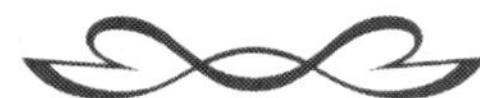

## Cleft Palate

# Case 27

# Zachary: Blowing Bubbles and Rubbing Lips: No Cure in Sight

*Eileen Marrinan and Robert J. Shprintzen*

## Conceptual Knowledge Areas

Cleft lip and palate occur in the very early stages of embryonic development when the facial tissue and bone fail to grow toward each other and fuse. This is one of the most common congenital anomalies. The lip is surgically repaired in the first few months of life and the cleft palate is typically repaired before 1 year of age. Most children develop normal speech after the cleft palate repair. A small percentage of children require another operation at about 4 or 5 years of age if air continues to leak through their nose during speech. Some children develop compensatory speech articulation patterns secondary to this velopharyngeal insufficiency. It is the speech-language pathologist's role and responsibility to identify these problems and refer the child to a specialist for further evaluation, when indicated.

## Description of the Case

### Background Information

One year ago, the Wallace family moved to an upscale college community with a superb school system. Dr. Wallace and Dr. Wright-Wallace had recently completed their PhD degrees and were excited to begin their careers as university professors. The past several years had not been easy. In addition to the stress of completing and defending their dissertations they juggled child care and later preschool and kindergarten schedules for their 7-year-old son, Zachary. Zach was born with a left-sided cleft lip and palate, which already had required several operations with more to come. The shock and strain of giving birth to a child who was not physically perfect was eased by the loving support of their extended families. They had a premier health insurance policy enabling them to receive care from a major cleft center with an excellent reputation. These early years had been a challenge but they adored their son and learned to advocate for his needs quite effectively. They were very pleased with the result of his lip repair. Zach's nose was well aligned and the lip scar was barely noticeable. In fact, few people had any realization that Zach was born with a cleft lip. However, speech problems had been evident since he began talking. A speech-language pathologist (SLP) from their local early intervention program came to their home once weekly when Zach was a baby. Subsequently, Zach received therapy services during his preschool and kindergarten enrollment. At the time of this study, the Wallaces were concerned that he was not progressing and managed to convince the school district to increase his speech therapy from twice weekly to daily sessions.

## Reason for Referral

Zach's parents entered his first grade classroom for the year-end teacher conference brimming with pride. Their previous two conferences with his teacher were met with high accolades. Zach was enthusiastic about entering first grade and quickly made new friends and excelled academically. This time, however, his teacher was not smiling. "I'm concerned about Zach" was not the opening statement his parents expected to hear. The teacher had observed a change in Zach's behavior. He had become reticent, often refusing to participate in class discussions and playing alone at recess. He was not the sociable boy he had been. She had observed several occasions when other children from his own and other grades had teased him about his speech. She had hoped this would pass but his withdrawal seemed to be even more pronounced.

Later that morning, Zach's parents met with an SLP who had already been made aware of his recent social difficulties in the classroom. She admitted that Zach had shown little, if any, progress in his speech since the beginning of the school year. However, she explained that this was not uncommon for children with dyspraxia. The Wallaces were familiar with this diagnostic label as it had been used in reference to Zach's speech disorder since he was a baby. Zach was a precocious baby who spoke his first words before his palate was repaired at 13 months of age. While he was able to clearly say *Mama* and *Nana* (in reference to his grandmother), he typically "omitted" the consonants in other early words such as *bye-bye*, *Dada*, *car*, and *baba* (bottle). Thus, it appeared to the SLPs who had treated him that most of Zach's words were comprised of vowels only. They were impressed by the early intervention SLP whom they remembered as earnest and committed. In fact, she had attended an oral motor conference to learn more effective therapy techniques for dyspraxia. The Wallaces appreciated and adopted her can-do attitude. They purchased many of the "tools of the trade" used by the SLP to treat his dyspraxia including the Jiggler™ Facial Massager and the Nuk® Massage Brush. Another goal was to optimize his velopharyngeal function by encouraging Zach to blow bubbles and cotton balls. Still, he continued to produce primarily "vowels." As his vocabulary expanded rapidly and his mean length of utterance increased, it was increasingly difficult to understand him. The Wallaces, in conjunction with Zach's SLP, redoubled their efforts to stimulate his oral muscles by adding range of movement and what had been referred to as "strengthening exercises" to his therapeutic repertoire. This included sucking a lollipop without holding it and licking bits of peanut butter dabbed on the outer corner of his lips and even on the tip of his nose. This, however, did not result in the desired effect of using his lips and tongue to produce consonants.

When Zach transitioned from early intervention services to preschool, he worked with a new and equally enthusiastic SLP during his preschool and kindergarten years. She agreed with the dyspraxia diagnosis but suggested a different approach in treatment. Rather than focus on nonspeech activities she advised teaching Zach how to use his lips and tongue to make speech sounds. She also incorporated coactive movement and melodic intonation therapy as a means to facilitate his ability to control the temporal and spatial properties of speech, which is the underlying problem in dyspraxia. Rapid repetitions and transitions were aimed at helping articulatory coordination. He did show improvement, which bolstered everyone's resolve. He began to include consonants made with his lips (/p/and /b/) and his tongue tip (/t/ and /d/), though they did not sound quite right. However, he continued to omit fricative consonants and the velar plosives.

The manner in which services were delivered had changed also. Zach's parents were not present during the therapy sessions, which were conducted during his school day. They received regular updates that praised Zach for his diligence. They also learned which sounds were being addressed in therapy. Pictures of words containing those sounds were brought home for practice. The Wallaces complied with instructions to hold the picture close to their mouths as they modeled the words for Zach to repeat.

At the beginning of first grade, Zach's current SLP laid out a new plan for speech therapy. Zach's parents were eager to help, but she explained that the PROMPT© Therapy (Prompts for

Restructuring Oral Muscular Phonetic Targets) approach discourages parents from using the prompts. She explained that she had received specialized training in PROMPT© and that Zach could become confused and frustrated if PROMPT© was used incorrectly by persons who did not have the proper training. The Wallaces were surprised but also somewhat relieved. There was increasing tension between Zach and his parents when they asked him to repeat target sounds. He was unable to do so and they could see that he was dispirited. Zach's parents were encouraged to communicate regularly with his SLP and to ask Zach what he did in therapy (e.g., crafts made, words and sounds practiced). The Wallaces were impressed by the program description, which involved a tactile-kinesthetic to reshape individual sounds and sound sequences. They were told that this would maximize his neuro-motor system potential, ultimately improving his ability to speak clearly.

## Referral to the Cleft Palate Team

The SLP no longer held the same optimism using this approach for Zach. She stated that Zach was not responding as she had hoped. She had now come to the conclusion that Zach's speech problem had a physical base. She suspected that his palate was not working properly and pointed out the nasal quality of his speech. The SLP advised the Wallaces to make an appointment at the cleft palate center located at their city's children's hospital. She provided the family with contact information.

The Wallaces were crestfallen when they returned home from Zach's parent-teacher conference. Above all, they wanted their son to be happy. The realization of his social withdrawal at school broke their hearts. They called the local cleft palate center to schedule a full team evaluation. They also contacted the cleft palate center where he originally received care as a baby and asked them to forward all records to the new center.

Though the Wallaces had been advised to bring Zach for annual visits to the cleft palate center where his lip and palate were repaired, they had not complied. They knew Zach would likely not need another operation until he was 9 or 10 years old when his permanent teeth were ready to erupt into the alveolar (gum) cleft. A graft of bone would be harvested from his hip and packed into his gum. His pediatrician provided annual well-child checks, and his speech needs were well managed by his community speech-language pathologist.

## Cleft Palate Team Evaluation

The Children's Hospital Cleft Palate Center team members warmly greeted the Wallace family. They met separately with the plastic surgeon, otolaryngologist, dentist, orthodontist, audiologist, SLP, genetic counselor, and psychologist. While this was a bit overwhelming, they were grateful for the wealth of information they gleaned. They concluded their morning by meeting with the full team for a summary of their findings and recommendations while Zach played in the waiting room. They learned that while the expected alveolar bone graft was several years off, Zach had a crossbite that could be treated now with palatal expansion. The otolaryngologist and audiologist reported that Zach had eustachian tube dysfunction with middle ear effusion that resulted in a mild hearing loss. A bilateral myringotomy with placement of ear tubes to aerate the middle ears was recommended. The plastic surgeon was pleased with the lip and nose and stated that further revision was not necessary.

The team psychologist had separate interviews with Zach and his parents and also administered validated psychological measures to determine Zach's psychosocial status. She relayed a concerning profile. Zach had confided to her that he hated his speech and children at school often teased him. He had expressed his frustration about trying so hard in speech therapy to no avail and stated that while he enjoyed schoolwork, he wished he did not have to go to school. The psychologist explained that studies have shown having been teased about speech or appearance is the main predictor of psychosocial problems for children born with cleft lip/palate (Gibbons, 2006; Hunt, Burden, Hepper, Stevenson, & Johnston, 2007; Millard & Richman, 2001). In addition, psychosocial issues in childhood often predict similar problems in adulthood (Hunt et al., 2006). She suggested family counseling to help Zach develop positive strategies to prevent or negate peer teasing.

The genetic counselor took a thorough family history. Zach's paternal grandmother had been born with an incomplete cleft lip. It was the family's understanding that this familial clefting slightly increased their risk of having another child with cleft lip and palate, but they did not plan to have more children. Thus, they did not see the need to follow through on a recommended genetic evaluation after Zach's birth. The counselor noted small mounds on Zach's lower lip and lip pits (slight depressions) in his father's lower lip and concluded that Zach, his father, and his grandmother had profiles consistent with a diagnosis of Van der Woude syndrome (OMIM ®). He explained that 1% to 2% of all patients with cleft lip or palate have this genetic condition, associated with a mutation of genetic material on the long arm of chromosome 1, and that it is an autosomal dominant condition. This means that there is a 50% chance for affected individuals to pass it on to their children. A genetic evaluation and molecular genetic testing was recommended to confirm the diagnosis of Van der Woude syndrome.

The team SLP was thorough in her explanation of Zach's speech disorder and confident and positive about the outcome following appropriate management. First, using a diagram of the human vocal tract, she described how normal speech is produced, with special emphasis on the role of the vocal folds and the sphincteric nature of velopharyngeal closure. The Wallaces now understood that resonance is a vowel phenomenon and that the consonants would sound weak as a result of decreased intraoral pressure if some air escaped through the nose during speech. It was explained that Zach's resonance was hypernasal. The SLP pointed out that Zach did not omit consonants in words as was previously thought. He made those sounds in his larynx by forcefully closing his vocal folds, which results in a slight cough-like sound called a glottal stop. She further explained that when the velopharyngeal valve leaks air, some children compensate for the decrease in intraoral pressure by substituting the glottal stop for sounds made by the lips, tongue or teeth. This substitution bypasses the faulty velopharyngeal valve to create subglottic pressure with laryngeal articulation. For the few consonants that he produced such as /p/, /b/, /t/, and /d/, he had been shown how to place his lips and tongue to make the sound, but had never been shown how to eliminate the glottal stop. Therefore, he coarticulated forceful vocal fold closure deep in his throat over the placement higher in his vocal tract. Once the SLP demonstrated this sound herself, Zach's parents immediately recognized it and understood that their son had been using this sound since he said his very first words. She said that the glottal stop required very specific speech therapy techniques to eliminate it. "Children who begin to speak before the palate is repaired are more likely to make sounds at the level of the glottis," she explained (Chapman et al., 2008). The Wallaces were encouraged to hear that when the appropriate techniques were applied, Zach would learn to make the sounds correctly in his mouth rather than his larynx. The SLP stated, "Zach has not progressed in speech therapy focused on techniques to resolve speech dyspraxia simply because he does not have dyspraxia. What's more, oral motor exercises have been shown to be ineffective in resolving any speech disorders," (Braisli & Cascella, 2005; Forrest, 2002; Lass & Pannbacker, 2008; Lof & Watson, 2008; Ruscello, 2008). While all of his SLPs had been well intentioned, the therapeutic techniques used since infancy were ineffective.

The SLP reviewed the recorded video results of the nasopharyngoscopic evaluation that documented Zach's velopharyngeal structure and function. She had soaked a small bit of cotton in a local anesthetic and inserted it into one of Zach's nostrils. After a few minutes, she removed the cotton and slowly inserted a flexible endoscope (tube) about the width of spaghetti into Zach's nose. During speech, Zach's soft palate moved but did not reach his adenoid, and the lateral pharyngeal walls (sides of throat) did not move at all. A gap, referred to as velopharyngeal insufficiency, remained that accounted for his hypernasal resonance. Moving down below the velopharyngeal port, the larynx was viewed. The glottal stops for most all consonants were now clearly seen as well as heard.

Finally, the team summarized their findings and discussed the optimal treatment plan with Zach's parents. The surgeon and the SLP agreed that it would be best to apply appropriate therapeutic techniques to resolve the glottal stops prior to making a definitive surgical plan. The SLP explained that it is possible for movement of the palate and pharynx to increase as children eliminate glottal stops. Thus, Zach's velopharyngeal function would be reevaluated after he demonstrated progress in speech therapy. The need for surgical management would be made at that time. Zach's parents understood that an operation to correct velopharyngeal insufficiency would change only his resonance and intraoral pressure—not his laryngeal articulation errors.

## Presurgical Speech Therapy

The Wallace family returned home a bit drained but empowered by the knowledge they had acquired. They had multiple follow-up appointments scheduled with the geneticist, otolaryngologist, orthodontist, psychologist, and SLP.

The first appointment was with the SLP. The Wallaces were grateful that Zach's school SLP enthusiastically agreed to come in for this demonstration of speech therapy techniques to eliminate glottal stops. The team SLP reviewed the nature of glottal articulation with the adults and outlined her goal for the session: teaching Zach the difference between glottal and oral articulation and using techniques to eliminate the glottal stops. Next, she explained to Zach in a simple yet factual way how speech sounds are made, beginning with the air breathed in and out of the lungs. She demonstrated how the airflow can be stopped in the throat or mouth when speaking. She demonstrated a "neck sound" (i.e., glottal stop) and a windy mouth sound made by stopping the mouth wind with the lips ("Pah"). Zach demonstrated he could easily perceive the difference between laryngeal and oral articulation when produced by the SLP. Subsequently, she asked Zach to make the windy sound "Hhhhaaa." At first, Zach stopped the air in the larynx, but when this was pointed out as a neck sound with a reminder to keep the wind blowing up and through his mouth, he was successful. This new skill was quickly transitioned to the word level (e.g., home, ham, hi, hoe, etc.). Zach was delighted with his mastery of this task. Next, the adults were surprised and concerned when the SLP asked Zach to make the neck sound rather than the windy H sound at the beginning of these words. She explained that negative practice is an effective technique to teach children they can turn the glottal stop on and off. Indeed, Zach seemed to understand and enjoy this task. He soon progressed to using continuous airflow without glottal interruptions at the beginning and end of a nonsense word (e.g., "hamp"). The SLP asked him to whisper "ham" and then blow his lips apart at the end with his mouth wind. She explained that by instructing him in the *process* of making a bilabial plosive rather than saying "say hamp," he would be less likely to default to his deeply engrained pattern of producing the P as a bilabial plosive and a glottal simultaneously (i.e., coarticulation). She further stated that whispering can facilitate the process of keeping the glottis open during speech.

During the session, Zach placed a penny in a piggy bank for each correct response and he happily counted $1.58 by the end of the session. The team SLP explained that she did not use toys or games during the therapy session in order to maintain a focus on speech. While she quickly rewarded Zach with a penny for each correct response, she stated that the primary reinforcement for children is not the penny but the feeling of mastery in using the therapy techniques to produce the sound correctly. She explained that there are four stages of learning: (1) unconscious incompetence (e.g., not knowing you are producing glottal stops); (2) conscious incompetence (e.g., the realization you are making glottals); (3) conscious competence (e.g., with great effort you modify the airstream orally rather than in the larynx); and (4) unconscious competence (e.g., the brain acquires a new memory to produce the sounds correctly without conscious effort). She asked Zach to summarize what he had learned. He recounted his understanding of the neck sound and windy sound and asked when he would come back for another visit. A follow-up appointment was scheduled for 1 month later. In the interim, she gave Zach her business card and asked him to call her once weekly to update her on his progress at home (i.e., "conscious competence"). She asked Zach, "Who is the boss of your mouth?" Zach sheepishly replied "You?" Zach smiled when she told him that he alone was in charge of how his sounds were made.

The SLP outlined a school and home therapy program for Zach. She proposed that his school therapy program change from daily group therapy to individual sessions. Recognizing the school SLP's large caseload, she suggested that even with less frequent individual sessions, given the appropriate techniques, Zach should progress rapidly. She detailed outcome research that shows children with language disorders attain their goals more quickly in group therapy (since language is a social phenomenon), whereas children with speech articulation disorders are discharged sooner from therapy when individual therapy is provided (ASHA, 2010).

Further, research has shown that children who have daily home programs incorporated in everyday routines resolve their speech problems much more quickly (ASHA, 2009; Pamplona et al. 2005). In fact, progress should be evidenced at each session at home and school. In order for Zach's parents to understand the techniques and level of expected proficiency, she suggested they attend one of Zach's therapy sessions each week. It was explained that unlike other practiced skills (e.g., piano, skating, tennis) when a child only has an opportunity to make errors when engaged in those activities, a child practices the "wrong" speech patterns throughout each day. The more opportunities a child has engaged in "conscious competence," the faster the problem will resolve. Zach's parents and school SLP left with a newfound understanding of the nature of Zach's speech disorder and the initial steps to be taken on the path to normal speech.

## Re-evaluation of the VP Valve

Following 4 months of thrice weekly individual speech therapy at school coordinated with a daily home program and monthly guidance sessions by the cleft palate team SLP, Zach showed rapid progress in producing all oral consonants with the correct placement and manner in the absence of glottal stops—at the conscious level of competence. He was ready for reevaluation of his velopharyngeal function. Nasopharyngoscopic evaluation was repeated. As was hoped, Zach's lateral pharyngeal wall movement increased in the absence of glottal stops. However, a small velopharyngeal gap remained, accounting for his persistent hypernasal resonance and slightly reduced intraoral pressure for oral consonants.

## Surgical Management of VPI

Zach's parents learned that approximately 10% of all children born with a unilateral cleft lip and palate will not achieve velopharyngeal competency following palate repair and will require a secondary surgical procedure (Marrinan, LaBrie, & Mulliken, 1998; Sullivan, Marrinan, Rogers, & Mulliken, 2009).

The Wallaces remembered that the adenoidal tissue plays an important role in velopharyngeal function and were thus surprised that prior to the construction of a pharyngeal flap to resolve Zach's velopharyngeal insufficiency, tonsillectomy and adenoidectomy were recommended. They were informed that the flap would be raised from the posterior pharyngeal wall and inserted into the soft palate, leaving two air portals on each side of the flap (for nasal breathing and the nasal speech sounds). They learned that research had shown that the greatest risk factor for developing obstructive sleep apnea after a pharyngeal flap was the presence of the tonsils, structures that played no role in normal velopharyngeal function. Adenoid removal was necessary so the flap could be raised sufficiently high to further decrease the risk of obstructive breathing (Chegar, Shprintzen, Curtis, & Tatum, 2007; Shprintzen, Singer, Sidoti, & Argamaso, 1992).

The tonsillectomy and adenoidectomy were uncomplicated. For the time being, Zach's hypernasality increased. He continued to show steady gains in speech therapy. Four months following the tonsillectomy and adenoidectomy, Zach returned for another nasopharyngoscopic evaluation and a multiview videofluoroscopy study to plan for his pharyngeal flap that was scheduled for the following week. The SLP explained that the pharyngeal flap was not a "one size fits all" procedure, but was carefully "tailored" based on the results of the visualization studies. The multiview videofluoroscopy study was described as a motion picture X-ray taken in several different positions while Zach was talking. This provides important information about how the muscles in the soft palate and lateral pharyngeal walls move. The width of the pharyngeal flap would be based on the movement of the lateral pharyngeal walls toward midline. Following Zach's success in therapy, his lateral pharyngeal walls moved more than halfway toward midline. The nasopharyngoscopy study showed that the pharynx was well healed. The results of the visualization studies were reviewed with the surgeon and the Wallaces. It was decided that a moderately wide pharyngeal flap would be raised.

## Postsurgical Outcomes

Following the pharyngeal flap, Zach sounded stuffy and snored, as they had been warned. However, as the swelling decreased, the hyponasality subsided and he breathed quietly during sleep.

During these months, Zach's parents complied with all other team recommendations. A bilateral myringotomy and tube procedure was performed at the time of the tonsillectomy and adenoidectomy. A postoperative visit with the otolaryngologist and audiologist documented clear ears and normal hearing. A geneticist evaluated Zach and his father and reviewed the family history. She concurred with the diagnosis of Van der Woude syndrome, which was subsequently confirmed by molecular genetic testing. Zach was near completion of his palatal expansion, which had corrected his crossbite.

Zach and his parents had been seeing the team psychologist on a regular basis. The social and emotional difficulties related to Zach's speech disorder were made very clear at the onset of the process. The focus of the therapy program was on developing strategies to effectively deal with teasing. Zach learned that children who tease often feel insecure themselves. Another contributor to teasing is the discomfort one feels when a situation is unfamiliar. Ignorance begets fear and fear can beget acting out. Given this insight, Zach himself proposed a stellar solution: "My second grade science project will be on Van der Woude syndrome!" Indeed, this was an effective strategy in enlightening both peers and teachers about his genetic condition and the possible speech ramifications associated with cleft palate. Zach even showed video copies of his nasopharyngoscopy and multiview videofluoroscopy studies, which both informed and impressed. By the time Zach returned for his 6-month post–pharyngeal flap visit, he had eliminated all glottal stops and his resonance and intraoral pressure were normal. The last phase of his speech therapy program was eliminating glottal stops in conversational speech. A secret code word spoken by his teachers and parents that brought him back to a conscious competent level in the classroom and home was successful in completely eliminating glottals. For the first time, Zach's speech was entirely normal!

By the end of second grade, Zach's confidence was unmistakable. This was achieved through a combination of normal speech and the empowerment Zach developed in effectively dealing with teasing, which no longer occurred. It was clear to Zach's family that normal speech is as important to a child's well-being as a normal-appearing face. Zach could now just be a kid.

## Author Note

This case represents a common scenario—it was not based on a single patient but is a composite of several.

## References

American Speech-Language-Hearing Association. (2010). *Does service delivery model influence speech language pathology outcomes in preschoolers?* Retrieved from http://www.asha.org/uploadedFiles/members/research/NOMS/PreKinderNOMSoutcomesFactSheet.pdf.

Braisli, M. A. G., & Cascella, P. W. (2005). A preliminary investigation of the efficacy of oral motor exercises for children with mild articulation disorders. *International Journal of Rehabilitation Research, 28*(3), 263–266.

Chapman, K. L., Hardin-Jones, M. A., Goldstein, J. A., Halter, K. A., Havlik, R. J., & Schulte, J. (2008). Timing of palatal surgery and speech outcome. *Cleft Palate-Craniofacial Journal, 45*(3), 297–308.

Chegar, B. E., Shprintzen, R. J., Curtis, M. S., & Tatum, S. A. (2007). Pharyngeal flap and obstructive apnea: Maximizing speech outcome while limiting complications. *Archives of Facial Plastic Surgery, 9*, 252–259.

Forrest, K. (2002). Are oral-motor exercises useful in the treatment of phonological/articulatory disorders? *Seminars in Speech and Language, 23*(1) 15–25.

Gibbons, C. (2006). You talk like a monkey: Reflections on a teacher's personal study of growing up with a cleft palate. *Pastoral Care in Education, 24*(2), 53–59.

Hunt, O., Burden, D., Orth, D., Hepper, P., Stevenson, M., & Johnston, C. (2006). Self-reports of psychosocial functioning among children and young adults with cleft lip and palate. *Cleft Palate-Craniofacial Journal, 43*(5), 598–605.

Hunt, O., Burden, D., Hepper, P., Stevenson, M., & Johnston, C. (2007). Parents' reports of the psychosocial functioning of children with cleft lip and/or palate. *Cleft Palate Craniofacial Journal, 44*(3), 304–311.

Lass, N. J., & Pannbacker, M. (2008). The application of evidence-based practice to non-speech oral motor treatments. *Language, Speech, and Hearing Services in Schools, 39*(July), 408–421.

Lof, G. L., & Watson, M. M. (2008). A nationwide survey of nonspeech oral motor exercise use: Implications for evidence-based practice. *Language, Speech, and Hearing Services in Schools, 39*(July), 392–407.

Marrinan, E. M., LaBrie, R. A., & Mulliken, J. B. (1998). Velopharyngeal function in nonsyndromic cleft palate: Relevance of surgical technique, age at repair, and cleft type. *Cleft Palate-Craniofacial Journal, 35*(2), 95–100.

Millard, T., & Richman, L. C. (2001). Different cleft conditions, facial appearance, and speech: Relationship to psychological variables. *Cleft Palate-Craniofacial Journal, 38*(1), 68–75.

OMIM ®—Online Mendelian Inheritance in Man. Retrieved March 2009 from http://www.ncbi.nlm.nih.gov/entrez/dispomim.cgi?id=119300

Pamplona, C., Ysunza, A. C. Patino, C., Ramifrez, E., Drucker, M., & Mazon, J. (2005). Speech summer camp for treating articulation disorders in cleft palate patients. *International Journal of Pediatric Otolaryngology, 69*(3) 351–359.

Shprintzen, R. J., Singer, L., Sidoti, E. J., & Argamaso, R. V. (1992). Pharyngeal flap surgery: Postoperative complications. *International Anesthesiology Clinics, 30*, 115–124.

Sullivan, S. R., Marrinan, E. M., Rogers, G. F., & Mulliken, J. B. (2009). Palatoplasty outcomes in nonsyndromic patients with cleft palate: A 29-Year assessment of one surgeon's experience. *Journal of Craniofacial Surgery* (20) Suppl. 1, 612–616.

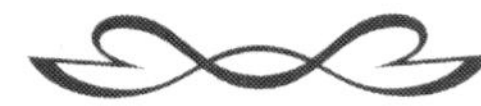

# DYSARTHRIA

## CASE 28

# James: Acquired Childhood Dysarthria in a School-Age Child

*Petrea L. Cornwell and Louise M. Cahill*

## Conceptual Knowledge Areas

The dysarthrias, as a group of speech disorders resulting from disturbances in the neuromuscular execution of speech, have been widely written about since the modern definition of dysarthria was provided in 1969 by Darley, Aronson, and Brown's seminal works (1969a; 1969b). Much of the focus, however, has been on describing dysarthria in adult populations and outlining assessment and treatment procedures for this population. Far less attention has been given to developmental dysarthria, a general diagnostic label that encompasses both *congenital* (prior to speech development) and *acquired* (during speech development) speech disorders (Crary, 1993; Thompson, 1988). Developmental dysarthrias, like their adult counterparts, are exemplified by disturbances in the speed, strength, range, and timing of speech movements that ultimately affect speech intelligibility (Duffy, 2005). The types of developmental dysarthria, as with adult dysarthrias, can be differentiated based on the site of neurological damage, the expression of this neuromuscular impairment in the speech muscles, and subsequently speech production (Hodge & Wellman, 1999). However, conjecture exists within the literature as to the suitability of applying the dysarthria classification system proposed by Darley and colleagues to the developmental population (Cornwell, Murdoch, & Ward, 2003). The issues that surround the use of the adult dysarthria classification system are similar to those that complicate the treatment planning for developmental dysarthria. The first consideration relates to the interaction between emerging cognitive-linguistic skills and neuromuscular disruption of speech, and how this impacts the expression of dysarthria as well as the course of treatment. Second, motor control of speech during childhood differs from that of adults (Sharkey & Folkins, 1985) and continues to develop throughout childhood to young adulthood (Clark, Robin, McCullagh, & Schmidt, 2001). This relates to beliefs that neural recovery/plasticity is greater in children than adults (Johnston, Nishimura, Harum, Pekar, & Blue, 2001). Further complicating the decision-making processes surrounding the treatment of developmental dysarthria and in particular acquired childhood dysarthria is the lack of research evidence available to guide evidence-based practice.

This case provides an overview of the planning for and treatment of developmental dysarthria, with a focus on acquired childhood dysarthria. Treatment planning requires a thorough understanding of the nature of the dysarthria and its impact on the child, and knowledge of treatment approaches that could optimize communication. An overview will be provided of a management framework that can be used to guide assessment and treatment. The applicability of this management framework to clinical practice will be demonstrated using the case of a school-age child who developed dysarthria following the surgical excision of a brainstem tumor.

## Management Framework

The World Health Organization (WHO) first developed a model of chronic disorder in the 1990s that has subsequently been applied to a treatment framework for dysarthria (Yorkston, Strand, & Kennedy, 1996). Clinically, this framework has proven useful in directing assessment, reporting assessment findings, planning treatment, evaluating change due to treatment, and monitoring change in children's speech with age. There are five levels to this model: pathophysiology, impairment, functional limitation, disability, and societal limitation, with the middle three levels the areas addressed most commonly in current clinical practice. Societal limitation is also often an area that clinicians address through education of family, friends, and others involved in the child's life. For greater detail see Yorkston et al. (1996), or within the context of developmental dysarthria, Hodge and Wellman (1999).

- ***Impairment*** refers to the pathophysiological basis for the dysarthria and reflects the neurological deficits within the speech production process (respiratory, laryngeal, velopharyngeal, and articulatory function).
- ***Functional limitation*** is the inability or limited ability to carry out the actions associated with speech production and is reflected in the perceptual characteristics of speech (e.g., speech intelligibility, vocal quality, speaking rate, articulatory precision).
- ***Disability*** represents the limitations experienced by a child in communicating effectively due to dysarthria across a range of physical and social contexts.
- ***Societal limitation*** is the level within the model that relates to factors external to the child such as physical and attitudinal barriers, as well as social policy.

WHO reviewed the model on which this dysarthria treatment framework is based and in 2001 released the International Classification of Functioning, Disability, and Health (ICF; WHO, 2001). This revised WHO model[1] extends the original framework, explicitly incorporating factors that health professionals have long known to influence the management of their patients. In this new framework *health condition/disorder*, *environmental factors*, and *personal factors* are seen to moderate and interact with the three areas that are primarily the focus of treatment. Therefore, they should be considered in both the process of treatment planning and the ongoing management of the child. An example of how this conceptual framework can be used to organize information obtained from the assessment phase of treatment planning is provided in Figure 28.1.

## Assessment Procedures

The purpose of assessing a child with acquired dysarthria is essentially to guide treatment planning through gaining a comprehensive understanding of the child's communicative difficulties. This includes: (1) determining the nature and extent of any speech, language, and swallowing disorder, (2) understanding the impact of that diagnosis on the child's communicative abilities across a range of environments, and (3) obtaining a holistic view of the child and factors that may influence the disorder and progress in treatment.

The conceptual framework described provides a sound basis for assessment and should be used to guide assessment procedures chosen. There are four essential components to a comprehensive examination of speech in children with an acquired dysarthria (Strand & McCauley, 1999):

- The case history
- Structural examination of the speech musculature
- Motor speech examination
- Inventory of the child's sound system

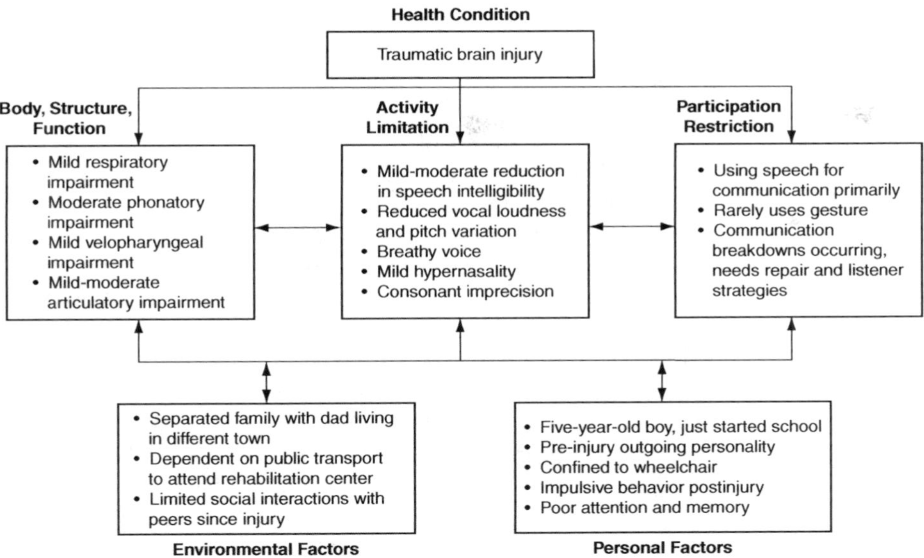


FIGURE 28.1 Utilizing the ICF Framework to Organize Information Obtained Through Assessment Procedures for a School-Age Child with Dysarthria

The *case history* completed by the clinician involves accessing a number of different sources and may be dependent on the environment (e.g., hospital medical chart, health professional reports, child and family). The aim of the case history is to obtain information across all areas of the ICF dysarthria treatment framework, but will initially be a primary source of information on the *health condition, participation restrictions* experienced as a result of the disorder, and *environmental and personal factors* that may influence treatment. A standard case history should be obtained through talking with the parents and child (dependent on age) to gain a picture of the child's development up to the point of neurological injury. This should be supplemented by the parents' and child's (where possible) understanding of current medical, physical, cognitive, and communication status, as well as information from the child's medical chart and health reports.

The *structural examination of the speech musculature* and *motor speech examination* have both been comprehensively described within the adult dysarthria literature (Duffy, 2005), as well as in texts on childhood motor speech disorders (Caruso & Strand, 1999). These examinations provide specific information on the *body, structure, and function*, and *activity limitation* levels of the ICF framework. The structural examination of the speech musculature is completed to identify the specific areas and severity of deficit within the motor speech subsystems (respiratory, laryngeal, velopharyngeal, and articulatory) using nonspeech tasks. Results of this examination may in some cases be supplemented by instrumental measures of subsystems depending on the availability of these tools. The application of instrumental techniques in the assessment of dysarthrias has been described (Yorkston, Beukelman, Strand, & Bell, 1999); however, these descriptions have focused more on the adult dysarthria populations. A range of techniques are available from low-technology evaluations of adequacy of respiratory support using a glass of water and straw (Hixon, Hawley, & Wilson, 1982) to evaluation of articulatory dynamics using electromagnetic articulography (Caarstens Medizinelektronik). Instrumental assessments provide an objective record of subsystem impairment that is beneficial in quantifying treatment outcome, and where clinically possible should be considered as a component of the structural examination.

The motor speech examination incorporates speech-like and speech tasks that allow clinicians to assess how the structural impairments affect motor speech production, which occurs in parallel with language formulation. Therefore, tasks included should vary the utterance length and linguistic complexity of the task (i.e., range from CV syllables to sentences to connected speech). This enables the clinician to determine overall communication efficiency and prosody in the child with dysarthria and exclude an apraxia of speech through increasing linguistic complexity. Specific information to be obtained from a motor speech examination includes a measure of speech intelligibility and an evaluation of perceptual speech characteristics such as respiration in speech, pitch characteristics, vocal quality, loudness, articulatory accuracy, and prosody. All tasks chosen should be appropriate for the age and developmental stage of the child (e.g., imitation and picture description for younger children; mix of imitation, picture description, and reading for older, literate children).

Collection of information about the child's *sound inventory* is where the assessment of dysarthria differs between adults and children. In assessing adults with dysarthria it is assumed that they have developed a mature speech sound system; however, when dysarthria is acquired during childhood it is important to distinguish between developmental and acquired sound errors (i.e., age-appropriate sound substitutions or articulatory impairment such as consonant imprecision or phoneme prolongation).

## Treatment Considerations

Communication that is effective and optimal for the child is the ultimate goal of intervention with a child with acquired dysarthria. Depending on age at the time of onset of dysarthria, a child may have experienced communicative success to varying degrees. An adolescent child not only will have used speech to meet basic communicative needs (e.g., getting food), but also will know its importance in meeting social and educational needs (e.g., chatting with friends, participating in the classroom). Therefore, it is important to determine where the child sits along this communication continuum and distinguish between preinjury and postinjury communicative behaviors and needs. Prior to the sudden onset of the neurological event causing the dysarthria, many of these children will have had normally developing motor speech skills, and therefore management goals are similar to those for adults with acquired dysarthria (Hodge & Wellman, 1999). That is, management goals seek to restore lost function (*body, structure, and function*), maximize the use of residual function (*activity limitation*), and compensate for lost function (*participation restriction*). Importantly, it is in the health conditions and environmental and personal factors where the major point of difference exists between the groups. In particular, the neurological causes of dysarthria in adults include a range of progressive neurological disorders not seen in children, while stroke and traumatic brain injury are etiologies common to both age groups. Brain tumors are a cause of dysarthria in both populations, but the incidence of primary brain tumors is more frequent in the pediatric population.

Individual planning is required for each child with acquired dysarthria, but in all cases it is important to consider the central aspects of the ICF framework (the dysarthria) and factors influencing the dysarthria (external factors). The external factors influencing treatment include medical diagnosis and prognosis, environment and communication partners, associated problems (e.g., motor, cognitive, and behavioral), patient motivation, adjustment to the neurological injury, and treatment availability and accessibility. Each of these factors lies within the ICF realms of *health condition, environmental factors,* and *personal factors*, and individually and collectively affect the treatment goals set, treatment approaches chosen, and timing and frequency of treatment sessions. Factors related specifically to the dysarthria also need to be considered in developing the treatment plan and choice of specific treatment approaches. In particular, dysarthria severity will influence the focus of treatment within the ICF dysarthria treatment model of *body, structure, and function, activity limitation*, and *participation restriction*, while dysarthria type will affect the treatment tasks used.

The effectiveness of the treatments provided for dysarthria is not well researched. Recent reviews of the dysarthria treatment literature (Sellars, Hughes, & Langhorne, 2005) have highlighted the paucity of research evidence to guide clinical practice with emphasis on the treatment of child dysarthria, as the majority of treatment studies address adult and not child populations. Consequently, clinical practice in the area of acquired childhood dysarthria tends to adopt treatment approaches used in adult dysarthria. General consensus exists among clinicians that treatment for dysarthria improves speech intelligibility and communication participation (Duffy, 2005). There are also a number of case study reports, case series, and some small group studies that have documented gains from dysarthria treatment across a range of treatment approaches.

Treatment approaches can be broadly described as either speech-oriented or communication-oriented (Duffy, 2005), with the former addressing the ICF framework at the levels of *body, structure, and function* and *activity limitation* and the latter focused at reducing *participation restriction*. Working at the level of speech-oriented treatment requires clinicians to understand the principles of motor learning, which can be divided into two variables to manipulate: (1) practice conditions, and (2) feedback conditions. Practice conditions include intensity of sessions, variability of tasks, saliency of tasks, scheduling of tasks, and task complexity, while type, frequency, and timing of feedback can all be manipulated within treatment plans. It is beyond the scope of this case to provide a detailed explanation of these factors: however, Duffy (2005) and Maas et al. (2008) provide guidelines for including these principles in treatment sessions.

Clinicians developing a child's treatment plan to address acquired dysarthria would also consider how the impact of dysarthria severity can guide short- and long-treatment goals. For example, where the child presents with severe dysarthria, initially the clinician may need to provide an augmentative and alternative communication (AAC) system to overcome communication barriers experienced (*participation restriction*), while a parallel treatment goal is to reduce the physiological impairments evident in the speech mechanism (*body, structure, and function*). Conversely, in a child with mild dysarthria the treatment goals may be about maximizing the residual function through both speaker (*activity limitation)* and listener (*participation restriction*) strategies. Individual session goals and treatment activities should therefore consider first the purpose of the task within the context of the dysarthria treatment framework, and second how the neuropathological basis for the dysarthria will affect the types of tasks chosen to address speech-oriented treatment goals. Key to individual session treatment planning is the clinician integrating medical information and results of the examination of speech to know whether muscular weakness, increased muscular tone, or muscular incoordination is contributing to the acquired dysarthria seen in the child.

Treatment planning for the child with acquired dysarthria is thus multifactorial, and the importance of integrating the information gained through assessment procedures cannot be overestimated. The needs of the child and the family for improved communication should always be considered and integrated within the context of the child's medical condition and overall rehabilitation program. Acquired dysarthria does not usually occur in isolation but follows the sudden onset of neurological injury. The benefits of the ICF framework as a way to conceptualize the child's dysarthria within the overall picture of the child's *health condition*, *environmental factors*, and *personal factors* become evident when participating in treatment planning at the level of the rehabilitation team.

## Description of the Case

Acquired childhood dysarthria, as opposed to congenital dysarthria, refers to a motor speech disorder whose onset is at a point in a child's life when there has been some degree of speech and language skill development prior to the neurological event. Epidemiological data about the causes of acquired childhood dysarthria are scarce. The most common neurological etiologies include traumatic brain injury, stroke, hypoxia, and brain tumors. The case study presented here is that of a school-age child with acquired dysarthria subsequent to the excision of a midbrain pilocytic astrocytoma. A brief overview of medical information such as epidemiology, clinical signs and symptoms, medical management, and prognosis for brainstem tumors is presented in Figure 28.2.

| | |
|---|---|
| Epidemiology | • Central nervous system (CNS) tumors are the second most prevalent childhood cancer (Giles & Gonzales, 1995)<br>• Brainstem tumors account for 10–20% of all pediatric CNS tumors (Recinos, Sciubba, & Jallo, 2007)<br>• Range of classification systems used; most recent includes four types: Type I—diffuse, Type II—intrinsic, focal, Type III—exophytic, focal, Type IV—cervicomedullary (Choux, Lena, & Do, 2000) |
| Clinical signs & symptoms | • Varies with respect to tumor location and pattern of growth; however, triad of findings indicative of brainstem tumors include: (1) cranial nerve neuropathies; (2) long-tract signs; (3) ataxia (Cohen & Duffner, 1984)<br>• Most frequently occurring symptom is cranial nerve palsy, with more than one cranial nerve implicated in more than 70% of cases (Lassman, 1983)<br>• Disturbances of gait and hemiparesis causing clumsiness, unsteadiness, and dragging of one foot have all been documented symptoms (Atac & Blaauw, 1979) |
| Medical management | • Dependent on tumor type<br>• Diffuse lesion—no benefit from surgery, may gain temporary benefit from corticosteroids or radiotherapy (Albright & Pollack, 2004)<br>• Focal lesions—surgical resection is treatment of choice (Tomita & Cortes, 2002)<br>• Surgical resection comes with the risk of cranial nerve dysfunction (Recinos et al., 2007) |
| Prognosis | • Dependent on tumor type/location<br>• Pontine tumors more likely to be Type I and survival rates are low (Recinos et al., 2007)<br>• Tumors of medulla and midbrain more likely to be benign, undergo surgical resection, have long-term survival (Recinos et al., 2007) |

FIGURE 28.2 Medical Information Relating to Brainstem Tumors

## Background Information

James, a 12-year-old boy, had been living in a rural town with his parents and younger sister. He was attending the local school prior to onset of general symptoms of tiredness and clumsiness, and seemed to be tripping over his own feet more regularly. An initial examination by the local physician indicated that these symptoms had been progressively worsening over the last 5 months. A CT scan at his local hospital revealed an infratentorial tumor (exact tumor site not stated) and moderate obstructive hydrocephalus. Consequently, a referral was made to a pediatric neurosurgeon in the state capital (4 hours drive from home). MRI scans completed at this time revealed a focal brainstem lesion arising from the midbrain region with neurological examination identifying a right-sided hemiparesis. Due to the focal localization of the tumor, surgical excision was considered the most appropriate method of medical management and James underwent surgery 1 week later. Gross tumor resection was achieved and an external ventricular drain (EVD) inserted to manage postoperative hydrocephalus. Pathology results postsurgery revealed the tumor to be low-grade (pilocytic astrocytoma), and its origin was at the level of the cerebral peduncle. Postsurgery, the right-sided hemiparesis had worsened and he had developed dysarthria and dysphagia. The dysphagia resolved within the first weeks postsurgery but the dysarthria and hemiparesis persisted, resulting in referral to a Pediatric Rehabilitation Center (in the state's capital city). Discharge from the acute care hospital was delayed due to postoperative complications 1 month postsurgery, with extradural hemorrhages evacuated by craniotomy twice, 3 days apart. The EVD was removed 2 months postsurgery and James's medical condition stabilized, facilitating transfer to the Pediatric Rehabilitation Center to begin inpatient rehabilitation.

## Reason for Referral

James had a significant right-sided hemiparesis impacting his ability to walk independently and complete activities of daily living (e.g., personal care), as well as a moderate dysarthria that reduced his ability to communicate effectively. He was referred to the Pediatric

Rehabilitation Center for a comprehensive assessment of physical, cognitive, and communication abilities, and treatment to enable him to return home and to formal schooling.

## Findings of the Evaluation

### Case History

Case history details were obtained by consulting medical reports from the referring hospital and an interview with James and his mother, supplemented by information provided by other rehabilitation team members. Prior to the onset of the symptoms that led to the diagnosis of the brainstem tumor, James's mother reported no significant medical history and said that all developmental milestones (gross and fine motor and communication) had been achieved within normal time frames. She also indicated that there was no family history of speech and/or language disorder. Prior to the diagnosis of the brainstem tumor, James had many friends, was actively involved in sports (including tennis and football), and enjoyed school. Educational performance was reported to be above average.

The prognosis for James was good, with his tumor benign and requiring no further treatment. Reports given by other members of the rehabilitation team indicated that the right-sided hemiparesis required James to walk with the assistance of a frame and made activities such as dressing himself and writing difficult. James's general cognitive abilities appeared to be intact. The impact of the surgery in terms of James's physical limitations and speech difficulties caused him frustration, particularly at losing the independence he had developed prior to the surgery. James and his parents were very focused on him regaining his physical abilities so that he could return home, but they also wanted his speech to "be normal again." James's mother noticed that it was difficult for her to understand his speech in noisy environments, and that she needed to ask him to repeat words and slow down. James's father and sister had difficulty understanding him over the phone, and unfamiliar people had a great deal of difficulty understanding James's speech. The impact of the tumor was reported by James's mother to extend beyond the physical and speech difficulties, with the family unit having to split up while James, his mother, and sister lived in the capital city during the treatment, and James's father remained in their home town. Emotionally, James's mother felt isolated from her husband as a support person. The family also experienced financial strain as they had earned two incomes prior to this event.

### Structural Examination of Speech Musculature

James's speech musculature was examined using the Frenchay Dysarthria Assessment (Enderby, 1983), which revealed moderately impaired respiration, palatal, lip, tongue, and laryngeal function. Jaw function at rest and in speech displayed normal function. James demonstrated occasional coughing on thin fluids and swallowing was slower than premorbidly. Table 28.1 details the results of the initial assessment from the Frenchay Dysarthria Assessment.

Respiratory function was impaired, with James demonstrating marked interruptions of inspiration and expiration and requiring 4 breaths to count from 1 to 20. Laryngeal function was moderately impaired, with James able to maintain clear phonation for only 5 seconds. He was only able to demonstrate minimal change in volume and pitch, and frequent pitch and phonation difficulties were observed during speech. Velopharyngeal function was moderately impaired, with minimal movement of the soft palate observed during the production of "ah" and speech noted to be moderately hypernasal. James also reported that fluids occasionally came out of his nose.

James demonstrated a slight facial droop at rest, which became more obvious during the lip spread task where there was minimal retraction on the right side. Alternate lip rounding and spreading was also moderately impaired, with no spread on the right and poor lip rounding. James's ability to maintain lip seal was affected by nasal emission and his inability to maintain intraoral pressure. When his nose was pinched he was able to maintain a lip seal for an appropriate amount of time, suggesting adequate lip strength.

TABLE 28.1 Results of the Frenchay Dysarthria Assessment at Baseline and Posttreatment

| | Baseline Assessment | Posttreatment Assessment |
|---|---|---|
| **Reflex** | | |
| Cough | Occasional coughing with thin fluids | No coughing reported on thin fluids |
| Swallow | Mildly delayed swallow; care taken when drinking | Care still required when drinking |
| Dribble | None reported | None reported |
| **Respiration** | | |
| At rest | Marked interruptions of inhalation and expiration | Inhalation much improved, but still shallow |
| In speech | Required 4 breaths to count to 20 | Only 2 breaths required when counting to 20 |
| **Lips** | | |
| At rest | Slight asymmetry with right facial droop | No abnormality |
| Spread | Severely distorted smile with elevation on left only | Slight asymmetry |
| Seal | Lip seal observed, but auditorily weak—affected by nasal air escape | Improved plosion, but occasional air leakage |
| Alternate | Lip spread severely distorted; rounding mildly distorted | Mild variability in rounding and spread of lips |
| In speech | Poor movement; acoustically weak | Occasional weakness and variable acoustic presentation |
| **Jaw** | | |
| At rest | No abnormality | No abnormality |
| In speech | No abnormality | No abnormality |
| **Palate** | | |
| Fluids | Occasional difficulty | No difficulty |
| Maintenance | Minimal palatal movement | Improved, but full movement |
| In speech | Moderate hypernasality | Mild-moderate hypernasality and some nasal emission |
| **Laryngeal** | | |
| Time | Clear phonation for 5 sec | Clear phonation for 15 sec |
| Pitch | Minimal change in pitch | Able to represent four distinct pitch changes |
| Volume | Only limited change in volume | Uneven progression in volume change |
| In speech | Frequent pitch and phonation difficulties | Occasional inappropriate use of pitch |
| **Tongue** | | |
| At rest | Involuntary movements | Occasional involuntary movements |
| Protrusion | Deviates to right; slow (8 sec), tremor | Tongue still deviates to right, but task completed in less time (5 sec) |
| Elevation | Elevation poor; laborious | Moves well both directions, but slow |
| Lateral | Slow (7 sec), laborious, and incomplete | Still slow (5 sec), but full range |
| Alternate | Sounds poorly represented; task deteriorates; slow (10 sec) | Slight incoordination; task slightly slow (6 sec) |
| In speech | Slow alternating movements; omissions of consonants | Tongue movement slightly inaccurate; occasional mispronunciation |

Tongue fasciculations were noted at rest, but no atrophy or asymmetry was evident. Tongue movements were generally slow, labored, and poorly coordinated. On protrusion James's tongue deviated to the right. Lateral tongue movements were reduced in range, strength, and speed. Tongue elevation was minimal and tongue depression was limited. Alternate tongue movements during the production of "kala" were poorly represented, and the task was slow and deteriorated across repetitions.

### Motor Speech Examination

Perceptual evaluation of James's speech revealed a moderately decreased rate, moderately impaired pitch and loudness variation, and breath support. Consonants and vowels were noted to be moderately imprecise, phonemes were prolonged to a mild-moderate degree, and moderate hypernasality was evident. Sentence intelligibility was 63% on the Assessment of Intelligibility of Dysarthric Speech (AssIDS) (Yorkston & Beukelman, 1981). James had a moderate flaccid dysarthria according to the criteria of Darley, Aronson, and Brown (1975).

James's nasalance level was assessed on the Nasometer™ II (KayPENTAX). His average nasalance over three readings of the non-nasal sentence "Look at this book with us" was 46%, confirming the perceptual rating of moderate hypernasality. The Visi-Pitch™ IV (KayPENTAX) was utilized to evaluate various phonatory values. James's maximum phonation time was 8 seconds, pitch range on the production of a glide was 124 Hz, and pitch variability (SD in Hz) during the reading of two sentences of "The Grandfather Passage" (Darley et al., 1975) was 12.77. The posttreatment motor speech examination results are summarized in Table 28.2.

## Treatment Options Considered

The results of a team planning meeting to discuss the rehabilitation to be offered to James and his family were that he remain at the center for 6 weeks of treatment before returning home. At the completion of this treatment block the team would evaluate whether subsequent treatment was required at the center, or whether his rehabilitation could be managed in his hometown.

Research evidence to guide the optimal time to commence treatment for James's dysarthria is lacking, although it is generally considered that early treatment is preferred to deferred treatment (Duffy, 2005). A true understanding of what constitutes "early" treatment is not evident; however, commencing impairment-based therapy is considered appropriate once a person is medically stable. The limited research available in the area of rehabilitation for pediatric brain tumor means that we need to look to other areas of neurological rehabilitation, such as stroke rehabilitation, to guide when and how much intervention should occur. In general, the stroke rehabilitation literature suggests that early and intense intervention is preferable and more strongly linked to treatment success than duration of intervention (Kwakkel, Wagenaar, Koelman, Lankhorst, & Koetsier, 2002). It should also be noted that deferred intervention, although not considered preferable, can still be effective (Abkarian & Dworkin, 1993; Keatley & Wirz, 1994). Early intervention, at this point in James's recovery (2 months post-surgery), would therefore seem appropriate and likely to be linked with successful treatment outcome. James and his mother also identified his speech difficulties as an area for rehabilitation, and clinically it is known that motivation to work on an area increases the potential for positive treatment outcomes.

TABLE 28.2 Results of the AssIDS, Visipitch and Nasometer Assessments at Baseline and Posttreatment

| | Baseline Assessment | Posttreatment Assessment |
|---|---|---|
| **AssIDS** | | |
| Sentence Intelligibility | 63% | 84% |
| **Visipitch™ IV** | | |
| Maximum phonation time | 8 sec | 15 sec |
| Pitch range—glide | 124 Hz | 284Hz |
| Monotone | SD = 12.77 | SD = 21.53 |
| **Nasometer™ II** | | |
| Nasalance | 46% | 39% |

N.B. AssIDS = Assessment of Intelligibility of Dysarthric Speech

The stroke rehabilitation research raised the issue of intensity of treatment as a key factor in treatment success, in accord with the principles of motor learning. The Pediatric Rehabilitation Team provides a 5-day a week inpatient therapy service; therefore it was possible for James to receive frequent therapy sessions, one component of practice intensity. Practice intensity refers to the number of trials of a task completed during a session. The literature suggests that high practice intensity (large numbers of repetitions) for nonspeech tasks is beneficial (Park & Shea, 2005); however, there is no clear evidence to suggest that the same is true for speech tasks (Maas et al., 2008). James's speech pathology treatment was part of the overall rehabilitation program, including physical therapy and occupational therapy, which were his and his family's priority areas of treatment. James was still easily fatigued and the combination of other therapy sessions for physical impairments and high practice intensity and frequent sessions for speech pathology might have led him to fatigue quickly in sessions. Therefore, it was important to consider how to optimize speech pathology intervention and distribute practice across the week. Currently there is no evidence to support or refute the benefits of massed versus distributed practice sessions (Maas et al., 2008), and consequently clinical experience and organizational constraints should guide decision making. Clinical experience in combination with research evidence guided James's treatment plan in terms of the frequency and intensity of sessions. In particular, to limit the effect of fatigue, clinical experience with rehabilitation in patients has shown that success in treatment can be achieved through scheduling two shorter treatment sessions (20 minutes long), 3–4 times per week. The issue of practice intensity arises where the focus of treatment is speech-oriented.

James's dysarthria was diagnosed as moderate flaccid due to muscular weakness using adult dysarthria classifications. In determining levels within the ICF framework to direct treatment, consideration was given to the severity of the impairment, the length of time post-onset, and the long-term goal of maximizing communication effectiveness, efficiency, and naturalness. Given the moderate severity of James's dysarthria, regaining "normal speech" through speech therapy was not considered realistic (Duffy, 2005); however, given the early point in his recovery at which treatment was being initiated, three levels of the ICF framework were considered: *body, structure and function*, *activity limitation*, and *participation restriction*. Addressing all three areas of the ICF requires the treatment plan to incorporate both speech-oriented and communication-oriented approaches to intervention. Including approaches across all aspects of communication can be beneficial in that it helps to maximize the communicative abilities of the person and increase the number of successful communicative interactions; however, disadvantages include the complexity of the treatment sessions and carry-over activities to be completed. Specifically targeting one or another of the approaches can therefore reduce the complexity of treatment sessions and allow the child and family to be more focused in carry-over tasks outside therapy sessions. Conversely, it may reduce communicative success outside the therapy setting in the initial stages. The current research evidence focuses on the outcomes obtained from individual treatment approaches, both speech- and communication-oriented (Helm-Estabrooks, Yorkston, Spencer, & Duffy, 2003; Helm-Estabrooks, Yorkston, & Beukelman, 2004), but does not guide the mix of treatment goals that clinically results in the best overall outcomes for either adults or children with dysarthria. Clinical experience suggests that developing a treatment plan that incorporates both speech- and communication-oriented approaches into intervention and education sessions is the most successful. Treatment goals were therefore planned to (1) reduce impairment by increasing physiological support for speech, (2) introduce behavioral compensations that modify particular aspects of his speech, and (3) educate family, friends, and health staff about listener strategies that could reduce communication breakdowns. James and his mother were involved in the goal setting process and were keen for the three areas to be addressed; however, they rated the first goal as the most important to them. They felt that despite being informed that "normal speech" might not be a realistic expectation of therapy, they wanted to do everything they could.

Addressing the goal of *reducing impairment by increasing physiological support for speech* requires the clinician to identify the deficits within the speech production mechanism where change is possible and will increase physiological support for speech, thereby improving speech production (Yorkston et al., 1996). James's assessment results indicated that all aspects of speech production were impaired (respiratory, laryngeal, velopharyngeal, and articulatory function) but, upon closer examination, impairments in respiratory and velopharyngeal function were thought to impact most significantly on his speech intelligibility. Treatment at the level of respiratory support for speech is often a priority as both research studies and clinical experience have shown that improvements at this level can have a positive effect on other components of the speech mechanism and speech intelligibility (Hayden & Square, 1994). The results of the assessment of velopharyngeal function revealed minimal to no movement of the velum, suggestive of incomplete closure of the velopharyngeal port, which was supported perceptually through the finding of hypernasality of speech and nasal emission and nasometry findings documenting high levels of nasalance. Poor velopharyngeal closure compounds respiratory insufficiency and potentially contributes to shorter breath groups, as well as impacting the ability for adequate intraoral air pressure for phoneme production. The evidence to support treatment tasks within these motor speech subsystems was recently reviewed (Yorkston et al., 2001), and while high levels of evidence are not available for treatment focused at respiratory function, there is clinical consensus that these treatments are beneficial. Similarly, the majority of behavioral approaches to velopharyngeal impairment (VPI) are founded on expert opinion (Yorkston et al., 1999), with the exception of continuous positive airway pressure (CPAP), where small studies have shown this technique to be beneficial (Kuehn, 1997). Evidence-based practice guidelines for management of VPI in dysarthria (Yorkston et al., 2001) have indicated that a prosthetic palatal lift is the most effective means of treating VPI. There are, however, problems involved in fitting the prosthesis, hyperactive gag responses, lack of cooperation and acceptance, and the growing oral cavity that would require monitoring of fit.

Overall treatment planning with James and his mother revealed that goals for therapy were distributed across three areas; reducing impairment, reducing *functional* limitation, and reducing *participation restriction.* The treatment goals for each of these areas are detailed in Table 28.3. Initial treatment sessions goals for James focused heavily in the area of impairment-based intervention, focusing on improving respiratory-phonatory support for speech and strengthening the velopharyngeal mechanism.

## Course of Treatment

Initial treatment focused on improving James' breath support for speech. The Visi-Pitch™ IV was used to provide both visual and auditory biofeedback on productions of prolonged "ah." James was required to sit upright and produce the longest prolonged "ah" that he could into the microphone attached to the Visi-Pitch™ IV. Visual feedback was obtained from the Visi-Pitch™ IV to encourage him to increase the length of each "ah" produced. Posture was monitored during these tasks and James was encouraged to use abdominal breathing and limit clavicular breathing. Work also concentrated on increasing James's pitch range, once again utilizing the Visi-Pitch™ IV to provide visual and auditory feedback to assist him to reach upper and lower pitch targets. After numerous repetitions (this varied depending on his fatigue level), James was given the opportunity to play one of the Visi-Pitch™ IV games that focused on maintaining phonation and/or changing pitch as a reinforcement of his participation in treatment sessions.

After 2 weeks of therapy focusing on respiratory-phonatory control James's breath support for speech was much improved. CPAP therapy commenced, with the goal to help strengthen the velopharyngeal musculature and increase palatal movement. The CPAP device delivers air pressure by means of a hose and nasal mask assembly to the nasal cavities. CPAP therapy is based on the principal that the resistance exercise program will strengthen the muscles involved in velopharyngeal closure and thereby help to reduce hypernasality (Kuehn, 1997). During CPAP therapy the person is required to repeat a series of single-word utterances of the form VNCV, where V = any vowel, N = any nasal consonant (/m/, /n/, /ng/), and C = any

TABLE 28.3 Itemized Treatment Goals for James

| Goals | Strategies |
|---|---|
| **Reduce Impairment** | |
| *Respiratory-phonatory function* | |
| • Improve breath control for speech | • Vowel prolongation tasks<br>• Increasing syllables per breath in phrases of increasing length |
| *Velopharyngeal function* | |
| • Improve strength of soft palate and increase range of movement during speech | • Use of Continuous Positive Airway Pressure (CPAP) therapy |
| *Articulatory function* | |
| • Increase lip and tongue strength | • Incidental strengthening during CPAP therapy, which requires accurate production against nasal pressure during speech tasks |
| *Laryngeal function* | |
| • Increase vocal fold range of movement | • Visual feedback via Visi-Pitch$^{TM}$ IV to increase pitch range |
| **Reduce Functional Limitation** | |
| *Improve speech intelligibility* | |
| • Improve intonation patterns to maximize speech naturalness | • Visual feedback of intonation via Visi-Pitch$^{TM}$ IV during production of utterances of increasing length |
| • Improve breath group phrasing during speech | • Optimal phrasing practiced during reading of common sentences and short paragraphs, with visual and auditory feedback via Visi-Pitch$^{TM}$ IV |
| • Improve articulation of pressure consonants | • Speech drills to facilitate optimal consonant production during connected speech |
| **Reduce Participation Restriction** | |
| • Increase participation in everyday activities | • Conversational activities with family and other therapists utilizing strategies learned in therapy sessions to increase communication effectiveness<br>• Excursions to practice functional phrases and strategies learned in therapy sessions |

pressure consonant (stop, fricative, affricate), stressing the second syllable (eg. um*pee*). The rationale for this particular phoneme sequence is that the nasal consonant induces a lowered velar position, and the pressure consonant initiating the stressed syllable enhances the likelihood of a rigorous velar elevation. Such activity in the presence of heightened nasal air pressure theoretically takes advantage of the resistance exercise situation.

At the beginning of the CPAP treatment session an appropriately sized mask was placed over James's nose, ensuring an airtight seal. The pressure for the session was then set on the CPAP machine. James was required to repeat a series of single-word utterances of the form VNCV, as described previously. The pressures used in each session and the duration of each session gradually increased over the 4-week period. The initial pressure selected was 3 cm $H_2O$, which James tolerated well. This pressure was gradually increased to a maximum of 6.5 cm $H_2O$ by the fourth week of the CPAP therapy program. The initial duration of treatment was 5 minutes, increasing to 12 minutes by the end of the program. James received CPAP therapy 4 days per week for 4 weeks (16 sessions in total).

In addition to the CPAP therapy, James continued to work on improving his breath support for speech and pitch range. Functional phrases were utilized to work on increasing pitch variation, with visual and auditory feedback provided via the Visi-Pitch$^{TM}$ IV. Reading tasks and later conversational speech tasks were also utilized to practice use of appropriate breath grouping and clear production of all consonants. These tasks were tape-recorded and James was able to replay and then re-record, improving his production if possible. This technique was also used for homework tasks.

During initial sessions James and his mother were provided with education on speaker and listener strategies that could be used to improve conversational interactions. This information was also provided in written format, so that James's father was also aware of ways that he could increase James's success during conversations with him. Toward the end of James's block of therapy, several outings were organized so that he could practice his functional speech skills in a more natural conversational environment.

## Analysis of Client's Response to Treatment

James made gains in many areas during his 6-week therapy block (see Tables 28.1 and 28.2 for details), which were collectively seen to contribute to increased sentence intelligibility (from 63% to 84%) as measured on the AssIDS. All measures on the Frenchay Dysarthria Assessment improved to some degree, maximum phonation increased from 8 to 15 seconds, and both pitch range and pitch variation showed substantial improvements. Interestingly, although palatal movement improved and speech was perceived to be less nasal, nasalance values obtained from the Nasometer™ II were only slightly reduced posttreatment. James and his family reported that they knew that progress had been made, but that there were still times and environments where it was difficult for James to get his message across. In particular, the mother indicated that when James was tired his speech became far less intelligible, and he was easily frustrated when people asked him to repeat what he had said.

## Further Recommendations

James demonstrated good outcomes from intensive therapy and was able to return to school with much improved speech intelligibility. Local speech-language pathology services were not available in his hometown to continue his rehabilitation. Information was provided to educate James's teachers and fellow students about the communication difficulties James might experience and strategies that listeners could utilize to improve communicative interactions. It was suggested that James should return to the rehabilitation center for another block of therapy in the future to further improve all speech subsystems, particularly targeting velopharyngeal function.

## Author Note

The case presented is not based on an actual patient but is drawn from the clinical experiences of the authors.

## Endnote

1. The terms *impairment, functional limitation,* and *disability* are no longer used in WHO's revised model of chronic disorder. These conceptual terms have been replaced by the terms impairment = *body, structure, and function;* functional limitation = *activity limitation;* and disability = *participation restriction* (WHO, 2001).

## References


Abkarian, G. G., & Dworkin, J. P. (1993). Treating severe motor speech disorders: Give speech a chance. *Journal of Medical Speech-Language Pathology, 1*, 285–287.

Albright, A. L., & Pollack, I. F. (2004). Brainstem gliomas. In H. R. Winn (Ed.), *Youmans neurological surgery*, Vol. 3 (pp. 3663–3669). Philadelphia: Saunders.

Atac, B., & Blaauw, G. (1979). Radiotherapy in brainstem gliomas in children. *Clinical Neurology and Neurosurgery, 84,* 281–290.

Caarstens Medizinelekronik (2009). Articulography—Electromagnetic systems for visualization of speech movement inside the mouth. Retrieved April 2010 from http://www.articulograph.de/.

Caruso, A. J., & Strand, E. A. (1999). *Clinical management of motor speech disorders in children*. New York: Thieme.

Choux, M., Lena, G., & Do, I. (2000). Brainstem tumors. In M. Choux, C. Di Rocco, & A. Hockley (Eds.), *Pediatric neurosurgery* (pp. 471–491). New York: Churchill Livingstone.

Clark, H., Robin, D. A., McCullagh, G., & Schmidt, R. A. (2001). Motor control in children and adults during a non-speech oral-task. *Journal of Speech Language and Hearing Research, 44*, 1015–1025.

Cohen, M.E., & Duffner, P.K. (1984). *Brain tumors in children: Principles of diagnosis and treatment*. New York: Raven Press.

Cornwell, P. L., Murdoch, B. E., & Ward, E. C. (2003). Perceptual evaluation of motor speech following treatment for childhood cerebellar tumor. *Clinical Linguistics and Phonetics, 17*, 597–615.

Crary, M. (1993). *Developmental motor speech disorders*. San Diego: Singular Press.

Darley, F. L., Aronson, A. E., & Brown, J. R. (1969a). Clusters of deviant speech dimensions in the dysarthrias. *Journal of Speech and Hearing Research, 12*, 462–496.

Darley, F. L., Aronson, A. E., & Brown, J. R. (1969b). Differential diagnostic patterns of the dysarthrias. *Journal of Speech and Hearing, 12*, 246–269.

Darley, F. L., Aronson, A. E., & Brown, J. R. (1975). *Motor speech disorders*. Philadelphia: Saunders.

Duffy, J. R. (2005). *Motor speech disorders: Substrates, differential diagnosis, and management*. St Louis: Elsevier Mosby.

Enderby, P. M. (1983). *Frenchay Dysarthria Assessment*. San Diego: College-Hill Press.

Giles, G. G., & Gonzales, M. F. (1995). Epidemiology of brain tumors and factors in prognosis. In A. H. Kaye & E. R. Laws (Eds.), *Brain tumors* (pp. 521–532). Boston: College-Hill Press.

Hayden, D. A, & Square, P. A. (1994). Motor speech treatment hierarchy: A systems approach. *Clinical Communication Disorders, 4*(3), 162–174.

Helm-Estabrooks, N., Yorkston, K. M., & Beukelman, D. R. (2004). Speech supplementation techniques for dysarthria: A systematic review. *Journal of Medical Speech-Language Pathology, 12*, ix–xxix.

Helm-Estabrooks, N., Yorkston, K. M., Spencer, K. A., & Duffy, J. R. (2003). Behavioral management of respiratory/phonatory dysfunction: A systematic review of the evidence. *Journal of Medical Speech-Language Pathology, 11*, xiii–xxxviii.

Hixon, T., Hawley, J., & Wilson, J. (1982). An around-the-house device for the clinical determination of respiratory driving pressure. *Journal of Speech and Hearing Disorders, 47*, 413–415.

Hodge, M. M., & Wellman, L. (1999). Management of children with dysarthria. In A. J. Caruso & E. A. Strand (Eds.), *Clinical management of motor speech disorders in children* (pp. 209–280). New York: Thieme.

Johnston, M.V., Nishimura, A., Harum, K., Pekar, J., & Blue, M. E. (2001). Sculpting the developing brain. *Advances in Pediatrics, 48*, 1–38.

Keatley, A., & Wirz, S. (1994). Is 20 years too long?: Improving intelligibility in long-standing dysarthria—A single case treatment study. *European Journal of Disorders of Communication, 29*, 183–201.

Kuehn, D. P. (1997). The development of a new technique for treatment of hypernasality: CPAP. *American Journal of Speech Language Pathology, 6*(4), 5–8.

Kwakkel, G., Wagenaar, R. C., Koelman, T. W., Lankhorst, G. J., & Koetsier, J. C. (2002). Effects of intensity of rehabilitation after stroke. *Stroke, 28*, 1550–1556.

Lassman, L. P. (1983). Tumours of the pons and medulla oblongata. In L. V. Amador (Ed.), *Brain tumors in the young* (pp. 546–564). Springfield, IL: Charles C Thomas.

Maas, E., Robin, D. A., Austermann Hula, S. N., Freedman, S. E., Wulf, G., Ballard, K. J., et al. (2008). Principles of motor learning in treatment of motor speech disorders. *American Journal of Speech-Language Pathology, 17*(3), 277–298.

Park, J. H., & Shea, C. H. (2005). Sequence learning: Response structure and effector transfer. *Quarterly Journal of Experimental Psychology, 58A*, 387–419.

Recinos, P. F., Sciubba, D. M., & Jallo, G. I. (2007). Brainstem tumors: Where are we today? *Pediatric Neurosurgery, 43*, 192–201.

Sellars, C., Hughes, T., & Langhorne, P. (2005). Speech and language therapy for dysarthria due to non-progressive brain damage. *Cochrane Database of Systematic Reviews* 2005, Issue 3. Art. No.: CD002088. DOI: 10.1002/14651858.CD002088.pub2.

Sharkey, S. G., & Folkins, J. W. (1985). Variability of lip and jaw movements in children and adults: Implications for the development of speech motor control. *Journal of Speech and Hearing Research, 28*, 8–15.

Strand, E. A., & McCauley, R. J. (1999). Assessment procedures for treatment planning in children with phonologic and motor speech disorders. In A. J. Caruso & E. A. Strand (Eds.), *Clinical management of motor speech disorders in children* (pp. 73–108). New York: Thieme.

Thompson, C. K. (1988). Articulation disorders in the child with neurogenic pathology. In N. Lass, L. McReynolds, J. Northern, & D. Yoder (Eds.), *Handbook of speech language pathology and audiology* (pp. 548–590). Toronto: BC Decker.

Tomita, T., & Cortes, R. F. (2002). Astrocytomas of the cerebral peduncle in children: Surgical experience in seven patients. *Child's Nervous System, 18,* 225–230.

World Health Organization. (2001). *ICF: Introduction.* Retrieved June 15, 2008 from http://www.who.int/classifications/icf/site/icftemplate.cfm?myurl=introduction.html%20&mytitle=Introduction.

Yorkston, K. M., & Beukelman, D. R. (1981). *Assessment of intelligibility of dysarthric speech.* Austin, TX: PRO-ED.

Yorkston, K. M., Beukelman, D. R., Strand, E. A., & Bell, K. R. (1999). *Management of motor speech disorders in children and adults.* Austin, TX: PRO-ED.

Yorkston, K. M., Spencer, K. A, Duffy, J. R., Beukelman, D. R, Golper, L., Miller, R., et al. (2001). Evidence-based practice guidelines for dysarthria: Management of velopharyngeal function. *Journal of Medical Speech-Language Pathology, 9,* 257–274.

Yorkston, K. M., Strand, E. A., & Kennedy, M. R. T. (1996). Comprehensibility of dysarthric speech: Implications for assessment and treatment planning. *American Journal of Speech-Language Pathology, 5,* 55–66.

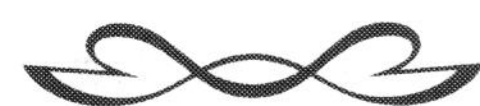

# FLUENCY

## CASE 29

## Francesca: Syllable-Timed Speech to Treat Stuttering in a School-Age Child

*Cheryl Andrews, Natasha Trajkovski, and Mark Onslow*

### Conceptual Knowledge Areas

Stuttering is a speech disorder that begins in the early years of life and involves disruptions to normal verbal behavior, such as (1) repeated movements of whole or part-words, (2) fixed postures with or without audible airflow, and (3) superfluous behaviors such as grimacing (Teesson, Packman, & Onslow, 2003). A recent prospective, community-ascertained cohort study found the cumulative incidence of stuttering to be 8.5% of children by the age of 3 years (Reilly et al., 2009). If left untreated, stuttering may be associated with serious consequences. These may include social phobia (social anxiety disorder), perturbed peer interactions, and occupational underachievement (Craig & Calver, 1991; Hayhow, Cray, & Enderby, 2002; Menzies, Onslow, & Packman, 1999; Stein, Baird, & Walker, 1996).

Consequently, early stuttering intervention is critical. It is generally agreed that stuttering is tractable during the preschool years; however, tractability decreases in direct proportion to age, presumably as neural networks for speech become established (Wohlert & Smith, 2002). The transitional period prior to the point where stuttering becomes intractable appears to be between the ages of 7–12 years. Accordingly, treatment in this age group is seen as one of the final opportunities to resolve stuttering in childhood. Nevertheless, clinical management of this population is fraught with difficulty (Conture & Guitar, 1993). As a child advances through school, there is an increase in the demand for social communication, which may impact the child's ability to generalize and maintain stutter-free speech. As a result, issues such as motivation and anxiety can become a problem. By the time a child who stutters reaches the school-age years there may have been many unsuccessful attempts at treatment or several relapses after successful treatment. Both these scenarios will almost certainly decrease motivation to comply with further attempts at treatment.

## Description of the Case

### Background Information

Francesca presented as a quiet and sometimes hesitant 11-year-old at the time of the assessment. She lived with her parents who supported her when she requested further intervention for her stuttering. During the assessment she spoke with interest about animals, sports, and movies. Francesca was in Grade 6 at a local public primary school.

The parents brought Francesca to the Australian Stuttering Research Centre (ASRC). Francesca and her mother explained that she began stuttering consistently at 7 years of age. Her mother noted that the stuttering might have developed earlier but remained unnoticed because, at the age of 7 years, 6 months, Francesca moved from Italy to Australia and was acquiring a second language. When Francesca moved to Australia, her dominant language was Italian.

At the assessment Francesca expressed specific concerns about participating in class discussions and talking on the phone. She explained that she attempted to control her stuttering by stopping and starting again but that this technique was not helping.

### Reason for Referral

This was Francesca's second presentation at the clinic. Several years previously she presented with moderate stuttering consisting of repeated movements and fixed postures. She was treated by the first author using the Lidcombe Program of Early Stuttering Intervention (Jones et al., 2005; Onslow, 2003). To deal with language issues, Francesca's mother was instructed to conduct treatment in English and her father was instructed to conduct treatment in Italian. After seven clinic visits, Francesca had reached the criteria for entry into Stage II (maintenance). Francesca progressed through the criterion-based Stage II of the Lidcombe Program. Against the advice of the clinician, treatment stopped after 7 months because Francesca's parents were satisfied with the outcome. Francesca maintained stutter-free speech for 3 years post-treatment; however, she had gradually relapsed by the time she was 11 years. Treatment was not sought immediately after relapse because her stuttering was mild and infrequent. Francesca's stuttering progressively worsened and 5 months after relapse, treatment was sought.

### Findings of the Evaluation

Francesca's parents reported a normal birth and developmental history, and there were no signs of any other speech or language problems. Her speech was assessed using a standard two-button electronic counter during a discussion with the clinician. Francesca's mean pretreatment stuttering rate was 9.0% syllables stuttered (%SS), consisting of repeated movements and frequent fixed postures without audible airflow. What appeared to be word-finding difficulty was in fact word-avoiding behavior. Because of the effort she was putting into avoiding stuttering, Francesca's conversation was characterized by frequent pausing, which made it difficult to follow the content of her conversation. Francesca reported that stuttering made her feel anxious and that the "blocking" (fixed postures) stutters were particularly frustrating. Before treatment began, the clinician ensured that Francesca understood that her stuttering was not a result of an emotional disorder, but rather was a problem associated with neural speech processing (Packman & Attanasio, 2004).

## Treatment Options Considered

Despite, or perhaps because of, the complex issues in the treatment of school-age children who stutter, the amount of published evidence available for treating this population is limited. Onslow, Jones, O'Brian, Menzies, & Packman (2008) argued that a reasonably loose definition of a clinical trial is a prospective study involving speech measures beyond the clinic with at least 3 months follow-up. Using that definition, there have been clinical trials published of four treatments for this age group (7–12 years): (1) *speech restructuring* (Boberg & Kully, 1994; Craig et al., 1996; Hancock et al., 1998[1]; Kully & Boberg, 1991; Ryan & Van Kirk Ryan, 1995), (2) *EMG biofeedback* (Block, 2004;[2] Craig et al., 1996; Hancock et al., 1998), (3) *regulated breathing* (De Klinder & Boelens, 1998), and (4) *verbal response contingent stimulation* (Lincoln, Onslow, Lewis & Wilson,1996[3]; Ryan & Van Kirk Ryan, 1983, 1995).

On balance, this body of clinical trials evidence is weak (Onslow et al., 2008) because it does not include any trials that contain the watershed methodology of randomization, and because it provides reasonable evidence only for *speech restructuring* and *verbal response contingent stimulation.* There has been no replication of the De Klinder & Boelens (1998) report on *regulated breathing,* and the findings about *EMG biofeedback* are subject to contention, with a failure to replicate findings. A further limitation of this body of evidence is that all these treatments were developed for either older or younger populations and applied to school-age children; there has been no treatment designed specifically for the needs of school-age children.

On balance, in Francesca's case, the only treatments that the clinician considered to have a believable clinical trials evidence base were verbal *response contingent stimulation* and *speech restructuring.* A treatment from the former category—the Lidcombe Program—had controlled stuttering for some years. However, after a brief trial resuming that treatment, the clinician formed the view that Francesca's stuttering was no longer tractable to this type of treatment. Hence, the only treatment with trials evidence that would be viable was *speech restructuring.* However, in addition to the limitation that *speech restructuring* was developed for adults and adapted for children, the clinician noted that the bulk of the clinical trials evidence involved an intensive group format, which was not a viable option for Francesa. Additionally, *speech restructuring* treatments involve quite extensive changes to speech, such as reduced rate, extended vowel duration, gentle vowel onsets, and continuous voicing. Although able to control stuttering, it is well known that such treatments may result in unnatural sounding speech, and the clinician did not feel that to be suitable for Francesca.

The limitations of available clinical trials evidence for treatments during the school years may well compel researchers and clinicians to look for other types of clinical research with this age group to guide their practices. One such line of research that has been overlooked in recent years is Syllable Timed Speech (STS). Syllable Timed Speech involves saying each syllable in time to a regular beat. The technique has been used extensively in the past as the basis of treatment for adults (Ingham, 1984; Packman, Onslow, & Menzies, 2000); however, it has fallen from favor during recent years. This is primarily because the reduction in stuttering that is associated with STS use does not appear to generalize when a person reverts to customary speech.

There have been three reports of STS being used with school-age children. Greenburg (1970) exposed 20 stuttering children age 9 to 11 years to a metronome beat for 5 minutes. One group was instructed to pace speech to the beat of the metronome, while the other group was not given any instructions to do so. Results indicated that both groups reduced the number of "dysfluencies" by a similar amount, whether instructed to pace speech or not.

In a clinical study, Alford and Ingham (1969) treated 9 children between the ages of 7 and 11 years with a combination of token reinforcement, negative practice, and STS in an intensive speech therapy program. Follow-up data were collected for 4 participants who had experienced a reduction in stuttering ranging from 1.3 to 10.6 %SS at post-treatment. In another clinical study, Andrews and Harris (1964) used STS to treat stuttering in various age groups ranging from 11 to 44 years. At 9 months posttreatment, the school-age group showed the best treatment response as compared to the adolescent or adult groups.

Although they do not qualify as clinical trials according to a liberal definition of a clinical trial (Onslow et al., 2008), these studies suggest that STS has considerable potential to warrant further development as a treatment for school-age children. Consequently, the authors incorporated STS into a treatment protocol to specifically target stuttering in the simplest way possible for Francesca without using speech changes such as reduced rate, extended vowel duration, gentle vowel onsets, and continuous voicing. This protocol was tested and outcomes for Francesca's case are reported. This initial clinical trial of the protocol was the first stage in a program of clinical trials development of STS for school-age children undertaken by the authors and colleagues.

## Course of Treatment

The treatment involved training Francesca and her parents to regularly practice using STS in conversation beyond the clinic. The treatment process required 15 weekly treatment sessions lasting 45 minutes and a 12-month maintenance program.

At the initial treatment visit, the clinician taught Francesca and her parents to use STS through demonstration, imitation, and instruction. STS was used at normal speech rate and with normal intonation. No emphasis was placed on speed and a metronome was not used. After Francesca demonstrated that she could imitate the clinician's model of STS consistently, she was required to engage in a series of short-answer questions with the clinician. To do this, both Francesca and the clinician used STS in a picture description task.

As Francesca became more proficient at using STS, she quickly proceeded to using STS in conversation with the clinician. Her parents were also trained to use STS in a similar manner. By the end of the initial clinic visit, Francesca and her parents maintained STS in conversation with each other. The clinician recommended that the family practice speaking in conversation with STS at home for 10 minutes 4 to 6 times per day. If Francesca stopped using STS, a short prompt was given to remind her to resume doing so. A simple reward system was developed to encourage Francesca to participate in the treatment sessions with her parents. Although Francesca was fully aware that she was receiving treatment for her stuttering, at no point was feedback contingent on her stuttering.

The family returned to the clinic after one week of practice and reported an immediate decrease in stuttering severity (see Figure 29.1). After the clinician observed Francesca's parents demonstrating STS practice with Francesca, it was recommended that treatment continue as specified, with a minimum of four practice sessions per day. The clinician also recommended that Francesca's parents occasionally prompt her to use STS briefly, for one or two sentences, between the 10-minute practice sessions. Weekly clinic visits continued until the clinician was satisfied that treatment was being conducted consistently at home, after which clinic visits were spaced 2 weeks apart. Francesca was moved into a criterion-based maintenance program after 15 clinic visits when her stuttering had reached a very low level. The aim of maintenance was to gradually withdraw the STS practice and still maintain a low level of stuttering while the family attended the clinic less frequently.

## Analysis of Client's Response to Intervention

In order to measure change, the clinician used a dual-button electronic counter to measure %SS at the start of each clinic visit. This measure was based on a conversational speech sample that was a minimum of 300 syllables or 10 minutes in duration. Figure 29.1 presents the within-clinic %SS measures collected by the treating clinician during each clinic session. The

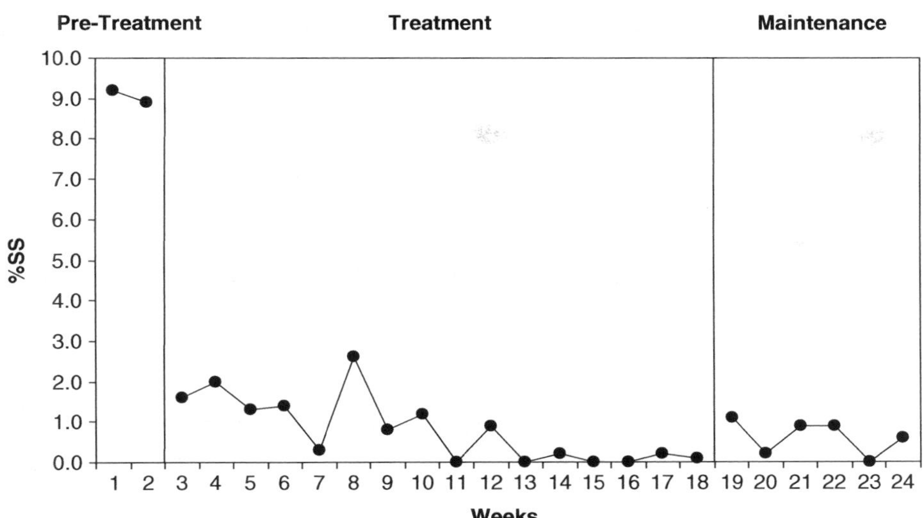


FIGURE 29.1 Weekly Within-Clinic Percent Syllables Stuttered (%SS) Scores Collected by the Treating Clinician

first 2 measures were made at pretreatment, the following 15 measures were made during treatment, and the final 7 measures were made during the maintenance phase.

The clinician trained Francesca and her parents to measure average stuttering severity each day in everyday speaking situations, using a 10-point severity rating (SR) scale where 1 = no stuttering, 2 = extremely mild stuttering, and 10 = extremely severe stuttering. The clinician explained these severity ratings during the first clinic visit. At each subsequent clinic visit, after making the %SS measure, the clinician also assigned Francesca's stuttering in that speech sample an SR score and asked her parents to do the same. In this way, ratings were compared and discussed until reasonable agreement occurred. Reasonable agreement occurred when SR scores differed by no more than 1 scale value. Figure 29.2 presents the mean weekly SR scores collected by Francesca's parents. The first 3 measures were made at pretreatment, the following 23 measures were made during treatment, and the final 15 measures were made during the maintenance phase.

FIGURE 29.2 Mean Weekly Beyond-Clinic Severity Rating (SR) Scores Collected by Francesca's Parents

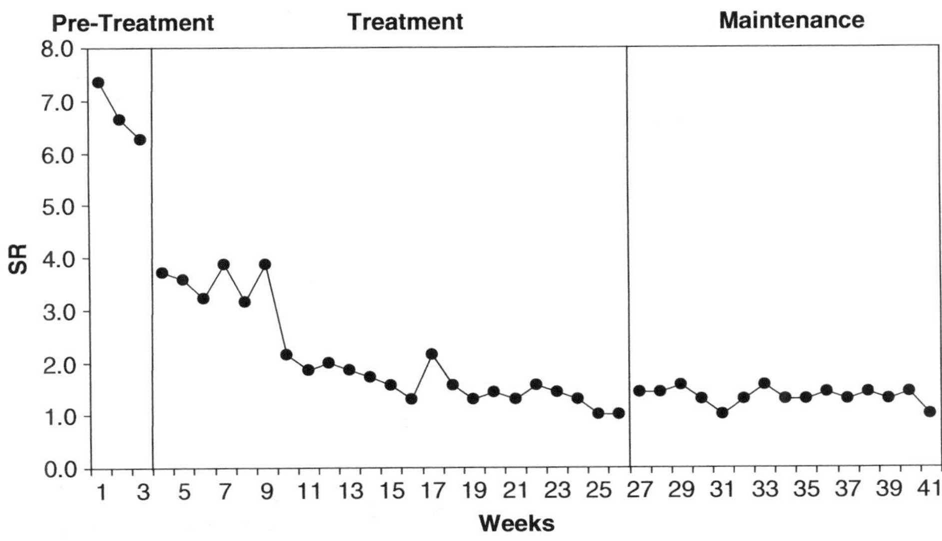

TABLE 29.1 Francesca's Outcome Questionnaire Responses Collected at Pretreatment, Entry into Maintenance, 9-months Post–start of Treatment, and 18-months Post–start of Treatment

| | **Pretreatment** | | | **Entry Into Maintenance** | | | **9 Months Post** | | | **18 Months Post** | | |
|---|---|---|---|---|---|---|---|---|---|---|---|---|
| How happy are you with your speech at the moment? Use a 1 to 9 scale: 1 = extremely happy; 9 = extremely unhappy | | 7 | | | 3 | | | 2 | | | 2 | |
| Situation | Avoidance Never, Sometimes, Usually | Typical Severity 1 = no stutters; 9 = severe stuttering | Worse Severity 1 = no stutters; 9 = severe stuttering | Avoidance Never, Sometimes, Usually | Typical Severity | Worse Severity | Avoidance Never, Sometimes, Usually | Typical Severity | Worse Severity | Avoidance Never, Sometimes, Usually | Typical Severity | Worse Severity |
| Talking with a family member | Never | 5 | 6 | Never | 1 | 4 | Never | 1 | 4 | Never | 1 | 2 |
| Talking with your best friend | Sometimes | 6 | 7 | Never | 2 | 6 | Never | 2 | 5 | Never | 1 | 2 |
| Talking with a group of friends | Sometimes | 6 | 7 | Sometimes | 2 | 6 | Sometimes | 4 | 4 | Never | 1 | 2 |
| Talking to your teacher | Never | 5 | 6 | Never | 1 | 5 | Never | 1 | 3 | Sometimes | 2 | 2 |
| Talking to other grownups | Never | 5 | 7 | Never | 2 | 4 | Never | 2 | 4 | Never | 1 | 2 |
| Reading aloud in class | Usually | 7 | 9 | Sometimes | 2 | 5 | Never | 2 | 2 | Sometimes | 1 | 2 |
| Talking in front of the class | Usually | 7 | 9 | Sometimes | 1 | 5 | Never | 1 | 3 | Never | 1 | 2 |
| Talking on the phone | Sometimes | 6 | 7 | Never | 1 | 3 | Never | 1 | 4 | Never | 1 | 2 |

Francesca completed four outcome questionnaires that required her to allocate two SRs to various speaking situations beyond the clinic. The first SR was allocated to her typical severity and the second SR was allocated to her worst severity under each speaking situation. Francesca completed the questionnaire at pretreatment, entry into maintenance, 9 months post–start of treatment, and 18 months post–start of treatment. Table 29.1 presents a table of Francesca's outcome questionnaire responses.

Francesca's within-clinic %SS decreased from 9.0 to 0.1 after 15 clinic visits over 23 weeks. Francesca progressed to a criterion-based maintenance program after she achieved 3 consecutive weeks of within-clinic %SS scores below 1.5 and beyond-clinic SR scores averaging 2.0 or below. Francesca maintained this low level of stuttering for the duration of her 12-month maintenance schedule. Interestingly, toward the final stages of maintenance, Francesca's perception of her own speech improved significantly (see Table 29.1). This highlights the importance of having a structured and supportive maintenance program to bolster the treatment of school-age children who stutter.

Francesca's case illustrates some potential advantages of using STS to treat school-age children who stutter. First, the treatment was simple. In contrast to other treatments for school-age children, the STS treatment involved little effort apart from practicing STS in conversation for 10 minutes four to six times per day. As such, the compliance issues that are known to relate to this age group could potentially be overcome. Second, the treatment was efficient. Only 15 clinic visits were required to reach the criteria set for maintenance. Third, Francesca's everyday speech was judged to sound quite natural by her parents and the treating clinician.

Of course, it is not possible to generalize from Francesca's case to the population of school-age children who require treatment for their stuttering. Further, systematic clinical trials will be needed with a cohort of school-age children. Nonetheless, the results of this single case are encouraging and the authors and colleagues are currently conducting such trials.

## Author Note

The trialing of this protocol was cleared by the Human Ethics Committee of The University of Sydney, and Francesca and her parents gave written consent to participate. The name of the client has been changed for the purposes of confidentiality.

## Endnotes

1. This study failed to replicate the positive findings of the Craig et al. (1996) and Hancock et al. (1998) trials for EMG biofeedback.
2. This study failed to replicate the positive findings of the Craig et al. (1996) and Hancock et al. (1998) trials for EMG biofeedback.
3. The treatment in this report was the Lidcombe Program.

## References


Alford, J., & Ingham, R. J. (1969). The application of token reinforcement system to the treatment of stuttering in children. *Journal of the Australian College of Speech Therapists, 19,* 53–57.

Andrews, G., & Harris, M. G. (1964). *The syndrome of stuttering.* London: Spastics Society Medical Education and Information Unit in association with William Heinemann Medical Books.

Block, S. (2004). The evidence base for the treatment of stuttering. In S. Reilly, J. Douglas, & J. Oates (Eds.), *Evidence based practice in speech pathology.* London: Whurr.

Boberg, E., & Kully, D. (1994). Long-term results of an intensive treatment program for adults and adolescents who stutter. *Journal of Speech & Hearing Research, 37*(5), 1050–1059.

Conture, E., & Guitar, B. (1993). Evaluating efficacy of treatment of stuttering: School-age children. *Journal of Fluency Disorders, 18,* 253–287.

Craig, A. R., & Calver, P. (1991). Following up on treated stutterers: Studies of perceptions of fluency and job status. *Journal of Speech and Hearing Research, 34*(2), 279–284.

Craig, A., Hancock, K., Chang, E., Shepley, A., McCaul, A., & Costello, D. (1996). A controlled clinical trial for stuttering in persons aged 9 to 14 years. *Journal of Speech and Hearing Research, 39*(4), 808–826.

De Klinder, M., & Boelens, H. (1998). Habit-reversal treatment for children's stuttering—Assessment in three settings. *Journal of Behavior Therapy and Experimental Psychiatry, 29*(3), 261–265.

Greenburg, J. B. (1970). The effect of a metronome on the speech of young stutterers. *Behaviour Therapy, 1*(2), 240–244.

Hancock, K., Craig, A., McCready, C., McCaul, A., Costello, D., & Gilmore, G. (1998). Two- to six-year controlled-trial stuttering outcomes for children and adolescents. *Journal of Speech, Language, and Hearing Research, 41*(6), 1242–1252.

Hayhow, R., Cray, A. M., & Enderby, P. (2002). Stammering and therapy views of people who stammer. *Journal of Fluency Disorders, 27*(1), 1–17.

Ingham, R. J. (1984). *Stuttering and behavior therapy: Current status and experimental foundations.* San Diego, CA: College-Hill Press.

Jones, M., Onslow, M., Packman, A., Williams, S., Ormond, T., & Schwarz, I. (2005). Randomised controlled trial of the Lidcombe programme of early stuttering intervention. *British Medical Journal, 331*(7518), 659–661.

Lincoln, M., Onslow, M., Lewis, C., & Wilson, L. (1996). A clinical trial of an operant treatment for school-age children who stutter. *American Journal of Speech-Language Pathology, 5*(2), 73–85.

Kully, D., & Boberg, E. (1991). Therapy for school-age children. *Seminars in Speech and Language, 12*(4), 291–300.

Menzies, R., Onslow, M., & Packman, A. (1999). Anxiety and stuttering: Exploring a complex relationship. *American Journal of Speech-Language Pathology, 8*(1), 3–10.

Onslow, M. (2003). Evidence-based treatment of stuttering: IV. Empowerment through evidence-based treatment practices. *Journal of Fluency Disorders, 28*(3), 237–244.

Onslow, M., Jones, M., O'Brian, S., Menzies, R., & Packman, A. (2008). Defining, identifying, and evaluating clinical trials of stuttering treatments: A tutorial for clinicians. *American Journal of Speech Language Pathology, 17,* 401–415.

Packman, A., & Attanasio, J. S. (2004). *Theoretical issues in stuttering.* London: Taylor & Francis.

Packman, A., Onslow, M., & Menzies, R. (2000). Novel speech patterns and the treatment of stuttering. *Disability and Rehabilitation, 22*(1), 65–79.

Reilly, S., Onslow, M., Packman, A., Wake, M., Bavin, E., Prior, M., et al. (2009). Predicting stuttering onset by age 3 years: A prospective, community cohort study. *Pediatrics, 123,* 270–277.

Ryan, B., & Van Kirk Ryan, B. (1983). Programmed stuttering therapy for children: Comparisons of four establishment programs. *Journal of Fluency Disorders, 8,* 291–321.

Ryan, B. P., & Van Kirk Ryan, B. (1995). Programmed stuttering treatment for children: Comparison of two establishment programs through transfer, maintenance, and follow-up. *Journal of Speech and Hearing Research, 38*(1), 61–75.

Stein, M. B., Baird, A., & Walker, J. R. (1996). Social phobia in adults with stuttering. *American Journal of Psychiatry, 153*(2), 278–280.

Teesson, K., Packman, A., & Onslow, M. (2003). The Lidcombe behavioral data language of stuttering. *Journal of Speech, Language, and Hearing Research, 46*(4), 1009–1015.

Wohlert, A., & Smith, A. (2002). Developmental change in variability of lip muscle activity during speech. *Journal of Speech Language and Hearing Research, 45,* 1077–1087.

# CASE 30

# Paul: Treatment of Cluttering in a School-Age Child

*Kathleen Scaler Scott, David Ward, and Kenneth O. St. Louis*

## Conceptual Background Areas

Cluttering is a much misunderstood and underresearched disorder, a fact that stands in sharp contrast to the extensive literature that exists for its more famous relative, stuttering. In contrast to stuttering, cluttering lacks visibility to (a) the cluttering client, wherein lack of awareness is actually regarded as a strong diagnostic feature, (b) the public, and (c) even most clinicians, many of whom report that they are uncertain how to identify, diagnose, and treat this disorder. There is no single known cause for cluttering, although many believe it reflects genetic and/or physiological differences (see St. Louis, Myers, Bakker, & Raphael, 2007). There has been continuing evidence that cluttering has a strong relationship with stuttering, with which it commonly co-occurs.

### Onset and Development

Like stuttering, cluttering is considered a developmental disorder, although there have been occasional reports of cluttering arising following neurological trauma (e.g., Lebrun, 1996; Thacker & De Nil, 1996). Cluttering typically is not diagnosed until 7 or 8 years of age (Diedrich, 1984). Reasons for late diagnoses include lack of awareness of the disorder and the fact that cluttering often becomes salient in more complex, later developing language or motor achievements (Pitluk, 1982; St. Louis, Hinzman, & Hull, 1985). It may also be that, because the difficulties with speech motor control, language, or fluency that a young clutterer might experience are usually at a high level, many children go either undiagnosed or unseen by speech-language pathologists. Ward (2006) noted that cluttering is often diagnosed after a referral for stuttering, with older children and adults often expressing surprise when they find that they not only stutter, but have cluttering as well.

Two core reasons may account for the lack of understanding of cluttering: (a) differences of opinion as to which features may be regarded as essential to the disorder versus those that are merely incidental to it, and (b) the reality that cluttering (particularly severe cluttering) rarely occurs in isolation and most commonly is seen in combination with stuttering or other disorders (Freund, 1952; Preus, 1996; St. Louis et al., 2007; Weiss, 1964). Although more data are needed to establish a firm prevalence of coexisting cluttering and stuttering, a recent review of the literature suggests that between one-third and two-thirds of those who stutter also clutter (Ward, 2006). Cluttering has also been found to co-occur with other language and nonlanguage disorders such as Down syndrome, autism spectrum disorders, learning disabilities, and attention-deficit/hyperactivity disorder (ADHD) (Blood, Blood, & Tellis, 2000; Farmer & Brayton, 1979; Grewel, 1970; Molt, 1996; Scott, Grossman, Abendroth, Tetnowski, & Damico, 2006; St. Louis et al., 2007; Van Borsel & Vandermeulen, in press; Ward, 2006). Some of the speech characteristics inherently seen in these disorders are somewhat similar to those identified in cluttering, thus lending ambiguity as to whether these may be attributed exclusively to cluttering.

Despite these difficulties, there are some features of cluttering that are apparently readily recognized by clinical practitioners. In a recent survey of the opinions of 60 expert clinicians, Daly and Cantrell (2006) observed high interrater agreement for six features: fast and irregular speech rate, telescoped words, imprecise articulation, poor intelligibility, and word finding difficulties. Other characteristics thought important included a lack of pausing, lack of awareness, lack of self-monitoring skills, and disorganized language.

### Assessment

There is now an emerging consensus that cluttering is a multifaceted disorder, and as such requires comprehensive assessment in order to arrive at an informed diagnostic decision (Daly & Burnett, 1999; St. Louis et al., 2007; Ward, 2006). In addition to a thorough case history, a comprehensive assessment is needed to gain a secure diagnosis. Depending on the age of the client, the clinician may need to assess (formally or informally) overall speaking rate, fluency, language function, motor speech, articulation, and rhythm (smoothness versus jerkiness). Cluttering checklists (e.g., Daly, 1992–1993, 2006; Daly & Burnett, 1997; Daly & Cantrell, 2006; Ward, 2006), which also include sections on nonverbal behaviors (e.g., handwriting) that may be associated with the disorder, can assist in this process. When assessing a suspected clutter in a young child, the clinician may also need to consider related disorders, such as tachilalia (excessively rapid speech), stuttering, ADHD, developmental language disorder, dyspraxia, and autism spectrum disorders. For younger clients, input from teachers, special educators, and psychologists may be sought; for older clients, a neurologist's report may be required, together with brain scan evidence in order to rule out the possibility of neurological trauma or disease as a causal factor. See St. Louis et al. (2007) and Ward (2006) for comprehensive assessment protocols.

## Description of the Case

### Background Information

Paul was a 10-year-old, fifth-grade boy whose mother, Mrs. R, contacted the first author for a speech-language evaluation. She indicated that Paul tended to speak quickly and at a low volume, making it difficult for others to understand him. In her judgment, Paul's speech problem had worsened within the previous year.

Paul had been diagnosed with Asperger's disorder (AD) in the second grade. He suffered from anxiety, for which a selective seratonin reuptake inhibitor had been prescribed. At the time of the evaluation he had been receiving individual counseling biweekly. Within the previous year, Paul's family had relocated from a suburban to a rural area after Paul's father, whose job required frequent travel, was transferred by his employer. The family was in temporary housing awaiting a final decision about staying in the area. Paul's mother was a nonemployed speech-language pathologist who cared for Paul and his first-grade younger brother at home.

Paul's birth and medical histories were unremarkable. There was a familial history of stuttering (maternal grandmother and great-uncle). Paul stuttered for approximately 6 months when he was 4 years old. The stuttering, consisting of repetitions and prolongations, reportedly resolved spontaneously.

### Reason for Referral

Paul enjoyed school and participated in gifted and talented programs both within school and elsewhere. Paul's second grade teacher reportedly could not read his handwriting because of improper letter spacing, but this later resolved in grade 2 when he easily mastered cursive writing. Paul received occupational therapy to address such fine motor difficulties as handwriting and tying his shoes, and physical therapy to increase speed and coordination for gross motor activities, for example, running and jumping rope. His mother had noticed improvement in both fine and gross motor skills, but described Paul as "slower" and "slightly less coordinated" than normal in gross motor skills. At the time of the evaluation, Paul commented that he enjoyed his current participation in karate, swimming, and spinning classes, but he did not enjoy team sports.

Paul indicated that he had had a best friend in his neighborhood prior to the recent move, but had no friends at his new school. Paul's mother noted that he spoke with a few girls in his current class, and sometimes a friend (who also has social difficulties) from his new school came to his home, which she regarded as positive for Paul.

## Findings of the Evaluation

As children with AD are often found to exhibit at least average performance on formal speech and language measures (Shriberg et al., 2001; Tager-Flusberg, 1995), and to have greatest difficulty integrating language skills appropriately in context (Barnhill, 2001; Szatmari, 1991), language skills were assessed informally in conversational speech rather than through standardized testing. Accordingly, for the evaluation, samples of conversation and oral reading were videotaped and later analyzed for speaking rate, intelligibility, and disfluencies. Paul's mother, a speech-language pathologist, raised no concerns about his grammatical skills or vocabulary, nor were any such difficulties observed during the evaluation.

Table 30.1 summarizes the evaluation findings. Using Yairi's (1996) criteria, Paul exhibited 2% stuttering-like disfluencies (SLDs) (i.e., mostly blocks/tense pauses plug one prolongation and occasional part-word repetitions), and 11% nonstuttering-like disfluencies (NSLDs) (i.e., revisions, interjections, and phrase repetitions) during the 5-minute conversation speech sample. Paul's blocks/tense pauses and prolongations were brief, that is, up to 1 second in duration and less than 1 second, respectively. The Stuttering Severity Instrument for Children and Adults, Third Edition (SSI-3; Riley, 1994), administered for both conversation and reading, placed Paul in the mild range of stuttering. On the Communication Attitude Test, Revised

TABLE 30.1 Summary of Pretherapy Evaluation Findings

| Area | Measures Used | Data |
|---|---|---|
| Fluency | Conversation sample | SLDs: 2%<br>NSLDs: 11% |
| Fluency | Reading sample | SLDs: 1%<br>NSLDs: 0.5% |
| Fluency | Combined reading and conversation | SSI-3 score: 10<br>SSI-3 severity rating: mild |
| Articulation | Examiner judgment | Intermittent weak syllable deletion<br>Decreased vocal intensity |
| Speech Rate | Examiner judgment<br>*Overall speaking rate: 4.7 syllables/sec<br>**Articulation rate: 5.1 syllables/sec | Rapid, irregular |
| Language Usage | Examiner judgment | Excessive use of fillers and mazing<br>Decreased inclusion of background information |
| Attitudes | CAT-R | ***$z = -2.06$ |
| Parent Ratings | Ward Cluttering Checklist | ****68 |

* Number of syllables per second *including* disfluencies, pauses, hesitations; i.e., rate of message transmission

** Number of syllables per second *excluding* disfluencies, pauses, hesitations; i.e., rate of motor movements of mouth

*** As compared to school-age children with no speech/language issues, where average $z = 0.00$

**** See Table 30.3 for comparison of pre- and postscores, with decrease in score indicating movement toward more normalized speech.

(CAT-R; Brutten & Vanryckeghem, 2007), Paul scored more than 2 standard deviations below children his age who do not stutter, and within the same range as children his age who do stutter, indicating considerable negative attitudes toward speaking.

Speech intelligibility was judged by the first author to be "fair to poor" in unknown contexts and "fair" in known contexts. Rate and articulation contributed to the difficulty in understanding Paul. His rate tended to increase as he went on with a sentence or topic. He intermittently failed to pronounce word endings and/or weak syllables fully (i.e., weak syllable deletion), which gave the impression of words blending into one another. Additionally, he sometimes exhibited tense pauses between his words or phrases, producing an atypical rhythm (i.e., an irregular rate of speech). Finally, Paul's frequent low intensity further compromised his intelligibility.

While formulating language, Paul did not always include the necessary background information. At times he appeared to become "lost" in the content of what he was saying, going into specific details before giving general information or realizing he was veering from the main topic. Such "lost" or empty speech is known as *mazes* (Loban, 1976; Ward, 2006). It was speculated that Paul's decreased awareness precluded him from "tuning in" to the listener's nonverbal feedback to assist him in regulating his speech. When the clinician directly asked him for clarification, he responded, "Never mind," even when told the clinician wanted to hear what he had to say.

On occasions when Paul had difficulty formulating his ideas, he tended to insert filler words (e.g., "like," "um," "uh"), use nonspecific language (e.g., "stuff"), or revise or restart his utterance, all making his message difficult to follow. He also seemed to insert phrases as a means of getting himself started, such as "Okay, well," "Okay," or "You see." The following represents a sample of Paul's speech in which these patterns were noted:

"So like then we had to figure out this pro—, group project that we wanted to do. And then well, like, it was one of us, I don't know, it was me. I came up with like, you see we went to Bixby Village in like the fall it's like this historical place where there were like all, all it's like, back in li—, it's like, like, it was like, in New Ham—, yeah it's in New Hampshire like Sussex County. There's like this Buffalo Village. Of course that's not what it's all about. I don't remember what time period it was but it was long ago."

## Diagnostic Hypotheses

Paul was diagnosed with coexisting disorders of cluttering, stuttering, and Asperger's disorder (AD). Knowing that individuals with AD tend to have difficulties with executive functioning skills (Hill & Bird, 2006), the role they were suspected to play in Paul's speech and language could not be overlooked.

Executive functioning skills, such as self-regulation, planning, organizing, and problem solving, control and affect the outcome of performance in everyday tasks. They allow a child to plan an action, hold that plan in memory and sequence, and inhibit irrelevant responses (Denckla, 1996; Singer & Bashir, 1999). Although Paul presumably possessed the language *information* to formulate messages clearly and concisely, his difficulties with executive functioning skills likely resulted in verbal planning and organizing difficulties. Accordingly, although some of Paul's excessive nonstuttered disfluency may have been habitual (e.g., excessive use of the filler word "like"), that such disfluencies significantly decreased during reading tasks when language formulation was not required, suggested that most of these disfluencies were the result of language formulation issues. It was hypothesized that he first had difficulty formulating a message, followed by weaknesses in regulating and problem solving to compensate effectively for this language formulation difficulty. Although he appeared to be compensating for this difficulty by inserting excessive disfluencies or frequently revising his message to hold his conversational turn, he did not employ the most effective compensatory strategies that would make it easy for listeners to follow his ideas. Therefore, the difficulty lay not in his language skills alone, but in integration of language and executive functioning skills that is necessary for efficient and effective communication to take place.

The combination of rapid and/or irregular rate with decreased intelligibility and excessive use of NSLDs confirmed a diagnosis of cluttered speech, following the current working definition of cluttering (St. Louis et al., 2007):

> Cluttering is a fluency disorder characterized by a rate that is perceived to be abnormally rapid, irregular, or both for the speaker (although measured syllable rates may not exceed normal limits). These rate abnormalities further are manifest in one or more of the following symptoms: (a) an excessive number of disfluencies, the majority of which are not typical of people who stutter; (b) the frequent placement of pauses and use of prosodic patterns that do not conform to syntactic and semantic constraints; and (c) inappropriate (usually excessive) degrees of co-articulation among sounds, especially in multisyllabic words. (pp. 299–300)

There is currently debate as to whether language formulation issues are obligatory or incidental features of cluttering. Therefore, formulation issues were not used to diagnose cluttered speech, but would be addressed in treatment of overall effective communication. Paul also exhibited mild stuttering. Because the stuttering was mild and Paul did not engage in such behaviors as communication avoidance, tension, or struggle in relation to these moments of stuttering, it was determined that addressing cluttering should be the first treatment priority. Treatment would determine whether once cluttering was addressed, stuttering might worsen. Scaler Scott, Tetnowski, Roussel, and Flaitz (in press) found increased stuttering in a young clutterer-stutterer taught to use pausing to decrease rate of speech. The investigators hypothesized that because stuttering often involves difficulty with initiation of voicing, reducing speaking rate in cluttering via pausing. This area would need to be monitored during treatment with Paul and stuttering strategies introduced if and when appropriate.

## Treatment Options Considered

### Therapy Model

At present, there is a serious lack of an evidence base for the treatment of cluttering, and well-controlled trials on treatment efficacy are lacking. Strategies currently endorsed by clinicians experienced in dealing with cluttering appear to reflect their own personal experiences.

From a clinical perspective, cluttering can be thought of as a modular disorder, with separately identifiable components that nonetheless interrelate; for example, excessive coarticulation is likely to correlate with an overrapid speech rate. A synergistic model was adopted, that is, the idea that successful intervention within one area may have positive effects in another (Myers & Bradley, 1992; St. Louis et al., 2007). It can provide the maximal benefit with minimal clinical time if treatment goals are based on interrelated or hierarchically organized skill deficits. Therefore, in this model, individualized treatment plans must be individually tailored, using information gained from a careful evaluation. In addition to disfluency, therapy may well address such areas as awareness, speech rate, speech rhythm, articulation, and language formulation.

## Course of Treatment

Because Paul had an active after-school schedule, he was seen for 10 two-hour therapy sessions over the course of a two-week period. Most sessions occurred in the evenings after a full day of activities. In spite of initial concerns that Paul might be too fatigued from his day to focus on an area of challenge such as his speech, he sustained sufficient attention for all sessions.

## Goals, Principle, and Sequence of Treatment

Initial goals were:

1. To increase awareness of specific speech difficulties (i.e., fluency, articulation, rate, and language usage) and effective vs. ineffective responses to these difficulties.
2. To increase use of effective executive functioning strategies when communication breakdowns occur, and to:
   a. Identify the potential source of communication breakdown ("hypothesis");
   b. Respond with a repair strategy related to this hypothesis;
   c. Self-evaluate and debrief in structured conversations with the clinician and mother; and
   d. Use pausing and language strategies in functional contexts by progressing through a hierarchy from more- to less-structured language.

Three specific principles of treatment were applied to ensure effective therapy. First, to build Paul's self-esteem regarding his speech, the approach needed to be supportive rather than confrontational. His score on the CAT-R indicated that he was not comfortable as a speaker and had negative feelings associated with speaking. Two hours of nightly focus upon something about which Paul had negative feelings could easily become demoralizing. Paul needed to know that in spite of speech difficulties, he had many other assets. Second, to foster Paul's enthusiastic participation in therapy, the approach needed to be light-hearted and fun, building on his interests and strengths. Paul was a gifted child who, like many children with AD, enjoyed intellectual activities. Therefore, he was frequently assigned the role of "teacher" and/or "researcher" when examining how changes in one's speech result in changes in listener reactions. Third, to help ensure carryover, goals needed to be incorporated as soon as possible into everyday contexts, and, whenever possible, Paul's family needed to be involved. To accomplish this, Paul was given assignments such as explaining things he had learned to family members, designing and administering quizzes on strategies and information he learned, and reporting the results back to the clinician. These activities enhanced Paul's sense of empowerment in therapy and allowed the clinician to address any misperceptions as they occurred.

Within the context of these three principles, the long-term goals were addressed in a sequence of specific therapy focus areas. Table 30.2 summarizes the sequence.

### Awareness

Experience indicates that although many with cluttered speech are unaware of how they come across to others, they may be somewhat aware that something is not "right" about their speech, if only because of vague feedback they have received from listeners (Dewey, 2005). Paul's CAT-R score seemed to suggest that he was not completely unaware of his speech. Over the years, he had received feedback from professionals and his family about his rapid rate of speech. Therefore, in introducing the concept of awareness, it was decided to take the conversation beyond Paul and apply it to everyone's speech in general. Children with social

TABLE 30.2 Summary of Therapy Session Structure

| Focus area | Activities |
|---|---|
| Awareness | Identify potential errors that impact intelligibility; negative practice; games to identify errors in self and others; flowcharts; practice "tuning in" to and responding to nonverbal communication |
| Pausing | Insertion of pauses in structured hierarchy |
| Language | Expediter and Pyramid strategies |
| Home Carryover | Designing, administering, and reporting on family quizzes; e-mail assignments with clinician for accountability |

and/or severe communication issues such as Paul's are often ignored, teased, or reminded about their speech by others (Gertner, Rice, & Hadley, 1994). Because communication occurs throughout a child's day, reminders can be frequent. The feedback can become quite tiring and can lead to feelings of guilt and shame, especially when a child knows that he or she should change his or her speech (based upon what others are saying) but does not know how to do so effectively (Murphy, 1999). Often by school age, students have developed defense reactions and unwanted feedback about their speech. Many assert that there is "nothing wrong" (Weiss, 1964). Paul responded exactly in this way during baseline measurement. This denial suggested that a "back door" approach might be more effective than even gentle confrontation about Paul's speech. As often happens, when brainstorming with Paul reasons that people might not understand a speaker in general—rather than himself specifically—he volunteered that several of the options presented were characteristic of him (e.g., "I do that one all the time").

### Desensitization

Next, therapy involved identifying and experiencing through negative practice different types of less-than-intelligible speech segments, for example, mumbling or deleting syllables. Much of this was done in a game context, client and clinician competing for points for correctly identifying the types of the other's unintelligible speech. This fostered desensitization to the negative connotations that might surround drawing attention to Paul's speech. Rather than regarding his speech as a weakness or failure, it helped Paul become an "expert" at identifying and producing unintelligible speech (Murphy, Yaruss, & Quesal, 2007). Paul gradually became more aware of his compromised intelligibility and open to discussing it. For example, when commended for accurately identifying mumbling combined with rapid speech during a game, Paul commented, "That's easy for me to guess. I do it all the time!"

### Pausing

Paul was taught to use pauses to improve the clarity of his speech. Visual markers, that is, slash marks, were inserted into oral reading passages. The clinician explained that pausing would help him both in slowing down and in having time to think about what he wanted to say (St. Louis & Myers, 1995). A science experiment was designed whereby Paul read 10 sentences to his mother, 5 during which he used pausing, and 5 during which he did not use pausing. He scored the number of words his mother could correctly repeat for each sentence and compared her overall combined accuracy for sentences with and without pausing. Paul repeated this task with his father. In the case of both parents, Paul was able to see how accuracy scores dropped dramatically when pauses were not used. This activity focused on his intellect and motivated him to use the pausing strategy in the future. Once he was "hooked," Paul practiced pausing in a speech hierarchy, progressing through sentences, paragraphs, book chapters, short structured conversations (i.e., 1–2 sentence answers), and spontaneous conversations.

### Language Strategies

As Paul became proficient at pausing, he learned how to use the strategy in response to nonverbal feedback from others. Paul had developed a flowchart of "hypotheses" about the source of listener confusion and corresponding repair strategies. The strategies were applied to two broad categories of listener confusion: confusion because of "what I said" (e.g., omitted background information), or "how I said it" (e.g., too soft). At this point, the "what" of Ward's (2004, 2006) "Pyramid Approach" and Scaler Scott's (2002) "Expediter Rules" were introduced (see Figure 30.1). It is important to note that Paul, like many children with AD, frequently was unaware of feedback from others because he often found speaker-listener eye contact aversive. As a desensitizing activity, Paul and the clinician played games wherein each took turns identifying when the listener's face looked confused. Once desensitized, Paul was ready to use

FIGURE 30.1 Summary of Language Strategies

* Highlights of the program used with Paul; for a full program description, see Ward (2006), pp. 371–372.

* Principles adapted from the "Pyramid Approach" (Ward, 2006):
    - Progress from the "big picture" to small details in descriptions.
    - Resist providing additional information or asides before the "big picture" is explained.
    - Resist using fillers.
* Principles adapted from "Expediter Rules" (Scaler Scott, 2002):
    - Use short sentences.
    - Get right to the point.
    - Do not use too many examples.
    - Do not use nonspecific pronouns.
    - Give the listener background information.

eye contact to apply what he had learned about identifying listener confusion and making the appropriate repair. During games, Paul and the clinician practiced guessing the source of listener confusion and making the necessary speech repairs. In this activity, Paul again was engaged in the game and not focused upon his shortcomings, that is, how difficult eye contact could be for him. He began to regard feedback as valuable rather than aversive, and as something over which he had control (Ward, 2006).

### Self-Monitoring and Carryover

As therapy progressed, Paul became more and more successful in self-monitoring his speech: (a) proactively, to speak intelligibly in the first place (through use of pausing, "Pyramid," and "Expediter" strategies), and (b) reactively, to respond either to his own knowledge that he was unclear, or to feedback from others. He was praised for attempts at all of these levels.

By the seventh session, Paul was typically able to utilize all strategies effectively and independently in structured communication situations, including such structured daily situations as conversing with his mother in the car. In order to increase distraction and thereby make speech monitoring more challenging, the last three sessions focused solely on spontaneous speech involving Paul, his mother, and his younger brother. In Session 8 the trio and the clinician played several games ("Game Night") and Paul was required to use clear speech, even when excited. Session 9 involved one of Paul's interests, a cooking activity. In Session 10, Paul ordered lunch at a restaurant and was asked to speak to his server in a loud and clear voice.

To foster carryover, the clinician helped Paul construct a hierarchy of 10 speaking situations, arranged from least to most challenging. Additionally, she asked Paul to e-mail her nightly with his commitment for the following day's practice, and then follow up the following night with an evaluation of how it went. In this way, treatment would continue beyond structured therapy.

## Analysis of Client's Response to Treatment

Paul's speech was reevaluated 2 days following his last therapy session and again at 3 weeks posttherapy. At all follow-up sessions, Paul's mother indicated that she felt he was more aware of his lack of speech clarity and made more efforts to self-correct. She also indicated that Paul was much less defensive when she intermittently reminded him to repeat or slow his rate. Parent training was implemented for Mrs. R to avoid "overdoing" her reminders, and to remember to praise Paul for independent attempts at his speech.

Table 30.3 shows that in a posttherapy repeat conversation sample, Paul's NSLDs decreased from 11% to 5%. Without any cueing from the clinician, he made concerted efforts to use pauses in his speech. He did the same during a repeat oral reading task, in which his NSLDs decreased from 0.5% to 0%. His SLDs remained at 2% in conversation and increased

TABLE 30.3 Summary of Pre- and Postdata

| Area | Pre | Post | 3-Week Follow-up |
|---|---|---|---|
| Disfluencies | | | |
| Conversation | SLDs: 2%<br>NSLDs: 11% | SLDs: 2%<br>NSLDs: 5% | SLDs: 3%<br>NSLDs: 13% |
| Reading | SLDs: 1%<br>NSLDs: 0.5% | SLDs: 2%<br>NSLDs: 0% | SLDs: 1%<br>NSLDs: 0.5% |
| Fluency | SSI-3 score: 10<br>SSI-3 severity rating: very mild | SSI-3 score: 12<br>SSI-3 severity rating: mild | SSI-3 score: 10<br>SSI-3 severity rating: very mild |
| Articulation: Examiner Judgment | Intermittent weak syllable deletion; frequent instance of decreased vocal intensity | Fewer instances of weak syllable deletion and decreased vocal intensity | Intermittent weak syllable deletion continues; increased regularity of vocal intensity maintained |
| Speech Rate | Examiner judgment: rapid, irregular<br>*Overall speaking rate: 4.7 syllables/sec<br>**Articulation rate: 5.1 syllables/sec | Examiner judgment: Deliberate pauses used and increased regularity<br>*Overall speaking rate: 3.1 syllables/sec<br>**Articulation rate: 3.0 syllables/sec | Examiner judgment: pauses and regularity maintained<br>*Overall speaking rate: 3.8 syllables/sec<br>**Articulation rate: 4.6 syllables/sec |
| Language Usage | Informal observations: Excessive use of fillers, mazing and decreased inclusion of background information | Informal observations: Decreased use of fillers and mazing; increased inclusion of background information | Informal observations: Fillers increase; increased provision of background information; increased cohesion of message |
| Attitudes | ***$z = -2.06$ | ***$z = -2.65$ | ***$z = -0.88$ |
| Parent Ratings | ****68 | ****60 | ****62 |
| Executive Functioning | Examiner judgment: Decreased self-monitoring of clarity and persistence when not understood | Examiner judgment: Increased self-monitoring and persistence when not understood | Examiner judgment: Slightly decreased self-monitoring when excited but persistence when not understood maintained |

* Number of syllables per second including disfluencies, pauses, hesitations; i.e., rate of message transmission

** Number of syllables per second excluding disfluencies, pauses, hesitations; i.e., rate of motor movements of mouth

*** As compared to school-age children with no speech/language issues, where average $z = 0.00$

from 1% to 2% in oral reading. On the CAT-R, Paul's negative scores increased in comparison to children who do not stutter (i.e., 2.65 standard deviations below this group). This increase in score is likely related to increased speech awareness after therapy. In addition, Paul's comments on the CAT-R indicated that he moved closer toward more positive feelings, but given the opportunity on the test to select only "true" or "false," his score did not change for several items. For example, in response to "I don't talk like other children," Paul responded "true" in both pre- and posttesting, but on posttesting qualified this answer with "sometimes." At 3-week follow up, Paul's score on the CAT-R had decreased dramatically to –0.88, suggesting his positive feelings about his speech were continuing to increase over time. His mother's rating on Ward's (2006) "Checklist of Cluttering Behavior" showed that Paul's speech ratings changed in the direction of normal scores, that is, from 68 to 60, and increased only slightly at 3-week follow-up to 62.

Overall Paul responded favorably to intensive intervention and showed increased clarity of speech in structured situations. He became more comfortable with his speech and with monitoring it. He was empowered in being able to modify his speech so that others could understand him. He demonstrated a desire to use these strategies to be more clear to his listener, evidenced by numerous examples of modifying and repeating his message when unclear rather than saying, "Never mind." Paul either initiated modifications on his own or in response to the nonverbal feedback of listener confusion. Three weeks after therapy had ended, he had carried out the aforementioned e-mail assignments approximately one to two times weekly, rather than every day as assigned. At 3-week follow-up, Paul indicated that he was having difficulty remembering to do the e-mail assignments. At his mother's suggestion, Paul agreed to make the e-mail a part of his daily routine after dinner and before homework; however, even with this plan in place, Paul continued to complete assignments only once or twice weekly.

## Further Recommendations

Initial evaluation results revealed stuttering and cluttering. As previously mentioned, it was possible that as Paul decreased his cluttered speech, stuttering might increase (Scaler Scott et al., in press). His overall score on the SSI-3 did reflect a slight increase at posttesting, with a return to baseline level 3 weeks later. Given the variability of stuttering behaviors, this slight fluctuation is not surprising. However, possibly because they were not directly addressed in this intervention plan, Paul's SLDs also did not *decrease* with therapy. As the clinicians became increasingly familiar with Paul, his typical stuttering pattern became apparent. The majority of the SLDs were "tense pauses," that is, minor blocks of less than 1 second in duration with no impact upon his willingness to communicate. Throughout treatment, Paul repeatedly denied other symptoms of stuttering, such as feelings of words getting "stuck" in his mouth. Given his dramatic improvement in attitude toward himself as a speaker even though SLDs were not addressed, it seems valid to state that the SLDs have negligible impact upon Paul as a communicator. Therefore, it was felt that giving Paul another strategy to use in response to his SLDs would only result in an unnecessary additional self-monitoring load. As a next step, the clinicians recommended that Paul receive continued assistance and coaching with current cluttering strategies through daily situations on his hierarchy. They also recommended that his SLDs continue to be monitored for signs that further intervention is warranted (such as increased tension, struggle, or word or communication avoidance).

Paul's NSLDs also increased to baseline level at 3 weeks posttesting. Qualitatively, however, a difference was noted in the functional use of his NSLDs. That is, at 3-week follow-up, he did make frequent revisions in his speech (which are coded as NSLDs), but often did so as a means of revising an unclear message. This functional use of NSLDs was in contrast with his baseline use of NSLDs as empty time fillers. Nonetheless, although Paul had maintained many of his gains in self-monitoring by 3 weeks posttesting, he also was demonstrating some slips in self-monitoring when regular therapy sessions ceased. One such slip was decreased monitoring of speech when excited. Paul's data demonstrate that although therapy can result in great improvement in the short term, consistent therapy in the long term is required for maintenance of gains. Finally, since Paul's clarity of speech improved after introduction of language strategies and pausing—notably *without* specific exercises to address motor speech—a synergistic approach to treatment was validated.

## Author Note

The author wishes to acknowledge the participation of "Paul" (all names and identifying information changed to maintain confidentiality) and his family. This case is based upon a real client and has met the requirements for IRB exemption.

## References


Barnhill, G. P. (2001). Social attributions and depression in adolescents with Asperger syndrome. *Focus on Autism and Other Developmental Disabilities, 16,* 46–53.

Blood, G. W., Blood, I. M., & Tellis, G. (2000). Auditory processing and cluttering in young children. *Perceptual Motor Skills, 90,* 631–639.

Brutten, G., & Vanryckeghem, M. (2007). *Behavior Assessment Battery for Children Who Stutter.* San Diego, CA: Plural.

Daly, D. A. (1992–1993). Cluttering: A language-based syndrome. *Clinical Connection, 6,* 4–7.

Daly, D. A. (2006). *Predictive Cluttering Inventory.* Ann Arbor, MI: Author.

Daly, D. A., & Burnett, M. L. (1997). Checklist for Identification of Cluttering—Revised.

Daly, D. A., & Burnett, M. L. (1999). Cluttering: Traditional views and new perspectives. In R. F. Curlee (Ed.), *Stuttering and related disorders of fluency* (2nd ed.). New York: Thieme.

Daly, D. A., & Cantrell, R. P. (2006, July). *Cluttering: Characteristics identified as diagnostically significant by 60 fluency experts.* Presentation at the Fifth World Congress of Fluency Disorders, Dublin, Ireland.

Denckla, M. B. (1996). A theory and model of executive function: A neuropsychological perspective. In G. R. Lyon & N. A. Krasnegor (Eds.), *Attention, memory, and executive function* (pp. 263–278). Baltimore, MD: Paul Brookes.

Dewey, J. (2005). *My experiences with cluttering.* Eighth Annual International Stuttering Awareness Day (ISAD) On-line Conference.

Diedrich, W. M. (1984). Cluttering: Its diagnosis. In H. Winitz (Ed.), *Treating articulation disorders: For clinicians by clinicians* (pp. 307–323). Baltimore: University Park Press.

Farmer, A., & Brayton, E. R. (1979). Speech characteristics of fluent and dysfluent Down's syndrome adults. *Folia Phoniatrica, 31,* 284–290.

Freund, H. (1952). Studies in the interrelationship between stuttering and cluttering. *Folia Phoniatrica, 4,* 146–168.

Gertner, B. L., Rice, M. L., & Hadley, P. A. (1994). Influence of communicative competence on peer preferences in a preschool classroom. *Journal of Speech and Hearing Research, 37,* 913–923.

Grewel, F. (1970). Cluttering and its problems. *Folia Phoniatrica, 22,* 301–310.

Hill, E. L., & Bird, C. M. (2006). Executive processes in Asperger syndrome: Patterns of performance in a multiple case series. *Neuropsychologia, 44,* 2822–2835.

LeBrun, Y. (1996). Cluttering after brain damage. *Journal of Fluency Disorders, 21,* 289– 295.

Loban, W. (1976). *The language of elementary school children.* Champaign, IL: National Council of Teachers of English.

Molt, L. F. (1996). An examination of various aspects of auditory processing in clutterers. *Journal of Fluency Disorders, 21,* 215–225.

Murphy, W. P. (1999). A preliminary look at shame, guilt, and stuttering. In N. Bernstein Ratner & E. C. Healey (Eds.), *Stuttering Research and Practice: Bridging the Gap* (pp. 131–143). Mahwah: Lawrence Erlbaum Associates.

Murphy, W. P., Yaruss, J. S., & Quesal, R. W. (2007). Enhancing treatment for school-age children who stutter. I. Reducing negative reactions through desensitization and cognitive restructuring. *Journal of Fluency Disorders, 32,* 121–139.

Myers, F. L., & Bradley, C. L. (1992). Clinical management of cluttering from a synergistic framework. In F. L. Myers & K. O. St. Louis (Eds.), *Cluttering: A clinical perspective* (pp. 85–105). Kibworth, Great Britain: Far Communications. (Reissued in 1996 by Singular, San Diego, CA.)

Pitluk, N. (1982). Aspects of the expressive language of cluttering and stuttering schoolchildren. *The South African Journal of Communication Disorders, 29,* 77–84.

Preus, A. (1996). Cluttering upgraded. *Journal of Fluency Disorders, 21,* 349–357.

Riley, G. D. (1994). *Stuttering severity instrument for children and adults* (3rd ed.). Austin, TX: PRO-ED.

Scaler Scott, K. (2002). Expediter strategies. Unpublished research.

Scaler Scott, K., Tetnowski, J. A., Roussel, N. C., & Flaitz, J. R. (in press). Impact of a pausing treatment strategy upon the speech of a clutterer-stutterer. *Proceedings of the First World Conference on Cluttering.* Razlog, Bulgaria.

Scott, K. S., Grossman, H. L., Abendroth, K. J., Tetnowski, J. A., & Damico, J. S. (2006). Asperger syndrome and attention deficit disorder: Clinical disfluency analysis. In J. Au-Yeung & M. M. Leahy (Eds.), Research, treatment, and self-help in fluency disorders: New horizons. *Proceedings of the Fifth World Congress on Fluency Disorders.* Dublin, Ireland: International Fluency Association.

Shriberg, L. D., Paul, R., McSweeny, J. L., Klin, A., Cohen, D. J., & Volkmar, F. R. (2001). Speech and prosody characteristics of adolescents and adults with high-functioning autism and Asperger syndrome. *Journal of Speech, Language, and Hearing Research, 44*, 1097–1115.

Singer, B. D., & Bashir, T. S. (1999). What are executive functions and self-regulation and what do they have to do with language-learning disorders? *Language, Speech and Hearing Services in Schools, 30*, 265–273.

St. Louis, K. O., Hinzman, A. R., & Hull, F. M. (1985). Studies of cluttering: Disfluency and language measures in young possible clutterers and stutterers. *Journal of Fluency Disorders, 10*, 151–172.

St. Louis, K. O., & Myers, F. L. (1995). Clinical management of cluttering. *Language Speech and Hearing Services in Schools, 26*, 187–195.

St. Louis, K. O., Myers, F. L., Bakker, K., & Raphael, L. J. (2007). Understanding and treating cluttering. In E. Conture & R. Curlee (Eds.), *Stuttering and related disorders of fluency* (3rd ed., pp. 297–325). New York: Thieme.

Szatmari, P. (1991). Asperger's syndrome: Diagnosis, treatment and outcome. *Psychiatric Clinics of North America, 14*, 81–92.

Tager-Flusberg, H. (1995). Dissociation in form and function in the acquisition of language by autistic children. In H. Tager-Flusberg (Ed.), *Constraints on language acquisition: Studies of atypical children* (pp. 175–194). Hillsdale, NJ: Erlbaum.

Thacker, R. C., & De Nil, L. F. (1996). Neurogenic cluttering. *Journal of Fluency Disorders, 21*, 227–238.

Van Borsel, J., & Vandermeulen, A. (in press). Cluttering and Down syndrome. *Folia Phoniatrica.*

Ward, D. (2004). Cluttering, speech rate and linguistic deficit: A case report. In A. Packman, A. Meltzer, & H. F. M. Peters (Eds.), Theory, therapy and research in fluency disorders. *Proceedings of the 4th World Congress on Fluency Disorders* (pp. 511–516), Nijmegan, Nijmegan University Press.

Ward, D. (2006). *Stuttering and cluttering: Frameworks for understanding and treatment.* New York: Psychology Press.

Weiss, D. A. (1964). *Cluttering.* Englewood Cliffs, NJ: Prentice Hall.

Yairi, E. (1996). Applications of disfluencies in measurements of stuttering. Letter to the Editor. *Journal of Speech and Hearing Research, 39*, 402–403.

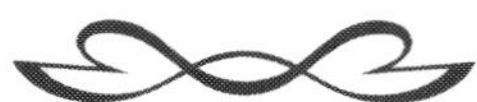

## HEARING

# CASE 31

# Sid: Using the Multisensory Syllabic Unit Approach to Treat the Fricative Productions of a Child with Moderate-to-Severe Hearing Loss

*Sheila Pratt*

## Conceptual Knowledge Areas

Hearing loss has a notable effect on speech development and production when the loss is congenital or occurs in early childhood. The treatment of speech impairment secondary to hearing loss typically is viewed from a sensory modality perspective—whether speech production should be stimulated and treated via the impaired auditory system or through multiple modalities, including the auditory system. Unisensory approaches argue for strengthening the auditory system, whereas multisensory approaches argue for training flexibility in access and use of the best available set of speech cues across modalities.

## Description of the Case

### Background Information

This report describes a child with a moderate-to-severe hearing loss who had difficulty with fricative production and was treated with the Multisensory Syllabic Unit Approach. The Multisensory Syllabic Unit Approach was first used at the Central Institute for the Deaf and described by Carhart (1947, 1963) and later by Silverman (1971). It was subsequently adapted and incorporated into other treatment approaches for children with speech impairment secondary to hearing loss.

#### History

Sid was a 6-year-old boy with a genetic bilateral hearing loss that was identified at 1 year of age, so by current standards he was considered late-identified (Yoshinaga-Itano, 2003). He was fitted bilaterally with behind-the-ear hearing aids at approximately 3 years of age, and enrolled in intervention through a local day-school program for deaf and hard-of-hearing children. He continued there through elementary school. The school used an auditory-oral approach to education and treatment, although students were allowed to use sign language in casual conversation outside the classroom. American Sign Language was Sid's native language in the home but he used oral English at school and when communicating with oral-aural communicators. During school his speech production was promoted through auditory stimulation and training, and not through direct speech production intervention.

### Reason for Referral

Sid was referred by his parents for treatment because he had difficulty producing fricatives and affricates. He also was not making substantive gains in speech intelligibility. There was concern that because of his age further gains in speech production skills would be limited without direct intervention.

### Findings of the Evaluation

Sid presented clear ear canals upon otoscopic inspection and normal tympanograms bilaterally (ASHA, 1997). Pure-tone thresholds revealed a moderate-to-severe sensorineural hearing loss in both ears (Figure 31.1). The hearing loss configuration was symmetrical across ears and relatively flat. Word recognition was measured with the Northwestern University-Children's Perception of Speech (Elliott & Katz, 1980a) presented at 30 dB HL. Performance was 82% correct in the right ear and 74% correct in the left. These results were consistent with his age and hearing loss severity, yet over 2 SD below that expected by normal-hearing children of the same age (Elliott & Katz, 1980b).

Sid's oral-aural language skills were consistent with his age and hearing loss but substantively delayed when compared to normal-hearing children. On the Peabody Picture Vocabulary Test-Revised (Dunn & Dunn, 1981) he produced a standard score of 59 and percentile rank of 1. On the Rhode Island Test of Language Structure (Engen & Engen, 1983), which was administered in oral English, his percentile rank was 49.2 when compared to children with hearing loss but < 1 when compared to normal-hearing children his age. With sign language considered, his mother reported that he was at age-level on the expressive and receptive language subtests of the Child Development Inventory (Ireton, 1992), as well as on the inventory overall. These results suggested that Sid's fundamental ability to comprehend and produce language was intact but that oral-aural language was constrained by his hearing loss.

Sid's auditory verbal memory span was assessed with the Digit Span subtest of the Wechsler Intelligence Scale for Children-Third Edition (Wechsler, 1991), and the results were

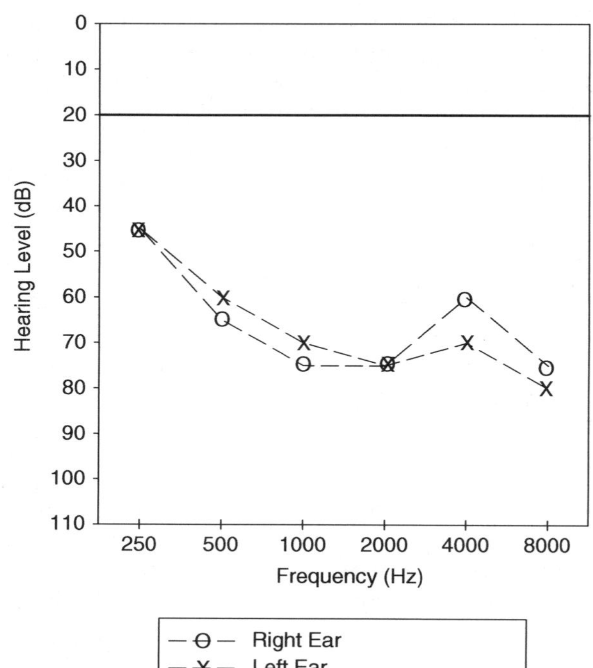


FIGURE 31.1 The Child's Unaided Pure-Tone Thresholds Obtained with Insert Earphones

borderline with a subtest scaled score of 5 (Kramer, 1993). This result was not unexpected because auditory working memory often is depressed in children with prelingual hearing loss and oral-aural language delay (Cleary, Pisoni, & Kirk, 2000; Dillon, Burkholder, Cleary, & Pisoni, 2004). In contrast, Sid's performance on the Motor-Free Visual Perception Test (Colarusso & Hammill, 1972) was at age-level (standard score of 95). These results confirmed that the impact of his hearing loss was limited to auditory dependent skills.

Consistent with this argument, Sid's speech production was impaired but his oral-motor function appeared to be normal. An oral peripheral examination revealed intact oral structures and normal movement and coordination for speech (Robbins & Klee, 1987). The Goldman-Fristoe Test of Articulation (Goldman & Fristoe, 1986) was administered at the single-word level and most of his errors were on fricative and affricate sounds, /r/, and blends. Fricatives and affricates in the final word position were typically omitted, while those in the initial and medial position were substituted with plosives of comparable place and voicing. For example, /f/ was replaced by /p/ and /v/ was replaced by /b/; /s/ was substituted with /t/ and /z/ was substituted with /d/. The /r/ sound was usually replaced with /w/ and most blends were reduced. Other speech sounds were correctly produced at the single word level. However, in conversational speech his consonant inventory primarily consisted of stops, nasals, and early emerging liquids and glides. Fricatives were globally affected and were either stopped or omitted. Affricates were omitted in conversation. In addition, some inconsistent voicing distortions (shifts toward the perceptual boundary) were common and indicated issues with coarticulatory timing. Voice quality, resonance, and prosody were normal in ongoing speech, which was somewhat surprising given the severity of the child's hearing loss. Single word intelligibility, as assessed with the CID Picture SPINE (Monsen, Moog, & Geers, 1988), was 60%, but in conversation Sid was understood most of the time, especially when he reduced his speaking rate. He was quite social and talkative, and his speech production problems did not appear to interfere substantially with casual communication with his peers and teachers in the school setting.

## Representation of the Problem at the Time of Evaluation

Sid presented a speech production disorder secondary to prelingual hearing loss that was characterized by omission of fricatives in the final word position, and the substitution of initial and medial fricatives with plosives. Affricates followed this same pattern in single words but tended to be omitted in all word positions in conversational speech. Of particular notice was the substitution of /f/ and /v/, because these sounds are highly visible continuants and typically produced correctly by children with moderate-to-severe hearing loss. With the mix of substitutions, omissions, and inconsistent voicing, it was difficult to determine whether the disorder was solely a phonological or a sensorimotor one. The consistent stopping of initial and medial fricatives was suggestive of a phonological disorder, but the omissions and inconsistent control of voicing was more characteristic of a sensorimotor disorder. It is likely that both levels were affected. A primary motor impairment was not indicated.

Sid's hearing loss also was associated with delayed auditory vocabulary and immature oral-aural language structure, both of which probably impacted speech and language intelligibility adversely, but manual communication skills were age-appropriate. As stated previously, auditory verbal memory span was borderline normal, and visual processing skills were typical for his age.

## Treatment Options Considered

### Well-Established Knowledge and Scientific Evidence

The nature and severity of speech impairments secondary to hearing loss in the pediatric population vary substantively across children. The variability largely relates to differences in hearing loss severity, age of identification and treatment, and the quality of treatment (Paatsch, Blamey, Sarant, & Bow, 2006). The impact of hearing loss on speech is most pronounced in children with profound and severe hearing losses, especially those children who are identified and enrolled into treatment after 6 months of age (Yoshinaga-Itano & Sedey, 1998). Profound and severe hearing losses in childhood can affect the entire speech production mechanism from respiration to coarticulation and prosody, but even children with mild-to-moderate hearing loss are at a risk for resonance and segmental speech problems (see Pratt & Tye-Murray, 2008).

Most children with hearing loss require some type of intervention in order to speak intelligibly and in a manner acceptable to the average listener. Intervention usually begins shortly after diagnosis and typically is a long-term process that continues through early childhood. Despite an acknowledged need, well-controlled studies documenting speech treatment effectiveness and efficacy are limited for this population. Little has been published on which behavioral treatment approaches work best for the range of speech impairments that occur in children with hearing loss. Nearly all speech treatment approaches used with children with hearing loss optimize the use of residual hearing and/or compensate for the hearing loss by using other sensory modalities for input and feedback (Pratt, 2005; Pratt & Tye-Murray, 2008). Concentrating on the auditory modality typically is preferred if the auditory system itself can be treated (i.e., sensory devices and auditory training) and sufficient sensory input and feedback can be made accessible. However, if children with hearing loss are unable to develop and interface with a complete internal auditory representation of speech, production will be impaired. As a result, a substantive number of children with hearing loss fail to develop normal phonological and sensorimotor speech production skills despite proper and early fitting of sensory aids and appropriate behavioral intervention (Blamey et al., 2001; Serry & Blamey, 1999, 2001; Uchanski & Geers, 2003). For some children, augmenting or supplementing speech information through other sensory modalities is required for speech skill acquisition or correction to occur. The visual modality frequently is used to provide supplementary sensory input and feedback during speech treatment, although this is not without controversy.

Ling (1976, 2002) and others have argued that nonauditory input and feedback, especially if artificial, can interfere with the retention and generalization of speech sound acquisition. Ling acknowledged that visual and other forms of nonauditory sensory information can benefit some children when initially learning to produce particular sounds, but that a dependency can develop. He warned that visual and other nonauditory cues and feedback should be withdrawn as quickly as possible once a child has acquired a sound. This argument has not been tested in children with hearing loss, but is supported by the motor-learning literature (Lintern,

Roscoe, & Sivier, 1990). During motor learning tasks, a dependency can result during practice as the artificial cues and feedback become a part of the motor memory and interfere with the weaker intrinsic cues of the target movement (Proteau & Cournoyer, 1990; Proteau, Marteniuk, Girouard, & Dugas, 1987). This dependence on nonintrinsic cues and feedback is particularly problematic when the task and feedback are simple and feedback is provided with every trial (Weinstein & Schmidt, 1990; Wulf, Shea, & Matschiner, 1998). Behaviors that are complex and have multiple characteristics, such as speech, might be less affected by feedback frequency.

In contrast, Carhart (1947, 1963) advocated teaching speech production to children with hearing impairment through a multisensory approach. He suggested speech production should be improved by optimizing auditory performance through auditory training and appropriate amplification, especially with children who have substantial residual hearing. However, Carhart also argued that children should be taught to focus on the face of speakers, first for gestural information and then speech articulation cues. Furthermore, kinesthetic and vibrotactile information should be integrated into speech production training to promote the development of self-monitoring. That is, children should be taught to monitor their speech production by how it sounds and by how it feels. Carhart's description of what has been referred to as the Multisensory Syllabic Unit Approach or the Traditional Approach was expanded by Silverman (1971). He included the use of other visual and tactile systems such as orthography, graphic displays, visual displays of acoustic signals, fingerspelling, cued speech, and tactile aids.

The Multisensory Syllabic Unit Approach is largely analytic. As its name implies, the basic unit of treatment is the syllable. Phonemes are taught in a predetermined sequence, with most children beginning with bilabial consonants in combination with mid and back vowels (Davis & Hardick, 1981, p. 272). During treatment, the visual cues and feedback typically associated with the targeted sounds are highlighted, as is other sensory information. More artificial information is added as needed. The targeted phonemes are taught first in isolation or consonant-vowel (CV) and vowel-consonant (VC) syllables. The training then advances to more complex syllable combinations such as CVC, CCVC, and CVCCC syllables. Although treatment starts at the syllable level, natural voice and prosody are promoted. However, prosody is directly treated in an analytic fashion once the children have acquired a sizable phoneme repertoire. Finally, the social act of speech, not the precise articulation of segments, is the ultimate goal of the approach, so children are encouraged to use newly acquired speech skills in context.

### Clinical Experiences

Previous work by the author has shown that visual information, such as visual feedback from computer-based feedback systems, improves the speech of children who have limited auditory function, although a large number of sessions are needed to reach criterion and for the behaviors to stabilize and generalize (Pratt, 2003, 2007; Pratt, Heintzelman, & Deming, 1993). Other investigators have observed similar findings (e.g., Dagenais, Critz-Crosby, Fletcher, & McCutcheon, 1994; Ertmer & Maki, 2000).

### Client Preferences

Sid and his parents did not have a preferred treatment approach and were comfortable with the treatment implemented. He was very willing to attend the sessions and was engaged in the treatment process.

## Course of Treatment

Sid was seen for individual treatment two times a week for approximately 30 minutes a session, with the sessions conducted at least two, but no more than five days apart. The treatment was conducted at his school by an ASHA-certified speech-language pathologist who had experience treating speech and language disorders in children who have hearing loss. A single-subject multiple-baseline design was used with /f/ (and later /s/) as the targeted sound in

CV syllables. The vowels were limited to /a/, /o/, /u/, and /i/. Probes of /f/ in CV syllables were used to monitor and document treatment effects. The criterion for acquisition was 80% correct production on the CV probes for four consecutive sessions. Also probed were /v/, /s/, and /z/ in CV syllables. These syllables were monitored to assess generalization to related sound and developmental effects. The production of /f/ and /v/ in words was probed to assess generalization to larger linguistic units. The words were probed by having Sid label pictures. All of the probes were conducted at the beginning of the subsequent session to document learning and retention from the previous treatment session.

The treatment was an adaptation of the Multisensory Syllabic Unit Approach and consisted of a multisensory syllabic imitation task preceded by an auditory identification task. The auditory identification task consisted of the clinician presenting the targeted sound or its common substitution in a CV syllable (e.g., /fo/ vs. /po/) to Sid live-voice but without visual lip cues. Sid was then asked to indicate by pointing to one of two letters whether the /f/ or /p/ sound was heard. This was followed by the clinician modeling the /f/ in the CV syllable combination for Sid while pointing to her lips. He was then required to produce the syllable. This sequence was completed 10 times for each of the CV combinations with the order of the combinations randomized for each session. Performance was judged online by the clinician as correct or incorrect, and feedback was provided by the clinician for both the identification and imitation tasks on 80% of the treatment trials. Sid did not receive any concurrent speech therapy while receiving this treatment.

## Analysis of Client's Response to Treatment

The treatment results were assessed visually by the clinician from graphic display of the data and with the *C*-statistic. Jones (2003) previously demonstrated that the *C*-statistic is a reasonable statistical test for assessing clinical treatment data that is serially dependent, especially when associated with a flat pretreatment baseline. The statistical analyses of the treatment and generalization results are displayed in Table 31.1. The judgments of the clinician agreed

TABLE 31.1 Tests of Treatment and Generalization Effects

| Effects | *C*-statistic | *z*-score | *p*-value |
|---|---|---|---|
| **Treatment** | | | |
| /f/ Treatment 1 | 0.554 | 3.507 | .001** |
| /f/ Treatment 2 | 0.655 | 4.095 | .001** |
| /s/ Treatment 2 | 0.816 | 5.716 | .001** |
| **Generalization of /f/ Treatment 1** | | | |
| /v/ CV | 0.363 | 2.439 | .007* |
| /s/ CV | 0.166 | 1.053 | .146 |
| /z/ CV | –0.043 | –0.287 | .612 |
| /f/ Words | 0.769 | 0.045 | .001** |
| /v/ Words | 0.626 | 3.865 | .001** |
| **Generalization of /f/ Treatment 2** | | | |
| /v/ CV | 0.657 | 4.361 | .001** |
| /s/ CV | 0.110 | 0.692 | .244 |
| /z/ CV | 0.029 | 0.194 | .422 |
| /f/ Words | 0.802 | 2.821 | .002* |
| /v/ Words | 0.742 | 4.580 | .001** |
| **Generalization of /s/ Treatment 2** | | | |
| /z/ CV | 0.694 | 4.505 | .001** |

Note: * $p \leq .01$

** $p \leq .001$

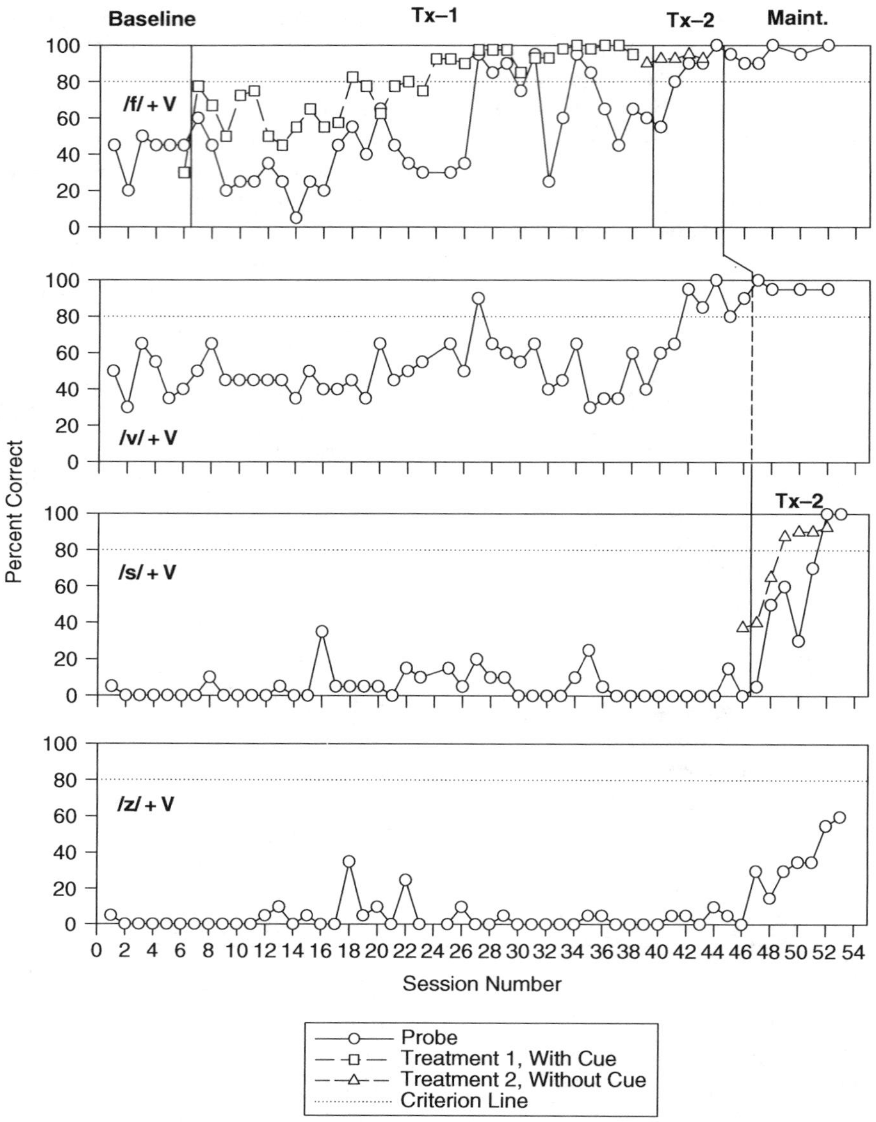


FIGURE 31.2 Treatment and Generalization Results at the CV Level

perfectly with the statistical results and are therefore not presented separately. Sid's auditory identification was 80 –100% correct after the first treatment session, so it will not be reported further.

The results of the treatment upon /f/ production in CV syllables are illustrated in Figure 31.2. The figure displays Sid's production accuracy for the treatment session and the probes collected during the following session. However, determination of treatment effects, generalization, and maintenance were based only on probe data (open circles). With the treatment, Sid appeared to acquire the /f/ sound but had difficulty stabilizing performance sufficiently to meet criterion. So, starting at session 39 it was decided to remove the finger pointing cue from the treatment. This was done because he appeared to focus excessively on the finger point and also because of cautions associated with using artificial visual cues (Ling, 1976, 2002). The removal of the finger point did facilitate stabilization of the /f/ production as well as generalization to the /v/ syllables (which met criterion without treatment) and /f/ and /v/ words. After reaching criterion, correct /f/ production maintained during the treatment of /s/ production. Although the treatment of /s/

was not completed due to the onset of Sid's summer break from school, it too showed a positive response to the treatment and generalization to /z/.

Despite the generalization of the treatment of /f/ to the production of /v/ in CV syllables (especially after removal of the finger cue), there was no generalization to /s/ and /z/ syllables, indicating that the effects of the treatment were not only limited to /f/ and /v/, but also that there was no general improvement in Sid's speech production that could be attributed to development or educational activities. That is, the initial flat /s/ and /z/ baselines supported the notion that the significant changes in /f/ and /v/ production were caused by the treatment and not by some other uncontrolled influence.

In addition to generalization at the CV level, the treatment of /f/ was associated with generalization to /f/ and /v/ at the CVC and multisyllabic word level (Figures 31.3 and 31.4). Somewhat surprising was that generalization to the word level was a bit more pronounced for the /v/ than the /f/ words. The /f/ words might have been more difficult linguistically or phonetically than the /v/ words. It also is possible that for Sid, producing a voiceless fricative at the word level was more difficult than producing a voiced fricative. It is not unusual for children with hearing loss to demonstrate difficulty turning the voice on and off in coordination with the upper airway articulators.

FIGURE 31.3 Generalization to /f/ in Words

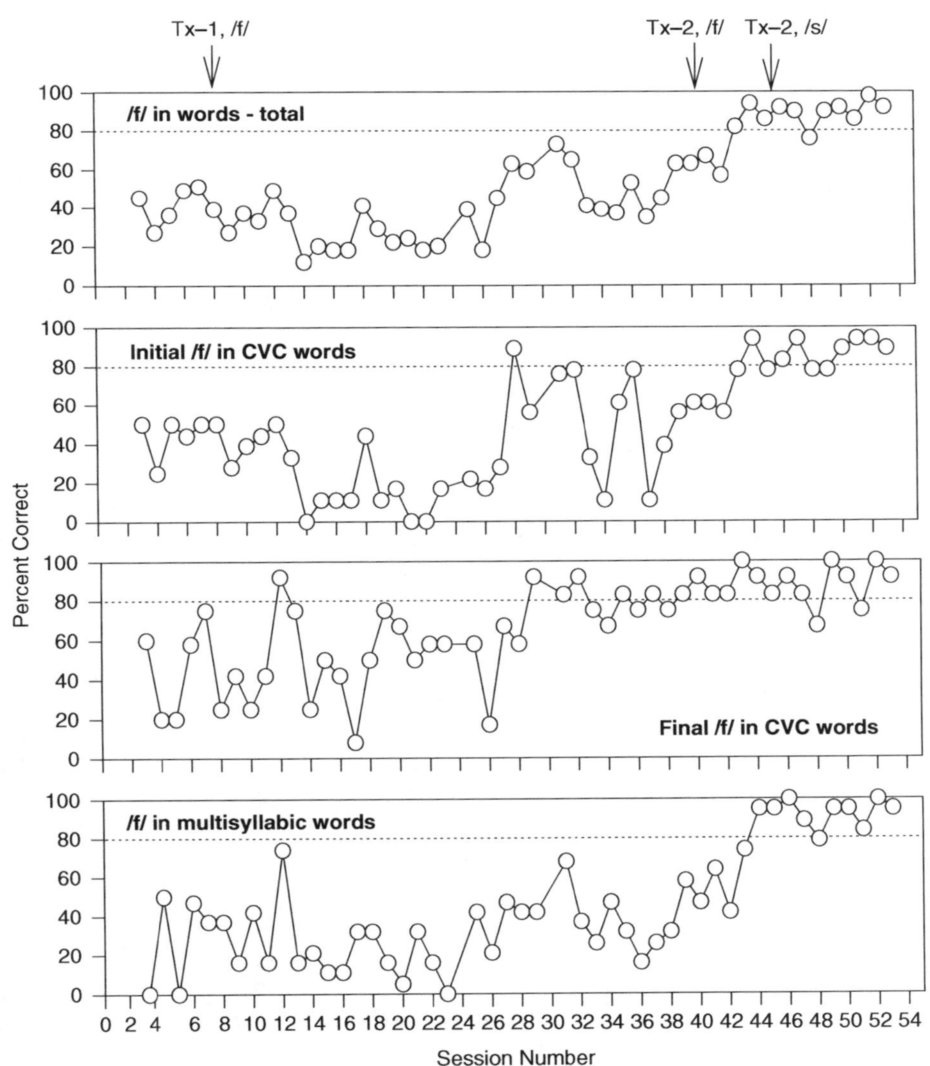

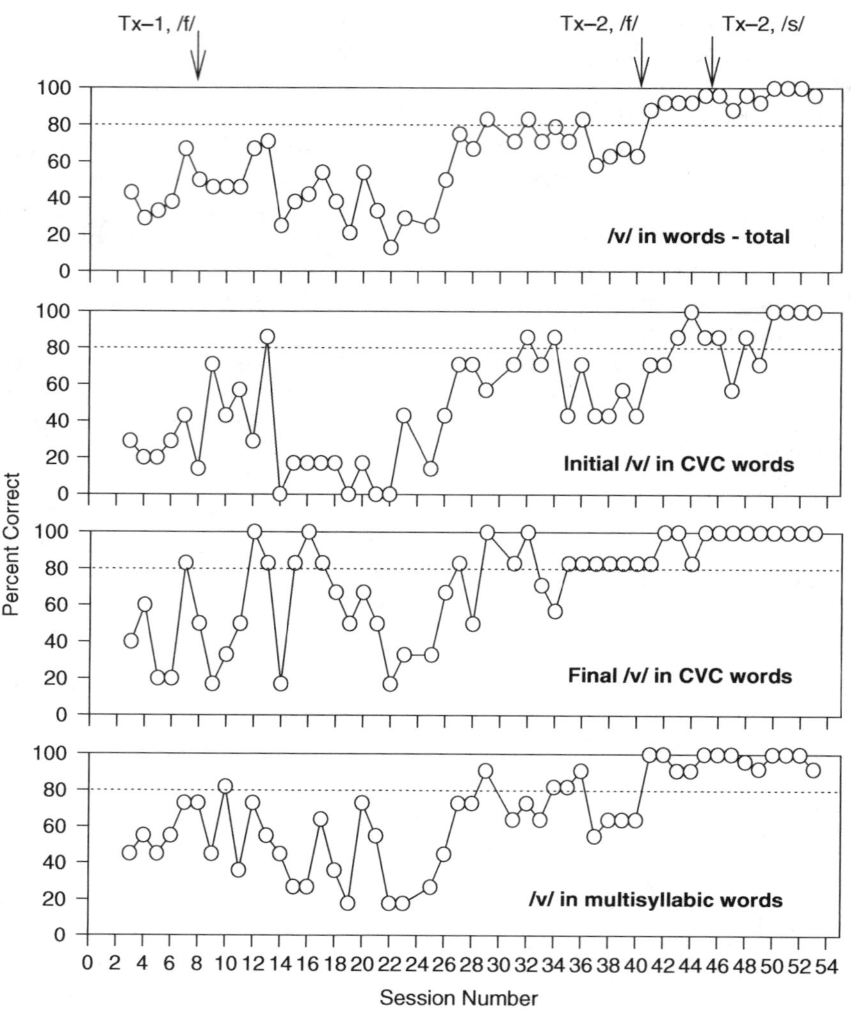


FIGURE 31.4 Generalization to /v/ in Words

Single word intelligibility on the CID Picture SPINE improved from 60% to 84% correct over the course of the treatment. Sid was producing /f/ and /v/ correctly in conversation and in the classroom by the time treatment was terminated. In addition, his teachers and parents expressed approval of his progress.

## Further Recommendations

The treatment produced a positive and significant response in Sid with substantive generalization to the voiced cognate and to more complex linguistic levels. It was concluded that with Sid in particular, a structured multisensory treatment approach at the syllabic level was effective, although the use of an artificial visual cue interfered with stabilization and generalization. The auditory task might have facilitated the treatment, but because he was near ceiling levels after one session, it was difficult to ascertain its role in the treatment. It was recommended that Sid continue speech treatment when school resumed.

## Author Note

This paper describes a real case. The treatment was provided gratis by the author and permission was previously obtained to present this case for instructive purposes. Identifiable information was excluded, and the child's name was changed to protect his identity.

## References


American Speech-Language-Hearing Association. (1997). *Guidelines for audiologic screening.* Available from www.asha.org/policy.

Blamey, P. J., et al. (2001). Relationships among speech perception, production, language, hearing loss, and age in children with impaired hearing. *Journal of Speech, Language, & Hearing Research, 44*, 264–285.

Carhart, R. (1947). Conservation of speech. In H. Davis (Ed.), *Hearing and deafness, a guide for laymen* (pp. 300–317). New York: Murray Hill Books.

Carhart, R. (1963). Conservation of speech. In H. Davis & S. R. Silverman (Eds.), *Hearing and deafness* (rev. ed., pp. 387–302). New York: Holt, Rinehart and Winston.

Cleary, M., Pisoni, D., & Kirk, K. I. (2000). Working memory spans as predictors of spoken word recognition and receptive vocabulary in children with cochlear implants. *Volta Review, 102*, 259–280.

Colarusso, R., & Hammill, D. (1972). *Motor-Free Visual Perception Test.* Novato, CA: Academic Therapy Publications.

Dagenais, P., Critz-Crosby, P., Fletcher, S., & McCutcheon, M. (1994). Comparing abilities of children with profound hearing impairments to learn consonants using electropalatography or traditional aural-oral techniques. *Journal of Speech and Hearing Research, 37*, 687–699.

Davis, J., & Hardick, E. (1981). *Rehabilitative audiology for children and adults.* New York: John Wiley & Sons.

Dillon, C. M., Burkholder, R. A., Cleary, M., & Pisoni, D. B. (2004). Nonword repetition by children with cochlear implants: Accuracy ratings from normal-hearing listeners. *Journal of Speech, Language, and Hearing Research, 47*, 1103–1116.

Dunn, L., & Dunn, L. (1981). *Peabody Picture Vocabulary Test-Revised.* Circle Pines, MN: American Guidance Service.

Elliott, L., & Katz, D. (1980a). *Northwestern University-Children's Perception of Speech.* St. Louis, MO: Auditec of St. Louis.

Elliott, L., & Katz, D. (1980b). *Development of a new children's test of speech discrimination.* St. Louis, MO: Auditec of St. Louis.

Engen, E., & Engen, T. (1983). *Rhode Island Test of Language Structure.* Austin, TX: PRO-ED.

Ertmer, D. J., & Maki, J. E. (2000). A comparison of speech training methods with deaf adolescents: Spectrographic versus noninstrumental instruction. *Journal of Speech, Language, and Hearing Research, 43*, 1509–1523.

Goldman, R., & Fristoe, M. (1986). *Goldman-Fristoe Test of Articulation.* Circle Pines, MN: American Guidance Service.

Ireton, H. (1992). *Child Development Inventory.* Minneapolis, MN: Behavior Science Systems.

Jones, W. P. (2003). Single-case time series with Bayesian analysis: A practitioner's guide. *Measurement and Evaluation in Counseling Development, 36*, 28–39.

Kramer, J. H. (1993). Interpretation of individual subtest scores on the WISC-III. *Psychological Assessment, 5*, 193–196.

Ling, D. (1976). *Speech and the hearing-impaired child: Theory and practice.* Washington, DC: A.G. Bell Association for the Deaf.

Ling, D. (2002). *Speech and the hearing-impaired child: Theory and practice* (2nd ed.). Washington, DC: A.G. Bell Association for the Deaf.

Lintern, G., Roscoe, S. N., & Sivier, J. (1990). Display principles, control dynamics, and environmental factors in pilot training and transfer. *Human Factors, 32*, 299–317.

Monsen, R., Moog, J., & Geers, A. (1988). *CID Picture SPINE.* St. Louis, MO: Central Institute for the Deaf.

Paatsch, L. E., Blamey, P. J., Sarant, J. Z., & Bow, C. P. (2006) The effects of speech production and vocabulary training on different components of spoken language performance. *Journal of Deaf Studies & Deaf Education, 11*, 39–55.

Pratt, S. R. (2003). Reducing voicing inconsistency in a child with severe hearing loss. *Journal of the Academy of Rehabilitative Audiology*, 36, 45–65.

Pratt, S. (2005). Aural habilitation update: The role of auditory feedback on speech production skills of infants and children with hearing loss. *ASHA Leader, 10*(4), 8–9, 32–33.

Pratt, S. (2007). Using electropalatographic feedback to treat the speech of a child with severe-to-profound hearing loss. *The Journal of Speech & Language Pathology—Applied Behavior Analysis, 2*, 213–237.

Pratt, S., Heintzelman, A., & Deming, S. (1993). The efficacy of using the IBM SpeechViewer Vowel Accuracy Module to treat young children with hearing impairment. *Journal of Speech and Hearing Research, 36*, 1063–1074.

Pratt, S. R., & Tye-Murray, N. (2008). Speech impairment secondary to hearing loss. In M. R. McNeil (Ed.), *Clinical management of sensorimotor speech disorders* (2nd ed., pp. 204–234). New York: Thieme Medical Publishers.

Proteau, L., & Cournoyer, L. (1990). Vision of the stylus in a manual aiming task: The

effects of practice. *Quarterly Journal of Experimental Psychology, 42B*, 811–828.
Proteau, L., Marteniuk, R. G., Girouard, Y., & Dugas, C. (1987). On the type of information used to control and learn an aiming movement after moderate and extensive training. *Human Movement Science, 6*, 181–199.
Robbins, J., & Klee, T. (1987). Clinical assessment of oropharyngeal motor development in young children. *Journal of Speech and Hearing Disorders, 52*, 271–277.
Serry, T. A., & Blamey, P. J. (1999). A 4-year investigation into phonetic inventory development in young cochlear implant users. *Journal of Speech, Language, and Hearing Research, 42*, 141–154.
Silverman, S. (1971). The education of deaf children. In L. E. Travis (Ed.), *Handbook of speech and language pathology* (pp. 399–430). Englewood Cliffs, NJ: Prentice Hall.
Wechsler, D. (1991). *Wechsler Intelligence Scale for Children-Third Edition.* San Antonio, TX: Psychological Corporation.
Weinstein, C. J., & Schmidt, R. A. (1990). Reducing frequency of knowledge of results enhances motor skill learning. *Journal of Experimental Psychology: Learning, Memory and Cognition, 16*, 677–691.
Wulf, G., Shea, C. H., & Matschiner, S. (1998). Frequent feedback enhances complex skill learning. *Journal of Motor Behavior, 30*, 180–192.
Uchanski, R. M., & Geers, A. E. (2003). Acoustic characteristics of the speech of young cochlear implant users: A comparison with normal-hearing age-mates. *Ear and Hearing, 24* (Suppl.), 90–105.
Yoshinaga-Itano, C. (2003). Early intervention after universal neonatal hearing screening: Impact on outcomes. *Mental Retardation & Developmental Disabilities Research Reviews, 9*, 252–266.
Yoshinaga-Itano, C., & Sedey, A. (1998). Early speech development in children who are deaf or hard of hearing: Interrelationships with language and hearing. *Volta Review, 100*, 181–211.

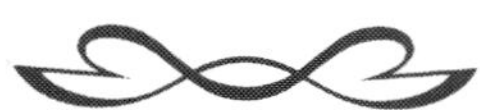

LANGUAGE

# CASE 32

# Jessica: A School-Age Child with Specific Language Impairment: A Case of Continuity

*Amy L. Weiss*

## Conceptual Knowledge Areas

To be well prepared to understand this case, it is necessary to have a thorough knowledge of the definition and characteristic profiles of children diagnosed with specific language impairment (SLI). Just as important as an understanding of what SLI is, is an appreciation of what it is not. That is, there are several etiological factors that disqualify children with language problems from being diagnosed with SLI (e.g., hearing impairment, mental retardation, autism). Most typical of individuals diagnosed with SLI is their difficulty in learning and consistently using the grammatical morphemes of their language, although disruptions in the learning and use of other language areas, both receptively and expressively, are frequently observed (Leonard, 1998). In addition, it is critical to understand that SLI is a disorder that may underlie both the learning of oral language comprehension and production and written language comprehension and production (i.e., reading and writing.) Given the bridging between oral and literate language learning, the speech-language pathologist (SLP) must also be well versed in foundations of typical development in both of these communication modes, and a number of texts do a fine job of providing this information (Stone, Silliman, Ehren, & Apel, 2004). In particular, see Paul (2007, pp. 433–442) for a very useful set of definitions delineating differences among learning disabilities, language-learning disabilities, reading disabilities, and dyslexia. In terms of course work, graduate students are advised to have completed courses in language development, language disorders in school-age children, assessment and diagnosis, as well as a course covering the principles of intervention prior to beginning practicum with a school-age client diagnosed with SLI. Further, because federal, state, and local jurisdictions mandate specific requirements for service delivery (e.g., eligibility, accountability), SLPs should frequently check appropriate websites for updated information (e.g., Department of Education, www.ed.gov; American Speech-Language-Hearing Association, www.asha.org).

## Description of the Case

### Background Information

Jessica was referred by her parents to a local university speech and hearing clinic that served as a training site for speech-language pathology students. At this time Jessica was 10 years, 3 months of age and enrolled in the fourth grade. The child's parents wanted to know why their daughter was struggling to keep up with her classmates in terms of academic achievement. More specifically, Jessica demonstrated deficient oral language skills characterized by immature grammar that immediately set her apart in conversations from her same-age peers. That is, she often omitted grammatical morphemes that were obligatory in the contexts used. For example, although Standard American English represented both home and school dialect for Jessica, she often omitted third person singular verb forms as in "Lester walk to school but Henry ride the bus." Her ability to follow multistep directions, necessary for successful completion of classroom tasks, was also well below grade-level expectations, perhaps indicating a concomitant comprehension problem. Likewise, when considering Jessica's ability to meet the reading and writing expectations for her grade, her parents reported their daughter demonstrated problems with decoding, reading comprehension, and spelling. Their daughter was reading at the second-grade level; "reading for pleasure" was not an activity that Jessica willingly selected.

When asked about Jessica's history of speech and language development, her parents noted that their daughter began receiving speech and language therapy at 28 months of age. Although some early progress had been made, they were certain that their child remained behind her classmates in her language competencies when she entered kindergarten. Jessica's parents appeared to have served as good advocates for their daughter's special needs both within their local school district and by securing outside service providers (e.g., a home-based tutor for reading). They explained that their concerns about Jessica's language had escalated over the last several years as literacy-learning expectations exponentially increased. Jessica's parents indicated that they had two goals for the present evaluation: They were seeking advice for ways to help their daughter catch up through working with her at home, and they also wanted recommendations for the appropriate services Jessica should be provided in school.

#### History Information

The following information was gleaned from a combination of direct interview and medical reports released to the clinic. Jessica was born at 36 weeks gestation, the product of an otherwise unremarkable pregnancy. During her first 2 years of life, Jessica was reported to have had frequent upper respiratory infections, occasionally accompanied by ear infections with mild hearing loss. A diagnosis of allergies to spring grasses and tree pollen was also made. Jessica's ear infections were typically treated with antibiotics; for her seasonal allergies an antihistamine that caused drowsiness was administered as needed. Although her early motor milestones appeared within the typical age-expected range, all of her speech and language milestones—both receptive and expressive—were delayed. Jessica was enrolled in an early intervention (EI) home program at her parents' insistence when she was 2 years, 4 months of age. At that time the most remarkable characteristic about Jessica's communication was the presence of multiple misarticulations that made the speech she did produce highly unintelligible. Once Jessica was no longer eligible for EI services, she was transitioned to speech therapy services through her local school district where she received once-weekly therapy for 30-minute sessions during the next 2 years of preschool. It was apparent from the parents' report that the focus of therapy was on increasing Jessica's intelligibility, although standardized testing indicated that along with multiple misarticulations, Jessica exhibited a more global deficit in both receptive and expressive language. During these 2 years Jessica also attended a mainstreamed preschool program 5 mornings each week. When Jessica entered kindergarten, she continued to receive one weekly, 30-minute session of speech therapy as well as one 30-minute session of resource support per week that targeted phonological awareness skills, according to Jessica's parents. When she entered first grade, her individual pull-out therapy was terminated (i.e., Jessica's speech sound production was judged to be intelligible enough for classroom success), although in second grade Jessica began receiving some additional reading support in the classroom. For the next 2 years, Jessica failed to meet eligibility requirements for SLP services in school; results of annual screenings conducted by the school's SLP demonstrated oral language skills that were within normal limits. Jessica has remained in the lowest achieving reading group in her class, and although the resource teacher works with this group twice weekly, the child's parents have not observed appreciable changes in their daughter's ability to understand what she has read. In third grade, a neighbor's daughter, who attended a local college and was completing a degree in special education, was hired by the family to help Jessica with her homework twice a week after school.

According to Jessica's mother, her daughter enjoys attending school despite the child's awareness that she is struggling academically. Jessica excels in both art class and physical education activities and was described by her mother as someone who enjoys interacting with her friends and is a bright, fun-loving, and social child. The mother did express her fear that Jessica's continued frustration with reading might result in her deciding not to continue her education beyond high school. It was clear to me that Jessica's parents were very concerned about the impact her current difficulties would have on her future endeavors.

## Reason for the Referral

It appeared that Jessica's mother's chief concern was that she did not understand why her daughter's problems with language and literacy learning had continued for so long in spite of the many years of therapy and other supports received. Because Jessica's language problems had transcended oral language understanding and production to reading and writing, her mother expressed urgency in finding an effective therapy program. Her mother also noted that Jessica appeared to be falling farther behind in her schoolwork. She stated that what was once a year's lag in development had become a two-year lag and that now her daughter was almost three years behind in reading comprehension.

In order to better describe Jessica's speech and language understanding and performance as well as investigate some of the underlying competencies that supported that performance, several standardized tests and two nonstandardized assessment tools were employed. More specifically, my intent was to be sure to cover the areas of language learning that supported reading and writing development. The following standardized tests were administered over two 90-minute evaluation sessions:

- Peabody Picture Vocabulary Test (Fourth Edition) (Dunn & Dunn, 2007) to evaluate the student's receptive vocabulary.
  - Jessica's receptive vocabulary as measured by the PPVT-4 (Form A) yielded a standard score of 75, placing her between 1 and 2 standard deviations below the mean for her age.
- Comprehensive Test of Phonological Processing for Ages 7 through 24 (Wagner, Torgesen, & Rashotte, 1999) to determine the student's ability to manipulate the phonological system as it may relate to literacy learning.
  - Only the seven core subtests were administered. Although Jessica's phonological awareness composite (i.e., elision and blending words subtests) placed her in the low-normal range, her phonological memory composite (i.e., memory for digits, nonword repetition subtests) and rapid naming composite (i.e., rapid digit naming and rapid letter naming subtests) both placed her performance in the lowest quartile when compared with other students her age.
- Test of Narrative Language (Gillam & Pearson, 2004) to determine both the student's comprehension (i.e., inferencing) and production of narrative text.
  - A comparison of Jessica's understanding and production of stories clearly showed that the student's performance in both modalities was significantly below age-expected levels. As the amount of support for storytelling diminished (i.e., retelling, to sequence pictures, to one stimulus picture), Jessica demonstrated increased difficulty including story grammar elements in a logical manner. Her ability to accurately respond to questions that evaluated her understanding of narratives consistently revealed problems with inferencing.
- Test for Auditory Comprehension of Language (Third Edition) (Carrow-Woolfolk, 1999) to evaluate the student's comprehension of grammatical morphemes and elaborated sentence types.
  - Scores for the vocabulary, grammatical morphemes, and elaborated phrases and sentences subtests consistently placed Jessica in the below-average range (standard scores ranged from 8 to 6).
- Comprehensive Assessment of Spoken Language for Ages 7 to 21 (Carrow-Woolfolk, 1999) to evaluate more advanced pragmatic, lexical, and syntactic language understanding and use.
  - The five core subtests appropriate for Jessica's chronological age (e.g., antonyms, syntax construction, paragraph comprehension, nonliteral language, pragmatic judgment) were administered. Jessica had the least difficulty providing opposites for the words in the antonyms subtest and the most difficulty with the pragmatic judgment task, often remaining silent when given the task prompt. With the exception of the antonym subtest, the remaining subtests placed Jessica in the lowest quartile of performance.
- A 100-utterance spontaneous language sample was also collected and subjected to Systematic Analysis of Language Transcripts (SALT) (Miller & Chapman, 2003).
  - Jessica was not easy to engage in conversation. Thus, the language sample used for analysis was pieced together from incidental language output gathered throughout the test sessions. Having noted this, the results of the language sample analysis should not be considered representative of her best language performance. However, the utterances that were collected substantiated the inconsistencies observed in Jessica's use of grammatical morphemes.
- To look at Jessica's written language competencies, she was asked to use the picture stimuli from Task 4 of the Test of Narrative Language (TNL) (Gillam & Pearson, 2004) to write a story.
  - This nonstandardized probe was administered approximately 30 minutes after the TNL was administered to prevent contamination of the results. It was difficult to motivate Jessica to attempt the story. She wrote one sentence for each picture, characterized by

frequent misspellings, use of nonspecific words (e.g., that, it), and lack of cohesion. It was not clear that Jessica was using the pictures to support a story with a beginning, a logical middle, and an end.

- Given Jessica's history of ear infections with documented episodes of hearing loss, information about her hearing status was sought before beginning an evaluation.
  - A hearing evaluation was scheduled just prior to the speech and language evaluation. The results demonstrated that her hearing thresholds were within normal limits bilaterally and tympanometry revealed normal middle ear pressure in both ears. There were no concerns about the child's peripheral hearing at the time of testing. Note that this evaluation did not include any tests specific to a central auditory processing evaluation.

## Findings of the Evaluation

### Observations

Jessica was compliant during both of the test sessions; although testing covered concepts that were clearly difficult for her, Jessica appeared to try her best. However, it was noted during the testing sessions that the she was reticent and reluctantly engaged in conversation with the examiner despite the use of a number of attractive and provocative materials. As had been stated by the child's mother, it was also the examiner's opinion that Jessica was acutely aware of her difficulties communicating.

### Interview Revelations

During the evaluation sessions, it was necessary to remind Jessica's mother several times that some of the material presented to her daughter would likely be too difficult for her to handle successfully. The child's mother expressed concern that repeated frustrations with testing would result in her daughter not wanting to continue trying her best. The examiner did not share this opinion.

## Representation of the Problem at the Time of Evaluation

Jessica's test results confirmed her mother's impression that Jessica did indeed have a significant delay in both age-expected receptive and expressive language competencies in the absence of any obvious cognitive deficit, peripheral hearing loss, social-emotional difficulties, or oral motor problems (i.e., there was no indication of either dysarthria or apraxia.) Given the absence of any disqualifying etiological factor, and the presence of multiple areas of language learning that were below age expectations, a working diagnosis of SLI was supported. In addition to the results gleaned from formalized testing, Jessica's long history of problems with speech and language learning pointed to a diagnosis of SLI. Although speech sound errors were discerned through testing and observation, they did not negatively affect Jessica's intelligibility. However, long-standing problems with the speech sound system may be indicative of a problem with phonological memory that can impact new word learning and word retrieval, concerns that are not foreign to many children with the diagnosis of SLI. In addition, the problems with the phonological processing component of language learning also would contribute to a diagnosis of dyslexia, a particular type of reading disability.

It appeared that Jessica was at risk for falling farther behind without a significant, team-based approach to working on her underlying language-learning issues. Although Jessica might not have qualified for speech and language services based on early oral language screening results, she did now as indicated by her test performance. In fact, given the student's poor reading performance and the long-standing nature of her difficulties, service delivery was felt to be a high priority. Her Individualized Education Plan (IEP) would specify the objectives, therapy approach, the intensity of the therapy received, and who would be providing the services. The plan was not only to recommend services but to provide some guidance about the type of program thought best given what was known about Jessica's needs and available therapy approaches.

## Treatment Options Considered

### Clinical Experiences

Clinical experiences led to the belief that any successful treatment program for Jessica would have to include all of the following features:

- Selection of specific goals for Jessica would need to be developmental, functional, and classroom curriculum based. The continuity between oral language understanding and production and successful literacy learning (i.e., learning to read and write) would have to be exploited.
- Both the classroom teacher and the school SLP would be included as integral parts of the planning and implementation of the treatment program to enhance carryover of language-learning strategies.
- Multiple modalities would be utilized to maximize learning.
- Evidence-based data supporting the success of the program for students with language-learning needs like Jessica's were available.

### Description of Two Approaches

Two specific treatment approaches for meeting Jessica's language-learning needs were selected for discussion because they could be compared across the four parameters delineated above. One of the treatment approaches considered was the Fast ForWord Language (FFWL) program as described by Agocs, Burns, De Ley, Miller, & Calhoun (2006). The second approach was the Writing Lab Approach (WLA) as described by Nelson and Van Meter (2006).

The FFWL program purports to be effective in improving the oral and written language competencies of children diagnosed with SLI by "attempting to remediate underlying cognitive and perceptual disorders and providing focused language stimulation" (Agocs et al., 2006, p. 478). The treatment is delivered via a set of software lessons in an intensive, computer-based program spanning as long as 2 months, 5 days per week for almost 2 hours per day. Specifically, the software is designed to provide extensive experience to improve three fundamental levels of receptive skills: the student's phoneme discrimination, speech perception, and finally listening comprehension competencies. Provision of the program requires provider education for the SLP, classroom teacher, and/or parent. The outcomes of studies assessing the effectiveness of FFWL have yielded mixed results. Several studies supported by the Scientific Learning Corporation, which publishes the FFWL software, have shown significantly improved scores for students on several standardized tests that are routinely used for evaluating receptive and expressive oral language as well as reading when they have completed this program. That is, the progress shown by the majority of children far surpassed what would have been expected in the time of treatment alone. Note that there was no control group used for the National Field Trial reported by Agocs et al. (2006). Other researchers (Agnew, Dorn, & Eden, 2004; Gillam et al., 2008; Pokorni, Worthington, & Jamison, 2004) have presented data suggesting that FFWL is not as globally effective in terms of population diagnosis or modalities improved as indicated in studies reported by Agocs and colleagues (2006).

The WLA, as described by Nelson and Van Meter (2006; see also Nelson, Bahr, & Van Meter, 2004), also involves the use of computer technology but is more integrated into the classroom curriculum than the FFWL program just described. This language program focuses on the enhancement of writing competencies by providing frequent opportunities to produce and receive feedback on written assignments. Although the products are primarily written, the authors note that the underlying targeted features of language development include both the oral and written modalities from words and sounds at the most basic level of discourse (p. 384). There are three main portions of the WLA: (1) writing process instruction, (2) computer support, and (3) inclusive instructional practices. Students are presented with writing projects that are "authentic" (p. 384). That is, a specific genre is practiced (e.g., narrative, expository) related to the intended audience of the product. Fulfillment of the program requires collaboration between SLPs and general and/or special education teachers as appropriate to ensure that the objectives are curriculum based.

Nelson and Van Meter (2006) claim that support for the WLA program can be traced to studies that have demonstrated the efficacy of "process-based approaches to writing" (p. 389) such as 4th-, 8th-, and 12th-grade students' results on the National Assessment of Educational Process exams taken in 1992, when the students who were most successful on the exam described their teachers as providing them with frequent writing exercises accompanied by practice with strategies that encouraged organization of writing products. The authors also cited work by MacArthur and colleagues (Graham, MacArthur, & Schwartz, 1995; MacArthur, Graham, & Schwartz, 1993; MacArthur, Schwartz, & Graham, 1991) demonstrating that computer-based and process instruction models of intervention were effective in improving the maturity of essays produced by the students in the experimental groups. Research aimed at evaluating the WLA is preliminary in nature (Nelson & Van Meter, 2003; Nelson, Van Meter, & Bahr, 2003) but reveals impressive growth for students with language-learning disabilities at all three levels of writing assessed: the word, sentence, and discourse. In addition, the majority of students made appreciable gains in written word production fluency and in production of well-formed stories, although less far-reaching were positive changes in the production of more complex sentences.

### Selection of Treatment Approach

It was decided that the WLA program was the better choice for Jessica for several reasons. First, the WLA program was founded on the principle of the continuity between oral and literate language. It is a flexible program. That is, the specific written projects can more easily be altered to fit within the boundaries of the student's curriculum (e.g., creating a diary as if written by an explorer to the New World would be appropriate for a social studies unit about explorers). Second, the WLA, by design, is implemented with collaboration between the SLP and the classroom teacher to maximize functionality and carryover. Third, the WLA includes a computer instructional portion but is not completely reliant upon this modality. Jessica most likely would benefit from inclusion of visual cuing (e.g., graphic organizers) in addition to activities based on computer instruction. Last, the evidence-based practice data for the WLA, although not completed as of this time, show at least as much promise as that for the FFWL approach. The foundational skills on which the program is based (e.g., the continuity between oral and literate language learning) are accepted as viable instructional principles.

Another important factor in the decision making was Jessica's parents' preferences to institute a program that kept their daughter as integrated within the general curriculum as possible. They expressed concerns about the time Jessica would miss from the general education curriculum if she were to begin the FFWL program. In addition, given that none of the SLPs in the school district had access to the FFWL program or training, they were concerned that adoption of the FFWL would result in a further delay in implementation of a new approach to teaching their daughter.

## Course of Treatment

The clinician was asked to work with the school in determining the treatment program to be implemented. After careful consideration, a consensus was reached on the WLA. According to Nelson and Van Meter (2006), implementation of the WLA requires that the SLP be involved in the daily, hour-long intervention sessions conducted in the classroom 2–3 times per week. In order to use the school SLP's time most beneficially, it was decided that the 7 children in the fourth grade who were in similar need of language-learning instruction/writing instruction would be assigned to meet together for 1 hour daily. The resource room teacher was designated as the expert who would be trained in the WLA model and would meet with the children; one of the three fourth-grade classroom teachers was always present, rotating through the program on a weekly basis. The school SLP also participated 3 times a week. All of the professionals met weekly to discuss goals, lesson plans, and the students' progress. Because the WLA approach was as new to the school personnel as it was to the fourth-grade students, everyone went through a period of adjustment. Fortunately, the elementary school had a strong history of administrative support for both continuing education and preparation time for its faculty, and thus the personnel involved had ample time to prepare what for them was a new service delivery model. The plan was to begin the program by November 1 and to informally assess the students' classroom performance six weeks prior to the beginning of the December break. Because all of the activities that were employed as part of the WLA could be very useful for enhancing the writing competencies of all of the children in the fourth grade, the teachers decided that after December they would make the program more inclusive and each of the fourth graders participated in the program at least once weekly. The role of the SLP was to provide additional assistance with feedback to Jessica and her cohorts and in analyzing the individual lessons to maximize the learning benefits for the children with IEPs. Jessica thrived in this environment.

## Analysis of the Client's Response to Intervention

According to her mother and the classroom teachers, Jessica enjoyed the activities planned for her and her group. Because of the care taken by the school personnel involved in the WLA to individualize the program for each of the students with IEPs, Jessica was provided with sufficient support to be successful most of the time. She appeared to gain confidence in her ability to complete the writing tasks presented. Jessica also became more willing to offer information in class. When the typical language-learners were incorporated into the WLA context, the teachers began to develop writing projects that fostered collaboration between Jessica and her classmates who were not having difficulty with language learning. The SLP facilitated these group endeavors to be certain that Jessica was not left out of the decision-making process. At the end of the school year, standardized testing revealed that Jessica had gained approximately one and one half grade levels in her reading and writing performance. There was also a notable change in the maturity of the sentences she produced in conversation. It appeared that the use of frequent orthographic cuing had made the presence of obligatory morphemes more salient to Jessica, and she was consistently including regular plurals, past tense verb forms, and third person singular verb forms, among other grammatical morphemes. The WLA had also had a positive effect on Jessica's vocabulary; it was noted by her classroom teacher that her use of nonspecific words had also noticeably diminished.

## Further Recommendations

As hoped, the WLA made an appreciable difference in providing Jessica the support she needed to learn the foundational skills for achieving grade-level reading and writing competencies. Her success in the WLA program substantiated the belief that Jessica's difficulty with the oral language modality was inextricably tied to her difficulties with reading and writing. At the next IEP meeting, the SLP suggested that Jessica receive an additional session per week of SLP services to specifically address some of her remaining problems with the formulation of complex sentence structures (e.g., adverbial clauses, noun + post modification).

## Author Note

Jessica's case study is not based on an actual client. Rather, her case represents a composite of several hundred school-age clients the author has worked with in more than 30 years as an SLP.

## References


Agnew, J., Dorn, C., & Eden, G. (2004). Effect of intensive training on auditory processing and reading skills. *Brain and Language, 88*, 21–25.

Agocs, M., Burns, M., De Ley, L., Miller, S., & Calhoun, B. (2006). Fast ForWord language. In R. McCauley & M. Fey (Eds.), *Treatment of language disorders in children* (pp. 471–508). Baltimore: Paul H. Brookes Publishing.

Carrow-Woolfolk, E. (1999). *Test for auditory comprehension of language*-3. Austin, TX: PRO-ED.

Carrow-Woolfolk, E. (1999). *Comprehensive assessment of spoken language.* Circle Pines, MN: American Guidance Service.

Dunn, L., & Dunn, L. (2007). *Peabody picture vocabulary test-IV.* Circle Pines, MN: American Guidance Service.

Gillam, R., Loeb, D., Hoffman, L., Bohman, T., Champlin, C., Thibodeau, L., et al. (2008). The efficacy of Fast ForWord language intervention in school-age children with language impairment: A randomized controlled trial. *Journal of Speech, Language, and Hearing Research, 51*, 97–119.

Gillam, R., & Pearson, N. (2004). *Test of narrative language.* Greenville, SC: Super Duper Publications.

Graham, S., MacArthur, C., & Schwartz, S. (1995). Effects of goal setting and procedural facilitation on the revising behavior and writing performance of students with writing and learning problems. *Journal of Educational Psychology, 87*, 230–240.

Leonard, L. (1998). *Children with specific language impairment.* Cambridge: MIT Press.

MacArthur, C., Graham, S., & Schwartz, S. (1993). Integrating strategy instruction and word processing into a process approach to writing instruction. *School Psychology Review, 22*, 671–681.

MacArthur, C., Schwartz, S., & Graham, S. (1991). Effects of a reciprocal peer revision strategy in special education classrooms. *Learning Disabilities Research and Practice, 6*, 201–210.

Miller, J., & Chapman, R. (2003). *SALT: Systematic analysis of language transcripts v. 8.* Madison, WI: Language Analysis Laboratory, Waisman Center, University of Wisconsin-Madison.

Nelson, N., Bahr, C., & Van Meter, A. (2004). *The writing lab approach to language instruction and intervention.* Baltimore: Paul H. Brookes Publishing.

Nelson, N., & Van Meter, A. (June, 2003). *Measuring written language abilities and change through the elementary years.* Poster presented at the Symposium for Research in Child Language Disorders, University of Wisconsin-Madison.

Nelson, N., & Van Meter, A. (2006). The writing lab approach for building language, literacy, and communication abilities (pp. 383–422). In R. McCauley & M. Fey (Eds.), *Treatment of language disorders in children.* Baltimore: Paul H. Brookes Publishing.

Nelson, N., Van Meter, A., & Bahr, C. (2003, July). *Written language development and writing lab instruction: Growth for students with and without language-learning difficulties.* Poster presented at the International Academy of Learning Disabilities, University of Wales, Bangor.

Paul, R. (2007). *Language disorders from infancy through adolescence* (3rd ed.). St. Louis: Mosby Elsevier.

Pokorni, J., Worthington, C., & Jamison, P. (2004). Phonological awareness intervention: Comparison of Fast ForWord, Earobics, and LIPS. *Journal of Educational Research, 97*, 147–157.

Stone, C., Silliman, E., Ehren, B., & Apel, K. (Eds.), (2004). *Handbook of language & literacy: Development and disorders.* New York: The Guilford Press.

Wagner, R., Torgesen, J., & Rashotte, C. (1999). *Comprehensive test of phonological processing (CTOPP).* Austin, TX: PRO-ED.

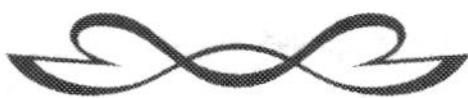



CASE 33

# Kevin: A School-Age Child with Behavior Disorders and Language-Learning Disabilities: Applying Contextualized Written Language and Behavioral Support Intervention

*Robyn A. Ziolkowski and Howard Goldstein*

## Conceptual Background

The co-occurrence of language disabilities and emotional and behavior disorders has been well documented in the research literature (e.g., Aram, Ekelman, & Nation, 1984; Beitchman, Wilson, Brownlie, Inglis, & Lancee, 1996; Benner, Nelson, & Epstein, 2002). Findings from a recent synthesis of emerging research indicates that approximately three out of four children (i.e., 71%) diagnosed with emotional and behavioral disabilities (EBDs) have significant receptive, expressive, and/or pragmatic language impairments (LIs), and one out of two children (57%) diagnosed with LI have also been identified as having EBD (Benner, et al., 2002). Moreover, in children with EBD, these language impairments are stable across age (Nelson, Benner, & Cheney, 2005).

In addition to the connection between LI and EBD, Beitchman and colleagues (1996) expanded this relation to include evidence of a joint association among LI, EBD, and learning disabilities. They found that children who demonstrated concomitant LI and psychiatric conditions also had school learning problems. In fact, research indicates that most children with EBD function below grade level when compared to peers without disabilities (Trout, Nordness, Pierce, & Epstein, 2003), have lower graduation rates, lower reading and math scores, and are less likely to attend postsecondary school (Kauffman, 2001). Many students with EBD become involved in criminal activity and are involved in the justice system at an early age (U.S. Department of Health and Human Services, 1999).

There is considerable consensus that language, reading, and behavioral deficits of students with EBD become harder to remediate as these children become older (Nelson, Brenner, Lane, & Smith, 2004). Of particular importance is to attend to the underlying skills and processes required for a student to become a better, more independent learner and to identify effective intervention strategies that can have an effect on the multiple deficit areas (Lovett et al., 2000). Speech-language pathologists (SLPs) who work with school-age children should be familiar with the ASHA (2001) guidelines for providing literacy-focused language intervention, understanding that interventions should focus on improved spoken and written language proficiency. Further, intervention objectives should be relevant to the expectations of the general education curriculum, including aligning literacy-focused language intervention goals to state and district achievement standards and benchmarks and to the district curriculum. Standards and benchmarks can be found by contacting state Department of Education offices or by simply perusing the state website. District information can be garnered by contacting the curriculum and instruction departments or on websites as well. One must keep in mind that standards and benchmarks are normative and are set for students with typically developing skills. They serve as guidelines for the skill sets that students should possess at a specific grade level.

Students with LI and EBD are at high risk for developing academic deficits, particularly in the area of written language (Snow, Griffin, & Burns, 1998). In fact, some students may appear to be fairly proficient in handwriting in earlier grades, but begin to experience difficulties as they progress into the later academic grades. These difficulties have been attributed to the increased complexity of the classroom content (Westby, 2004), the expectation to produce more complex written discourse (Scott, 2002), and the need to self-regulate, or independently manage their own learning and behavior (Zimmerman & Schunk, 2001).

In addition to language and academic difficulties, children with LI, reading disabilities (RD), and EBD typically exhibit delays in their ability to self-regulate (Westby, 2004). Zimmerman (1986) indicates that self-regulated learners are metacognitively, motivationally, and behaviorally active participants in their own learning process. Moreover, self-regulation contributes to one's systematic effort to direct thoughts, feelings, and actions toward the attainment of one's goals. Upper elementary students with EBD and LI often have difficulty organizing their time, completing assignments, and doing independent seat work. These students often hold negative opinions about themselves and their ability to gain control over their academic environment. It is difficult for these students to formulate, work toward, and attain goals. However, well-designed interventions can accommodate and support development of self-regulated learning (Harris & Graham, 1998). One area where extant literature has begun to support self-regulated strategy development for school-age students with EBD and LI is through improving literacy skills (Lane, Graham, Harris, & Weisenbach, 2006).

Students with EBD and LI who struggle academically often have depressed vocabulary levels when compared to peers without difficulties (Ebbers & Denton, 2008). Numerous encounters with new words facilitate greater word knowledge through these experiences (Nagy & Scott, 2000). However, students with literacy difficulties spend less time engaged in literacy activities, subsequently limiting encounters with new words and inhibiting their vocabulary growth (Baker, Simmons, & Kame'enui, 1998). Intervention researchers have developed a number of strategies to facilitate word learning, including (1) teaching word study strategies that fuse root words and affixes (Reed, 2008), (2) using semantic maps (Kim, Vaughn, Wanzek, & Wei, 2004), and (3) providing numerous exposures to the new word in different contexts (Beck, McKeown, and Kucan, 2002).

Children with LI and EBD also have difficulty with written language (Lane et al., 2006; Lane et al., 2008). The writing of these students typically contains more mechanical errors and is less expansive, coherent, and effective (Moxley, Lutz, Ahlborn, Boley, & Armstrong, 1995). These difficulties may exist secondary to students with disabilities engaging in writing tasks with little or no planning, limiting revisions to minor corrections, and having problems with punctuation, spelling, or handwriting (Gersten & Baker, 2001). Students with LI and EBD may increase their writing proficiency when taught in an explicit and direct manner using a basic framework of planning, writing, and revision as exemplified by the Self-Regulated Strategy Development (SRSD) approach (Lane et al., 2008).

The SRSD model (Graham & Harris, 1999) is an empirically validated instructional approach designed to improve students' strategic thought processes. It has been used to teach strategies for improving academic skills such as reading, writing, and math to students with attention-deficit/hyperactivity disorder (ADHD) or students with learning disabilities, and it appears to be a promising intervention for children with EBD (Lane et al., 2008). To date, more than 25 studies have been conducted using SRSD to teach planning and drafting strategies for narrative and expository text with strong treatment effects and maintenance of skills over time (Rogers & Graham, 2008). Students are taught self-regulatory strategies such as self-monitoring, goal setting, and self-instructions in conjunction with specific writing task strategies. These self-regulatory strategies help students manage any undesirable behaviors that interrupt task performance. The use of self-monitoring is very motivating because it provides a visual account or record of performance over time (Goddard & Sendi, 2008).

The following case study is a descriptive account of how the SLP can play a significant role in establishing and implementing a contextualized language and self-regulated writing intervention for a student diagnosed with LI and EBD.

## Description of the Case

### Background Information

Kevin was an 11.3-year-old Caucasian male student who had just completed the fourth grade. He presented with a history of oppositional defiant disorder (ODD), attention deficit/hyperactivity disorder (ADHD), receptive and expressive language impairment (specific language impairment, SLI), and a reading disability (RD) (American Psychiatric Association, 2000). He had just returned home after spending two weeks in a residential treatment center where he was receiving psychiatric intervention after threatening bodily harm to his previous fourth-grade teacher and running away on the last day of school. He was taking Ritalin for ADHD management and was enrolled in individual psychotherapy to develop effective anger management and daily coping skills. He had a history of explosive temper tantrums, active defiance, and refusal to comply with adult requests and rules. To avoid certain tasks, he would make deliberate attempts to get into trouble and annoy others around him. He often talked about "seeking" revenge when he became angry. Kevin lived with his maternal grandparents, who had been his primary caregivers and custodial guardians since he was 5 years old and his mother gave up her custodial rights due to ongoing substance abuse issues, resulting in social services intervention for neglect. Kevin's mother had minimal contact with him. Unfortunately, his grandparents were not able to provide much history on his development from birth to age 5 because of his mother's transient lifestyle. Kevin's father, an artist, died when he was an infant.

Kevin's psychiatrists referred him to the examiner in the summer between his fourth- and fifth-grade school years because of concerns that his language impairment and reading disability were contributing factors in the sudden exacerbation of his psychiatric condition. The report from the psychologist indicated that Kevin's nonverbal IQ was in the average range. History and background information were obtained from an in-depth interview with Kevin's grandparents and review of Kevin's medical records. Kevin was diagnosed with a receptive/expressive language disorder at 6 years of age and received ongoing language therapy through the school system provided by the speech-language pathologist. Kevin was retained in kindergarten secondary to not meeting school benchmarks and his grandparents' insistence. His reading disability was diagnosed at the end of his third-grade school year. Kevin also demonstrated difficulty with written language. At the end of the fourth grade he received grades of C, D, and F and did not pass the state competency exam for reading or writing. Even though Kevin did not meet the entire fourth-grade requirements for promotion, Kevin's school decided that he would be passed on to fifth grade based on his special education status. No additional information related to Kevin's current level of language or reading level was available from the school at the time of his referral.

Kevin's grandparents stated that Kevin was an exceptional artist and loved to draw people and animals. They indicated that the only time Kevin would complete his homework without arguing was when the teacher assigned some type of art project. In fact, many times they resorted to hiding Kevin's sketch paper, paints, and special drawing pencils so he would complete his homework.

## Assessments

Before intervention, baseline measures of receptive and expressive language, reading, and writing were obtained. The Clinical Evaluation of Language Fundamentals-4th Edition (Semel, Wiig, & Secord, 2003) was used to evaluate Kevin's receptive and expressive language. Kevin obtained a receptive language standard score of 72 and an expressive language standard score of 62. Overall, his total language standard score was 65, confirming a severe receptive/expressive language disorder. In addition, the Peabody Picture Vocabulary Test-III (PPVT-III; Dunn & Dunn, 1997) was administered to assess receptive vocabulary. Kevin's yielded a standard score of 80, indicating his receptive vocabulary was in the below-average range.

After completing the language assessments and reviewing the results, it appeared that Kevin's difficulty with writing might have been due to underlying language impairment. However, records could not be obtained from the school district in a timely manner, and as per his grandparents' report, district placement testing was completed during the last semester of Kevin's third-grade year. This would make the evaluation results over one year old. Subsequently, an informal writing assessment was administered.

### Writing

Prior to the assessment session, Kevin was asked to provide two handwritten writing samples. His grandparents were given written instructions for Kevin to complete two forms of writing, one story and one essay. As per his grandmother's report, Kevin refused to complete the written sample task and threatened to run away from home if they made him do it. After they provided a rationale for the assessment, Kevin complied with the request to complete a 3-minute Writing Curriculum-Based Measure (WCBM). A WCBM is a short, simple measure of writing skill that has been used successfully with students with and without disabilities (Watkinson & Lee, 1992). Students write for 3 minutes after they are given an instructional-level story starter. Several components of written communication can then be evaluated, including fluency, syntactic maturity, vocabulary, content, and conventions (e.g., spelling, punctuation, and capitalization) (Epsin, Scierka, Skare, & Halvorson, 1999). Norms are available for certain components such as Total Number of Words and Correct Writing Sequences (Powell-Smith & Shinn, 2004). In addition to the WCBM, Kevin completed a checklist of indicators assessing his ability to apply self-regulation strategies during the writing process (modified version of Harris and Graham's [1998] full checklist) and a Motivation to Write Survey tool developed by the clinician.

Kevin's timed WCBM samples were scored for (1) total number of words written (TWW), (2) total number of different words (NDW), (3) total number of correct writing sequences (CWS; i.e., "two adjacent, correctly spelled words that are acceptable within the context of the phrase to a native speaker of the English language" [Videen, Deno, & Martson, 1982]). Samples were further analyzed for syntax and vocabulary. Kevin's writing sample included: (1) short length for his age and grade level based on published norms from Merkin and colleagues (1981), (2) minimal diversity in word use or inclusion of novel vocabulary, (3) fragmented sentences and incorrect writing sequences. Punctuation and capitalization were judged as generally proficient, although errors in grammar use were observed. Kevin's writing scores were similar to the scores of a student in the middle of the third-grade school year. In addition, the checklist indicated that Kevin demonstrated poor self-regulation during the writing process, particularly in the areas of planning, organizing information, and revising. The motivational survey results were not surprising: Kevin had significantly depressed motivation to engage in and complete writing tasks.

### Hypothesis

It was clear from the outcome of the standardized language assessments that Kevin's receptive and expressive language difficulties, specifically in the areas of grammatical understanding, language production, and semantic understanding, were likely affecting his ability to perform proficiently in the areas of expressive language and writing. Further, it was hypothesized that Kevin's ability to self-regulate and apply metacognitive strategies when engaging in reading and writing tasks was decreased, and this difficulty was impacted further by his decreased motivational level. He would likely benefit from direct and explicit instruction aimed at increasing his ability to formulate and utilize more complex grammatical structures, improve his understanding of unknown vocabulary, and increase his written expression. It was hypothesized that Kevin's ability to self-regulate would improve if he could effectively implement self-regulating strategies while engaging in language formulation and written expression tasks, such as planning, organizing, and revising written material. Likewise, intrinsic motivation to engage in these tasks would likely increase if Kevin could monitor his own progress and visually determine that his efforts were successful.

## Treatment Options

Three different treatment options were considered and discussed with Kevin's grandparents and with Kevin. All of the options were based on research found to be effective for children with EBD, LI, and RD. Two of these options incorporated the same treatment goals (stated above); however, the instructional delivery and session time differed.

### Option 1: Individualized Treatment

The first treatment option was to begin individualized treatment specific for Kevin's language impairment and difficulties with writing. Intervention would utilize direct and explicit instruction to increase grammar and vocabulary and elements of SRSD to increase written language. Weekly data would be taken and ongoing intervention goals would be determined by data outcomes. Kevin would be seen in 2 individual hour-long treatment sessions for 10 weeks, for a total of 20 hours of intervention. The advantages of this treatment option included individualized attention, ongoing assessment for treatment planning, and convenient session blocks for the grandparents. The greatest disadvantage of this treatment plan was that Kevin would not have multiple opportunities to engage in collaborative learning with fellow students with the expected outcome of improved social and emotional skills.

### Option 2: Intensive Small Group

The second treatment option considered was in an intensive small group (i.e., 4 students) program for school-age students, all of whom were diagnosed with EBD. Programming would be designed to develop literate language skills within purposeful academic contexts and, in addition to the self-regulation component, would focus on developing appropriate peer relationships and social skills. Explicit/direct intervention, small group instruction, positive emotional support, and repeated practice has led to powerful student outcomes (Foorman & Torgesen, 2001) and would be incorporated into the planning of this group and implemented in a strategic manner that responded to Kevin's language level, reading level, and EBD needs. Weekly data would be taken and ongoing intervention goals determined by data outcomes. The group would meet for 90 minutes 3 times a week for 10 weeks, for a total of 45 hours of intervention. The advantages of this option included the small group format, with embedded social and emotional learning opportunities. Further, Kevin would be engaged in practice with peers as opposed to just the clinician. The disadvantage was that Kevin's behavior problems might prevent his full participation.

### Option 3: Consultation and Home-Based Intervention

The third treatment option considered was a combination of consultation and home-based intervention using the home computer. It was proposed that Kevin's grandparents would consult with the clinician once every week to review the previous week's outcomes, preview the coming week's instruction, and complete a weekly WCBM. Kevin would independently work on his writing, grammar, and vocabulary goals via the computer. The clinician would give the grandparents a series of interventions to be completed during the week. Although this model has not been validated for teaching SRSD, utilizing word processing has been shown to have moderate effects on writing outcomes (see Bangert-Drowns, 1993) and is a recommended strategy for students with ADHD (Simonson, Fairbanks, Briesch, Myers, & Sugai, 2008). The recommended instructional time for this model was 3 times per week for half an hour via computer for 10 weeks, for a total of 15 hours of instruction. The advantages of this program were minimal: it was convenient for Kevin's grandparents. The disadvantages included potential poor home participation and follow-through with minimal scaffolding support and social encouragement during intervention.

Kevin's grandparents chose the second option (i.e., small group) based on the premise that he would be able to interact and learn with peers his own age. They felt that Kevin's challenging behaviors would be less likely to occur in the presence of a peer group and that this option would be the most motivating to Kevin in the long run. Kevin indicated that he "didn't care one way or the other because either way he would not do anything anyway."

## Intervention Approach and Activities

### Developing Treatment Goals

Kevin's school district website was reviewed and language, reading, and writing content standards and benchmarks and curriculum matrix were easily obtained for intervention goal planning. The following content standards were incorporated: "Students write and speak for a variety of purposes"; "Students write and speak using formal grammar, usage, sentence structure, punctuation, capitalization, and spelling"; and "Students apply thinking skills to their reading, writing, speaking, listening, and viewing." Third-grade and fourth-grade curriculum map goals were utilized secondary to Kevin's language and writing assessment results that indicated he demonstrated difficulty with many of the skill areas targeted. Intervention was planned to include the following treatment goals: (1) Increase production and application of more complex grammatical forms, focusing on those targets that would support growth in Kevin's writing; (2) increase understanding and use of novel vocabulary, including recognizing meaning of select prefixes and suffixes; (3) improve written expression in TWW (baseline = 39 words), NDW (baseline = 17 words), and CWS (baseline = 23) when writing narratives; (4) independently incorporate self-regulating strategies during each stage of writing (criterion for each stage = 5 based on self-reported checklist). Further, the clinician would be able to clearly delineate the main idea and supporting details and elements of story grammar.

### Developing the Therapeutic Community

On the first day of intervention, students were introduced to each other and intervention commenced. Kevin and the other three group members created a series of rules and group expectations that the small group would abide by and named the expectations "The Cooperation Code." The Cooperation Code was posted in the intervention area and systematically reviewed by the students at each session. Student and clinician roles and responsibilities were clearly defined, as were the cooperative learning procedures (i.e., interactive dialogue procedures such as turn-taking and asking for help) and the specific negotiating actions that were to be implemented when group members did not agree. This type of behavioral management strategy has been shown to decrease off-task behavior and increase academic engagement, leadership, and conflict resolution (see Simonsen et al., 2008). Further, the clinician and group members agreed to use positive statements and praise during interactions, including when feeling discouraged or unsuccessful. Kevin did not demonstrate any challenging behavior and fully participated. The students appeared to enjoy setting up their own therapy "community."

The students were also expected to develop their own management hierarchy related to how the independent practice center would run. The students decided to create a leadership role and determined that "what the boss says goes." This role was to be rotated each week so each student had the opportunity to be "the boss." This strategy appeared to be a positive motivator for group participation as well as a facilitator of self-regulated behavior when in the boss role. The leadership rules became part of the Cooperation Code.

### Self-Monitoring

Kevin (and his group members) completed one baseline assessment at their first evaluation appointment. To determine whether this baseline measure was stable, three more 3-minute samples were completed. On the first day of intervention, the self-monitoring strategy was introduced. Kevin and his fellow group members learned how to count and graph the Total Words Written (TWW) and the Number of Different Words (NDW). Procedures used were modeled after Goddand and Sendi (2008), who found significant increases in writing quantity and quality after students began self-monitoring. Students would then graph their own data from the WCBM on the TWW and NDW that were administered at the end of every week.

### General Intervention Procedures

Students with EBD appear to require increased structure, minimal distractions, decreased transition time, and active engagement with multiple opportunities to respond to promote academic and social behaviors (Simonson et al., 2008). Subsequently, the structure of the therapy session was consistent and, although the content and intervention targets were data driven, the form of delivery did not change for the 10 weeks. Separate "centers" were developed in order to structure each intervention component. Centers ran as follows: (1) 2 minutes for reviewing rules and garnering materials, (2) 15 minutes of direct grammar and vocabulary instruction, (3) 13 minutes of partner pairs for reviewing vocabulary words and practicing newly learned grammatical forms, (4) 5 minutes for planning, (5) 10 minutes for organizing, (6) 15 minutes for writing (varied among direct clinician instructional time, collaborative peer work, independent work), (7) 15 minutes for revising (varied among direct clinician instructional time, collaborative peer work, independent work), (8) 10 minutes for drawing illustrations to complete the narrative, and (9) 5 minutes for wrap-up. The centers were timed with a 2-minute warning for transitions between the 8 phases.

Based on recommendations from extant research, the following instructional components were implemented during the intervention sessions: (1) reviews of previously covered material, (2) clearly stated purpose of the new lesson, (3) explicit and direct strategy instruction, (4) active modeling, (5) scaffolding of student responses, (6) guided practice in collaborative groups or pairs, (7) motivating and culturally sensitive corrective feedback, and (8) practice to mastery (Swanson, 1999).

Strategies were first introduced via direct, explicit instruction and supported through clinician models. The students were required to attempt the strategies presented with clinician support. The self-monitoring data were used to determine when the students required less support. As the students demonstrated increased proficiency, the level of support was decreased.

### Strategic Programming

The program was designed to address goals in a comprehensive manner. Intervention was delivered in units. The unit components were thoughtfully chosen so the grammar/vocabulary elements would be utilized and included in the writing product.

Each unit was comprised of the following components:

1. A theme intended to target a social emotional area (e.g., making friends)
2. A story starter that was tied to the theme and would guide the choice of grammar and vocabulary targets (e.g., One fine day, ____________ )
3. Grammar targets (examples):
   a. Adjectives (bright, sunny, dark, gloomy)
   b. Adverbs (quickly, tearfully, happily)

c. Auxiliary verbs (are, will, have, has, can, does)
d. Homophones (their, there, they're)
e. Cohesive units (and, but, also, even though)
f. Prefix (re-)
g. Simple vs. compound sentences

4. Vocabulary: words that assist with providing rich, colorful, accurate, and precise language and descriptions (e.g., pal [n], enemy [n], respect [v], entice [v], loyal [a], reluctant [a])

## Task-Specific Strategy for Planning and Writing

The "3-5-3" model of story writing, a modified version of the Think, Plan, and Write—SPACE approach (Graham & Harris, 1999), was introduced and utilized over the course of the 10 weeks. It is based on the SRSD model (Graham & Harris, 1993), which incorporates six stages of instruction that can be reordered, combined, revisited, or modified if required by the students' individualized needs. These stages are *develop background knowledge, discuss it, model it, memorize it, support it,* and *independent performance.* Each will be noted as it occurs during the following instructional sequence for the 3-5-3 model of writing. (In addition to the Think, Plan, and Write—SPACE approach, De La Paz [1999] has developed an empirically supported approach called PLAN—WRITE as well as DARE—STOP [De La Paz & Graham, 1997] for essay construction.)

***Develop Background Knowledge*** During the first session, the purpose of the small group intervention and potential outcomes were discussed with Kevin and the other group members. Each group member provided a reason for becoming a better writer (e.g., to pass tests, to get better grades, to earn my art supplies back, so I can go to the sixth grade). Each reason was written on construction paper and posted to serve as a reminder of their personal goals.

***Discuss It*** Next, the clinician discussed what mnemonics are and why it is important for Kevin to apply these strategies to his writing. The clinician introduced the 3-5-3 model as the steps needed to construct a well-written story. The strategies were introduced as follows:

1. ***Prompt***—Pay attention to the prompt! Underline it. Is this story going to be funny? Happy? Scary?
2. ***Plan***—Visualize! Brainstorm! Who is the main character? What are some of the attributes you want to make sure the reader understands? What is the setting? What is the action or problem in the story? What are the consequences? How did the character feel?
3. ***Put (in order)***—Visualize what happens first.

Step 5 included the 5 elements of story grammar. SPACE was described to Kevin as the time to write his ideas for the most common or basic parts of a story. After each part was defined, as suggested by Graham and Harris (1999), the clinician and the group went through numerous picture books and short stories to learn how to identify these elements in well-known stories. The students were taught how to visualize as well as to brainstorm when thinking about ideas that fit into the SPACE elements. The students were taught to write all of the elements using the SPACE acronym. The strategies were introduced as follows:

1. ***Setting***—the character(s), place, and time
2. ***Problem***—the problem or conflict faced by the main character
3. ***Action***—the actions or events the main character completes in order to overcome the problem
4. ***Consequence***—the resolution or consequences of the actions taken by the main character
5. ***Emotions***—the feelings of the characters in the story

The final step in the 3-5-3 model of story writing was described to Kevin as the time to write and create the story. The clinician and Kevin discussed how to create the whole story in the mind as if it were a movie, to use a graphic organizer if needed, and then to write it down to ensure all the SPACE elements were included. Finally, the clinician discussed how Kevin needed to go back into the story to look for the elements of grammar and the vocabulary words previously taught to see if they were included. The strategies were introduced as follows:

1. ***Create***—the story on paper
2. ***Count***—the new vocabulary words and grammar that were learned and ask, "Are all of the elements of story grammar included?"
3. ***Create again***—another version. Revise—Make sure elements of story grammar are clear; include more words; elaborate and expand on what is already written. Can you sequence the story in frames? What happened first, second, next, and then last?

***Model It*** The clinician used the 3-5-3 model for writing by implementing each strategy using a story from one of the picture books used. Kevin was shown how to begin writing the story on paper after he visualized the complete story sequence in his mind. The clinician then modeled the self-monitoring process and charted the TWW.

***Memorize It*** Kevin and the other students put on a presentation for their grandparents/parents, modeling the different components of the 3-5-3 model. The family members were informed that each student must memorize the strategies used in the model, including the mnemonics, and that this was very important to the group's success. Kevin's grandparents agreed to help Kevin memorize the strategies. During the presentation, Kevin appeared very proud after his grandfather indicated that he (i.e., the grandfather) "was learning a thing or two about writing too."

***Support It*** Kevin demonstrated full awareness of the 3-5-3 strategies after the first two weeks. He did not require support to verbally state the steps; however, he did require ongoing support to write all of the SPACE elements during implementation. He wanted to skip this step and just write his story. The importance of clearly defining each story grammar piece before composing the full story was discussed. At the end of each intervention week, Kevin's progress was monitored using the 3-minute WCBM. He charted his own progress at the end of each week. After the first few times, Kevin became independent at charting and proudly showed his scores to his grandparents.

***Independent Performance*** To help facilitate independent use of the new grammatical elements and vocabulary learned, a word wall was developed and served as a visual prompt during the first 4 weeks of intervention. This prompt was then faded in the fifth week and totally removed by the sixth week. When the word wall was taken down, Kevin developed a personal goal, which was to include at least 5 different, newly learned grammatical elements in his weekly WCBM. To facilitate this, he made up a rap that contained all of the new words learned during the grammar/vocabulary center. This caught on quickly, and Kevin and the group members took this approach further and made up a rap that included the 3-5-3 strategies. Each week, during the independent learning center, Kevin and the other group members created a new rap that incorporated the 3-5-3 elements and the new grammar and vocabulary. It was clear that they were utilizing this strategy independently during their writing; each was observed quietly restating key elements (i.e., rapping) during the 3-minute weekly CBM.

## Peer Revising Strategy

Prior to participation in the revising center, Kevin and the other students were taught how to provide reciprocal peer revisions (MacArthur, Schwartz, & Graham, 1991). To aid in this process, they were given a checklist and a list of specific feedback messages. After 4 weeks, the list was faded out and the students completed peer feedback without the visual aid but with careful ongoing monitoring by the clinician. The revising strategy helped Kevin develop his ability to monitor others' written products, and subsequently he became more proficient at revising his own work. In addition, Kevin learned appropriate ways to deliver constructive criticism and how to incorporate others' feedback into his work.

## Intervention Outcomes

The activities and procedures implemented in this intensive intervention program appeared to advance Kevin's understanding and use of specific strategies when engaged in the writing process. Kevin was highly responsive to the intervention as evidenced by the postintervention scores. Postintervention was measured by another series (i.e., 3) of 3-minute WCBMs. During baseline, it was determined that Kevin's stories were incomplete and brief. After 10 weeks of intervention, the number of total words written increased from baseline mean of 37 words to postintervention of 48 words; this brought Kevin close to the fifth-grade norm of 49 (Mirkin et al., 1981). Kevin also increased the number of different words from baseline mean of 17 to postintervention of 25 words. The number of correct writing sequences increased from baseline mean of 23 to postintervention of 49, which indicated Kevin was beginning to close the gap to the fifth grade norm of 58 (Powell-Smith & Shinn, 2004). In addition, Kevin demonstrated a positive change in the number of story grammar elements from a mean of 2 in baseline (i.e., setting and problem) to including all 5. In addition, his 3 WCBMs contained clearly delineated main ideas. Further, he demonstrated increased use of auxiliary verbs, adjectives, and adverbs and was utilizing cohesive units correctly in his final stories. Although growth was observed in the use of novel vocabulary, Kevin did not demonstrate increased recognition of select prefixes and suffixes. The clinician was able to determine that Kevin was independently incorporating self-regulating strategies during writing by readministering the self-report checklist, and an increase in Kevin's motivation to write was evident based on clinician observation of Kevin's active engagement in the writing process and independent implementation of the 3-5-3 rap. This observation also was supported through comments and statements made by Kevin's grandparents, including that Kevin had started "writing some books at home."

Kevin's progress highlights the positive effect of intervention that incorporates self-regulated learning strategies into contextualized intervention planning for a child diagnosed with language-learning disabilities and EBD. Within a relatively brief amount of time, Kevin made significant growth in his writing abilities, as well as in his use of novel vocabulary and grammar in his writing. The behavioral and instructional principles applied to the intervention program represented strategies known to aid in increasing on-task behavior and student learning (Swanson, 1999). Direct, explicit instruction was provided in a highly concentrated manner with many opportunities for the students to engage and respond. Learning was based on modeling and scaffolding of new strategies and active employment of the SRSD model, including self-monitoring.

The assessment and current intervention approach used in this case study was implemented in a manner that reflected current research in writing instruction. Clinicians who practice in schools and clinic settings can utilize this case study as a model for intervening effectively with students who have language-learning disabilities, or as in Kevin's case, both language-learning disabilities and emotional behavior disorders.

Kevin will be attending a new elementary school in the fall secondary to the threat against his previous fourth-grade teacher. The school district has inclusive classrooms in place, and Kevin will be served in a general education classroom with support from the school psychologist, counselor, special education teacher, and the speech-language pathologist. The school SLP is excited to continue with Kevin's current programming.

## Author Note

Kevin is a fictional school-age client who was used to represent a student with a dual diagnosis of language impairment and emotional behavior disorder. Further depicted is the expected course of treatment and recovery for written language proficiency when taught in an explicit and direct manner utilizing strategic language instruction combined with the Self-Regulated Strategy Development approach.

## References


American Psychiatric Association. (2000). *Diagnostic and statistical manual of mental disorders* (4th ed., text rev.). Washington, DC: Author.

American Speech-Language-Hearing Association. (2001). *Roles and responsibilities of Speech-language pathologists with respect to reading and writing in children and adolescents* [Position statement]. Available from http://www.asha.org/docs/html/PS2001-00104.html.

Aram, D. M., Ekelman, B. L., & Nation, J. E. (1984). Preschoolers with language disorders: 10 years later. *Journal of Speech and Hearing Research, 22*, 232–243.

Baker, S. K., Simmons, D. C., & Kame'enui, E. J. (1998). Vocabulary acquisition: Instruction and curricular basics and implications. In D. C. Simmons & E. J. Kame'enui (Eds.), What reading research tells us about children with diverse learning needs: Bases and basics (pp. 219–238). Mahwah, NJ: Erlbaum.

Bangert-Drowns, R. (1993). The word processor as an instructional tool: A meta-analysis of word processing in writing instruction. *Review of Educational Research, 63*, 69–93.

Beck, I. L., McKeown, M. G., & Kucan, L. (2002). *Bringing words to life: Robust vocabulary instruction.* New York: Guilford.

Beitchman, J. H., Wilson, B., Brownlie, E. B., Inglis, A., & Lancee, W. (1996). Long-term consistency in speech/language profiles: II. Behavioral, emotional, and social outcomes. *Journal of American Academy of Child and Adolescent Psychiatry, 35,* 804–814.

Benner, G. J., Nelson, J. R., & Epstein, M. H. (2002). The language skills of children with emotional and behavioral disorders: A review of the literature. *Journal of Emotional and Behavioral Disorders, 10,* 43–59.

De La Paz, S. (1999). Teaching writing strategies and self-regulation to middle school students with learning disabilities. *Focus on Exceptional Children, 31*, 3–16.

De La Paz, S., & Graham, S. (1997). Effects of dictation and advanced planning instruction on the composing of students with writing and learning problems. *Journal of Educational Psychology, 89,* 203–222.

Dunn, L. M., & Dunn, L. M. (1997). *Peabody Picture Vocabulary Test, 3rd edition.* Circle Pines, MN: American Guidance Service.

Ebbers, S. M., & Denton, C. A. (2008). A root awakening: Vocabulary instruction for older students with reading difficulties. *Learning Disabilities Research and Practice, 23*, 90–102.

Epsin, C. A., Scierka, B. J., Skare, S., & Halvorson, N. (1999). Criterion-related validity of curriculum-based measures in writing for secondary school students. *Reading and Writing Quarterly: Overcoming Learning Difficulties, 15*, 5–27.

Foorman, B. R., & Torgesen, J. K. (2001). Critical elements of classroom and small group instruction promote reading success in all children. *Learning Disabilities: Research and Practice, 16*(4), 203–212.

Graham, S., & Harris, K. R. (1989). A components analysis of cognitive strategy instruction: Effects on learning disabled students' compositions and self-efficacy. *Journal of Educational Psychology, 81*, 353–361.

Graham, S., & Harris, K. R. (1993). Self-regulated strategy development: Helping students with learning problems develop as writers. *Elementary School Journal, 94*, 169–181.

Graham, S., & Harris, K. R. (1999). Assessment and intervention in overcoming writing difficulties: An illustration from the self-regulated strategy development model. *Language, Speech, and Hearing Services in Schools, 30,* 255–264.

Gersten, R., & Baker, S. (2001). Teaching expressive writing to students with learning disabilities: A meta-analysis. *Elementary School Journal, 101*, 251–272.

Goddard, Y. L., & Sendi, C. (2008). Effects of self-monitoring on the narrative and expository writing of four fourth-grade students with learning disabilities. *Reading and Writing Quarterly, 24*, 408–433.

Harris, K. R., & Graham, S. (1998). *Making the writing process work: Strategies for composition and self-regulation.* Cambridge, MA: Brookline.

Kauffman, J. M. (2001). *Characteristics of emotional and behavioral disorders in children and youth* (7th ed.). Upper Saddle River, NJ: Merrill/Pearson.

Kim, A., Vaughn, S., Wanzek, J., & Wei, S. (2004). Graphic organizers and their effects on reading comprehension of students with learning disabilities: A synthesis of research. *Journal of Learning Disabilities, 37*, 105–118.

Lane, K. L., Graham, S., Harris, K. R., & Weisenbach, J. L. (2006). Teaching writing strategies to young students struggling with writing and at-risk for behavioral disorders:

Self-regulated strategy development. *Teaching Exceptional Children, 39*, 60–64.

Lane, K. L., Harris, K. R., Graham, S., Weisenbach, J. L., Brindle, M., & Morphy, P. (2008). The effects of self-regulated strategy development of the writing performance of second-grade students with behavioral and writing difficulties. *The Journal of Special Education, 41*, 234–253.

Lovett, M. W., Lacerenza, L., Borden, S. L., Frijters, J. C., Steinbach, K. A., & DePalma, M. (2000). Components of effective remediation for developmental reading disabilities: Combining phonologically and strategy-based instruction to improve outcomes. *Journal of Educational Psychology, 92*, 263–283.

MacArthur, C., Schwartz, S., & Graham, S. (1991). Learning disabled students' composing with three methods: Handwriting, dictation, and word processing. *Journal of Special Education, 21*, 22–42.

Mirkin, P. K., Deno, S. L., Fuchs, L., Wesson, S., Trindel, G., Marston, D., et al. (1981). *Procedures to develop and monitor progress on IEP goals.* Minneapolis: University of Minnesota, Institute for Research on Learning Disabilities.

Moxley, R. A., Lutz, P. A., Ahlborn, R., Boley, N., & Armstrong, L. (1995). Self recorded word counts of free writing in grades 1–4. *Education and Treatment of Children, 18*, 138–157.

Nagy, W. E., & Scott, J. A. (2000). Vocabulary processes. In M. L. Kamil, P. Mosenthal, P. D. Pearson, & R. Barr (Eds.), *Handbook of reading research* (Vol. 3, pp. 269–287). Mahwah, NJ: Erlbaum.

Nelson, J. R., Benner, G. J., & Cheney, G. (2005). An investigation of the language skills of students with emotional disturbance served in public school settings. *The Journal of Special Education, 39*, 97–105.

Nelson, J. R., Brenner, G. J., Lane, K., & Smith, B. W. (2004). An investigation of the academic achievement of K-12 students with emotional and behavioral disorders in public school settings. *Exceptional Children, 71*, 59–74.

Powell-Smith, K. A., & Shinn, M. R. (2004). *Administration and scoring of written expression curriculum-based measurement for use in general outcome measurement.* Eden Prairie, MN: Edformation.

Reed, D. K. (2008). A synthesis of morphology interventions and effects on reading outcomes for students in grades K–12. *Learning Disabilities Research and Practice, 23*, 36-49.

Rogers, L. A., & Graham, S. (2008). A meta-analysis of single subject design writing intervention research. *Journal of Educational Psychology, 100*, 879–906.

Semel, E., Wiig, E. H., & Secord, W. H. (2003). *Clinical Evaluation of Language Fundamentals-Fourth Edition.* San Antonio, TX: Harcourt.

Scott, C. M. (2002). A fork in the road less traveled: Writing intervention based on language profile. In K. G. Butler & E. R. Silliman (Eds.), *Speaking, reading and writing in children with language learning disabilities* (pp. 219–237). Mahwah, NJ: Erlbaum.

Simonson, B., Fairbanks, S., Briesch, A., Myers, D., & Sugai, G. (2008). Evidence-based practices in classroom management: Considerations for research to practice. *Education and Treatment of Children, 31*, 351–380.

Snow, C. E., Burns, M. S., & Griffin, P. (1998). *Preventing reading difficulties in young children.* Washington, DC: National Academies Press.

Swanson, H. L. (1999). Instructional components that predict treatment outcomes for students with learning disabilities: Support for a combined strategy and direct instruction model. *Learning Disabilities Research and Practice, 14*, 12–140.

Trout, A. L., Nordess, P. D., Pierce, C. D., & Epstein, M. H. (2003). Research on the academic status of students with emotional and behavioral disorders: A review of the literature from 1961–2000. *Journal of Emotional and Behavioral Disorders, 11*, 198–210.

U. S. Department of Health and Human Services. (1999). *Mental health: A report of the Surgeon General.* Washington, DC: Author.

Videen, J., Deno, S., & Martson, D. B. (1982). Correct word sequences: A valid indicator of written expression (Rep. No. 84). Minneapolis, MN: Institute for Research on Learning Disabilities. (ERIC Document Reproduction Service No. ED 225112.)

Watkinson, J. T., & Lee, S. W. (1992). Curriculum-based measures of written expression for learning-disabled and nondisabled students. *Psychology in the Schools, 29*, 184–191.

Westby, C. E. (2004). Executive functioning, metacognition, and self-regulation in reading. In A. Stone, E. Silliman, B. Ehren, & K. Apel (Eds.), *Handbook of language and literacy development and disorders* (pp. 398–428). New York: Guilford.

Zimmerman, B. J. (1986). Development of self-regulated learning: Which are the key subprocesses? *Contemporary Educational Psychology, 11*, 307–313.

Zimmerman, B. J., & Schunk, D. H. (Eds.). (2001). *Self-regulated learning and academic achievement: Theoretical perspectives.* Mahwah, NJ: Erlbaum.

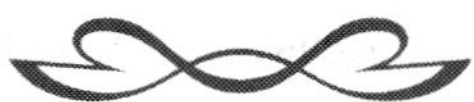

LITERACY

# CASE 34

# Annie: Treating Reading and Spelling Skills in an Elementary Student

*Deborah Cron and Julie J. Masterson*

## Conceptual Knowledge Areas

This case is based on Masterson and Apel's multilinguistic model of 5 factors involved in word-level reading and spelling (Masterson & Apel, 2007). The first component is *phonemic awareness,* which involves attention to the individual sounds within words. The second component is *orthographic knowledge* or *phonics*, and this involves the rules for translating speech into print. The next component is the *ability to store and use mental orthographic images (MOIs),* which are the images of words stored in memory. MOIs depend on adequate exposure to print, experience with phonemic analysis, and appreciation for sound-letter correspondences. The next component, *semantic knowledge*, affects the choice of an appropriate homonym (e.g., *bear* vs *bare*), and it is used in conjunction with the final component, *morphological awareness,* to decode and spell multimorphemic words involving inflections and derivations. Masterson and Apel (2000, 2007) suggest that a student's spellings can be analyzed to determine orthographic structures needing instruction and the type of instruction needed for each structure. Failure to represent a sound in spelling suggests a problem with phonemic awareness, use of illegal spellings suggest problems in orthographic or morphological knowledge, and legal, but incorrect, spellings suggest problems in adequate MOIs.

## Description of the Case

### Background Information

At the beginning of the spring semester, Annie B. was referred to the university clinic by her mother due to concerns about a lack of progress in reading. Graduate students supervised by clinical faculty conducted the evaluation and subsequent treatment. At the time of the initial evaluation, Annie was 9 years old and in the third grade at a private school. Developmental milestones, including speech and language, were achieved at expected ages. According to her mother, Annie's oral language skills had always been adequate. Mrs. B. indicated, however, that sometimes Annie would "transpose" phonemes (e.g., "ferrigerator" for refrigerator; "mazagine" for magazine; "aminal" for animal). Overall, Annie was described as easy to understand; good at expressing herself; able to understand and remember what was said to her; and good at following instructions. Annie attended nursery school before entering parochial school. In kindergarten, Annie was reportedly observed to transpose words when reading. Mrs. B. indicated that in preschool and kindergarten Annie would often "memorize" books and "read" them aloud.

Math and spelling grades were "low satisfactory," and reading was reported to be "below grade level." Although Annie did well on weekly spelling tests, she reportedly failed to retain the correct spellings. She had no school attendance problems. Annie had received tutoring to improve her reading skills. Annie's mother read textbooks aloud to help her with homework. No special education services were being provided through the school at the time of the evaluation.

## Reason for Referral

Annie's parents desired more information regarding her current reading level and information as to how to help Annie at home. Mrs. B. stated that Annie had difficulty "making sense of the written word" and consistently read below grade level. They were unsure about enrolling her for services at the university clinic.

## Findings of the Evaluation

### Speech, Oral Language, and Narrative Skills

Annie's articulation, fluency, voice, and hearing were within normal limits. Expressive oral skills in syntax, semantics, and morphology were observed during a conversation and also appeared to be typical. Conversational skills and pragmatics were excellent. Annie was able to retell a simple causal narrative with supporting details, listener friendly devices, and accurate sequence without difficulty. Additionally, she generated a story that contained a setting, a complication, a plan, indication of a result, and several descriptors including characters' feelings. Annie employed listener friendly devices such as "once upon a time" and exclamation points to draw attention and express strong feelings, as well as a conclusion ("The End").

### Spelling

The Test of Written Spelling-4 (Larson, Hammill, & Moats, 1999) was administered, and Annie's score was below normal limits. Her standard score (SS) was 76 (mean SS = 100; SD = 15). Multiple spelling errors were present in written narrative. Specifically, she misspelled 21% of the words written during the evaluation session. Incorrect capitalization was evident throughout, as was missing or incorrect punctuation. In contrast, Annie's handwriting was neat and legible. Her writing (typewritten) sample appears in Figure 34.1.

### Reading

Subtests from the Woodcock Diagnostic Reading Mastery Test-Revised (Woodcock, 1987) were administered to assess Annie's word-level reading skills. The Word Identification subtest was administered to measure Annie's ability to identify sight vocabulary. Annie scored within normal limits on this subtest (SS = 95; [mean SS = 100; SD = 15]). The Word Attack subtest, which measures the ability to apply phonic and structural analysis skills used to decode nonsense words, was also administered. Annie's standard score was 85 on this subset indicating borderline performance. The Passage Comprehension subtest was administered to evaluate

FIGURE 34.1 Annie's Generated Narrative with Original Spellings and Punctuation

*Once upon a time there was a turtle named shelly. shelly Loved egvenchers Once shelly pretened she was a piret with a long black beard. and once she wasa spy. She never thot of a real egvencher and one day she was in the pond and sudinly!!!!! A huge net came uround her she was stond she trid to screem but nothing came out she fanted she was so scarde when she yockup she didn't know where she was it looked like one of those things that in a newspaper that was by the pond she looked over a bruck wall a and lion the lion said. HI! My is lary, what is your name I am selly and were am I. lary said your're at the zoo [reversed z]. The ZOO [reversed z] we've got to exap!!! Lary and shelly made a plan it worked out great. THE END PS. if you whant to find out what happends next get the next book.*

Annie's reading comprehension skills through examining the ability to understand words and concepts. Annie's standard score was 86, again indicating borderline performance.

The Gray Oral Reading Test-4 (GORT-4; Weiderholdt & Bryant, 2001) was administered to further evaluate comprehension and to test reading fluency. Accuracy and Comprehension scores at that time were borderline average with standard scores of 8 (mean SS = 10; SD = 2). Rate and fluency were below normal limits with standard scores of 6 and 3 respectively. The overall oral reading quotient was 73 (mean = 100; SD = 15).

## Treatment Options Considered

Annie appeared to have significant deficiencies in word-level literacy skills, as evidenced by low performance on fluency, spelling, and reading nonsense words. Her scores in real word reading and comprehension were slightly better, although still compromised. Consequently, it was determined that treatment should focus heavily on word level reading and spelling, with additional support to increase fluency and improve comprehension. Annie's oral language and narrative skills and her high level of creativity were strengths.

Annie's parents initially desired that treatment focus on spelling with reading to be addressed through private tutoring. However, in addressing Annie's needs, the clinicians were mindful of current theory and research in combination with past clinical experiences. Annie's school, like most classrooms across the country, used the "Friday Test" as a strategy to teach spelling. This usually involved rote memory activities throughout the week. Students were asked to look up the meaning of each word and write it five times every day. The word list selection was often centered on classroom "themes." Rarely was any systematic attention paid to the lessons learned as time progressed and new lists were provided.

The main problem with the Friday Test method used in Annie's school was that only mental orthographic knowledge (MOI) was addressed, and it was felt that a multilinguistic approach would be better for Annie. Because spelling and reading have a reciprocal relationship, the clinicians planned to use Annie's spellings to determine the orthographic targets to use in focused word study to be supplemented with authentic reading and writing activities. To determine the initial targets and type of instruction needed, the Spelling Evaluation for Language and Literacy-2 (SPELL-2; Masterson, Apel, & Wasowicz, 2006) was administered. Annie's performance on SPELL-2 indicated needs in orthographic knowledge and the establishment of complete MOIs. Specific recommendations are illustrated in Figure 34.2.

## Course of Treatment

Treatment began immediately following the evaluation. Word study lessons came from SPELL-Links to Reading and Writing (SPELL-Links), (Wasowicz, Apel, Masterson, & Whitney, 2004), and the implementation procedures described in Masterson & Apel (2007) were used. Each lesson in SPELL-Links focuses on a particular orthographic target and emphasizes phonemic awareness, orthographic knowledge, morphological knowledge, semantic knowledge, or storage of mental orthographic images (MOIs). Annie's needs were primarily in orthographic knowledge and establishment of clear MOIs. Spell-Links activities such as Sort It Out establish two or three categories based on an orthographic pattern. A list of words representing the pattern to be learned along with a contrasting pattern was presented to Annie, who was encouraged to sort the words into two columns, one column of words that seem to be following one pattern and the other column for the other words/pattern. For example, the clinician addressed the spelling of long vowel 'a' and 'e' by explaining that there are many ways to spell the particular sound. Annie was given a pile of note cards with words containing the targeted long vowel sound and asked to underline the letters that spelled the vowel sound. If Annie underlined the wrong letters, she was asked to listen carefully as the word was produced and provided assistance. Other activities involved writing all possible spellings for a particular long vowel sound on a sheet of paper to form columns. Annie was then asked to write dictated words under the appropriate column. When applicable, words were selected from Annie's weekly school spelling lists to illustrate target patterns.

Develop clear and complete mental orthographic images of words containing the following spelling patterns for:

- consonants 'r, l'
- consonant digraph 'wh'

Develop clear and complete mental orthographic images of words containing spelling patterns for spelling of:

- short vowel /u/
- long vowel a̲ spelled as: 'ey, ay, ai'
- long vowel e̲ spelled as: 'ee, ea, y, ey, i, ie'
- long o̲ spelled as: 'oa, ough, ow'

Develop clear and complete mental orthographic images and orthographic knowledge sound symbol correspondence of:

- digraphs 'ch,' tch'

Develop clear and complete mental orthographic images and orthographic knowledge of sound symbol correspondence as well as long and short vowel principles for words containing the spelling pattern of:

- 'ck'
- Long o spelled as 'oCe'

Develop orthographic knowledge of sound-symbol correspondences for:

- Long vowel i̲ spelled as: 'y, ie, igh'

Develop ability to map letters to sound in words containing:

- Long u spelled as: 'uCe'
- Long u spelled as: 'ue, oo, o, ui'

FIGURE 34.2 Recommendations Generated from SPELL (Level 1)

High-frequency words were preferred stimuli to illustrate spelling patterns. Once Annie sorted the words successfully, she was asked to verbalize about the pattern (e.g., *when a vowel says its name, there are two vowel letters in the word*). The pattern description was added to a growing list of patterns and rules she wrote in her spelling journals.

An example of a SPELL-Links activity to facilitate Annie's establishment of complete MOIs was Picture This. This activity has both empirical and theoretical support (Glenn & Hurley, 1993; Richards et al., 2006). In the Picture This activity, Annie was first asked to look at a word and pay close attention to the specific parts it contained. The word was written, and strategies such as color (consonants in one, vowels in another), voice inflection (low voice for letters that drop below baseline, high for letters that go above), and backwards spelling were used to encourage her to form a complete mental picture of the word. As described by Masterson and Apel (2007), the Picture This activity takes quite a bit of time, considering that it is a strategy used to help develop MOIs for individual words. Annie was always encouraged to attempt to access other types of knowledge (phonemic awareness, orthographic knowledge, morphological awareness) first as most words do not need to be memorized completely. These techniques are based upon principles of optimal word study suggested by Masterson and Apel (2007); Apel and Masterson (2001); Masterson and Crede (1999); Bear, Invernizzi, Templeton, and Johnston (2000), Moats (2000), and Ehri (2000). Preliminary data indicate that these techniques result in increases in both spelling and word-level reading (e.g., Apel, Masterson, & Hart, 2004; Kelman & Apel, 2004; Masterson et al., 2005).

The transfer from word study to authentic reading and writing was addressed directly. Reading texts containing current word-study targets were used and the clinician called Annie's attention to those orthographic structures during guided reading. Later, she read passages in which the targeted patterns had been replaced by blanks in words. As she read, she determined the correct word and then spelled the word correctly in the passage. Additionally, authentic writing opportunities that involved targeted orthographic patterns were provided each session. Activities such as sentence dictation and generation were used, but for more fun, some sessions began with a Let's Pass Notes activity in which the only form of communication allowed was written. The student clinician ensured that targeted orthographic patterns were elicited by the topic selection and the nature of the questions asked. Narrative generation allowed additional instruction to facilitate good story structure, capitalized on Annie's creative thinking strengths, and incorporated story starters that encouraged targeted orthographic patterns. Academic writing skills such as essays and responses to compare and contrast questions were easy to load with target spelling patterns. Writing activities provided opportunities to facilitate correct use of capitalization and punctuation and were utilized for proofreading practice.

It is important to note that the orthographic targets were selected *first* and then authentic reading and writing activities were designed to provide opportunities to use these targets. As mentioned earlier, some of Annie's teachers, in an effort to make their spelling instruction meaningful, allowed their themes of instruction to drive the selection of spelling targets. For example, the teacher who was doing a unit on insects chose *cricket, moth, ant, caterpillar, mosquito, termite,* and *fly.* Because so many different orthographic patterns characterize these words, Annie was forced to resort to rote memorization as opposed to strategic use of spelling and word attack skills. Simply memorizing word lists so that the Friday spelling test will be passed does not result in optimal word-level knowledge (e.g., Scott, 2000).

Treatment continued by targeting syllable division rules for words containing r-controlled syllables, l-controlled syllables, accented and unaccented syllables, silent 'e,' and prefixes and suffixes. Spelling rules for doubling letters when adding suffixes and changing 'y' to 'i' when adding suffixes were also added. Over time, academic textbook reading was added to support study skills and monitor comprehension of more complex material. Care was also given to provide opportunities to read high-interest material. Proofreading skills were also addressed. In all, Annie received treatment for four 16-week academic semesters and two 8-week summer semesters.

### Reading Fluency

Reading fluency, the ability to read accurately at a normal rate with expression, is important for good comprehension. According to the *Report of the National Reading Panel: Teaching Children to Read* (2000), an independent panel formed by the U.S. Congress and led by the National Institute for Child Health and Development (NICHD) to evaluate evidence-based reading research in an effort to understand the best ways to teach reading, guided and repeated oral reading procedures improved word recognition, fluency, and comprehension skills across several grade levels. Guided oral reading involves providing opportunities for students to read out loud to someone who then provides feedback and corrects mistakes.

The guided oral reading and rereading activities used with Annie included clinician modeling of fluent reading, choral reading (reading in unison with the clinician), echo reading (in which the clinician read a portion of the material with Annie immediately rereading the same portion), and rereading (asking Annie to reread the passage after feedback had been provided). Children's acting monologues were used for repeated readings and to encourage expression. Although it is not known how many repetitions are optimal for individuals with reading problems, typical students reach maximum fluency levels with approximately four repetitions (NICHD, 2000). However, in a 2003 article in the *ASHA Leader*, summarizing the research on repeated oral readings, Kamhi stated, "Re-reading a text seven times is better than three times, which is better than one time" (p. 7). Consequently, the selected materials were either at or slightly below Annie's reading level, used all of the echo and rereading procedures, and could be repeated numerous times.

## Analysis of Client's Response to Intervention

Reevaluation of Annie's written language skills was completed at the end of her enrollment. Readministration of the Woodcock Diagnostic Reading Mastery Test (WDRMT), the Gray-Oral Reading Test-4 (GORT-4), and the Test of Written Spelling-4 (TWS-4) was conducted and comparison of pre- and posttreatment scores is shown in Table 34.1.

TABLE 34.1 Annie's Literacy Performance Pre- and Postintervention

| Test or Subtest | SS Pretreatment | SS Posttreatment |
|---|---|---|
| *WDRMT Word Attack* | 85 | 94 |
| *WDRMT Word Identification* | 86 | 95 |
| *WDRMT Passage Comprehension* | 86 | 103 |
| *GORT-4 Oral Reading* | 73 | 97 |
| *TWS-4* | 76 | 100 |
| SS = Standard score or quotient (mean = 100, standard deviation = 15) | | |

TABLE 34.2 Annie's Performance on the Individual Subtests of the GORT-4

| Profile | SS Pretreatment | SS Posttreatment |
|---|---|---|
| *Rate* | 6 | 6 |
| *Accuracy* | 8 | 8 |
| *Fluency* | 6 | 7 |
| *Comprehension* | 8 | 12 |
| *Fluency and Comprehension* | 14 | 19 |
| SS = Standard score (mean = 10, SD = 3) | | |

Annie's skills in applying phonic and structural analysis and her comprehension skills had improved from borderline to well within normal limits according to this measure. Annie's performance on the TWS-4 improved by almost two standard deviations to "average." Annie's oral reading had improved to the average range as well. It should be noted that Annie continued to exhibit a slower than average reading rate, however, her comprehension score had dramatically increased, likely contributing to the improvement in oral reading quotient. Individual profile scores on the GORT-4 are represented in Table 34.2.

In addition to repeating the tests administered pretreatment, the Written Expression Scale subtest from the Oral and Written Language Scales (OWLS; Carrow-Woolfolk, 1995) was administered to formally measure Annie's ability to use conventions such as letter formation, spelling/incorrect words, punctuation, capitalization, and other structures; to assess performance in the ability to use linguistic forms such as modifiers, phrases, question forms, verb forms, sentences, and complex sentence structures; and to test her ability to communicate meaningfully using appropriate content, details, coherence, supporting ideas, word choice, and unity. Annie's raw score was converted to two standard scores, one based on age and the other based on grade level (mean = 100; SD = 15). Annie's standard scores of 117 and 116 for age and grade, respectively, were both more than 1 standard deviation above the mean, indicating performance above expected levels.

## Parent Report

It has been a year since Annie stopped coming for services. She is now in Grade 6. Her mother reports that she is making grades of B in most classes and grades of C in reading and math. It should be noted that the parochial school that Annie attends requires percentages of 93 or better to receive a grade of A and 85 or better to receive a grade of B. Her parents feel Annie is happier in school compared to the frustration she was experiencing as a third grader. Her mother stated that she felt Annie was now more accepting of the extra time that she required for language arts and was willing to put forth the needed effort. Annie's parents also seemed very pleased to report that for the first time, Annie had recently begun reading silently for her own enjoyment.

## Conclusion

This case described an elementary student whose primary needs were in written language. Both her oral language and narrative skills were within normal limits and, in fact, were areas of strength that facilitated increased development of reading and spelling skills. The services delivered were beneficial, as evidenced by both assessment data and parental report. The information provided supports the benefits of speech-language pathologists' involvement in literacy intervention.

## Author Note

This case is hypothetical; however, it represents a composite of the characteristics, treatment, and outcomes that have been associated with the actual clients in the university clinic.

## References


American Speech-Language-Hearing Association. (2000). *Roles and responsibilities of speech-language pathologists with respect to reading and writing in children and adolescents: Position paper, guidelines, and technical report.* Rockville, MD: ASHA.

Apel, K., & Masterson, J. J. (2001). Theory-guided spelling assessment and intervention: A case study. *Language, Speech, and Hearing Services in the Schools, 32,* 182–195.

Apel, K., Masterson, J. J., & Hart, P. (2004). Integration of language components in spelling: Instruction that maximizes students' learning. In Silliman, E. R., & Wilkinson, L. C. (Eds.), *Language and literacy learning in schools* (pp. 292–315). New York: Guilford Press.

Bear, D., Invernizzi, M., Templeton, S., & Johnston, F. (2000). *Words their way: Word study for phonics, vocabulary, and spelling instruction* (2nd ed.). Upper Saddle River, NJ: Prentice Hall.

Carrow-Woolfolk, E. (1995). *Oral and Written Language Scales.* Circle Pines, MN: American Guidance Service.

Ehri, L. C. (2000). Learning to read and learning to spell: Two sides of a coin. *Topics in Language Disorders, 20,* 3, 19–36.

Glenn, P., & Hurley, S. (1993). Preventing spelling disabilities. *Child Language Teaching and Therapy, 9,* 1–12.

Kamhi, A. (2003, April). The role of the speech language pathologist in reading fluency. *The ASHA Leader,* p. 7.

Kelman, M., & Apel, K. (2004). Effects of a multilinguistic and prescriptive approach to spelling instruction. *Communication Disorders Quarterly, 25*(2), 56–66.

Larsen, S., Hammill, D., & Moats, L. (1999). *Test of Written Spelling-Fourth Edition.* Austin, TX: PRO-ED.

Masterson, J., & Apel, K. (2000). Spelling assessment: Charting a path to optimal instruction. *Topics in Language Disorders,* 20*(3),* 50–65.

Masterson, J., Apel, K., & Wasowicz, J. (2006). *SPELL-2: Spelling Performance Evaluation for Language & Literacy-2.* Evanston, IL: Learning By Design.

Masterson, J. J., Black, B., Ellman, K., Greig, A., Mooney R., & Wald, M. (2005). *Tailored reading-spelling instruction.* Poster presented at the annual convention of the American Speech-Language-Hearing Association, November, San Diego.

Masterson, J., & Crede, L. (1999). Learning to spell: Implications for assessment and intervention. *Language, Speech, and Hearing Services in Schools, 30*(3), 243–254.

Moats, L. (2000). *Speech to print: Language essentials for teachers.* Baltimore: Paul H. Brookes Publishing.

National Institute for Child Health and Development (NICHD). (2000). *Report of the National Reading Panel.* www.nationalreadingpanel.org/Publications/summary.htm; www.nichd.nih.gov/publications/nrp/smallbook.pdf.

Richards, T. L., Aylward, E. H., Berninger, V. W., Field, K. M., Grimme, A. C., Richards, A. L., et al. (2006). Individual fMRI activation in orthographic mapping and morpheme mapping after orthographic or morphological spelling treatment in child dyslexics. *Journal of Neurolinguistics, 19,* 5–36.

Scott, C. (2000). Principles and methods of spelling instruction: Applications for poor spellers. *Topics in Language Disorders, 20,* 3, 66–82.

Wasowicz, J., Apel, K., Masterson, J., & Whitney, A. (2004). *SPELL-Links to literacy.* Evanston, IL: Learning By Design.

Wiederholt, J. L., & Bryant, B. R., (2001). *Gray Oral Reading Test-Fourth Edition.* Austin, TX: PRO-ED.

Woodcock, R. (1987). *Woodcock Diagnostic Reading Mastery Test-Revised.* Circle Pines, MN: American Guidance Service.

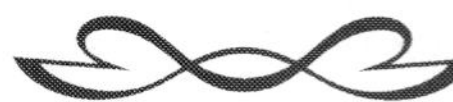

LITERACY/PHONOLOGY

# CASE 35

# Josh and Steve: Enhancing Phonological and Literacy Skills in Twins with Highly Unintelligible Speech

*Kathy H. Strattman and Barbara W. Hodson*

## Conceptual Knowledge Areas

By the time most children reach kindergarten, their understanding and productions in all domains of language typically have developed so that they are ready to learn. Language deficiencies, including expressive phonological impairments that are unresolved by the time children begin to learn to read and write, have a negative impact on literacy development (Bishop & Adams, 1990). Mental phonological representations remain "fuzzy" or not clearly established and adversely affect phoneme retrieval in decoding (Stackhouse, 1997). Once children begin to fall behind peers in reading they are likely to continue a downward spiral that Stanovich (1986) termed "Matthew effects," (i.e., the rich get richer, the poor get poorer). Good readers read more, gaining vocabulary and understanding about reading structures; poor readers read less and lose out on language and knowledge gained through reading. In addition, there is evidence (Bird, Bishop, & Freeman, 1995; Clarke-Klein & Hodson, 1995; Webster & Plante, 1992) that children with a history of unintelligible speech have poor phonological awareness skills important for literacy development.

Research results have shown that twins are at a higher risk for language delays and deficiencies (Lewis & Thompson, 1992) and evidence phonological deficiencies more frequently than single births (Dodd & McEvoy, 1994). What if twins continue to have phonological deficits beyond the critical age?

## Description of the Case

### Background Information

Josh and Steve, identical twin boys, were referred to the university clinic during their second semester of kindergarten at age 5 years,10 months. According to their speech-language pathologist (SLP), they had already participated in phoneme-oriented treatment for a couple of years, but gains had been minimal, and they were still extremely unintelligible. Typically fewer than 10% of their utterances in connected speech could be identified. The Hodson Assessment of Phonological Patterns-3 (HAPP-3; Hodson, 2004) was administered at this time (see Tables 35.1 and 35.2). Their initial scores on the HAPP-3 placed both boys in the profound severity interval. Table 35.3 provides some samples of their productions at age 5 years,10 months.

TABLE 35.1 Phonological Deviation Scores on the Hodson Assessment of Phonological Patterns-3 for Steve Prior to Phonological Treatment (age 5 years, 10 Months) and Following Each of Three Semesters

| | Percentages of Occurrences by Age | | | |
|---|---|---|---|---|
| | *5:10* | *6:5* | *6:10* | *7:5* |
| **Omissions** | | | | |
| Syllables | 25 | 0 | 0 | 0 |
| Consonant Sequences | 123* | 38 | 23 | 23 |
| Prevocalic Singletons | 21 | 0 | 0 | 0 |
| Intervocalic Singletons | 50 | 29 | 7 | 7 |
| Postvocalic Singletons | 100 | 6 | 6 | 0 |
| **Consonant Category Deficiencies*** | | | | |
| Liquids | 100 | 10 | 100 | 100 |
| Nasals | 62 | 5 | 14 | 0 |
| Glides | 90 | 20 | 20 | 20 |
| Stridents | 100 | 45 | 36 | 29 |
| Velars | 100 | 68 | 45 | 41 |
| Other Anterior Obstruents (Backing) | 43 | 6 | 3 | 3 |
| **TOMPD*** | 215 | 79 | 62 | 53 |

* Note 1: The formula for Consonant Sequences on the HAPP-3 represents dividing the number of total omissions of consonants in sequences by the number of possible "reductions" to one consonant.

* Note 2: Consonant Category Deficiencies are scored if the target consonant is omitted or if a consonant from another category as specified is substituted for the target.

* Note 3: TOMPD stands for **Total Occurrences of Major Phonological Deviations,** which is obtained by adding occurrences of Omissions and occurrences of Consonant Category Deficiencies.

Totals above 150 represent Profound; between 100 and 149, Severe; between 50 and 99, Moderate; below 50, Mild.

## Reasons for Referral

According to the critical age hypothesis (Bishop & Adams, 1990), children need to speak intelligibly by age 5 years, 6 months or literacy acquisition will surely be hindered. Josh and Steve were already past the critical age. The boys were to enter first grade in the fall (at age 6 years, 2 months). School personnel and parents were extremely concerned about their literacy abilities because of intelligibility difficulties.

### Birth and Medical History

Although they were born 6 weeks premature, prenatal and birth histories were relatively unremarkable. Josh weighed 3 lbs. 9 oz., and Steve weighed 4 lbs. 9 oz. They remained in the hospital initially to maintain body temperature and then to monitor growth and weight gain. The boys were raised in a two-parent, middle-income home. Their mother reported typical developmental milestones, except they used "some twin talk" but no real words until after they were 2 years of age. The boys had both undergone numerous surgeries for middle ear pathologies, vision, and polydactylism, but otherwise they were regarded as being generally healthy.

## Findings of the Evaluation

### Phonological Intervention

Beginning in first grade, both boys participated in individual weekly sessions for three semesters (approximately 35 contact hours). The emphasis at this time was on enhancing their phonological and metaphonological skills via the cycles phonological approach (Hodson, 2007).

TABLE 35.2 Phonological Deviation Scores on the HAPP-3 for Josh Prior to Phonological Treatment (age 5 Years,10 Months) and Following Each of Three Semesters

| | Percentages of Occurrences by Age | | | |
|---|---|---|---|---|
| | *5:10* | *6:5* | *6:10* | *7:5* |
| **Omissions** | | | | |
| Syllables | 6 | 0 | 0 | 0 |
| Consonant Sequences | 123* | 51 | 33 | 13 |
| Prevocalic Singletons | 18 | 0 | 0 | 0 |
| Intervocalic Singletons | 36 | 0 | 0 | 0 |
| Postvocalic Singletons | 100 | 22 | 3 | 0 |
| **Consonant Category Deficiencies*** | | | | |
| Liquids | 100 | 79 | 58 | 26 |
| Nasals | 62 | 14 | 0 | 0 |
| Glides | 90 | 20 | 20 | 20 |
| Stridents | 93 | 60 | 36 | 7 |
| Velars | 100 | 68 | 59 | 9 |
| Other Anterior Obstruents (Backing) | 43 | 7 | 7 | 0 |
| **TOMPD*** | 206 | 89 | 57 | 17 |

Note: See Table 35.1 for explanations.

TABLE 35.3 Phonetic Transcriptions of Sample Word Productions from HAPP-3 at age 5 Years, 10 Months

| Target Word | Productions by Both | |
|---|---|---|
| *clouds* | [taʊ] | |
| *square* | [tɛ] | |
| *candle* | [næ o] | |
| *string* | [nɪ] | |
| *rock* | [ɑʔ] | |
| *queen* | [ni] | |
| | **By Steve** | **By Josh** |
| *screwdriver* | [tudaɪ] | [dudaɪʊ] |
| *glasses* | [dæʔl] | [dædl] |

Their target patterns for the first semester/cycle included: (a) final consonants, (b) /s/ clusters (initial and final), (c) velars (final and initial), and (d) initial liquids. As the semesters progressed, velars, /s/ clusters, and liquids were recycled. Consonant clusters (e.g., medial /s/ clusters, velar clusters, liquid clusters, and 3-consonant clusters) were targeted. By the end of the third semester of phonological intervention, the boys were able to produce all consonants and consonant patterns in their production-practice words and considerable carryover into spontaneous utterances had occurred. Moreover, their severity intervals had decreased from profound to moderate or mild.

School personnel were expressing increasing concerns about literacy. Their second-grade teacher told the parents that she was considering retaining both boys at the end of the year. The two authors of this case visited the school and conferred with the teachers. It was evident that the boys were falling behind their peers because of their difficulties in literacy. The focus for the fourth clinic semester changed to literacy. Some phonology goals were still incorporated (e.g., multisyllabic word productions), but these were now secondary.

### Literacy Assessment and Intervention

Beginning in January of second grade, at age 7 years, 8 months, the boys were assessed for abilities affecting literacy. Reading and spelling abilities rely on phonological processing, which includes phonological awareness, speech sound production, and automatic components that facilitate comprehension (Catts & Kamhi, 2005). In a study of 75 typical second graders (Strattman & Hodson, 2005), children with good phonemic awareness skills demonstrated by deletion and manipulation tasks were better at decoding nonwords and spelling real words. Vocabulary understanding contributed positively to decoding performance. Improved phonological production as measured by productions of multisyllabic words contributed to spelling scores. Results of speech sound productions, receptive vocabulary, and reading assessment indicated new problems that could potentially interfere with reading and writing for Josh and Steve.

***Speech Sound Productions*** Although both boys were intelligible after three cycles of phonological treatment, speech sound errors were still noticeable. Results of the HAPP-3 demonstrated progress in phonology with a score in the high mild range for Josh and the low moderate range for Steve. The Assessment of Multisyllabic Words screening instrument (HAPP-3) revealed some consonant cluster reductions (e.g., *Seeping Beauty* for Sleeping Beauty), a few consonant singleton omissions within these more complex words, and also several word-specific assimilations.

***Receptive Vocabulary*** Receptive vocabulary was $1\frac{1}{2}$ to 2 years below expectation for chronological age (age equivalency 6 years, 2 months for Josh and 5 years, 11 months for Steve), according to results of the Peabody Picture Vocabulary Test-3 (Dunn & Dunn, 1997). Some believe that vocabulary increases reciprocally with reading skills. At this time, neither boy read for pleasure, although they enjoyed it when someone read to them. Their vocabularies were relatively simple with little variety in verbs and limited use of synonyms for nouns and adjectives.

***Reading and Spelling*** Sight word reading scores were within the typical range for second graders; however, decoding and reading comprehension were below age expectations. Reading real words was at grade level (2:6), as assessed by the Word Identification subtest of the Woodcock Reading Mastery Test (Woodcock, 1998). Scores on the Word Attack subtest indicated that decoding of nonwords was more difficult for Steve (grade equivalency 1:6) than for Josh (2:2). Results of the Passage Comprehension subtest demonstrated a significant problem for both boys (grade equivalency 1:3 for Josh; 1:4 for Steve). Spelling scores were at or just below 1 standard deviation from the mean. Josh scored 59 and Steve scored 56 on the spelling subtest of the Wide Range Achievement Test (mean = 69, SD =12) (Jastak & Jastak, 1993).

## Representation of the Problem at the Time of Referral

Reading comprehension was compromised by early phonological impairment that had not been fully resolved before learning to read and spell. Because reading was difficult, the boys did not want to read and did not develop strategies for learning from written text. More and more demand for independent reading and demonstration of comprehension is expected by third grade. Retention in second grade was not a guarantee of reading comprehension strategy development.

## Course of Treatment

Treatment focused on needs identified in assessment that contribute to reading and spelling success. To support decoding, some treatment was continued to facilitate the development of consonant sequences that contained liquids /r/ and /l/ and also included productions of multisyllabic words. In addition, phonemic manipulation tasks were utilized. The primary emphasis was on the development of reading comprehension strategies.

### Speech Sound Productions

The cycles phonological approach was continued. Target patterns for liquid clusters included more complex 3-consonant clusters (e.g., /spr/ *spring*, /spl/ *splash*). Active games (e.g., basketball, scavenger hunts) and table activities were alternated for motivation. Multisyllabic words from the stories were segmented by syllables, using felt squares. Letter tiles or plastic letters were placed on the felt squares to facilitate spelling any syllable that was deleted (e.g., *algator* for *alligator*) or contained an error (*agarium* for *aquarium*). No letters were placed on squares that were correct. After identifying the problem, correct syllable production was practiced, and then the entire word was rehearsed correctly and added to a list of "Really Long Words I Can Say."

### Reading Comprehension Strategies

Second graders often need help with strategies for understanding narrative stories and expository texts. Their reading textbook included both strategies. Explicit strategies facilitate comprehension but also help students engage in the story beyond just decoding the words. Josh and Steve often answered, "I don't know," when asked either an open-ended question (e.g., *What was that story about?*) or specific questions (e.g., *Who was the main character?*).

Strategies for narrative stories included identification of story grammar elements (characters, setting, initiating event, problem, problem-solving attempts, and resolution) within the story and using story grammar structure for answering questions, comparing stories, and retelling. Initially, narrative stories with school themes at the second-grade reading and interest level (e.g., *Arthur and the School Pet*, *Arthur's Valentine*) were chosen. Story grammar elements were labeled with Post-it® notes during reading. Graphic or visual organizers (e.g., story webs) were used to analyze the stories. Venn diagrams, two circles that overlap, were used to compare stories. Similarities between stories were listed in the overlapping part, and those that were unique to each story were listed in the part of the circles that did not overlap. (See Westby, 2005 for more information on graphic organizers.) Steve enjoyed narrative stories, but Josh preferred "real" stories.

Strategies for comprehension of expository texts were introduced as stories about real things included identification of elements: topic, main idea, and details. The same model used by the classroom teacher, a triangle with the topic at the top and the main idea in the middle, was adopted in the clinic. Details were listed on lines off the bottom of the triangle. Later, one boy read a narrative (e.g., *Shark tale*; Herman, 2004) and alternated with the other boy, who read an expository book (e.g., *Hungry, hungry sharks*; Cole, 1986). The books had a related theme, and they exchanged books the following week.

At school, they followed a program for monitoring reading comprehension of library books read on their own. Books were chosen from a specified list read at home and assessed via a computerized test. A variety of questions often followed story grammar or expository elements.

The hierarchical levels of language abstraction used in the Preschool Language Assessment Instrument-2 (Blank, Rose, & Berlin, 2003) were designed to assess preschoolers' abilities to answer questions that follow the language of instruction at school (e.g., *Which one is different? What do you think might happen next?*). This hierarchical structure of language is appropriate for school-age students because it is based on the premise of a perceptual-language continuum, which refers to the "distance" between what is immediately apparent (e.g., *How many sharks do you see?*) and an answer that requires more reasoning (e.g., Level 4—*How could fish breathe under water?*). Level 4 is the most abstract and requires the highest degree of reasoning. In Level 1 questions, what the child perceives matches what is seen or was just heard (e.g., *What color is this shark? How many sharks are there on this page?*). Level 2 requires some recall or reorganization (e.g., *What work did Lenny do at the Whale Wash? What lie did Oscar tell?*). Level 3 questions require reordering of information or inhibition of an anticipated response (e.g., *What swims in the ocean but is not a fish?*). Josh and Steve worked initially at Levels 1 and 2 followed by Levels 3 and 4. These questions were written on sticky notes throughout the books. The boys answered the questions as they were reading the story. Accuracy of answers was tallied. After the story was finished, some of the questions were asked again. They could look back in the book if they needed help recalling the answer.

Higher level narrative skill requires understanding the feelings and motivations of the characters. The boys' skills were compromised by their simple vocabulary (e.g., Arthur was *happy* when he got a Valentine. Lenny was *sad* not to be with his friends.). Other activities were designed to develop synonyms for feelings and emotions of the characters. The boys took turns with their clinicians drawing words from a bag and determining whether or not words meant the same thing (e.g., *happy, delighted, pleased*). Emotional thermometers were used to rank the degree of feeling (e.g., *pleased, happy, delighted, ecstatic*) (Westby, 2005).

## Analysis of the Client's Response to Intervention

By the end of the spring semester, both boys demonstrated progress. They could identify basic story grammar elements with minimal cuing. They generated the topic, main idea, and four details in high-interest nonfiction books with no cuing. Level 1 and 2 questions were answered accurately without cues. Each attempted to answer questions, even if unsure. Both boys were promoted to third grade because of their substantial gains in reading comprehension.

## Further Recommendations

Although the case was not closed, a solution was apparent—explicit treatment of deficit areas is necessary and has positive results. Although both boys were promoted, they continued to receive treatment and were learning additional strategies for reading comprehension and spelling. Steve was checking books out of the library, often choosing Arthur books (e.g., Brown, 1998, 2000). His mother reported that he read three books in one week. Children with histories of severe speech sound deficits are at risk for later literacy problems, and appropriate intervention makes a difference.

## Author Note

Real clients provided the basis for this study. Permission was obtained to present this information for instructional purposes. Names were changed and identifiable information was excluded.

## References


Bird, J., Bishop, D. V. M., & Freeman, M. H. (1995). Phonological awareness and literacy development in children with expressive phonological impairments. *Journal of Speech and Hearing Research, 38,* 446–462.

Bishop, D. V. M., and Adams, C. (1990). A prospective study of the relationship between specific language impairment, phonological disorders, and reading retardation. *Journal of Speech and Hearing Research, 38,* 1027–1050.

Blank, M., Rose, S. A., & Berlin, L. J. (2003). *Preschool language assessment instrument* (2nd ed.). Austin, TX: PRO-ED.

Catts, H. W., & Kamhi, A. G. (2005). *Language and reading disabilities* (2nd ed.). Boston: Pearson.

Clarke-Klein, S., & Hodson, B. W. (1995). Phonologically based analysis of misspellings by third graders with disordered-phonology histories. *Journal of Speech and Hearing Research, 38,* 839–849.

Dodd, B., & McEvoy, S. (1994). Twin language or phonological disorder? *Journal of Child Language, 21,* 273–289.

Dunn, L. & Dunn, L. (1997). *Peabody Picture Vocabulary Test-3.* Circle Pines, MN: American Guidance Service.

Hodson, B. W. (2004). *Hodson Assessment of Phonological Patterns* (3rd ed.). Austin, TX: PRO-ED.

Hodson, B. W. (2007). Enhancing children's phonological systems: The cycles remediation approach. In B.W. Hodson (Ed.), Evaluating and enhancing children's phonological system (pp. 87–113). Wichita, KS: PhonoComp Publishing.

Jastak, J. F., & Jastak, S. R. (1993). *Wide Range Achievement Test-3.* Wilmington, DE: Jastak & Associates.

Lewis, B. A., & Thompson, L. A. (1992). A study of developmental speech and language disorders in twins. *Journal of Speech and Hearing Research, 35,* 1086–1094.

Stackhouse, J. (1997). Phonological awareness: Connecting speech and literacy problems. In B. Hodson & M. Edwards (Eds.), *Perspectives in Applied Phonology* (157–196). Gaithersburg, MD: Aspen.

Stanovich, K. E. (1986). Matthew effects in reading: Some consequences of individual differences in the acquisition of literacy. *Reading Research Quarterly, 21*, 360–406.

Strattman, K. H., & Hodson, B. W. (2005). Variables that influence decoding and spelling in beginning readers. *Child Language: Teaching and Therapy, 24,* 1–26.

Webster, P.E., & Plante, A. S. (1992). Effects of phonological impairment on words, syllables, and phoneme segmentation and reading. *Language, Speech, and Hearing Services in Schools, 23,* 176–182.

Westby, C. (2005). Assessing and remediating text comprehension. In H. W. Catts & A. G. Kamhi (Eds.), *Language and reading disabilities.* Boston: Pearson.

Woodcock, R.W. (1998). *Woodcock Reading Mastery Test.* San Antonio, TX: Pearson.

*Children's Books*

Brown, M. (1998). *Arthur lost and found.* New York: Little, Brown.

Brown, M. (2000). *Arthur's valentine.* New York: Little, Brown.

Cole, J. (1986). *Hungry, hungry sharks.* New York: Random House for Young Readers.

Herman, G. (2004). *Shark tale: Lenny's fishy fib.* New York: Scholastic, Inc.

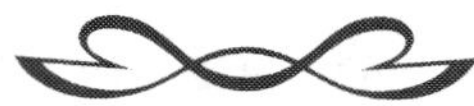

## SWALLOWING

# CASE 36

# Hannah: Dysphagia in the Schools: A Case Study

*Emily M. Homer and Dorothy Kelly*

## Conceptual Knowledge Areas

Children go to school to learn. In order for children to learn, they must not only be safe when eating at school, but they must have adequate nutrition and hydration (Homer, 2003). This case study profiles a student who has a primary classification of developmental delay with diagnosed impairments that include the following: cerebral palsy, encephalopathy, cortical blindness, and severe global developmental delays in motor, cognitive, self-help, language, and oral-motor skills.

## Federal and State Laws

When working within the school setting it is essential to understand that federal and state laws dictate the services provided to students with disabilities. The Individuals with Disabilities Education Act (IDEA, 2004) provides students with disabilities rights to special education and the protection of these rights. States must comply with IDEA but are able to set up their own policies and procedures. As a result each state's interpretation of IDEA may be somewhat different. IDEA is a funded law, which ensures that students with disabilities have access to a free and appropriate public education (FAPE). Children with disabilities are entitled to special education services including related services. According to IDEA, related services include speech-language therapy, occupational therapy, physical therapy, adapted physical education, health services, and so on. Medical services are included in IDEA as a related service; however, they must be provided by a physician and are limited to "diagnostic and evaluative purposes only." Health services are designed to enable a student with a disability to participate in school and as a result receive FAPE. A nurse or other qualified professional may provide health services.

## Educational Relevance

The educational goal for students with special needs is to optimize each student's developmental potential while maintaining adequate nutrition, hydration, and health so that he or she may access and benefit fully from the educational program (Arvedson, 2000). Health services are essential for some students to be able to access the curriculum. For example, a student with a seizure disorder may need the services of a nurse to train service providers to administer medication when the student has a seizure. Without this, the student would be unable to attend school. According to the guidelines for speech-language pathologists (SLPs) providing swallowing and feeding services in schools (ASHA, 2007), the following examples are arguments that support the educational relevance of addressing swallowing and feeding at school:

- It is the responsibility of the school system to ensure that students are safe while attending school. Appropriate personnel, food, and procedures must be provided to minimize risks for choking and for aspiration during oral intake.
- Students must have sufficient physical well-being and energy to function in the educational setting. Students who are undernourished or dehydrated due to swallowing and feeding problems cannot attend adequately to the learning environment, and consequently their performance at school may suffer.
- Students must have adequate health to attend school and to receive instruction. Students with swallowing and feeding disorders may miss school more frequently than other students due to related health issues. These may include repeated upper respiratory infections or other pulmonary problems related to aspiration during oral feeding or gastroesophageal reflux. In addition, students who have difficulty managing their saliva or who resist tooth brushing due to sensory-based disorders or autism spectrum disorders may have poor oral hygiene. Increased oral bacteria due to poor oral hygiene in adults is associated with greater risk of developing pneumonia (Langmore et al., 1998) and may be similar in children, although there are no published data.
- In order for students to participate fully in the educational program, they need to be efficient during regular meal and snack times, so that their meal and snack times are completed with their peers. Optimally, they should complete their meal or snack within 30 minutes or less. Prolonged mealtime is a major "red flag" for a swallowing and feeding disorder. Prolonged feeding times are indicative of excessive effort and energy that interfere with other activities important to a student's school day experiences. Prolonged mealtimes often are stressful for the student, and this stress can carry over into the remainder of the school day. Some students may require more frequent snacks or meals to maximize educational performance.

## Developmental Delay

The student profiled in this case study was diagnosed with developmental delay according to Louisiana Bulletin 1508 (Pupil Appraisal Handbook, 2004), which outlines eligibility criteria for special education classification in Louisiana. Developmental delay is a disability in which children ages 3 through 8 years old are identified as experiencing developmental delays in one or more of the following areas: physical development, cognitive development, communication development, and social, emotional, or adaptive development. According to Bulletin 1508 a child qualifies for services under developmental disability when he or she has met the following criteria: between the ages of 3 through 8 years and functioning significantly below age expectancy (i.e., exhibiting a delay of 25% or more on criterion-based measures or achieving a standard score greater than or equal to 1.5 standard deviations below the mean on norm-based measures) in one or more of the following areas:

1. Physical development, which includes:
   - Gross motor skills
   - Fine motor skills
   - Sensory (visual or hearing) abilities
   - Sensory-motor integration
2. Social, adaptive, or emotional development, which includes:
   - Play (solitary, parallel, cooperative)
   - Peer interaction
   - Adult interaction
   - Environmental interaction
   - Expression of emotions
3. Cognitive or communication development, which includes:
   - Language (receptive or expressive)
   - Concrete or abstract reasoning skills
   - Perceptual discriminations
   - Categorization and sequencing
   - Task attention
   - Memory
   - Essential developmental or academic skills, as appropriate (Pupil Appraisal Handbook, 2004)

## Cerebral Palsy

Cerebral palsy is a disorder of movement and/or posture, the result of a static encephalopathy with the insult to the brain occurring prenatally, perinatally, or during early childhood (Taft, 1987). Cerebral palsy is usually categorized by types and degree. Classification is typically identified as one of the following four: dyskinetic, rigid, atonic/hypotonic, or mixed. In addition, it is further described as mild, moderate, or severe as well as the area of involvement (Prontnicki, 1995). There are many symptoms and effects of cerebral palsy. The student in this study exhibited symptoms such as spasticity and rigidity of muscles, delayed motor development, history of cortical blindness, perceptual and attentional problems, dysarthria, language delays, decreased breath control, oral-motor deficits, and dysphagia.

## Dysphagia

This case profiles a student who had pediatric dysphagia secondary to cerebral palsy. A basic knowledge of the phases of dysphagia is essential to understand the issues surrounding this student's disorder. The phases of dysphagia include oral phase, oral preparatory, pharyngeal, and esophageal. According to Arvedson & Brodsky (2002), the oral and oral preparatory phases are under voluntary neural control. Students with oral and oral preparatory phase dysphagia have difficulty preparing the food for a swallow and propelling it to the pharynx. They often exhibit weak lip closure, poor mastication, pocketing of food in the oral cavity, and the inability to efficiently propel the food in a cohesive bolus to the back of the oral cavity, thus initiating the pharyngeal phase of the swallow. The pharyngeal phase of swallowing begins voluntarily with the beginning of a swallow. As the bolus travels down the pharynx the action becomes involuntary. Students with a pharyngeal phase dysphagia often have delays in the swallow, pooling in the valleculae and pyriform sinuses, and aspiration. The esophageal phase of dysphagia is the automatic movement, which carries the bolus through the esophagus and is completed when the food passes through the gastroesophageal junction into the stomach. Children with esophageal dysphagia may have gastroesophageal reflux disorder, which may result in a structural esophageal obstruction or a reflux-induced esophageal stricture. Esophageal dysphagia can lead to food aversion (Arvedson & Brodsky, 2002).

The reader may recall a choking experience or swallowing liquid that went "down the wrong way." These experiences relate to what the subject in this case goes through on a daily basis.

## Description of the Case

Hannah was a 5-years, 6-months-old female student with a primary exceptionality of developmental delay according to the Louisiana State Pupil Appraisal evaluation on July 15, 2005. Diagnosed impairments at that time included the following: cerebral palsy, encephalopathy, cortical blindness (originally, though vision has reportedly improved), and severe global developmental delays in motor, cognitive, self-help, language, and oral-motor skills.

### Background Information

Hannah was born prematurely at 26 weeks' gestation, weighing 3 pounds, 2 ounces. Ventilation was subsequently required for one and one half weeks due to underdeveloped lungs. She remained in the hospital for two months so that she could gain enough weight to be discharged. She went home weighing 5 pounds and was given an apnea monitor, though her biological parents apparently did not use it. At 5 months old, she contracted respiratory syncytial virus (RSV), which apparently went untreated until she became unconscious and her parents took her to the hospital. At that time, she sustained a severe anoxic brain injury associated with metabolic acidosis, and she remained in the hospital for one month. As a result of this neglect her biological parents lost custody of Hannah. Other pertinent health history included ear infections for which PE tubes were inserted at 1 year old as well as surgery for exotropia (divergent strabismus resulting in abnormal turning outward of one or both eyes) at the age of 2 years, 4 months. In addition, Hannah had seasonal allergies and reactive airway disease resulting in a compromised respiratory system. Medications included Xopenex regularly for respiratory difficulties, Zantac and Reglan for acid reflux, and Zyrtec for allergies.

Hannah wore glasses to correct her vision. Hearing was tested by her third birthday and found to be within normal limits. Hannah underwent 120 hyperbaric dives from 1 year, 2 months to 2 years of age as an adjunct therapy treatment to improve skills in multiple areas. Hyperbaric dives have been used to treat a variety of conditions such as autism, strokes, wounds, burns, and so on. Hannah's adoptive mother reported improvements in her vision and hearing following this treatment.

A long history of dysphagia was found with multiple modified barium swallow studies (MBSS) revealing silent aspiration. Her initial MBSS revealed that only honey-thick liquids could be safely swallowed without aspiration or penetration. Hannah received early intervention services for dysphagia as well as physical, occupational, and speech therapies. Subsequent MBSS revealed improvements with swallowing though dysphagia persisted. At the time that Hannah entered the school system, the most recent MBSS, conducted at 3 years, revealed aspiration with thin liquids and as a result, liquids were thickened to a nectar consistency.

## Reason for Referral and Findings of the Evaluation

Hannah participated in the Early Steps program that provided her with speech/language therapy, occupational therapy, and physical therapy. Due to the history of dysphagia from Early Steps, a referral was made for the school district's dysphagia team prior to Hannah's first day of school. The multidisciplinary dysphagia evaluation was conducted with the dysphagia case manager, Hannah's speech-language pathologist, and the occupational therapist on the first day of school. Input was also gathered from the special education nurse who wrote the emergency plan for Hannah. Oral motor difficulties consisted of labial, mandibular, buccal and lingual weakness, reduced range of motion, and incoordination, more prominent on the left side; oral hyposensitivity; and suspected apraxia. Based on these findings, symptoms that were suspected were the following: anterior loss due to decreased lip closure; oral residue and pocketing due to weakness, decreased coordination and range of motion; and decreased mastication and multiple swallows due to decreased bolus formation, oral hyposensitivity, and apraxia. The symptoms described were noted during the multidisciplinary swallowing and feeding evaluation. Based on these observations, Hannah's medical history, and previous MBSS, the following recommendations were made:

1. Positioning in a rifton chair (an adaptive chair designed to encourage normal sitting or standing posture for students with neuromuscular disorders) with cushion harness on the chest and shoulders to assist with sitting balance
2. Diet/food preparation:
   - Liquids should be thickened to 1.5 TBS per 8 ounces.
   - Soft foods such as vegetables should have crumbled crackers to add texture. (Hannah had oral hyposensitivity and thus has reduced tactile sensitivity; bland, smooth foods were difficult for Hannah to detect in her mouth.)
   - Dry foods such as cornbread should be slightly moistened to facilitate Hannah forming a more cohesive bolus.
3. Swallowing and feeding plan techniques/precautions:
   - Liquids taken one very small sip at a time and all liquids thickened to 1.5 TBS per 8 ounces
   - Chewable foods placed to her right side and on her molar table to encourage her to chew her food and give her visual cues to chew as needed
   - Pace slowed, allowing her to swallow 2–3 times per one bite of food or sip of liquid (she did this independently)
   - Mouth checked periodically for pocketing and a small sip of thickened liquid given if oral residue is noticed
   - Ensure she does not tilt her head back—give verbal and/or tactile cues to move head midline.

## Treatment Options Considered

Several treatment options were considered based on the results of the evaluation, including Beckman's (1986) oral-motor interventions as they do not require the child to follow oral-motor directions and thus can be passively performed on the child. In addition, these interventions target all oral-motor areas of difficulty. Hannah's speech-language pathologist (SLP) had attended the Beckman training and had witnessed the effectiveness of the treatment on numerous students of various ages. In addition, the SLP had used these interventions on several other children with good results. Hannah had good family support and it was hypothesized that these interventions would be trained for carryover at home. However, the SLP was unsuccessful in bringing in the adoptive mother for training with Beckman exercises with multiple attempts. Thermal/tactile stimulation was considered initially due to the delayed swallow reflex, though after attempts to train with Beckman were unsuccessful, this was not implemented as thermal/tactile stimulation needs to be done a minimum of 3 times daily to be effective (Logemann, 1998). Deep pharyngeal neuromuscular stimulation (DPNS) was not attempted, as it did not have research support at the time. Active oral-motor exercises could not be implemented due to difficulty following oral-motor directions. Chewing exercises and training utilizing the chewy tube was used with good success. The recommendations and swallowing precautions previously mentioned have been documented to facilitate improvements with areas of deficit as well as practice in swallowing various types and textures of foods. Hannah was followed by the dysphagia case manager (the school-based SLP) on a weekly basis, which included working with her during one of her lunch meals as well as consulting with the teachers and paraeducators who assisted with feeding.

## Course of Treatment

### Parent Perspective

Hannah's adoptive mother reported that the most difficult time for the family was in the initial stages of her dysphagia. Hannah was congested all the time and the mother was unable to keep her well. This fear was alleviated following the initial diagnosis of dysphagia and the cause of her frequent illnesses was determined. Initially, Hannah's dysphagia was severe and all liquids were reportedly thickened to pudding using an infa-feeder. It was two years before Hannah was able to eat baby food by spoon. Hannah's swallowing problems were among many that the family faced. Projectile vomiting and reflux were also significant problems for which Hannah reportedly was on two different medications. During this period of time, Hannah required breathing treatments every 3–4 hours. Hannah's adoptive father worked full-time and her adoptive mother did not have other family support as their families were upset with them for adopting a child with special needs. Furthermore, Hannah's adoptive mother reported that she and her husband fought with the Office of Community Services (OCS) for 8 months before the hyperbaric dives that Hannah needed were approved. The family also reportedly had to deal with negative medical comments, including that Hannah would never see or hear. Hannah's adoptive mother indicated that the hyperbaric dives significantly improved her hearing, sight, motor development, and swallowing. Hannah made much progress; however, the family continued to deal with medical and social issues such as wheelchairs and starting a baciofen pump to help with some persistent motor issues. Her swallowing and feeding improved significantly and Hannah was scheduled for an updated swallow study to see if she could handle thin liquids. Hannah's adoptive mother stated that Hannah's well-being is worth far more than the difficulties that the family has endured.

## Analysis of Client's Response to Intervention

Hannah made significant progress over the course of treatment. At the time of the study, Hannah fed herself and chewed her food, even soft chewable foods such as macaroni and cheese, with good success independently. Adding texture to foods was no longer required. The need for moistening foods was also minimized. Hannah placed the food to the side of her mouth independently by lateralizing her tongue. Pocketing and the use of a small sip of liquid were also significantly reduced. Only slight oral residue was noted to persist with certain chewable foods. Liquids continued to be thickened due to difficulty controlling thin liquids as well as to a delayed swallow reflex and reduced laryngeal sensation identified with the latest modified barium swallow.

## Author Note

This case study was based entirely on an actual student. The procedures and information provided reflect the actual treatment of this student by the school district's Interdisciplinary Dysphagia Team. Parents were aware of the case study and provided unconditional permission.

## References


American Speech-Language-Hearing Association. (2007). *Guidelines for the roles and responsibilities of the school-based speech-language pathologist. [Guidelines].* Retrieved from http://www.asha.org/docs/html/GL2000-00053.html.

Arvedson, J. C. (2000). Evaluation of children with feeding and swallowing problems. *Language, Speech, and Hearing Services in Schools, 31,* 28–41.

Arvedson, J. C., & Brodsky, L. (2002). *Pediatric swallowing and feeding: Assessment and management* (2nd ed.). Albany, NY: Singular Thomson Delmar Learning.

Beckman, D. A. (1986). *Oral motor assessment and treatment.* Winter Park, FL: Beckman and Associates.

Homer, E. M. (2003). An interdisciplinary team approach to providing dysphagia treatment in the schools. *Seminars in Speech and Language, 24,* 215–234.

Individuals with Disabilities Education Improvement Act of 2004. P.L. No. 108–446, 8 Stat. 2647 (2004).

Langmore, S.E., Terpenning, M.S., Schork, A., Chen, Y., Murray, J.T., Lopatin, D., et al. (1998) Predictors of aspiration pneumonia: How important is dysphagia? *American Journal of Otolaryngology, 13,* 69–81.

Logemann, J. (1998). *Evaluation and treatment of swallowing disorders* (rev. ed.). Austin, TX: PRO-ED.

Prontnicki, J. (1995). Presentation: Symptomatology and etiology of dysphagia. In S. R. Rosenthal, J. J. Sheppard, & M. Lotze (Eds.), *Dysphagia and the child with developmental disability. Medical, clinical and family interventions* (pp. 1–14). San Diego, CA: Singular.

Pupil Appraisal Handbook, Bulletin 1508. Title 28, Education Part CI. 31–32, Louisiana State Department of Education (2004).

Taft, L. T. (1987). Cerebral palsy. In H. M. Wallace, R. F. Biehl, L. T. Taft, & A. C. Oglesly (Eds.), *Handicapped children and youth* (pp. 281–297). New York: Human Sciences Press.


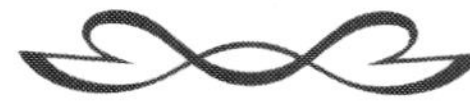

# VOICE

# CASE 37

# Adam: Vocal Cord Dysfunction in a Teenage Athlete


*Gail B. Kempster*


## Conceptual Knowledge Areas

### Knowledge of Vocal Fold Physiology in Breathing and Speech

The primary purpose of the structures of the larynx is for protection of the airway and the lower respiratory system. The true vocal folds (TVFs), also known as the vocal cords, are folds of tissue arising from the sides of the airway, protected by the cartilages of the larynx. The movements of the TVFs are controlled primarily by the intrinsic muscles of the larynx through innervation by branches of the vagus nerve. The posterior cricoarytenoid muscles open the TVFs, the lateral cricoarytenoid and interarytenoid muscles close the TVFs, and the thyroarytenoid and cricothyroid muscles tense and stiffen or elongate the TVFs. During quiet breathing, the TVFs remain open so that air may move through the respiratory tract for the exchange of oxygen and carbon dioxide (although small movements of the arytenoid cartilages are seen during breathing, toward abduction on inhalation and toward adduction on exhalation). The TVFs and other supraglottal sturctures close momentarily for a number of functions. These include protecting the airway from foreign substances such as during the act of swallowing, vomiting, coughing to expel material, allowing for the increase of intrathoracic pressure for lifting, defecation, birthing, and the like, and for producing voice (Hixon, Weismer, & Hoit, 2008).

## Knowledge of Typical Stresses of Adolescence, Especially Those of an Athlete

Stress is a significant problem for many teenagers. It is characterized by feelings of tension, frustration, worry, sadness, and withdrawal that may last anywhere from a few hours to days. While the majority of teenagers are not depressed, it is common for young people to experience life events involving friends or family that involve conflict or loss. Some of these events include the breakup with a boy- or girlfriend; increased arguments with parents, siblings, and friends; changes in a family's financial status; and parents experiencing relationship difficulties. The majority of teenagers face such negative life experiences with the resources to cope, but for others such stressors are overwhelming. For most adolescents, however, coping with life events involves learning skills to find positive ways to achieve peace of mind and assuming responsibility for oneself. These skills require practice and rely to a great extent on communication with others (Walker, 2002).

Athletics are one outlet for teenagers to learn positive coping skills and reduce stress. However, sports can promote both positive and negative stress. Researchers have found that adolescents' participation in competitive sports is linked with competition anxiety and self-centeredness. Also, balancing school and sports is not an easy task and can be very stressful. Some high-achieving teenagers are focused more on winning, on obtaining public recognition, and on their performance relative to others. This orientation and personality disposition may lead to additional stress on the teenager, which outweighs the positive benefits of the sports activity ("Sports-Related Stress").

## Knowledge of Signs, Symptoms, and Treatment for Vocal Fold Dysfunction

Vocal cord dysfunction (VCD) is a disorder in which the vocal folds move to an adducted or partially adducted position during inhalation and/or exhalation. This closure of the TVFs results in difficulty breathing, sometimes with stridor, with a resultant increase in anxiety. The etiology of VCD is unclear. It frequently co-occurs in individuals with asthma and has also been associated with allergies, reflux, and psychosocial stress. Some individuals with VCD have triggering symptoms such as exertion or being in an environment with a particular odor (e.g., perfume, gasoline, coffee). A patient experiencing VCD typically indicates that tightness is experienced in the throat area versus in the upper chest. The classic diagnostic finding related to VCD is a shortened inspiratory flow volume loop found on pulmonary function testing. Many individuals also present with a posterior, diamond-shaped glottal chink, even when not symptomatic (Mathers-Schmidt, 2001).

A patient with a diagnosis of VCD should be determined to have good control of asthma, allergies, and reflux symptoms. If these related disorders are being controlled, the treatment for VCD involves cognitive-behavioral therapy directed toward producing relaxed "abdominal breathing" (sometimes called "rescue breathing") and with attention diverted away from the area of tension in the throat.

## Knowledge of Characteristics of and Treatment for Tourette Syndrome

Tourette syndrome (TS) is a neurological condition characterized by repetitive, involuntary movements or vocalizations known as tics. The etiology of this disorder is unknown, but TS is thought to involve multiple brain areas with complex interactions. There is evidence to suggest that TS is inherited. TS is more common in males and is often diagnosed first in childhood. Although there is no known cure, the disorder appears at its worst during the early teen years and often improves in adulthood.

Individuals with Tourette syndrome frequently have a concomitant diagnosis of attention-deficit/hyperactivity disorder (ADHD) and may experience anxiety and depression. For those patients whose symptoms of TS interfere with daily functional activities, neuroleptic medications are commonly prescribed for tic suppression. These medications may have side effects and long-term use can lead to other movement disorders such as dystonia or even tardive dyskinesia (National Institute of Neurological Disorders and Stroke, n.d.).

## Description of the Case

### Background Information

The patient, Adam, a 15-year-old high school freshman, was referred to the Speech and Hearing Clinic at a large teaching hospital for evaluation. At the time of referral, Adam was active in several sports in high school as well as in church activities and scouting. He had two younger siblings, a brother with epilepsy and a sister diagnosed with central auditory processing disorder and dyslexia. His mother was a single parent who worked full-time at a local diner.

The family came to the medical center from a middle-class suburb some distance away. Adam attended a large high school with over 2,000 students. Despite his many activities, his grades were well above average, and he was on the honor roll almost every term. Adam's medical history included diagnoses of allergies, asthma, chronic otitis media, and ADHD. His current medications included Singulair, Advair, and Maxair for his asthma.

### Reason for Referral

About four years prior to this evaluation, Adam began exhibiting tics and other symptoms including sniffing, head jerks, and ear popping. He was evaluated by a neurologist and found to have Tourette syndrome. Clonodine and Concerta, prescribed for his ADHD, also seemed to help his symptoms of Tourette syndrome. The tics and other signs tended to recur when he was extremely anxious or tired. Sylvia, his mother, tried several homeopathic strategies to see if these relieved some of the symptoms. Based on trial and error, she and Adam believed a gluten-free diet had a positive effect.

Adam was monitored closely by his primary care physician and routinely by a consulting neurologist. Despite all of her children's many activities and their health issues, Sylvia was organized, knowledgeable, and proactive in dealing with their medical and educational needs. This attention was illustrated by her rousing all three of her children at 4:00 A.M. to come to the medical center on time for Adam's clinic appointment. Sylvia brought with her detailed records relating to Adam's medical history and supplemented his answers to our questions with specific information. She encouraged Adam to speak for himself and take ownership of the reason for his consult at our clinic.

### Findings of the Evaluation

Adam was previously evaluated by his primary care doctor and by a pulmonary specialist. The pulmonologist ordered pulmonary function testing and determined that Adam's asthma was under optimal control. His flow volume study, however, revealed a reduced inspiratory flow volume loop. This suggested an extrapulmonary source of constriction and is associated with a diagnosis of vocal cord dysfunction. Adam was referred to this medical center for confirmation of this diagnosis.

During the interview, Adam reported that he began experiencing difficulty breathing during exercise in fifth grade. He described these periods as having trouble getting air in or out and "feeling pain in the back of the throat." Unlike his asthma episodes when he typically experienced a feeling of tightness in his chest, which lasted an hour or two, the symptoms he experienced with exertion lasted only for a minute or two. Adam was active in multiple sports, including swimming and cross-country, and he noticed that episodes of breathing difficulty had been happening more and more frequently, sometimes during practice, but even more so during competitions. These episodes, which often occurred multiple times during a single workout session, had a significant effect on Adam's ability to perform and stay competitive. In fact, his coaches, his teammates, and even spectators became noticeably concerned and anxious whenever the situation occurred, and he was restricted from participation during competitions. Adam seemed matter-of-fact in discussing these episodes, but he had difficulty maintaining eye contact with the clinician and became somewhat agitated and less forthcoming when pressed for more details.

The evaluation protocol followed that recommended by Mathers-Schmidt (2001). After obtaining information related to the patient's medical and social history and his current symptoms, other elements—respiratory support and control, laryngeal valving efficiency and control, respiratory driving pressure control, laryngeal musculoskeletal tension, and structural/functional integrity of the speech structures—were assessed.

This assessment revealed that Adam had normal vocal pitch, loudness, and quality and had no difficulty with voiced and voiceless onsets and offsets in connected speech. His phonational range was 38 semitones, which is normal. He had no difficulty varying loudness as requested in specific tasks. Maximum phonation time on a prolonged vowel was normal at 15.3 seconds, although this value was judged to be below his maximum ability. Adam had no difficulty sustaining a steady respiratory driving pressure of 5 cm $H_20$ for 5 s. His oral mechanism exam was normal.

Palpation of the laryngeal area during quiet breathing and speech revealed musculoskeletal tension to be mildly elevated in the clinician's judgment. No episodes of difficulty breathing outside of the range of normal were elicited, despite having Adam run up five flights of stairs. Because Adam was asymptomatic during the evaluation, videoendoscopy was not completed.

Adam appeared mildly anxious during the assessment and intermittently exhibited signs of boredom, irritation, and embarrassment. These reactions were not, however, considered out of the ordinary for the patient's age and the evaluation environment. A few signs of Tourette syndrome were noted during the 90-minute session, including 2 facial tics on the patient's left side and 2 slight head jerks to the left.

The results of the evaluation supported the diagnosis of vocal cord dysfunction. In particular, the specific nature of the symptoms reported, their duration, and the context in which they occurred (in addition to the pulmonary function test results) clearly pointed to this diagnosis.

## Treatment Options Considered

Treatment for patients with vocal cord dysfunction consists of patient education, supportive counseling, and instruction in tension identification and control, and in relaxed open throat breathing (see Mathers-Schmidt, 2001). The clinician began by describing the anatomy of respiration, differences seen in quiet breathing versus speech breathing, and the function of the vocal folds. The primary purpose of the vocal folds, that of protection, was emphasized and examples provided. The etiology of vocal fold dysfunction is unclear, except in cases associated with neurologic origins. Movement disorders are one such neurologic etiology, and Tourette syndrome can be categorized in this way. However, Adam's shortness of breath symptoms did not seem correlated with episodes of tics. Rather, he reflected one common profile of patients with VCD, who typically are young, tend to be high achievers and have competitive natures, have a history of allergies and asthma, and experience specific triggering episodes.

Clinical experience has revealed that treatment for patients with VCD must first focus on achieving maximal control of conditions threatening the airway: that of asthma, allergies with chronic postnasal drip, and laryngopharyngeal reflux. Once the patient and his physicians assert that these conditions are well controlled medically, the patient is taught to recognize the initial, subtle signs of laryngeal tension during typical triggering activities. Some patients find that they need to cough, clear their throat, or swallow more in response to a kind of tickle, irritation, or tightness in the throat. It is shortly after experiencing such signs that tension in the throat builds and breathing becomes difficult on inspiration, expiration, or both.

## Course of Treatment

Adam acknowledged being aware of the change in feeling in his throat, so the clinician immediately taught him a relaxed, open throat breathing exercise (Blager, 1995). Many patients with symptoms of VCD recognize that if they force themselves to relax and breathe easily, the tension in the throat dissipates quickly. The difficulty, however, is in preventing the episodes from occurring.

Adam was instructed in the relaxed, open throat breathing exercise. Sitting quietly with his arms at rest and shoulders relaxed, he was taught to focus on relaxing his jaw with his lips closed and tongue resting on the floor of his mouth. After taking a moderately quick inhalation (a "sniff") through his nose, Adam was instructed to exhale slowly while quietly producing /s/, and to continue this exhalation focusing on the constriction at the front of the mouth until he had exhaled below resting expiratory level before inhaling again. This technique allowed two things to occur. First, his attention was distracted away from the tightness in the throat and drawn to the constriction in the front of the oral cavity during the exhalation. Second, exhaling below resting expiratory level promoted the need for an inhalation with a wide-open airway.

The clinician asked Adam to practice this exercise several times a day for a few weeks and to log any episodes of VCD, noting specific features about each episode, including the triggering situation, initial symptoms, and duration. Once Adam had experience with the exercise, his mother agreed to contact Adam's cross-country coach and the school nurse to inform them about this disorder and to see how support could be provided at school. Because the family lived so far from the medical center, the clinician recommended only a minimal amount of follow-up at the clinic with intervening telephone contacts as needed.

Adam returned for follow-up 1 month later. He said that he had been practicing the relaxed breathing exercise several times a day and demonstrated this. He continued to sit on the bench during athletic contests and reported no episodes of VCD in the last month. The mother had spoken with Adam's cross-country coach, and he was willing to monitor and support Adam. A packet of information about VCD, including the Mathers-Schmidt (2001) article and written instructions for the relaxed open throat breathing exercise, was prepared for the coach and the school nurse. It was agreed that the coach and nurse would contact the SLP with any questions. The plan was for Adam to begin jogging, slowing as needed, and using the breathing exercise whenever he felt the incipient tension beginning in his throat.

Ten weeks later, Adam returned to the clinic. He had practiced several times with his coach running with him. Each time the same thing happened: He would run 3 laps, would then sprint 100 yards, and then the VCD started. Adam described it this way: "I'll stop and breathe out, but then I choke and can't breathe in. It feels like someone's holding my head under water, and I need to breathe in, but I can't. Sometimes I almost feel like I'm gagging and need to throw up." Adam felt that the breathing exercise was not helping him. He was discouraged and stressed by what was occurring. At this session, signs of Tourette syndrome were more noticeable than before.

The clinician explored the pattern of the episodes thoroughly. Adam seemed to go from no problems to full-blown "choking" with almost no time in between despite his and his coach's best efforts. The clinician was convinced Adam was following the recommendations and had support there to help him. Although Adam received encouragement, he was clearly frustrated and felt any modifications of the strategy would be worthless. In a radical move, the clinician decided to recommend that Adam turn the breathing exercise "upside down"—that is, rather than using a quick inhalation and slow, controlled exhalation, he would try the opposite and use a slow, relaxed inhalation through pursed lips with a quicker, open-mouthed exhalation. Adam practiced this in the therapy room and reluctantly agreed to give it a try. The clinician asked him to test it and telephone with an update.

## Analysis of Client's Response to Intervention and Further Recommendations

The clinician did not hear from Adam, but the mother brought him back for a recheck visit 5 months later. Adam reported no episodes of VCD while at camp over the summer. He did, however, experience some episodes when starting cross-country practice again. But by now, Adam realized what to do and how to control the episodes. He needed to keep reminding himself to breathe and to maintain an even breathing rhythm, *not* to hold his breath during running. He was happy to report that he had had no episodes in the past 6 weeks.

The clinician discussed how to approach possible VCD episodes when Adam began swimming practice again. Adam's self-determined strategy seemed like a good one to stay with and he was encouraged to do this. Because of the humid and chlorinated environment of indoor pools, the clinician asked Adam to be especially vigilant in following his daily treatment plan for his asthma.

Adam was asked to call in 2 months to provide an update, but he did not follow through. Because the clinician believed that the mother would have continued to seek follow-up should Adam have problems, it was assumed that he was coping well and experiencing few, if any, episodes of VCD.

Clinical experience and evidence from the literature suggest that most student athletes with VCD typically do not continue to experience episodes long-term. It is unclear why this disorder appears to resolve in this population. In fact, evidence in support of the efficacy of behavioral treatment for VCD with breathing exercises is largely anecdotal in nature.

## Author Note

This case is based on the experiences of the clinician with patients with this disorder. All identifying characteristics have been altered to protect any individual patient's privacy. Content altered in this way was approved for publication by the Rush University Medical Center Privacy Office.

## References


Blager, F. (1995, September). Treatment of paradoxical vocal cord dysfunction. *Division 3 Newsletter.* American Speech-Language-Hearing Association.

Hixon, T., Weismer, G., & Hoit, J. (2008). *Preclinical speech science: Anatomy physiology acoustics perception.* San Diego, CA: Plural Publishing.

Mothers-Schmidt, B. (2001). Paradoxical vocal fold motion: A tutorial on a complex disorder and the speech-language pathologist's role. *American Journal of Speech-Language Pathology, 10*, 111–125.

National Institute of Neurological Disorders and Stroke. (n.d.). *Tourette syndrome fact sheet.* Retrieved December 30, 2008, from http://www.ninds.nih.gov/disorders/tourette/detail_tourette.htm.

*Sports-related stress in adolescents.* (n.d.). Retrieved December 30, 2008, from http://www.cedu.niu.edu/~shumow/iit/Sports-Related%20Stress.pdf

Walker, J. (2002). *Teens in distress series: Adolescent stress and depression.* Retrieved December 30, 2008, from University of Minnesota Extension, Center for 4-H Youth Development website: http://www.extension.umn.edu/distribution/youthdevelopment/DA3083.html

# Adult Cases

PART IV

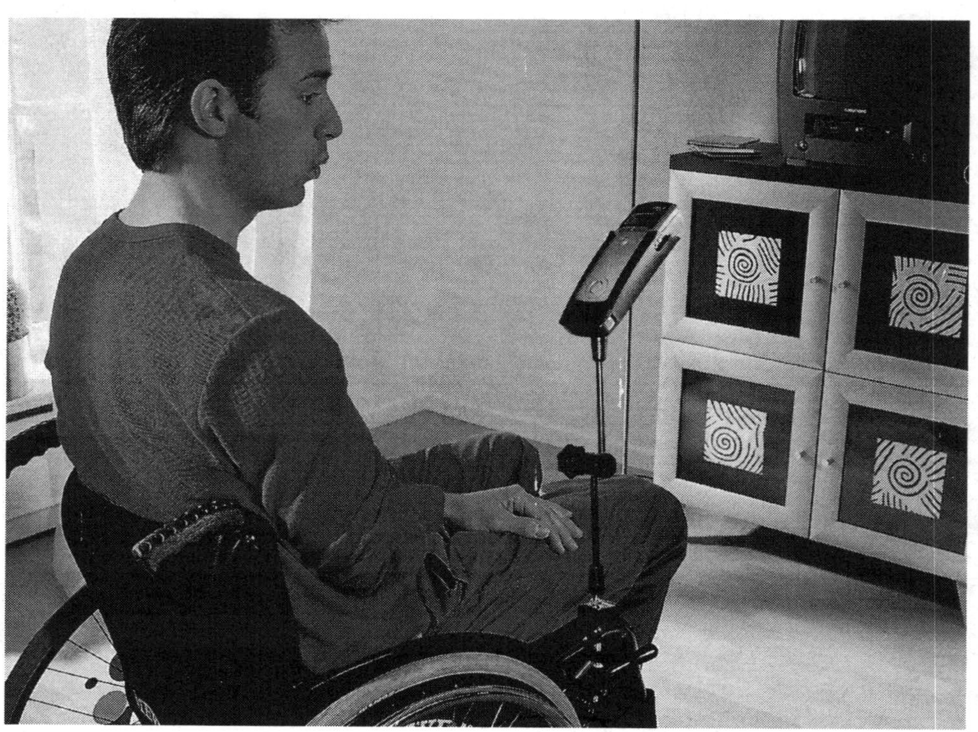

APHASIA



APRAXIA

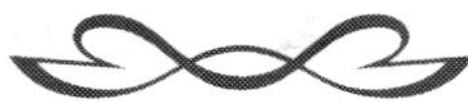

APHASIA

# CASE 38

# Andrew: A Case of Primary Progressive Aphasia in the Later Stages of the Disease

*Michael de Riesthal*

## Conceptual Knowledge Areas

This chapter describes the management of an individual with primary progressive aphasia (PPA). To understand this case, it is important to be familiar with the definition and presentation of PPA and how it differs from *nonprogressive* aphasia. This includes understanding the changes to language systems, speech motor systems, and cognitive systems that may occur in progressive diseases.

Aphasia is a disorder of language formulation and comprehension that results in deficits across input (auditory and reading comprehension) and output (speaking and writing) language modalities (Rosenbek, LaPointe & Wertz, 1989). Typically, nonprogressive aphasia results from a focal lesion in the cortical language areas due to a cerebrovascular accident and is abrupt in onset. Deficits are often maximal at onset of the stroke, and improvement in language function occurs during the acute and chronic stages of the disorder through the influence of spontaneous recovery and the implementation of treatment (Robey, 1998; Wertz et al., 1986). Definitions of aphasia often include exclusionary criteria to distinguish aphasia from communication disorders related to nonlinguistic physiologic, cognitive, and sensory deficits that differ with regard to diagnosis, prognosis, and management.

The definition and criteria for diagnosis of PPA differ from a nonprogressive aphasia. Weintraub, Rubin, and Mesulam (1990) define PPA as a neurodegenerative disease characterized by (1) a 2-year history of language decline, which may result in fluent or nonfluent aphasia, (2) no decline in other mental functions during this two-year time period, (3) maintenance of the ability to perform activities of daily living, (4) an etiology that is not typical of nonprogressive aphasia based on neurological evaluation, and (5) speech, language, and neuropsychological assessments that are consistent with the patient's presenting complaints. Typically, language decline begins with word-finding difficulty but often results in agrammatism and mutism later in the disease process (Marra et al., 2007). Auditory comprehension, reading comprehension, and written language skills decline as the disease progresses. Individuals with PPA may present with a coexisting dysarthria (McNeil, 1998) or apraxia of speech (AOS) (Kavrie & Duffy, 1994). For some, a progressive AOS may be the presenting symptom (McNeil & Duffy, 2001).

In addition to language and speech deficits, some individuals with PPA may also develop symptoms consistent with frontotemporal dementia (FTD; Neary et al., 1998) and corticobasal degeneration syndrome (CBDS; Kertesz, Blair, McMonagle, & Munoz, 2007); however, according to the criteria set by Weintraub, Rubin, & Mesulam (1990), these symptoms cannot be present within the first two years of onset. Kertesz and colleagues (2007) reported the clinical course of 101 individuals diagnosed with PPA. In their sample, 50% of individuals with PPA developed the core symptoms of the FTD behavioral variant, which include impaired social interpersonal conduct, impaired regulation of personal conduct, emotional blunting (i.e., lack of emotion), and loss of insight. In addition, 32% of the sample developed the core symptoms of CBDS, which include unilateral rigidity, apraxia, and "alien limb" (i.e., a syndrome in which the individual reports involuntary limb movement, as if it has "a mind of its own"). The average duration from the onset of illness to death was 7.5 years in Kertesz and colleagues' (2007) sample of individuals with PPA.

# Description of the Case

## Background Information

The patient, Andrew, a right-handed, native English speaker, was retired from a management position. He had an undergraduate degree in physics and a black belt in several forms of martial arts. When he was 55 years old, he began having difficulty with word finding and mathematical calculations. Concerned that these changes could be related to Alzheimer's disease (AD), he scheduled an appointment with his primary care physician, who referred him for psychological testing. Testing results were not consistent with AD, and it was felt that the changes could be due to depression and stress. He was prescribed Paxil and observed some improvement in speech and mathematical skill with an increased dose, but deficits persisted. He was referred to a neurologist for further assessment. Following the behavioral assessment and MRI, Andrew was diagnosed with AD. He and his wife, Sarah, were not satisfied with this diagnosis and continued their search for an accurate diagnosis. After Andrew and Sarah retired and moved to a new city, his new primary care physician felt that, although the MRI of the brain was negative, the symptoms were more consistent with a stroke. The physician referred Andrew for speech therapy. According to Sarah, Andrew became frustrated with speech therapy and was frequently emotional when he left a session. Eventually, Andrew was evaluated at a clinic that specialized in the assessment and diagnosis of individuals with progressive language and cognitive deficits. Following a thorough neuropsychological assessment, Andrew was diagnosed with PPA.

## Reasons for the Referral

Andrew was referred for speech and language assessment and training of "augmentative and alternative communication and aggressive speech and language therapy" by his primary care physician due to the diagnosis of PPA.

## Findings of the Evaluation

Neuropsychological testing was completed at another institution 11 months prior to Andrew being seen at Pi Beta Phi Rehabilitation Institute (PBPRI). Testing revealed a progressive, nonfluent language impairment characterized by single word utterances and echolalia in conversational speech, and severely impaired confrontation and generative naming. He demonstrated a moderate impairment in comprehension of narrative information and a moderate-to-severe impairment in comprehension of single and multistep commands. He was able to repeat some single words and high-probability phrases (i.e., Mother cooks dinner), but performance was poor with low-probability phrases (i.e., The pastry cook was elated). Andrew presented with a moderate impairment in visual immediate attention, conceptual reasoning, and immediate recall of visuospatial material. Evidence of motor perseveration was observed on the Luria 3-step motor sequence task. It was determined that Andrew's deficits were consistent with progressive nonfluent aphasia, with the primary symptom being the onset of word retrieval difficulty with progression of language dysfunction over the first three years of the disease.

At PBPRI, the Western Aphasia Battery-Revised (Kertesz, 2006) (language quotient subtests) and the Pyramids and Palm Trees Test (Howard & Patterson, 1992) were administered.

TABLE 38.1 Test Data for Andrew During Assessment at PBPRI

| **Western Aphasia Battery** | |
|---|---|
| **Spontaneous Speech** | |
| Information content | 3/10 |
| Fluency, grammatical competence, and paraphasia | 2/10 |
| **Auditory Verbal Comprehension** | |
| Yes/no questions | 33/60 |
| Auditory word recognition | 27/60 |
| Sequential commands | 39/80 |
| **Repetition** | 42/100 |
| **Naming and Word Finding** | |
| Object Naming | 22/60 |
| Word Fluency | 0/20 |
| Sentence Completion | 5/10 |
| Responsive Speech | 0/10 |
| **Reading** | |
| Comprehension of Sentences | 4/40 |
| Reading Commands | 3/20 |
| Written Word-Object Choice Matching | 0/6 |
| Written Word-Picture Choice Matching | 1/6 |
| Picture-Written Word Choice Matching | 3/6 |
| Spoken Word-Written Word Choice Matching | 2/6 |
| Letter Discrimination | 4/6 |
| Spelled Word Recognition | 0/6 |
| Spelling | 0/6 |
| **Writing** | |
| Writing Upon Request | 2/6 |
| Writing Output | 0/34 |
| Writing to Dictation | 0/6 |
| Writing Dictated Words | 1/10 |
| Alphabet and Numbers | 4/22.5 |
| Dictated Letters and Numbers | 2/7.5 |
| Copying a Sentence | 2/10 |
| **Pyramids and Palm Trees Test** | 29/52 |
| **ASHA FACS** | |
| Social Communication | 3.6/7 |
| Reading, Writing, and Number Concepts | 2.4/7 |
| Daily Planning | 2.0/7 |
| Communication of Basic Needs | 5.6/7 |

His wife Sarah completed the ASHA-Functional Assessment of Communication Skills for Adults (ASHA-FACS; Frattali, Thompson, Holland, Wohl, & Ferketic, 1995). The results (see Table 38.1), which were similar to those of previous neuropsychological testing, suggested a progressive, severe nonfluent aphasia. Andrew spoke in mostly single word utterances and tended to be more perseverative and echolalic on structured language and conversational tasks. Confrontation naming was severely impaired and was characterized by both paraphasic and perseverative errors. Generative naming was severely impaired, and naming-to-sentence-completion was moderately-to-severely impaired. Andrew was able to repeat single words and short phrases but was unable to repeat sentence-length material. His yes/no response was inconsistent. Auditory comprehension of sequential commands was moderately to severely impaired and variable across stimuli of increasing complexity. Reading comprehension was severely impaired.

Relative strengths were observed. Andrew demonstrated better performance on picture-to-written word matching than written word-to-picture matching, which suggested visual-picture information might be more useful in accessing the semantic system for communication. On informal testing, Andrew's auditory word-to-picture matching (field of two pictures) improved when the picture and written word stimuli were presented together. His accuracy also improved on a sentence description-to-picture matching task. Finally, Andrew demonstrated the ability to write a few single words to dictation and to copy simple words. Data from the ASHA-FACS revealed deficits in the areas of social communication, reading, writing, number concepts, and daily planning. However, according to Sarah, communication of basic needs was a relative strength.

Sarah reported that, recently, Andrew had experienced a change in social behavior and increased confusion. He was referred to a neurologist who confirmed the diagnosis of PPA and determined that the onset of behavioral symptoms was consistent with FTD.

During the initial interview, it was clear that the changes in Andrew's speech, language, and cognitive functioning due to PPA had had a significant impact on Andrew and Sarah. Their financial situation had become strained since the onset of the illness. He was not able to continue in his profession due to his speech and language issues, and Sarah was not able to work because she had to care for him. They were on a fixed income and had to make many lifestyle changes. They lived far from their respective families and did not have any routine social support. Both Andrew and Sarah were frustrated that many medical professionals, including speech-language pathologists, did not seem to have much experience with PPA. As Andrew's condition worsened, Sarah accepted more and more of the burden of communication and the completion of activities of daily living (ADLs). Andrew had always been a fiercely independent and capable person, and his loss of independence was demoralizing. At times, their situation left them feeling alone and, according to Sarah, as if "you are stranded on an island and the sun isn't shining."

## Representation of the Problem at the Time of Testing

Andrew's language function had declined significantly over the five years prior to the assessment, and this decline was the primary symptom experienced during the first few years post-onset. His moderately severe to severe oral-expressive language, writing, auditory, and reading comprehension deficits made it very difficult for him to communicate with others. In addition, the recent change in social behavior and increased confusion had resulted in difficulty performing ADLs. Andrew's history and the results of neuropsychological and speech and language testing were consistent with the diagnosis of PPA. Moreover, the neurological evaluation indicated the onset of FTD.

## Treatment Options Considered

As compared with published investigations of nonprogressive aphasia, the treatment literature for PPA is limited. Only a few studies have reported the therapeutic effect of specific treatment techniques for improving language function in individuals with PPA. Data suggest that individuals with PPA may benefit from a lexical-semantic treatment for word retrieval deficits (McNeil, Small, Masterson, & Fossett, 1995), an oral and gestural training of verb tense for sentence production deficits (Schneider, Thompson, & Luring, 1996), and a reading and constrained summarization treatment for discourse deficits (Rogalski & Edmonds, 2008). The degree of language impairment and length of time postdiagnosis of PPA for each participant varied across studies, and none of the participants were in the later stages of the disease. Thus, the existing treatment data suggest that individuals with PPA in the early to middle stages of the disease may improve on language tasks; however, given the small sample of patients involved in these treatments and the variability within the PPA population, the potential influence of each treatment on other individuals with PPA is unknown.

Despite the paucity of treatment data, several guidelines or recommendations for clinical practice have been promoted based on case studies and clinical expertise (e.g., Murray, 1998; Rogers & Alarcon, 1998). Rogers and Alarcon (1998) report a detailed case study of an individual with PPA who was followed over the course of his disease and whose treatment followed a set of principles that may be used to guide the management of other individuals with PPA. They suggest a proactive approach to the management of communication deficits, due to the progressive nature of the disease. In particular, they offer three principles to guide therapy. First, treatment goals must be implemented in anticipation of the patient's decline in oral-expressive language. They recommend training in the use of an alternative and augmentative communication (AAC) system *before* it is necessary, so there is an easier transition to using the system as the individual's language function declines. Second, the clinician must ensure that therapy is dyad-oriented, so that the patient and his or her communication partner learn the strategies necessary to promote accurate and efficient communication. As the individual's communication skills decline, there is increased burden on the communication partner to structure communicative interactions. Finally, therapy should be directed at the level of disability or activity limitation (i.e., limitation in performing global communication tasks, such as telling a story, engaging in conversation, understanding humor) within the current World Health Organization International Classification of Functioning, Disability, and Health (2001). Rogers and Alarcon (1998) advise against setting goals to restore or maintain function and suggest that developing strategies to decrease the individual's communication activity limitation is a more productive use of treatment time.

Thompson and Johnson (2005) provide a similar framework for managing the communication changes in PPA, including suggestions for the implementation of AAC early in treatment and the involvement of family and other conversational partners in education and training. However, they assert that in the early stages of the disease, treatment should focus on the impaired language systems with modification and adjustment of goals and treatment as the patient continues to decline. They suggest that some treatment approaches designed for nonprogressive aphasia following a stroke may be useful in treating PPA by slowing the decline in language function, enhancing communication ability, and promoting socialization and a sense of communicative independence.

After considering the literature on the management of PPA, it was determined that Andrew's treatment plan should include (1) educating patient and family, (2) training with an AAC system to improve communication, and, potentially, (3) implementing a behavioral treatment targeting a specific language impairment. Moreover, the treatment should be dyad-oriented to promote successful communication between Andrew and his wife. Given that Andrew was not diagnosed until he was in the middle to later stages of PPA and had no previous experience with an AAC system, it was unclear how he would respond to this type of treatment. Moreover, while there is evidence that individuals with PPA respond to impairment-based behavioral language treatment (e.g., Schneider et al., 1996), Andrew was in a later stage of the disease and had more severe language deficits than the participants included in published reports. Thus, the potential influence of such a treatment was unknown.

Lasker and colleagues (2006) recommended that the objectives of AAC in the later stages of PPA should be to help maintain personal connectedness and participation in communicative activities and to find alternative methods to achieve personal fulfillment. The goals for communication with Andrew's AAC system were based on this idea. Because he and Sarah were frustrated by the frequent communication breakdowns and the recent onset of difficulty performing certain ADLs, these concerns became the focus for designing the picture-based AAC system. In addition to this system, Andrew and Sarah were trained to use the techniques from the program Supported Conversation for Adults with Aphasia (SCA; Kagan, 1998) as another means of facilitating communication. Finally, given Andrew's limited ability to copy some words during the initial language assessment, the Copy and Recall Treatment (CART) program was implemented. The therapeutic effect of CART on written naming performance has been shown in individuals with severe nonprogressive aphasia (Beeson, Rising, & Volk, 2003) but not in individuals with PPA.

## Course of Treatment

Andrew was seen twice weekly for the first 2 months of treatment. However, due to the distance he and his wife traveled to treatment, session frequency was reduced to once each week. His wife, Sarah, participated in all sessions.

One of the first goals addressed in treatment was to improve the couple's knowledge and understanding of PPA. Andrew and Sarah entered treatment with some awareness of his disease: Prior to the diagnosis being made 11 months earlier, Sarah had suspected the diagnosis of PPA based on her own research. The speech-language pathologist was able to share his knowledge of the results of the assessment, the anticipated decline in function, and the treatment options available. Sarah was able to share her knowledge of PPA, verify the information, and ask questions. Education and counseling were incorporated throughout treatment during individual sessions and on the telephone. The speech-language pathologist shared literature regarding the expected course of the disease and the management of its associated communication deficits. Similarly, Sarah shared articles she found on the Internet and information she gathered from books. As Andrew's communicative function declined during treatment, the couple and the speech-language pathologist discussed changes with respect to the anticipated course of the disease and modified the treatment plan accordingly.

The AAC system was developed and introduced at the beginning of treatment. As mentioned, Sarah was concerned about Andrew's recent difficulty performing certain ADLs and the added burden this placed on her. In particular, Andrew was having difficulty carrying out the steps involved in organizing his clothes to get dressed in the morning, preparing his breakfast, washing his hands, brushing his teeth, and organizing his gym bag. Moreover, Sarah and Andrew were frustrated about their frequent communication breakdowns. To target these issues, a picture-based system was designed to facilitate Andrew's ability to perform certain ADLs and to communicate simple messages to his wife and other communication partners. The pictures were paired with printed words to provide multimodality input, which was found to aid comprehension during informal assessment. For each ADL identified, a set of pictures illustrating the steps in the process or the items needed to complete the process were printed and laminated. The pictures for each task were included on individual "storyboards" (using Velcro) that could be placed in the location where the activity took place (e.g., the kitchen counter, bathroom, closet). To improve communication of simple messages, picture/printed word cards were developed for yes/no responses, stores and restaurants, feelings/health, and frequently misplaced items.

The picture sets for the performance of ADLs and the communication of simple messages were introduced to Andrew one at a time during the treatment sessions. For the ADL picture sets, each picture was presented and the correct order of placement was demonstrated. He was asked to point to each picture on command in a field of 3 or 4. Errors were corrected, and cueing was provided. The pictures were then scrambled, and Andrew was asked to place the pictures in correct order. Again, errors were corrected and cueing was provided as needed. When possible, performance of the actual activity was practiced in the clinic. Training was similar for the use of the yes/no, store/restaurant, feelings/health, and frequently misplaced items picture sets. He and his wife were instructed on using the system at home and were asked to keep a log of his daily use of the system. Review of the picture sets during treatment sessions depended on Andrew's ability to perform the task at home.

Communication techniques from SCA (Kagan, 1998) were trained throughout treatment. In general, training focused on the three basic principles for revealing an individual's communicative competence during a conversation. These include (1) ensuring the individual with aphasia comprehends the conversation partner's message by having the partner use multiple input modalities and stimuli (e.g., gesture, written key words, drawings, and additional materials), (2) ensuring the individual with aphasia has a means for responding (e.g., yes/no or fixed-choice response, multiple response modalities), and (3) verifying that the conversation partner comprehends the aphasic individual's message by expanding upon that message and requesting additional information. Communication techniques based on these principles were modeled repeatedly by the clinician during treatment sessions. Andrew and Sarah practiced in the clinic and were encouraged to use the principles to communicate at home. Andrew understood information and responded best when provided with written words, pictures, and maps. Sarah organized a book of photos to use during conversations about parents, siblings, children, nieces and nephews, and close friends. Maps were used to aid communication about local trips, past travels, and details about Andrew's childhood. For example, Andrew was able to communicate how to get to the hardware store from his house using a local street map. Despite his significant communication deficits and the onset of cognitive deficits, Andrew maintained fairly well-preserved map- and route-finding skills and responded well to the use of maps in conversation.

Finally, Andrew was introduced to the CART program (Beeson et al., 2003). This program is a lexical-semantic treatment designed to improve single word spelling through repeated copying of target words while pairing the printed stimuli with the picture of the object or concept (Beeson et al., 2003). Typically, words are treated in groups of 5. The individual is provided with daily homework sheets that require him or her to copy each of the 5 words up to 20 times. Daily self-test sheets are provided to practice writing the word from recall. Five words were chosen for Andrew based on Sarah's input. He attempted to complete the homework task each week, but his attempts to copy the words were often unsuccessful. His initial attempt was the most accurate, but each successive attempt was further from the target, and some perseverative responses were observed. Andrew was not able to learn to write the words without copying them directly. The use of CART was discontinued after 2 weeks of treatment so that resources could be focused on more successful communication tasks.

## Analysis of Client's Response to Intervention

Andrew's response to intervention varied over the course of his treatment program. He and Sarah benefited from education and counseling. They became more knowledgeable of the deficits he was experiencing and what was expected in the future. Moreover, Andrew and Sarah had an opportunity to share their feelings of frustration regarding the challenges to communication and participated in "troubleshooting" the problems. Often, Sarah would describe her creative attempts to improve communication at home, and she appreciated having these ideas validated in the clinic. Communication at home continued to decline as Andrew's deficits worsened. However, having an outlet for discussion of these changes and frustrations beneficial.

Use of the AAC system as originally designed during the first 2 months of treatment proved useful. Initially, Andrew required occasional cueing from his wife to perform the ADLs targeted in the system. The log sheet indicated near daily use of the system to perform such tasks as preparing breakfast, dressing himself, brushing his teeth, washing his hands, and preparing popcorn. Moreover, Andrew and Sarah were able to use the system together to communicate feelings, plans to go to certain restaurants or shops, and misplaced items Andrew was trying to find (e.g., wallet, keys, etc.). During this time, Sarah reported that Andrew was exhibiting some increased independence in performing the ADLs targeted in treatment. This permitted Sarah to relax during the day for at least a short period of time (e.g., drink a cup of tea, read the newspaper, etc.).

After the first 2 months of treatment, Andrew began having more difficulty performing the tasks targeted in the AAC system. Sarah reported that he needed more cueing to perform many of the tasks, even when using the pictures as a guide. During treatment sessions, the system was changed to include more input from Sarah but still promote Andrew's independence. For example, Andrew still used the pictures to prepare his breakfast (bagel with butter), but Sarah placed the required materials (plate, knife, etc.) on the counter instead of having Andrew find the items in the kitchen. In addition, Sarah periodically modeled the task for Andrew and provided prompts to facilitate improved performance. Even with this change, Andrew required increased cueing from Sarah to perform the tasks.

Over the course of treatment, Andrew and Sarah benefited from using the principles of SCA to facilitate communication at home. As Andrew's communication skills deteriorated, Sarah accepted more responsibility during conversational interactions. At that point, supported conversation was the best means of communication, because Andrew required active participation by the listener. Having practiced utilizing the principles in the treatment sessions, Sarah was able to make this transition. Sarah used the picture stimuli from the AAC system, other referential graphics (e.g., picture book of family members, maps), and written key words to ensure that Andrew comprehended the information presented and had a means of responding.

## Further Recommendations

When treating patients with PPA, the clinical profile for the patient continues to change as his or her communication and (possibly) cognitive skills deteriorate. Hypotheses about the patient's deficits are continually revised, as are the format and goals of treatment. As previously discussed, clinicians, patients, and family members should prepare for these changes in advance so that there is a smooth transition to the next phase of language treatment and use of communication strategies. Andrew had already experienced a significant decline in his language skills and communicative function before he was first seen for treatment. During treatment, language and communicative function continued to decline, and he began to demonstrate increased confusion at home. Andrew's treatment continues, and he and Sarah are preparing for the next modification that will shift additional communication and activity burdens to her, while promoting his independence for as long as possible. Continued education and support has been a healthy coping mechanism for this client and his wife.

## Author Note

The case presented is of an actual client with PPA and his wife. He and his wife granted permission to the author to use their case in this text, and they actively participated in the creation of this manuscript through interviews and discussion. Both were excited to know that their experiences might help in the training of future clinicians.

## References


Beeson, P. M., Rising, K., & Volk, J. (2003). Writing treatment for severe aphasia: Who benefits? *Journal of Speech-Language Hearing Sciences, 46*, 1038–1060.

Frattali, C. M., Thompson, C. K., Holland, A. L., Wohl, C. B., & Ferketic, M. M. (1995). *The American Speech-Language-Hearing Association Functional Assessment of Communication Skills for Adults.* Rockville, MD: American Speech-Language-Hearing Association.

Howard D., & Patterson K. (1992) *Pyramids and Palm Trees: A test of semantic access from pictures and words.* Bury St. Edmunds, Suffolk, UK: Thames Valley Publishing.

Kagan, A. (1998). Supported conversation for adults with aphasia: Methods and resources for training conversational partners. *Aphasiology, 12*, 816–830.

Kavrie, S. H., & Duffy, J. R. (1994, November). *Primary progressive apraxia of speech.* Paper presented at the annual convention of the American Speech-Language-Hearing Association, New Orleans, LA.

Kertesz, A. (2006). *Western Aphasia Battery-Revised.* San Antonio, TX: Harcourt Assessment.

Kertesz, A., Blair, M., McMonagle, P., & Munoz, D. G. (2007). The diagnosis and course of frontotemporal dementia. *Alzheimer's Disease and Associated Disorders, 21*, 155–163.

Lasker J., King, J., Fox, L., Alarcon, N. B., & Garrett, K. (2006). *AAC decision-making in chronic and progressive aphasia.* Seminar presented at the American Speech-Language-Hearing Association Convention, Miami, FL.

Marra, C., Quaranta, D., Zinno, M., Misciagna, S., Bizzarro, A., Masullo, C., et al. (2007). Clusters of cognitive and behavioral disorders clearly distinguish primary progressive aphasia from frontotemporal dementia and Alzheimer's disease. *Dementia and Geriatric Disorders, 24*, 317–326.

McNeil, M. R. (1998). The case of the lawyer's lugubrious language: Dysarthria plus primary progressive aphasia or dysarthria plus dementia? *Seminars in Speech and Language, 19*, 49–57.

McNeil, M. R. & Duffy, J. R. (2001). Primary progressive aphasia. In R. Chapey (Ed.), *Language intervention strategies in adult aphasia* (4th ed.). Baltimore: Lippincott Williams & Wilkins.

McNeil, M. R., Small, S. L., Masterson, R. J., & Fossett, T. R. D. (1995). Behavioural and pharmacological treatment of lexical-semantic deficits in a single patient with primary progressive aphasia. *American*

*Journal of Speech-Language Pathology, 4,* 76–87.
Murray, L. L. (1998). Longitudinal treatment of primary progressive aphasia: A case study. *Aphasiology, 12,* 651–672.
Neary, D., Snowden, J. S., Gustafson, L., Passant, U., Stuss, D., Black, S., et al. (1998). Frontotemporal lobar degeneration: A consensus on clinical diagnostic criteria. *Neurology, 51,* 1546–1554.
Robey, R. R. (1998). A meta-analysis of clinical outcomes in the treatment of aphasia. *Journal of Speech, Language and Hearing Research, 41,* 172–187.
Rogalski, Y., & Edmonds, L.A. (2008). Attentive Reading and Constrained Summarisation (ARCS) treatment in primary progressive aphasia: A case study. *Aphasiology, 22,* 763–775.
Rogers, M. A., & Alarcon, N. B. (1998). Dissolution of spoken language in primary progressive aphasia. *Aphasiology, 12,* 329–339.
Rosenbek, J. C., LaPointe, L. L., & Wertz, R. T. (1989). *Aphasia: A clinical approach.* Austin: PRO-ED.
Schneider, S. L., Thompson, C. K., & Luring, B. (1996). Effects of verbal plus gestural matrix training on sentence production in a patient with primary progressive aphasia. *Aphasiology, 10,* 297–317.
Thompson, C. K., & Johnson, N. (2005). Language interventions in dementia. In D. K. Attix & K. A. Welsh-Bohmer (Eds.), *Geriatric neuropsychology: assessment and intervention.* New York: Guilford Press.
Weintraub, S., Rubin, N. P., & Mesulam, M. M. (1990). Primary progressive aphasia: Longitudinal course, neuropsychological profile, and language features. *Archives of Neurology, 47,* 1329–1335.
Wertz, R. T., Weiss, D., Aten, J. L., Brookshire, R. H., Garcia-Bunuel, L., Holland, A.L., et al. (1986). Comparison of clinic, home, and deferred language treatment for aphasia. *Archives of Neurology, 43,* 124–136.
World Health Organization. (2001). *International classification of functioning, disability, and health.* Geneva, Switzerland: World Health Organization.

# CASE 39

# Betty: Cognitive-Communication Impairments in a Woman with Right Hemisphere Disorder

*Scott R. Youmans*

## Conceptual Knowledge Areas

Right hemisphere disorder (RHD) arises from damage to the nondominant hemisphere of the brain. Until somewhat recently, the impact of lesions to the right hemisphere of the brain on communication was underestimated and, therefore, understudied. This was perhaps because communication impairments in persons with RHD are subtler than the communication impairments observed following language dominant hemisphere lesions (aphasia and/or apraxia). The communication impairments with which persons with RHD present are usually by-products of the cognitive problems that underlie them.

RHD is typically characterized by cognitive impairments of memory and attention and related difficulties, some of which also impair communication. Some of the more commonly reported impairments include the person's inability to recognize that he or she has a disorder (anosagnosia); an inattention to stimuli on the left side (left neglect); visuospatial and visuoperceptual impairments, which may also inhibit constructional abilities; an inability to recognize or convey emotions; impulsivity; difficulties with executive functions (problem solving, reasoning, judgment); problems with the social aspects of speech (pragmatics); and higher language use and comprehension (Brookshire, 1997).

## Description of the Case

### Background Information

In January 2008, Betty had a stroke in her right frontal lobe with mild residual left-sided weakness. When she was discharged from the hospital to her home, she was referred by her speech-language pathologist to our university clinic as an outpatient. Betty began coming to the clinic for an evaluation and subsequent treatment in March 2008.

#### History Information

At the time of her referral, Betty was a 57-year-old, right-handed, African American woman. Betty lived alone and identified herself as being in the low socioeconomic range. She was a Brooklyn native and English was her first and only language. Betty completed high school but never attended college. Prior to her hospitalization, she worked as an office manager for a local business office; due to her stroke-related difficulties, she was no longer employed. The loss of income reportedly made it difficult for Betty to make ends meet financially.

Betty was a widow; her husband died seven years prior to her referral. She had two unmarried adult sons, Ronnie and Peter, who lived locally. Ronnie visited his mother biweekly and called daily. Betty confided that Ronnie, the older of the two men, was supportive and tried to help her as much as he could, both financially and with household responsibilities. Peter was apparently frustrated by the limitations Betty exhibited following her stroke and expressed his impatience at her slow recovery. Peter visited her daily during her hospital stay following her stroke, but he visited and called less often following her discharge from the hospital.

Prior to Betty's stroke, she had never been hospitalized nor had she had any surgeries other than minor dental work. Her past medical history was significant for high cholesterol and hypertension. Betty had normal, corrected vision and stated that her hearing was within normal limits. Her premorbid reading and writing abilities were also reportedly average.

### Reasons for the Referral

Betty was originally referred to the speech-language pathologist by her primary hospital physician due to problems with swallowing. Upon Betty's release from the hospital, the speech-language pathologist reported that swallowing had returned to normal and that no further diet modifications or compensations were necessary, but expressed the need for a further evaluation of Betty's cognitive-communication abilities by an outpatient speech-language pathologist. Betty was referred to our clinic due to its "sliding scale" cost reduction for persons with low incomes.

#### Interview

When asked, Betty initially downplayed any problems with her cognition or communicative abilities resulting from her stroke. Upon further probing, Betty reported becoming confused during conversations, being easily distracted, and having difficulty concentrating during reading. Prior to concluding the interview, the examiner asked Betty if there was anything in particular that bothered her since her stroke. Betty again changed her response. This time she reported that it bothered her that she had difficulty reading because that was her favorite hobby prior to her stroke; however, she also reiterated that she really did not have any other difficulties.

Betty's son, Ronnie, who attended the evaluation, reported that his mother's personality seemed different since her stroke. He said she seemed "weird" and "like a different person."

When asked what, specifically, he noticed about her that was different, he responded that she was much more "literal" than she had been before; she was easily confused; and she talked on and on without conveying much information or getting to a point. He also mentioned that Betty's once dry, sarcastic sense of humor was no longer expressed.

### Observations

During the interview, the examiner noted that Betty exhibited a flat affect and showed little emotion. She did not initiate eye contact often and maintained it only briefly once it was established. Betty was distractible and frequently had difficulty maintaining and shifting topics. She answered questions with utterances that were excessive in length and somewhat empty of content. Receptively, Betty appeared to understand shorter, simpler utterances, but seemed to have more difficulty when the utterances became longer and more complex. She did not exhibit word finding difficulties, nor did she manifest any grammatical problems. A slight speech impairment was detected, which did not affect her intelligibility.

## Findings of the Evaluation

### Hearing

Although Betty reported that her hearing was normal, she was seen by the clinic audiologist to rule out a hearing loss that could explain some of her impairments. Hearing was within normal limits. Additionally, the audiologist reported that Betty could adequately perceive speech.

### Speech

An oral mechanism examination was conducted. The salient results were as follows: The client had slight tongue weakness and lower facial weakness on her left side in the absence of other abnormal findings. An analysis of her speech showed that Betty produced slightly distorted lingual and labial phonemes. Additionally, Betty's prosody during connected speech was observed to be flat; in other words, her speech was monotonous and somewhat robotic.

### Assessment of Abilities Associated with the Right Hemisphere

The Mini Inventory of Right Brain Injury-Second Edition (MIRBI-2; Pimental & Kingsbury, 2000) was administered to assess some of the cognitive and linguistic abilities that are commonly affected by damage to the right hemisphere.

Betty demonstrated difficulty visually scanning for letters (e.g., circling all of the A's in a particular row of letters). She did not exhibit left neglect. She made several errors during oral reading and was unable to answer a comprehension question. Betty was able to write to dictation with additional time, but made several errors when writing spontaneously. She had difficulty expressing emotion, exhibited a flat affect, demonstrated poor eye contact, and displayed distractibility. She also had mild difficulty with several higher language skills, such as understanding humor and comprehending oral narratives. Betty did not have difficulty comparing or contrasting items. She did have difficulty with oral expression at the narrative level that was described as disorganized, verbose, and tangential. Throughout the assessment, Betty frequently requested that items be repeated, and she appeared to require concentrated attention and effort to answer questions; however, she did not exhibit impulsivity in her responses.

### Conversation

Consistent with the observations made during her interview and on the MIRBI-2, Betty displayed moderate difficulty with verbal expression of her ideas when she was engaged in an unsupported, naturally paced conversation. Her verbal expression was frequently disorganized, fragmented, repetitive, irrelevant, and/or tangential to the topic at hand. She frequently used empty, nonspecific speech during conversation that was sometimes incomplete or ambiguous.

When conversation was supported with visual cues for the topic and sequencing of ideas, Betty performed somewhat better; however she continued to become confused and distracted. Betty's affect appeared flat throughout the exchange. She did not maintain eye contact and displayed some difficulty turn-taking. Also consistent with the results of the other assessments and observations, Betty appeared able to attend to and comprehend simple utterances, but appeared to get "lost" as listening and cognitive demands increased. The use of figurative language, abstract concepts, and humor by the examiner often elicited confused or inappropriate replies.

### Informal Writing Evaluation

Betty was able to write and sign her name and was able to write short sentences to dictation. She generated short, novel written sentences in response to pictorial stimuli but with obvious effort and significant delay. Spelling and letter formation were accurate during this brief screening.

### Informal Reading Evaluation

Betty was able to read short (5 to 10 sentences), seventh- to eighth-grade-level paragraphs orally, but with frequent errors. Her errors consisted of word omissions and word-ending omissions. She inconsistently recognized and self-corrected these errors. She spontaneously and inconsistently used the strategy of finger pointing, which seemed to aid her oral reading ability. In terms of comprehension, Betty interpreted meanings literally, failed to understand humor, and had difficulty assigning a central theme or moral to a story.

### Interpretation of the Findings

Betty presented with a mild unilateral upper motor neuron (UUMN) dysarthria. This type of dysarthria is typically mild, transient, and involves phonemic distortions due to tongue and lower facial weakness. UUMN dysarthria commonly occurs following a unilateral stroke in the cortex of the brain. Although Betty exhibited slightly abnormal speech due to these distortions, they were not significant enough to impair her intelligibility.

Additionally, based on the data obtained from the formal and informal evaluations of her cognition and communicative abilities, Betty exhibited a mild-moderate cognitive-communication impairment characteristic of right hemisphere disorder (RHD). Betty exhibited behavioral abnormalities, such as her flat affect and reduced prosody, which made her verbal output relatively free of emotion and animation. Betty also displayed some of the classic pragmatic impairments that often occur as a result of RHD, such as poor turn-taking, limited eye contact, and excessive verbal output with limited information content and no central point or theme. Betty also was concrete and had difficulty interpreting abstract meanings, including metaphors, and humor. Additional problems included reduced visuoperceptual abilities, comprehension of oral and written narratives, perseveration on a topic, and limited insight into her disorders.

Many of the problems individuals exhibit due to RHD are attributable to underlying problems with attention, including an individual's ability to sustain attention without becoming distracted, focus attention while other distractions are present, divide attention to multitask, and shift attention from one point of focus to another. These underlying problems with attention can obviously explain Betty's distractibility and difficulty maintaining or shifting topics during conversation. In addition, Betty's inability to attend to specific details can also be seen as the underlying cause of her lack of insight into her disorder, her visuoperceptual difficulties, disorganization of verbal and written expression, auditory and reading comprehension problems, and pragmatic impairments (e.g., inability to attend to the listener).

In conclusion, at the time of the initial evaluation, Betty appeared relatively linguistically intact; however, her underlying cognitive problems, primarily with attention, interfered with her ability to efficiently express herself orally or in writing or comprehend higher level oral or written language. Betty's strengths included her evident intelligence despite her stroke-related cognitive impairments, her ability to read and write premorbidly, her attempts to compensate for her impairments (i.e., finger pointing during reading and asking for repetitions when she did not understand a statement), her stimulability to treatment (i.e., conversation improved when conversation was supported), and her familial support. On the other hand, a major barrier to her treatment was Betty's lack of insight into her difficulties.

## Treatment Options Considered

The speech-language pathologist considered various goals and treatment options for this client. Upon reflection, he came to the conclusion that no matter what treatment avenue was pursued, it was imperative that Betty's lack of insight into her disorders be addressed either first or concomitantly while working on other goals. Without insight into her impairments, Betty would have difficulty understanding the purpose or necessity of treatment, and she might also have difficulty maintaining motivation to come to therapy and to complete home assignments or follow recommendations made by the speech-language pathologist.

The speech-language pathologist also considered whether to work directly on Betty's dysarthria. He concluded that directly treating Betty's dysarthria would probably not be a priority unless it was her primary concern. His reasoning was that UUMN dysarthria is often transient (i.e., resolves itself spontaneously as the acute effects of the stroke diminish); Betty's intelligibility was not affected, so communication would not be compromised by the dysarthria, and therapy did not involve extensive verbal output. By using the lip and facial muscles to speak, she would strengthen them and further improve her ability to speak.

Because attention underlies many of the cognitive abilities with which Betty was having difficulty, directly treating attention was considered. The therapist could generate specific treatments that targeted each of the types of attention (focused, sustained, divided, and alternating). By removing the underlying cause, the problem would be expected to diminish. Some researchers have suggested that this is the best approach to treatment (Tompkins, 1995); however, the speech-language pathologist was concerned that Betty might not understand how this treatment approach related to her other problems.

Therapy could also focus on Betty's conversational abilities, including her pragmatics, such as turn-taking, eye contact, and topic maintenance, and her inferential abilities, such as understanding humor, metaphors, incongruence, sarcasm, and implied meanings (Myers, 1990). Improving these abilities would help Betty to better express and comprehend language. Additionally, her son specifically mentioned that Betty's premorbid sense of humor was one of the characteristics that defined her personality. Many of these abilities can be worked on in a conversational context, which tends to be well received by clients due to its naturalness.

Finally, the speech-language pathologist considered direct work on Betty's reading ability because she had expressed a specific concern about this. To maintain motivation in therapy, it is wise to attempt to focus treatment on areas that would not only improve a client's communication abilities but would have the maximum effect on quality of life. Additionally, because Betty lacked some insight into her disorders, working on something she recognized as disordered and effectively remediating it could help her "buy into" therapy. As reading was a hobby of Betty's, she might find the home assignments and treatment activities enjoyable as long as they were ability-appropriate and not overly frustrating. Finally, focus on reading would facilitate work on visual scanning, reading comprehension, and underlying attention problems at the same time, while treating attention directly might seem to Betty to be unrelated to her concerns.

## Course of Treatment

The speech-language pathologist recommended that Betty attend individual 1-hour speech therapy sessions at the university clinic twice a week. The clinician also suggested that Betty attend an adult communication group that met for 1 hour a week and primarily included individuals with aphasia, apraxia, and RHD. It was further recommended that therapy focus on reading, conversational support strategies, and inferential abilities, and that strategy practice occur in structured and unstructured conversation and reading tasks.

The therapist discussed these recommendations with the client to obtain her input into the appropriateness and sufficiency of the goals. The client reported her understanding and approved of the goals without desire to modify or eliminate any of them or to add others. She reported that she was most interested in working on her reading, but she was willing to "try anything."

At first, Betty attended individual sessions sporadically and did not come to the communication group. She rarely completed home assignments and made limited progress. When asked how she liked speech therapy and the tasks on which we were working, she said that she really liked them, but she could not explain why she was doing them despite the speech-language pathologist's repeated attempts to explain this to her. Furthermore, she reported that the transportation van that she used to get to the clinic was always late and the driver was rude to her.

The speech-language pathologist telephoned Betty's son, Ronnie, and asked if he would encourage her to come to therapy more frequently. He agreed and offered to drive her to therapy personally when he was able. True to his word, Ronnie began to bring Betty to therapy.

As Betty began to attend therapy more consistently, she became more enthusiastic about it, and she particularly enjoyed the communication group. In the speech-language pathologist's experience, communication groups often have a powerful effect on clients, who often respond better to comments or redirection from other clients than they do to the speech-language pathologist. In addition, they appreciate hearing from other people who have overcome some of the communication problems that they are experiencing. Clients often share strategies that they have found successful in solving their communication problems, and they share their feelings about life after a neurological incident, such as a stroke or traumatic brain injury.

Betty also attended individual therapy sessions regularly. Therapy had two general focuses: reading and conversation. Betty read aloud paragraphs that increased in length and was encouraged to use her finger to point to every word and to read slowly in a distraction-free environment. She was also asked to recall details from the story and to explain the theme or point of the story to address her attention and reading comprehension abilities. As Betty's reading abilities improved, the speech-language pathologist planned to provide stories that included humor, incongruence, and figurative language to address those impairments as well.

Betty's conversation abilities were addressed by first showing videos of people having a conversation (generated by the speech-language pathologist and two graduate students) in which the conversational partners demonstrated both successful conversations and communication breakdowns due to pragmatic impairments. Betty was asked to first differentiate between the successful and unsuccessful conversations, and then to specifically identify what made the conversations successful or unsuccessful. The speech-language pathologist and Betty practiced conversing, and the speech-language pathologist provided feedback following each conversation. Betty was encouraged to practice her conversational goals during the group therapy sessions. Each group session was videotaped (written consent was obtained from all of the group members). During the subsequent individual therapy session, the speech-language pathologist and Betty watched the videotape together and analyzed her communication, discussing her strengths and the areas that still needed work. The goals included turn-taking, eye contact, topic maintenance, topic shifting, expressing her thoughts concisely and in an organized way, and comprehension of the listener's point. Again, as Betty's conversational abilities improved, the speech-language pathologist planned to provide stories that included humor, incongruence, and figurative language to address those areas as well.

## Analysis of Client's Response to Intervention

Betty continued to attend sessions regularly and reported that she liked coming. With the help of her son, she usually remembered to do her home assignments. She also practiced her conversational strategies with her son, who attended several of her therapy sessions and was informed of her goals. After 6 months, Betty was able to name all of her goals and to explain why they were important to successful reading and communication. She had begun to show slight improvement in reading comprehension, but continued to have difficulty with long passages. Betty's conversational skills had improved as well, including her ability to establish and maintain eye contact, and to maintain her topic; she still had difficulty with excessive and "empty" speech, but her comprehension had improved somewhat due to her improved attention to the listener. Betty carried a card to remind her of her goals throughout the day in case she needed to use it as a reference. She appeared to have "bought into" therapy, and the therapist was now considering adding goals to directly address the various components of attention.

## Author Note

The case described is not based on an actual client. All of the names, background, and diagnostic information are fictitious.

## References


Brookshire, R. H. (1997). *Introduction to neurogenic communication disorders* (5th ed.). St Louis, MO: Mosby-Year Book.

Myers, P. S. (1990). Right hemisphere syndrome. In L. L. LaPointe (Ed.), *Aphasia and related neurogenic language disorders* (2nd ed., pp. 201– 249). New York: Thieme.

Pimental, P. A., & Kingsbury, N. A. (2000). *The Mini Inventory of Right Brain Injury* (2nd ed.). Austin, TX: PRO-ED.

Tompkins, C. A. (1995). *Right hemisphere communication disorders: Theory and management.* San Diego, CA: Singular.


# CASE 40

# Patricia: A Case of Severe Wernicke's (Receptive) Aphasia Due to an Underlying Malignancy


*Elaine S. Sands*


## Conceptual Knowledge Areas

The term *aphasia* typically refers to a classification system credited to the Boston Aphasia Research group and the neurologist Dr. Norman Geschwind and his associates. This classification, upon which many testing and treatment methods are based, divides aphasia into two major categories: Nonfluent/anterior aphasia and Fluent/posterior aphasia. Nonfluent aphasia is characterized by lesions around Broca's area (third convolution of the frontal cortex), resulting in agrammatism or "telegraphic speech" in which syntax is impaired but information words (nouns and verbs) may be present. There is relatively good auditory comprehension. The most frequent classification is that of Broca's aphasia. In addition to Broca's aphasia, nonfluent aphasia also includes the relatively rare transcortical motor aphasia, which is like Broca's aphasia but with better ability to perform repetition tasks. Finally, global aphasia is generally viewed as an anterior aphasia with severe to complete impairment in all language modalities, affecting areas beyond the anterior cortex.

The second major classification is that of fluent/posterior aphasia. When this framework is used to look at fluent or "receptive" aphasia, it is not possible to have purely receptive difficulties without concomitant expressive difficulties. Therefore syndromes are examined that have strong receptive components (auditory comprehension difficulties) as fluent aphasias, typically caused by posterior lesions in the left cerebral cortex, usually around the area of the second temporal convolution. These are often classified as Wernicke's aphasia, conduction aphasia, anomic aphasia, transcortical sensory aphasia, and mixed aphasia. Conduction aphasia is generally found when there is a lesion in the area between Wernicke's and Broca's aphasia, known as the arcuate fasciculus. Transcortical sensory aphasia, a relatively rare phenomenon, is like Wernicke's aphasia but with preserved repetition. A complete discussion of these subtypes may be found in Davis, *Aphasiology* (2007, pp. 33–39). In general, the most frequently seen syndrome within the fluent aphasias is that of Wernicke's aphasia, which has as its major deficit poor auditory comprehension with speech that runs from jargon to real words interspersed with "paraphasic" utterances. Many of these patients have particular difficulties with verbal repetition tasks. Patients with these symptoms are generally among the most difficult to treat because of their frequent lack of awareness of their symptoms and difficulties with attention. Often, patients with Wernicke's aphasia may fail to comprehend even simple conversation or writing. Patients with somewhat better processing abilities may be able to get the main points of a conversation but not the details. An excellent description of this type of aphasia may be found in Brookshire's *Introduction to Neurogenic Communication Disorders* (2007).

## Description of the Case

### Background Information and Reason for Referral

The patient presented here, Patricia, is interesting in several ways. First, although she exhibited symptoms of what was clearly a fluent aphasia, her language problems were characteristic of two types of fluent aphasia: Wernicke's aphasia and conduction aphasia. This may seem paradoxical, but symptoms of both may be explained by the unusual etiology of multiple strokes (indicating more widespread insults to the brain) related to the medical precipitating factor of adenocarcinoma or lung cancer. Her young age (45 years) was another factor of interest. Despite the complex of symptoms, Patricia's case is a good example of how speech-language pathologists deal with these types of aphasia since they are generally thought of as the most difficult to treat.

### Findings of the Evaluation

Patricia was a 45-year-old woman referred to the university clinic for evaluation and possible treatment. She was married, had two children, and was a high school graduate. She was right-handed. Patricia had a history of hypertension and hypercholesterolemia and was a smoker. Approximately two years before she came to the clinic, she developed transient difficulty with speech and a right facial droop with impaired right-sided vision. She did not seek medical help. A month later she complained of chest pressure and was diagnosed with a myocardial infarction. Medical examination at that time indicated a right homonymous hemianopsia and a previous left occipital infarction. A week later she developed what is described as "global aphasia" and right hemiparesis. The MRI indicated that there was a new lesion in the left parietal area and a narrowing of the left middle and posterior cerebral arteries. There was occlusion of the left middle cerebral artery noted on cerebral angiography.

About a week later Patricia developed foot pain and was found to have left anterior and venous thromboses on the left. She also demonstrated tumor markers and a new area of infarction in the right pontine (cerebellum). Speech continued to deteriorate, and the patient developed severe dysphagia and required a gastrostomy tube for feeding. At this point she was diagnosed with lung adenocarcinoma and began a course of chemotherapy, which put her into complete remission (Cestari, Weine, Panageas, Segal, & DeAngelis, 2004). Swallowing improved and she was able to eat normally. The right hemiparesis appeared to have resolved as well.

In summary, this patient suffered multiple recurrent strokes over several months, although she was receiving anticoagulant therapy. Her physicians hypothesized that the hidden malignancy did not appear until it caused the strokes. Despite the relative rarity of this occurrence and the severity of her symptoms, Patricia had an excellent recovery from the cancer, but communication difficulties persisted.

Her responses during the "functional" portion of the evaluation consisted primarily of her use of an automatic phrase interspersed with appropriate use of syntax and intonation but without the information words (mainly nouns and verbs) necessary to make her an effective communicator. In addition, she sometimes used word substitutions, which either resembled the intended word or appeared to be random. The most impaired modality was clearly that of auditory comprehension. For the most part, she was unable to decode any verbal content unless frequent cueing (gestural, visual) was employed. However, in less formal situations, she was able to process some key words related to the context of the conversation. According to the family, this was similar to her limitations noted at home.

## Language Evaluation

Prior to the evaluation, this patient had already received speech therapy for 7 months at a local hospital with slight improvement. Therapy was terminated when health insurance benefits expired. This evaluation was performed approximately 3 months later.

Patricia exhibited symptoms of a moderately severe fluent aphasia (Wernicke's type). Her auditory comprehension was severely impaired, especially in response to direct questions. In a less formal and more functional context she could occasionally respond to conversation with gestures, single words, or phrases, which were sometimes appropriate. This indicated good nonverbal pragmatic abilities. She demonstrated ability to attend to the examiner and attempted to respond to conversation by using stereotypic utterances that were "subpropositional." For example, the utterance that she used during the evaluation and which was subsequently observed frequently was "a piece of them." She used this phrase to answer almost all questions, using appropriate intonation patterns and only partial awareness that she was not communicating.

Functionally, she could sometimes make herself understood with brief but appropriate single words or phrases, but not on a reliable basis and not in response to specific stimuli, rather, when she had something she wanted to express. Although she gestured for a pencil and paper, she was unable to use writing for purposes of communication. Writing was limited to printing her name and address. At one point while apparently trying to say the word "computer," she said the word "camper," a paraphasic response typical of this type of aphasia. When the examiner wrote the words "yes" and "no" on a piece of paper, she was only slightly better able to answer questions. She used gestures to indicate her needs or her understanding of the conversation. For example, when asked what she was going to do when she left the clinic she indicated through gestures that she would take a nap. In general the visual cue (picture, etc.) was found to be only slightly more helpful than the auditory or phonemic cue. Matching words with pictures was only inconsistently performed accurately. The patient appeared to be oriented, frustrated, yet motivated to improve her communication skills.

## Testing

The Bedside Evaluation Screening Test-Second Edition (BEST-2) was administered (Fitch-West, Sands, & Ross-Swain, 1998). This is a standardized screening test used to determine language abilities in speaking, understanding, and reading. On the conversational subtest she stated her nickname with cueing. She gave her age accurately and counted from 1–14, achieving a raw score of 7/30 on this subtest (16th percentile—severe). As expected, she was unable to name any objects, even with cues. She had similar difficulty on the test of describing objects (2/30 points, the 9th percentile). The patient was unable to repeat any single words. She pointed to some pictured objects inconsistently with repetition of stimuli, scoring 15/30, again indicating severe impairment (16th percentile). When a picture stimulus was used, she was able to point to some parts of a picture on command. In reading, she was generally unable to look at a printed word and find it in the picture. Test results indicated severe impairment in all language modalities tested.

Selected items from the Boston Diagnostic Aphasia Examination (Goodglass, Kaplan, & Barresi, 2001) were also attempted. On the "cookie theft" picture she seemed to understand the theme of the picture and used some appropriate gestures to indicate this. At one point she looked at the woman in the picture and stated, "I know she needs to—that's terrible" in response to an impending flood. She again performed poorly on auditory comprehension, unable to follow 1-step commands or point to her own body parts. She could count from 1–9 but was unable to perform other automatic sequences such as the days of the week, months of the year, or the alphabet. She was not able to replicate melodic line in singing familiar songs with the examiner. On one or two questions of responsive naming, for example, "what do you do with soap?" she used appropriate gestures. She performed oral movements in imitation of the examiner, although rate was slow. On verbal agility testing she was totally unable to repeat any words, that is, "mama, mama," after the examiner.

Speech was characterized by some semantic paraphasias, that is, "camper" for "computer." Vocal quality was somewhat loud and slightly hoarse at times. This could be related to stress on the vocal cords due to her many attempts to respond verbally. Possible mild dysarthria was noted but did not interfere with intelligibility and is probably the result of multiple infarctions and subsequent bilateral impairment of the speech mechanism.

In summary, during the evaluation, Patricia exhibited a moderately severe fluent aphasia with deficits in all language modalities. Most significant deficits were the inability to repeat verbal stimuli and severe auditory comprehension impairment. This is striking because the total lack of imitation skill is generally found in conjunction with conduction aphasia. However, persons with conduction aphasia typically have extremely good auditory comprehension. Patients with Wernicke's aphasia, however, typically do not have such a striking deficit with imitation. Again, this seems to be consistent with multiple infarctions causing atypical combinations of symptoms.

## Treatment Options Considered

In view of the nature and severity of symptoms as well as the time since onset (over a year), prognosis for improved language was felt to be guarded. However in view of Patricia's young age and apparent motivation, a period of therapy was instituted twice weekly. It was recommended that therapy focus on using a nonstructured, role-playing approach, supplemented by an attempt at Visual Action Therapy (Helm-Estabrooks, Fitzpatrick, & Barresi, 1982), designed to facilitate gestural communication. In addition, work on improving "yes-no" answers to auditory/visual stimuli was recommended, as was improving reading comprehension of single words.

## Course of Treatment

A speech-language remediation plan was developed shortly after the evaluation. Since Patricia's primary symptoms were severe auditory comprehension and language loss, therapy was directed at the use of gesture in lieu of speaking and the improvement of auditory comprehension in a low structured framework. A major goal was to try to provide Patricia with some means of conveying her everyday needs to friends and family. She received individual therapy twice weekly. The treatment goals were as follows:

1. Improving use of gesture and pantomime to indicate daily needs
2. Facilitating and reinforcing attempts at verbal expression
3. Improving auditory comprehension by using appropriate yes-no answers in conversational settings
4. Improving reading comprehension of single words

### Treatment Strategies

Speech and language therapy consisted of the following:

- Role playing during various functional-type situations such as going to the store, making a list of items to be purchased, eating at a restaurant, and going to the bank. The clinician used functional gestures to facilitate word-retrieval skills. This was generally not successful.
- Presenting gestures such as sleepy, tired, cold, and so on, along with their written counterparts, and asking to perform the associated gestures nonverbally after verbal presentation of the words to help the patient express emotion. This continued to be quite challenging for Patricia.
- Using Visual Action Therapy (Helm-Estabrooks et al., 1982) to facilitate use of gestures for communication. This is a nonverbal treatment program designed to help patients with severe aphasia produce symbolic gestures for visually absent pictured objects. It consists of 3 levels and uses 8 objects that can be represented with a specific gesture. It includes picture cards of the objects and action picture cards representing a person manipulating each object.
- Presenting pictures containing a missing object (e.g., a person sitting at a table without a chair) to facilitate the patient's use of a gestural, verbal, or written word to indicate which object was omitted from the picture. This was successful about 40–50% of the time.
- Answering "yes/no" questions was attempted briefly during each session to limit frustration while improving auditory comprehension.
- Engaging in reading exercises, such as silent reading of single words and matching these with corresponding pictures. There was some success with this task, although consistency was not established.

## Analysis of Client's Response to Intervention

### Language Reevaluation

After 7 months of individual therapy twice weekly, a language reevaluation was conducted. In general, results on the BEST-2 were largely unchanged. The only subtest score that improved was the reading task on which Patricia went from 4/30 to 18/30. Overall performance continued to fall in the range of severe impairment.

On the selected subtests of the BDAE, results were again consistent with earlier testing. On the "cookie theft" picture, her responses were characterized by appropriate syntax with significant impairment in the use of information words. For example, her initial response to the picture was, "She's on the . . . all things are—all the piece of them go and she knows about (jargon) and the other guys can't do them . . . ."

On the auditory word comprehension subtest she was able to point to several pictures on command but could not follow any of the strictly auditory commands except for "make a fist." On the automatized sequences she recited 4 consecutive days of the week and the numbers 1–8. This was similar to her earlier test performance. Again, she was unable to replicate the melodic line in singing familiar songs, repeat single words after the examiner, or name responsively. Reading and writing remained essentially unchanged with severe persistent impairment in both of these modalities.

### Informal/Functional Conversation

Despite the almost identical results on the formal tests, it was striking that during spontaneous conversation, Patricia was able to frequently use appropriate phrases and short sentences in her attempt to communicate. This was a marked difference from her performance 7 months earlier. In addition, there were fewer automatic perseverative phrases and many more appropriate utterances than on previous testing. Although there were no quantitative measures available in these areas, there was no question that functional language performance had improved.

## Further Recommendations

In summary, scores on formal testing and retesting remained essentially the same over a 7-month period. However, functional language use had improved. When not confronted with direct questions, and when conversation was less structured, Patricia seemed to communicate more effectively. Although she continued to exhibit symptoms of a moderately severe fluent aphasia, her ability to communicate functionally seemed to be more efficient than on previous occasions. It was possible that therapeutic efforts resulted in this type of improved function despite the lack of measurable improvement on the formal clinical testing. Patricia showed awareness that she communicated more effectively, demonstrated less frustration, and continued to show enthusiasm and motivation. For these reasons, prognosis for further improvement was fair, and continued therapy using a less structured and more functional approach was recommended.

When working with patients who have significant nonfluent aphasia, it is helpful to attempt to consider the possibility that low-structured treatment activities with decreased emphasis on auditory comprehension and increased emphasis on gesture and pantomime might be the most fruitful course. More observational evidence from the family about changes noted at home should be gathered. For example, the clinician learned that during this time period Patricia began to use the home computer to order groceries online. This was a major step toward increased independence and a source of great satisfaction. The results of this case would suggest that efforts should be directed more at actual real-life situations in as casual an environment as possible and to more actively include family members in the entire process of recovery from aphasia.

## Author Note

This report is based on an actual case. Patricia and her family enthusiastically agreed to share this information. A formal permission form was obtained from the patient at the recommendation of the Institutional Review Board at Adelphi University. I would like to thank my student Alyssa Scelfo for her assistance with this project.

## References

Brookshire, R. H. (2007). *Introduction to Neurogenic Communication Disorders* (7th ed., pp. 300–303). St. Louis, MO: Mosby Elsevier.

Cestari, D. M., Weine, D. M., Panageas, K. S., Segal, A. Z., & DeAngelis, L.M. (2004). Stroke in patients with cancer: Incidence and etiology. *Neurology, 62,* 2025–2030.

Davis, G. A. (2007). *Aphasiology, Disorders and Clinical Practice* (2nd ed., pp. 33–39). Boston: Pearson Education.

Fitch-West, J., Sands, E. S., & Ross-Swain, D. (1998). *Bedside Evaluation Screening Test* (2nd ed.). Austin, TX: PRO-ED.

Goodglass, H., Kaplan, E., & Barresi, B. (2001) *The Boston Diagnostic Aphasia Examination* (3rd ed.). Philadelphia: Lippincott, Williams and Wilkins.

Helm-Estabrooks, N., Fitzpatrick, P. M., & Barresi, B. N. (1982). Visual action therapy for global aphasia. *Journal of Speech and Hearing Disorders, 47,* 385–389.

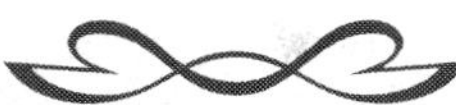

# CASE 41

# Deb: Compensation for Severe, Chronic Aphasia Using Augmentative and Alternative Communication

*Aimee Dietz, Miechelle McKelvey, Michele Schmerbauch, Kristy Weissling, and Karen Hux*

## Conceptual Knowledge Areas

Aphasia is an acquired disorder most commonly associated with left-hemisphere cerebrovascular accidents (CVAs). It impairs a person's comprehension and production of spoken, written, and gestural language. The clinical features of aphasia are not due to intellectual, sensory, or motor deficits; rather, a disruption of auditory and visual processing occurs along with verbal and written production challenges. In short, aphasia disrupts the symbolic processing associated with speaking, listening, reading, writing, and gesturing (McNeil & Pratt, 2001).

Over time and with restorative speech-language intervention, some people with aphasia can reestablish functional communication using natural speech. However, for approximately half the people with aphasia secondary to CVA, the severity and chronicity of impairment does not allow them to participate fully in conversational and information-transfer interactions (Laska, Hellblom, Murray, Kahan, & VonArbin, 2003). As such, people with aphasia often benefit from using augmentative and alternative communication (AAC) strategies, techniques, and devices to support their language comprehension and production. The type of AAC that people with aphasia find helpful is typically multimodal in nature and incorporates various strategies and techniques readily available to all people (e.g., gesturing, drawing) as well as low-technology (e.g., communication books) and/or high-technology (e.g., computer-based) materials.

This case study illustrates how one person with severe, chronic aphasia used multiple AAC strategies, including low-technology and high-technology materials, to support her interactions with a variety of communication partners and across a variety of communication settings and activities. A low-technology communication book and a high-technology AAC device employing visual scene displays (VSDs) incorporated a combination of contextually rich, personally relevant photographs, written words, and, when appropriate, synthesized voice output to support message formulation and system navigation (Dietz, McKelvey, & Beukelman, 2006; McKelvey, Dietz, Hux, Weissling, & Beukelman, 2007). Figures 41.1 and 41.2 provide example pages of low- and high-technology VSDs.

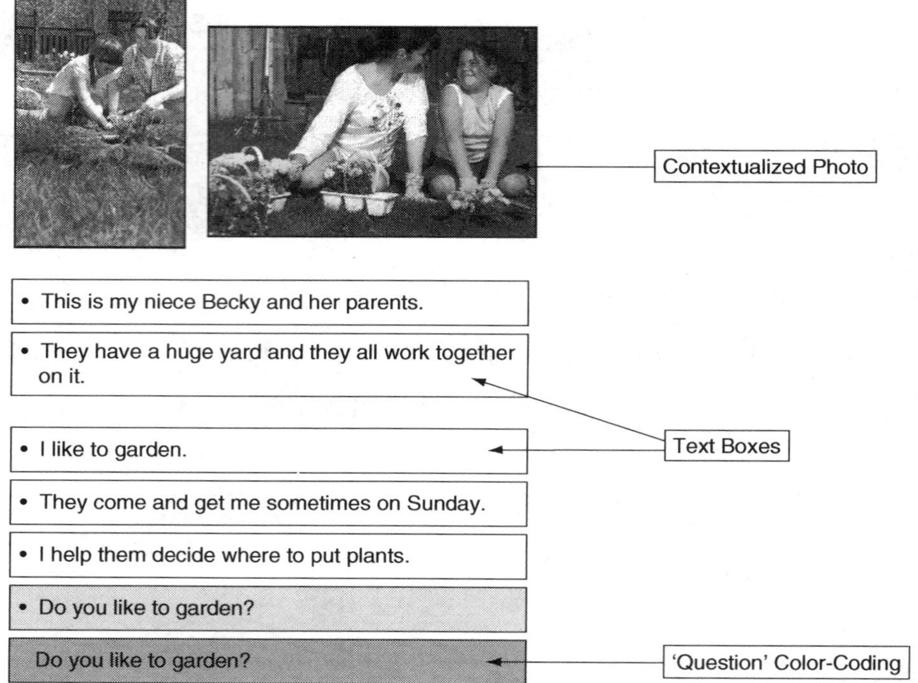


FIGURE 41.1 Example Visual Scene Display Page from a Low-Technology Communication Book

*Source:* Copyright © 2008 Kristy Weissling. Used with permission.

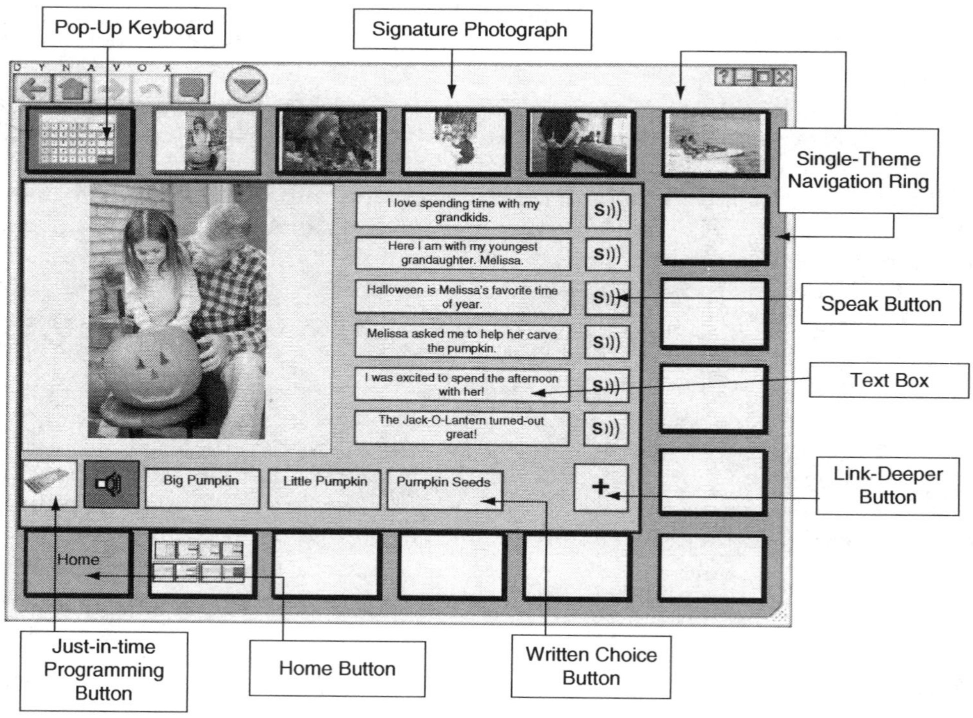


FIGURE 41.2 Example Visual Scene Display Screen from a High-Technology AAC Device

*Source:* Copyright © 2008 David R. Beukelman. Used with permission.

## Description of the Case

### Background Information

Deb was a 56-year-old, married mother of two and grandmother of four when she was referred to the speech-language pathologist (SLP). She had a high school education and her primary career focus was her family. Four years previously, Deb had sustained a left-hemisphere CVA resulting in severe aphasia. Following a stroke, Deb and her husband moved in with their adult daughter, son-in-law, and two grandsons due to financial strain. The family's socioeconomic status was lower middle class, and they resided in an urban area of a Midwestern state.

Prior to her stroke, Deb regularly attended women's meetings at her church, traveled with her husband, and attended family gatherings with her children and grandchildren. As often happens (Herrmann, Johannsen-Horbach, & Wallesch, 1993), Deb's participation in these activities ceased following her CVA. The family reported that Deb refused to attend functions due to embarrassment because of the challenges she faced when interacting with people outside her immediate family. The family reported that she "refused to leave the house [even though] extended family members wanted to see her." In response, Deb indicated that she was too uncomfortable to attend social functions, because she could not talk. Deb's adult daughter, son-in-law, and grandchildren expressed a strong desire for her to reestablish her social roles.

### Reason for the Referral

Deb received traditional speech-language intervention immediately following her stroke. The aim of this intervention was to facilitate Deb's recovery of speech and language skills (i.e., her ability to speak and to understand what others were saying). After several months of outpatient intervention, Deb's recovery reached a plateau, and she was discharged from therapy. After three years of increasing social isolation, Deb's family requested additional speech and language services. They were referred to a speech and language clinic for development of an AAC system. Intervention over the next several months focused on the development and use of AAC strategies including drawing, writing, use of a low-technology communication book that included contextually rich pictures and text, and use of a computerized, high-technology AAC device incorporating contextually rich pictures, written text, and synthesized speech. In addition to individual therapy sessions, Deb attended a weekly aphasia treatment group to increase her interactions with peers and to foster generalization.

### Findings of the Evaluation

Administration of the Aphasia Quotient (AQ) portion of the Western Aphasia Battery (WAB) (Kertesz, 1982) established the type and severity of Deb's aphasia. The WAB is a standardized test in which people with aphasia provide verbal answers to questions, describe pictures, manipulate and name common objects, follow directions, and repeat words. Scores on the AQ portion of the WAB range from 0 to 100, and distinct patterns of performance on various subtests correspond with different types of aphasia. Deb's AQ at the time of her referral to the clinic was 16.5, and she was diagnosed with severe Broca's aphasia. Her communicative repertoire included the use of vocalizations, a single stereotypy (i.e., [apapa]), simple gestures such as pointing and tapping, fragmented writing primarily in the form of single letters and partial words, and pointing to items in a low-technology communication book containing mostly printed words. Deb exhibited moderate auditory comprehension deficits.

### Representation of Problem at the Time of Evaluation

Deb was a partner-dependent transitional communicator (Garrett & Lasker, 2005). She interacted somewhat with familiar people during structured situations but was largely reliant on communication partners to verbalize her intended messages and repair communicative breakdowns. Deb's challenges in generating meaningful speech and in responding to others in novel contexts substantially limited her engagement in social interactions outside her home or speech-language intervention sessions. She needed communication strategies and techniques that would support her residual language processing skills but, at the same time, would provide her with a nonlinguistic manner of expressing ideas and messages. Deb's SLP hypothesized that her communicative effectiveness and willingness to participate in social interactions with others would improve if she could learn to implement a variety of AAC strategies. These techniques included the generation of simple drawings (Lyon, 1995), the writing of short words or partial words (Beeson, 1999), the use of a low-technology communication book that included VSDs (Weissling & Beukelman, 2006), and the use of a high-technology AAC system incorporating VSDs to support navigation and message formulation (Beukelman et al., 2007; McKelvey et al., 2007).

## Treatment Options Considered

A broad range of clinical practice methods exists to assist people with aphasia; hence, Deb's SLP had several options from which to choose when determining the best approach to intervention. The first decision was whether to pursue a language restoration or language compensation approach. Language restoration approaches—such as stimulation-facilitation (Schuell, Jenkins, & Jimenez-Pabon, 1964), constraint-induced language therapy (Pulvermuller et al., 2001), linguistic deficit reduction (e.g., Treatment of Underlying Forms, Thompson & Shapiro, 2005), and modality-specific training (e.g., Multiple Oral Reading, Beeson, 1998); Anagram, Copy, and Recall Therapy (Beeson, 1999); problem-solving approach for agraphia (Beeson, Rewega, Vail, & Rapcsak, 2000); and Melodic Intonation Therapy (Albert, Sparks, & Helm, 1973)—aim to re-establish natural speech and language processing. In contrast, the goal of language compensation approaches is to maximize a person's communicative effectiveness by providing supports to residual language competencies and, simultaneously, teaching multimodal strategies to supplement and serve as alternatives to natural speech and language comprehension and production. Language compensation approaches include instruction both to people with aphasia and their communication partners in the creation of aphasia-friendly environments (Howe, Worrall, & Hickson, 2004), the production of self-generated drawings (Lyon, 1995) and gestures, and the use of low-technology and high-technology AAC devices (Fox & Fried-Oken, 1996; Garrett & Huth, 2002).

Deb's SLP rejected language restoration approaches because of the chronic nature of her aphasia. Although some people with chronic aphasia achieve improved standardized test scores following the implementation of language restoration techniques (Aftonomos, Appelbaum, & Steele, 1999; Pulvermuller et al., 2001), these changes are insufficient to resolve persistent, unmet communication needs. Furthermore, Deb had already participated in several restoration-based approaches, and these resulted in minimal functional changes in her speech and language production and comprehension. Despite extensive language restoration therapy, Deb still could not communicate with multiple people about multiple topics and in multiple settings.

In keeping with the philosophy of multimodal support, Deb's SLP decided to pursue a combination of AAC-based language compensation approaches. These included providing Deb with (1) instruction in the production of self-generated drawings to clarify and expand her communicative intents; (2) reinforcement in the writing of simple words or partial words, because this was a relative strength for her and a strategy she already employed on occasion; (3) expansion of her low-technology communication book to include VSDs; and (4) exploration of high-technology AAC options.

The SLP's next decision concerned the type of high-technology AAC device she would recommend for Deb. Researchers have demonstrated that people with aphasia can use high-technology AAC devices to assist them in specific situations such as answering the phone, calling for help, ordering in restaurants or stores, giving speeches, saying prayers, and engaging in scripted conversations (Garrett & Lasker, 2005; Jackson-Waite, Robson, & Pring, 2003; Lasker & Bedrosian, 2001; Lasker, LaPointe, & Kodras, 2005). However, existing research also indicates that people with aphasia need months or even years to master such devices and that generalization to novel circumstances is difficult and often minimal at best

(Beck & Fritz, 1998; Jackson-Waite et al., 2003; Lasker & Bedrosian, 2001). Because one of the primary concerns of Deb's family was her loss of social interactions with multiple people both within and outside of her family, generalization issues were paramount; hence, Deb's SLP rejected AAC options that would only support specific situations.

The SLP also had concerns about existing high-technology AAC devices for people with aphasia that are not situation specific. Many of these devices rely on the substitution of a novel symbolic processing system for traditional written or spoken language. Hence, they require people with aphasia not only to learn symbols (i.e., icons or isolated pictures) that substitute for written or spoken words, but they force the sequential placement of those symbols in specific orders to form sentence-like structures. The symbolic processing challenges of people with aphasia limit mastery of such systems, and, given the severity and chronicity of Deb's aphasia, her SLP believed that introduction of such devices was unlikely to yield successful results.

To reduce the symbolic processing demands of existing AAC technology and facilitate interaction with multiple people on multiple topics and in multiple situations, the SLP employed a system using VSDs rather than abstract symbols to represent messages and support navigation (Dietz et al., 2006; McKelvey et al., 2007). VSDs can serve as the foundation either for low-technology or high-technology applications, so Deb's clinician decided to explore both options for her. High- and low-technology VSDs incorporate highly contextualized and personally relevant photographs and written words to represent situations, places, or experiences and to support message formulation. High-technology AAC devices incorporating VSDs have the additional benefits of providing synthesized voice output and providing a navigation structure also based on contextually rich images.

Using highly contextualized photographs in an AAC system has distinct advantages for people with aphasia over using other types of pictures or symbol sets. Most importantly, highly contextualized photographs depict elements in relation to the natural environment (e.g., people gathered at a church for a wedding ceremony or children skating on an ice rink during a hockey game) and provide support for referencing a wide variety of related information (e.g., family members and relationships; relevant locations and celebrations; ages, characteristics, hobbies, and likes and dislikes of depicted individuals). As such, they convey the gist of an event or experience with little external explanation or interpretation needed. In contrast, portraits (i.e., pictures of single or multiple people positioned in front of a plain background) or isolated pictures of objects provide limited and decontextualized information that typically supports only identification and labeling functions (e.g., granddaughter, chair). With portraits or isolated pictures, viewers must generate any additional, supportive, or contextual information related to the circumstances prompting the image capture. This spontaneous generation of specific and detailed linguistic information is precisely the task with which people with aphasia struggle. Hence, the use of highly contextualized images in VSD formats helps communication partners infer information and, thus, decreases the demands placed on people with aphasia during communicative interactions (Dietz et al., 2006).

An additional feature that made VSDs an appealing basis for constructing and organizing Deb's AAC system was the flexibility they allowed regarding content. By including multiple VSDs both in her low- and high-technology systems, Deb would have access to numerous, diverse themes (see Figure 41.2) from which to choose her communication topics. Furthermore, the low-technology communication book could serve as a backup system in the event of software or hardware failures or when a situation was not conducive to carrying or accessing the high-technology device. The SLP believed access to a variety of communication themes and maximal portability was crucial for Deb to initiate interactions with a variety of people and across a variety of communication situations. Furthermore, researchers have shown that AAC systems constructed with VSDs are relatively transparent to people with aphasia regarding organization and navigation; hence, people with aphasia master system use, theme expansion, and generalization to novel situations with relative ease (McKelvey et al., 2007). Again, this was important, because Deb's need for support was going to persist, and her AAC system had to be flexible, yet simple enough for her to use in virtually all communicative encounters.

## Course of Treatment

The SLP assisted Deb in developing her low-technology communication book during individual intervention sessions and introduced the high-technology AAC device during sessions at which her family was present. Topics in the initial versions of both communication supports included themes to facilitate communication about Deb's immediate family members and their activities.

Deb's family expressed a strong desire for her to use the high-technology AAC system, but Deb resisted. After 1 month of access to the system, Deb essentially refused to use it for any interactions occurring outside intervention sessions. Deb's family reported ongoing frustration with understanding her communication attempts and expressed concern about her persisting lack of social interactions.

Deb's SLP met jointly with her and her family at the beginning of a therapy session. Deb and each of her family members independently responded to statements presented with 5-point Likert scales (5 = strongly agree; 1 = strongly disagree) to indicate their perceptions about the effectiveness of Deb's communication strategies and their preferences for the various communication strategies available to her. Deb's ratings as well as the averaged ratings of her family members appear in Table 41.1. Of note, Deb and her family members agreed that use of the high-technology AAC device resulted in the greatest communicative effectiveness; they differed in their preferences regarding various strategies. Deb rationalized her preference for natural speech and writing by insisting she would eventually regain these functions and that her current communication strategies met her daily communicative needs. Only after the SLP shared with Deb her family members' effectiveness and preference ratings did she recognize the extent of their frustration with her current communicative strategies. Apparently, she had assumed her family understood her natural speech and writing attempts and, therefore, did not see the purpose of using the high-technology AAC device to supplement her natural speech and writing attempts.

As a result of this meeting, Deb's family suggested a compromise regarding the use of various communication strategies. Deb and her family agreed that she would first try to communicate using speech or writing; however, if her family did not understand her communicative intent, Deb would then use her low-technology communication book or her high-technology AAC device to resolve the breakdown. Deb also agreed that she would not persist with speech or writing attempts during these breakdowns. All parties felt this was an acceptable compromise, because it allowed Deb to use her preferred modes of communication and simultaneously facilitated a gradual move toward increased use of multimodal approaches to communication. For the first time since her stroke, Deb seemed to accept that full recovery of natural speech was an unrealistic goal and that she needed to take steps toward expanding her use of AAC options.

### Early VSD Content

After Deb and her family agreed on a strategy to repair communication breakdowns, Deb began using the low- and high-technology VSDs for a trial period. During her weekly intervention

TABLE 41.1 Likert-Scale Results from Deb and Her Family Members Regarding Communicative Effectiveness and Strategy Use Preferences

| | Communicative Effectiveness | | Preferences | |
|---|---|---|---|---|
| **Strategy** | ***Deb*** | ***Family*** | ***Deb*** | ***Family*** |
| High-tech AAC device | 5.0 | 4.25 | 3.0 | 4.25 |
| Communication book | 5.0 | 4.00 | 3.0 | 4.00 |
| Writing | 3.0 | 3.5 | 5.0 | 3.25 |
| Natural speech | 3.0 | 2.0 | 5.0 | 2.5 |

sessions, Deb's family continued to report struggles concerning the use of the high-technology VSDs. Often, these reports emerged during intervention sessions at which either Deb's husband or her adult daughter were present. The SLP promoted device use between Deb and a family member by demonstrating strategies or providing verbal cues when communication breakdowns occurred during conversations. The SLP used the last five minutes of each therapy session to summarize strategies as well as familiarize family members with new low- and high-technology AAC content. Additionally, Deb's family shared with the clinician notebook entries reporting successes and challenges they observed during the past week concerning Deb's use of multimodal communication strategies. This facilitated input from multiple family members even when they could not accompany Deb to therapy sessions, provided a means of idea exchange regarding development of new AAC content, and allowed the SLP to suggest alternative communication strategies and tips for Deb and her family to use outside the clinic setting.

As a result of family involvement in the intervention process, the SLP recognized an immediate need to create VSD pages to support Deb's communication at home. Themes that emerged included household communication topics such as doing laundry, cooking, washing dishes, going to the grocery store, watching television, and relaying messages regarding phone calls from and visits by people during the day when Deb was alone at home. The addition of these thematic pages alleviated a great deal of frustration for the family, and they reported less reliance on guessing when Deb communicated about these topics. This early success had the added benefit of encouraging Deb to consider participating in social activities beyond her immediate family.

### Content Organization and Continuing Intervention

As Deb gained confidence and skill using her low- and high-technology AAC devices and strategies, her primary intervention goal shifted to a pragmatic issue. Specifically, when using her high-technology device, Deb frequently selected speech output buttons in a sequential manner rather than a conversationally appropriate manner. For example, Deb often asked her communication partner a question even if the person had just asked her a question. Thus, Deb required coaching on how and when to ask appropriate questions when using the high-technology device. To address this, the SLP implemented a color-coding strategy to facilitate Deb's recall of the function of particular buttons on the VSD screens. Text boxes containing questions and corresponding speak buttons were color-coded with a blue background, and text boxes and speak buttons for statements had neutral backgrounds (see Figures 41.1 and 41.2). This strategy, combined with role-playing practice, facilitated a reduction in inappropriate question-asking. Similarly, the SLP used a color-coding scheme on Deb's social greetings VSD page, because she demonstrated difficulty distinguishing conversation starters from conversation closers. Having purple backgrounds for buttons associated with conversation closers alleviated this dilemma.

Another adjustment made by the SLP concerned the synthesized speech output of the high-technology AAC device. Deb's substantial auditory comprehension challenges were exacerbated by the quality and rate of the synthesized speech output. Degraded speech output also interfered with her communication partners' comprehension of synthesized messages, especially for the members of her aphasia support group. Through trial and error, the SLP identified an appropriate voice and speaking rate for the high-technology AAC device.

### Expansion of VSD Content to Support Social Engagement

The next area of focus involved reintegrating Deb into some of her former social roles. With encouragement from her SLP and family, Deb agreed to work on developing VSD themes to facilitate social interactions outside her home. Deb experienced several positive interactions with people in the speech and language clinic where she received services. In particular, participation in an aphasia support group facilitated her recognition of the potential offered by the use of high- and low-technology VSDs and other AAC strategies in expanding her communication repertoire. Several new VSD themes emerged. The first was a vacation theme regarding a trip she took with her husband several years before her stroke. Her use of this theme was a pivotal moment regarding her acceptance of the high-technology AAC device. She realized the potential for expanding her social networks, and became an active co-decision-maker regarding VSD content.

Following successful use of the vacation theme, Deb began requesting new themes. First, she asked for a speech and language clinic theme to facilitate socialization before and after intervention sessions; rather than sitting quietly and nodding her head at passers-by while waiting in the lobby prior to sessions, Deb wanted to interact with other clients and staff. Another new theme was about her hobbies. Using the high-technology device, Deb asked others about their hobbies in hopes that they, in turn, would ask about hers. Then she would use VSDs to show off her miniature cow collection; she shared information about the types of cows she had and where she displayed them in her home. Additional new themes addressed issues about her children and grandchildren, her extended family, her daughter's business, and her family's gatherings.

Deb's success led to a renewed interest in attending family gatherings. Six weeks after introducing the high-technology AAC device to Deb, she left her house to attend a social event—a family holiday gathering—for the first time since her stroke. Afterwards, she rated her communication satisfaction regarding the gathering as a 3 on a Likert-scale ranging from 1 to 3 (i.e., 1 = horrible, 2 = OK, 3 = great). Her daughter and son-in-law confirmed that Deb had communicative interactions with several people at the gathering and that her communication partners were consistently able to determine her intent. Furthermore, Deb did not give up when presented with challenges. For example, when a navigational link on one of her high-technology VSD pages did not work, she independently navigated to the story using another route.

Deb resumed her participation in women's meetings at church, on an intermittent basis. Initially, she appeared satisfied to interact with other women using small talk and sharing content from the themes already available in her low-and high-technology AAC materials. Over time, she expressed a strong desire to participate more actively in Bible study and prayer time. Her SLP identified someone at the church who could provide content, such as specific Bible passages, for advance programming into Deb's high-technology AAC system.

## Analysis of the Client's Response to Intervention

Initially, Deb resisted using the high-technology AAC device because of her belief that she could successfully communicate using natural speech. Once she realized the challenges associated with this communication approach, Deb became receptive to incorporating AAC strategies and device use into her communication repertoire. The SLP was instrumental in helping Deb and her family identify themes and use personal photos to create VSDs that would facilitate communication about daily activities and promote social closeness. As a result, she reestablished social roles within her family (e.g., attending family gatherings) and began to explore communication opportunities outside of her family (e.g., attending Bible study).

## Further Recommendations

Deb continued to live with severe, chronic Broca's aphasia; that is, her linguistic skills did not improve over the course of intervention and most likely will not improve substantially in the future. However, Deb's communicative competence improved greatly since the introduction of AAC strategies incorporating VSDs. Prior to development and implementation of a multimodal AAC system, Deb functioned as a partner-dependent transitional communicator; in contrast, with multimodal communication strategies and AAC support, she became a partner-independent generative communicator (Garrett & Lasker, 2005). Incorporation of multiple AAC strategies, techniques, devices, and materials prompted successful interactions with familiar and unfamiliar communication partners such that she could communicate with multiple communication partners, across multiple settings, and regarding multiple topics. Although she continued to experience communication breakdowns, she had a repertoire of multimodal approaches to resolve breakdowns. For example, when unable to communicate her intent, she had learned to switch with relative ease among gesturing, drawing, and using her low- or high-technology materials rather than repeating [apapa] as she did prior to intervention. At last report, Deb had over 185 images and 377 written statements paired with voice output and corresponding to 21 unique themes programmed into her high-technology AAC system. With continued practice, she is likely to refine further her communication techniques and materials to promote even greater success using a variety of strategies to support communicative interactions.

## Author Note

This case study was based on a true story; however, the client's name was changed to protect her privacy. The Institutional Board of the University of Nebraska–Lincoln approved performance of this work, and the client provided informed consent prior to her participation. Preparation of this chapter was supported in part by the Communication Enhancement Rehabilitation Engineering Research Center (AAC-RERC), which is funded by the National Institute on Disability and Rehabilitation Research of the U.S. Department of Education under grant number H133E980026. The opinions expressed in this chapter are those of the authors and do not necessarily reflect those of the Department of Education.

## References

Aftonomos, L., Appelbaum, M., & Steele, R. (1999). Improving outcomes for persons with aphasia in advanced community-based treatment programs. *Stroke, 30*, 1370–1379.

Albert, M., Sparks, R., & Helm, N. (1973). Melodic Intonation Therapy for aphasia. *Archives of Neurology, 29*, 130–131.

Beck, A., & Fritz, H. (1998). Can people who have aphasia learn iconic codes? *Augmentative and Alternative Communication, 14*, 184–196.

Beeson, P. M. (1998). Treatment for letter-by-letter reading: A case study. In N. Helm-Estabrooks & A. L. Holland (Eds.), *Approaches to the treatment of aphasia* (pp. 153–177). San Diego, CA: Singular.

Beeson, P. M. (1999). Treating acquired writing impairment: Strengthening grapheme representations. *Aphasiology, 13*, 767–785.

Beeson, P.M., Rewega, M., Vail, S., & Rapcsak, S. (2000). Problem-solving approach to agraphia treatment: Innovative use of lexical and sublexical spelling routes. *Aphasiology, 14*, 551–565.

Beukelman, D., Dietz, A., Hux, K., McKelvey, M., Wallace, S., & Weissling, K. (2007). *Training module: Visual scene displays: Case reports.* Pittsburgh, PA: DynaVox.

Dietz, A., McKelvey, M., & Beukelman, D. R. (2006). Visual scene display (VSD): New AAC interfaces for persons with aphasia. *Perspectives on Augmentative and Alternative Communication, 15*, 13–17.

Fox, L. E., & Fried-Oken, M. (1996). AAC Aphasiology: Partnership for future research. *Augmentative and Alternative Communication, 2*, 38–44.

Garrett, K. L., & Huth, C. (2002). The impact of graphic contextual information and instruction on the conversational behaviors of a person with severe aphasia. *Aphasiology, 16*, 523–536.

Garrett, K., & Lasker, J. (2005). Adults with severe aphasia. In D. Beukelman & P. Mirenda (Eds.), *Augmentative and alternative communication* (3rd ed., pp. 467–504). Baltimore, MD: Paul H. Brookes.

Herrmann, M., Johannsen-Horbach, H., & Wallesch, C.-W. (1993). The psychosocial aspects of aphasia. In D. Lafond, R. DeGiovani, Y. Joanette, J. Ponzio, & M. Taylor Sarno (Eds.), *Living with aphasia: Psychosocial issues* (pp. 187–206). San Diego: Singular.

Howe, T. J., Worrall, L. E., & Hickson, M. H. (2004). Review: What is an aphasia-friendly environment? *Aphasiology, 18*, 1015–1037.

Jackson-Waite, K., Robson, J., & Pring, T. (2003). Written communication using a Lightwriter in undifferentiated jargon aphasia: A single case study. *Aphasiology, 17*, 767–780.

Kertesz, A. (1982). *Western Aphasia Battery.* Austin, TX: PRO-ED.

Laska, A. C., Hellblom, A., Murray, V., Kahan, T., & VonArbin, M. (2003). Aphasia and acute stroke and relation to outcome. *Journal of Internal Medicine, 249*, 413–422.

Lasker, J., & Bedrosian, J. (2001). Promoting acceptance of AAC by adults with acquired communication disorders. *Augmentative and Alternative Communication, 17*, 141–153.

Lasker, J., LaPointe, L., & Kodras, J. E. (2005). Helping a professor with aphasia resume

teaching through multimodal approaches. *Aphasiology, 19*, 399–410.
Lyon, J. G. (1995). Drawing: Its value as a communication aid for adults with aphasia. *Aphasiology, 9*, 33–49.
McNeil, M. R., & Pratt, S.R. (2001). Defining aphasia: Some theoretical and clinical implications of operating from a formal definition, *Aphasiology, 15*, 901–911.
McKelvey, M., Dietz, A., Hux, K., Weissling, K., & Beukelman, D. (2007). Performance of a person with chronic aphasia using a visual scene display prototype. *Journal of Medical Speech Language Pathology, 15*, 305–317.
Pulvermuller, E., Neininger, B., Elbert, T., Mohr, B., Rockstroh, B., & Taub, E. (2001). Constraint-induced therapy of chronic aphasia following stroke. *Stroke, 32*, 1621–1626.
Schuell, H., Jenkins, J. J., & Jimenez-Pabon, E. (1964). *Aphasia in adults*. New York: Harper and Row.
Thompson, C. K., & Shapiro, L. P. (2005). Treating agrammatic aphasia within a linguistic framework: Treatment of Underlying Forms. *Aphasiology, 19*, 1021–1036.
Weissling, K., & Beukelman, D. (2006). Visual scene displays: Low tech options. *Perspectives on Augmentative and Alternative Communication, 15*(4), 15–17.

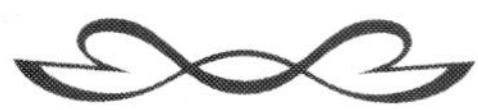

# CASE 42

# Faye: Acute Aphasia in Multiple Sclerosis

*Brooke Hatfield and Suzanne Coyle Redmond*

## Conceptual Knowledge Areas

Multiple sclerosis (MS) is defined by the MS Society as a chronic, unpredictable disease of the central nervous system (the brain, optic nerves, and spinal cord). It is thought to be an autoimmune disease that impacts white matter of the brain and can result in blurred vision, loss of balance, poor coordination, slurred speech, tremors, numbness, extreme fatigue, problems with memory and concentration, paralysis, and blindness as result of demyelination of the white matter of the central nervous system.

Speech-language pathologists (SLPs) are frequently involved in the management of cognitive-communication, speech, and swallowing impairments in clients with a medical diagnosis of multiple sclerosis. These deficits are most commonly associated with white matter involvement, including decreased episodic memory, slowed information processing, and decreased executive functions (Wallin, Wilken, & Kane, 2006), as well as sensorimotor impairments of dysarthria and dysphagia. The traditional understanding of MS is that language and intellectual function remain intact (Randolph, Arnett, & Freske, 2004), though the patient may be easily fatigued, which can impact performance.

The acute onset of aphasia is most commonly associated with gray matter involvement of the left hemisphere via cerebral vascular accident or focal trauma. Aphasia is not commonly a presenting complaint in those with autoimmune disease, which is associated with white matter lesions. As neuroimaging has advanced, however, magnetic resonance imaging (MRI) is detecting cortical *gray matter* lesions even in the earliest stages of MS (Kidd et al.,

1999) and may be its earliest clinical manifestation (Pirko, Lucchinetti, Sriram, & Bakshi, 2007).

Nevertheless, aphasia is rarely reported in the MS population, occurring in only 0.7–3% of cases (Devere, Trotter, & Cross, 2000; Erdem, Stalberg, & Calgar, 2001; Lacour et al., 2007). Even when specific language modality impairments such as alexia and decreased auditory comprehension are described, practitioners are reluctant to diagnosis or report aphasia, with one study noting, "It may be appropriate to consider difficulties with the semantic access the result of slowed processing of a single component of a language system" (Jonsdottir, Magnusson, & Kjartansson, 1998, p. 1474).

There are two primary proposed explanations for the presence of acute aphasia in patients with a primary diagnosis of MS. The first is diaschisis, which is described as damage occurring in white matter tracts connected to the cortical language centers, which results in a breakdown of message transmission (Devere et al., 2000). In other words, the message is formulated accurately but is interrupted as it travels to or from the eyes, mouth, or ears. The second proposed explanation is described as "giant plaques" that form in the white matter and present as cerebral tumors with mass effect (Achiron et al., 1992). In other words, large plaques form and displace cortical tissue, resulting in impairment at the site of the displacement.

A large-scale study of acute aphasia in MS (Lacour et al., 2004) reviewed cases of French patients with a primary diagnosis of MS. Of the 2,700 cases reviewed, only 22 (0.81%) were diagnosed with acute onset of aphasia. Of those 22 patients, 100% presented with nonfluent or unclassified aphasia, and 91% presented with a relapsing, remitting form of MS at onset. Aphasia was the *first clinical manifestation* of MS in 36% of the patients. Information regarding the prevalence of aphasia is not reported in the two other forms of MS, secondary-progressive and primary-progressive.

The anticipated course of recovery following the acute onset of aphasia from a stroke is mitigated by such anagraphical and neurolinguistic prognostic factors as age and severity (Basso, 1992). By comparison, recovery of communication impairments related to autoimmune disease is mitigated by periods of relapse and remission, and response to medication. Treatment strategies with MS frequently emphasize compensatory strategies and energy conservation, while treatment strategies for aphasia frequently address remediation of targeted, modality-specific language deficits and compensatory strategies to facilitate successful functional communication in the patient's environment (Greener, Enderby, & Whurr, 1999). The same study by Lacour et al. in 2004 revealed that of the 22 patients with acute aphasia as a result of MS, 86% of them were treated with methylpednisolone, a medication to suppress inflammation. A "full recovery" was reported in 64% of the cases, while in the remaining 36%, residual sequelae were "not severe." Details of SLP treatment interventions or whether or not subjects actively used compensatory strategies were not described. Mean recovery time was reported to be 15.7 weeks.

## Description of the Case

### Background Information and Reason for Referral

Faye is a 35-year-old right-handed female who was diagnosed with MS in January 2007 after developing both upper extremity and lower extremity weakness in the fall of 2006. In late February 2007 she presented to her local emergency room with speech difficulties and minimal unilateral right-sided weakness over a period of two days. An MRI on February 27, 2007 revealed a 4 cm lesion in the left centrum semiovale and small lesions in the left frontal subcortical white matter consistent with demyelinating disease. Faye was admitted to acute care for one week with the diagnosis of an MS exacerbation. She was not thought to have had a stroke despite the acute onset of both a speech impairment and unilateral weakness. Her medical team included radiologists, neurologists, and MS specialists, with all disciplines agreeing that there had been no cerebral vascular accident. Faye began a course of steroid treatment, which is a common management strategy for MS exacerbations. This steroid treatment resulted in significant improvement in motor function during her hospitalization, but speech difficulties persisted. She did not receive SLP services while in acute care; however, following one week of hospitalization, Faye was discharged to her home in the care of her husband with the recommendation to pursue outpatient SLP services.

Faye was employed as a government contractor and had a master's degree in literature. She lived with her husband and had a very supportive family and network of friends in the area. Prior to the recent MS diagnosis, her medical history had been unremarkable. Her husband described her as "very bright" and "a bookworm." She was active in her community and enjoyed many hobbies, including reading and participation in a book club, working out at her gym, and cooking.

Her job responsibilities included analysis and synthesis of information from multiple data sources and quickly consolidating and summarizing information. She needed to read, comprehend, and retain technical information and abstract theory. She also needed to verbally brief her staff and communicate effectively and efficiently via e-mail. Faye was very concerned about the severity of her language impairment and was highly motivated to return to work.

Faye's husband was employed full-time and was able to continue as such throughout Faye's rehabilitation, thus reducing the urgency with which Faye needed to return to work for financial reasons. However, she was interested in returning quickly because she loved her work and considered it a large part of her identity. Her manager was supportive of Faye's medical leave and rehabilitation, and was willing to provide any accommodations that Faye needed.

Both Faye and her husband had researched commonly linked changes in speech and cognitive-communication skills with MS and had also completed Internet research regarding aphasia. Faye's husband returned to work a few days after Faye returned from the hospital, as she appeared to be safe while unattended during the day. In his research regarding aphasia, he had read patient and family accounts that daily practice on structured tasks had resulted in improved language skills. He enlisted the help of friends who worked in education and gathered a variety of Internet resources to serve as practice materials. When he left for work in the morning, Faye went to what they called "boot camp" at the kitchen table, with Faye working on language-based activities for 3–4 hours/day with telephone check-ins from her husband.

In March 2007, Faye began outpatient SLP services at the recommendation of her physician to address residual communication impairments. She was accompanied to the initial evaluation by her husband.

## Findings of the Evaluation

No medical records were available at the time of the evaluation with the exception of the therapy order reading "speech and language therapy for MS exacerbation." Faye and her husband provided the medical history, relaying specific details and summarizing the results of neuroimaging and the impressions of her medical team. The information presented by the patient and her husband was judged to be accurate given their extensive notes and preparedness for this session.

A combination of objective and subjective measures were used to assess Faye's functional status, along with Faye's report and specific examples of difficulties/errors noted at home as Faye attempted to return to participation in her previous leisure activities.

In a cursory oral mechanism evaluation, Faye presented with facial symmetry at rest and in active movement. She denied changes in sensation. She was able to achieve and sustain all articulatory positions to command without groping or delay. Diadochokinesis was within normal limits.

In a spontaneous speech sample, Faye was greater than 90% intelligible in connected speech with no evidence of dysarthria. Vocal quality was WNL. She demonstrated occasional phonemic errors in her spontaneous speech, consistent with phonemic paraphasias versus apraxic errors (e.g., "skihorse" for "seahorse").

In conversation and structured diagnostic tasks, Faye was able to demonstrate comprehension of moderately complex auditory information when provided extended time and slightly reduced rate of presentation. She frequently requested repetition of auditory information to improve her comprehension; however, gestalt comprehension of both conversational and structured inferential paragraphs was intact. She followed multistep directions without difficulty. Faye reported that she felt that she "missed things" in conversations when there was more than one speaker.

Faye was able to demonstrate comprehension of factual written paragraphs such as brief newspaper articles with intact gestalt comprehension. Her oral reading of single paragraphs revealed rapid, efficient processing. However, Faye demonstrated difficulty as the abstract components and grammatical complexity of written material increased, and as a result her efficiency decreased. Prior to onset of this MS exacerbation, Faye had been an avid reader. She reported significant frustration with reading at the time of the evaluation. Faye reported and demonstrated that she was able to retain details from previously read information following a delay.

Expressive language skills appeared to be Faye's greatest difficulty. She relayed moderately complex novel information to an unfamiliar listener in nonfluent language with frequent assistance for clarification of her intended message. Her attempts at expressing thoughts were characterized by frequent hesitations and phonemic and semantic paraphasic errors. Faye demonstrated excellent awareness of her paraphasias, yet was generally unable to correct her errors. Attempts at narrative discourse generally resulted in a deletion of functors. Her spontaneous verbal expression included a higher percentage of nouns than verbs. Confrontation and generative naming were significantly reduced, which proved to be Faye's greatest frustration. She benefited equally from semantic and phonemic cueing. She frequently supplemented her attempts at verbal expression with gesture. Repetition was intact at both the single word and sentence level. Faye's pragmatic language skills (e.g., maintaining eye contact, maintaining topic, transitioning between topics, proxemics) were well within normal limits. In a structured picture description task, Faye produced the following: "Um, uh, the um, um, dishwasher, um is running out the, you know. Tea cups, no, not tea cups, and uh, um, now. I don't know. Cookie jar, um, and um, the um, the boy is um, tipping over. And, um the girl wants cookies."

Faye's written expression in a simple picture description task was semantically and syntactically accurate at a single sentence level. She continued to have weakness in her dominant right hand, which reduced the legibility of her writing and slowed her written output. Attempts at expressing abstract thoughts in writing resulted in significant frustration and reduced ability to accurately formulate complex written sentence structures, which somewhat mirrored her verbal expression.

Faye and her family reported no significant change in cognitive skills. Faye was an excellent historian of recent events and medical history. She was able to sustain attention to conversation and diagnostic tasks without redirection. Functional problem solving was not an area of concern for Faye or her family, as she had been managing her own medication and staying at home during the day unattended without incident. She consistently initiated alternative modes of communication when one method failed and revised her performance based on her communication partner's feedback. She reported feeling generally tired, but did not feel that her performance significantly deteriorated over the course of the day. Despite extensive probing, no cognitive deficits were indicated by Faye.

## Treatment Options Considered

Several management questions presented themselves given the constellation of cognitive-linguistic impairments including decreased sustained attention, organization, and short-term memory that are commonly associated with MS and the relapsing/remitting nature of the disease, in the face of the patient's presentation of impaired language in all modalities suggesting aphasia.

The first question was whether it was appropriate to provide treatment given the relapsing/remitting nature of MS and the client's anticipated response to medication. If the communication impairments present upon initial evaluation were likely to improve as the disease process remits or medication lessens its impact, it would be difficult to attribute change and progress to specific therapeutic interventions. There is little to no data to suggest or refute that when aphasia results from MS, it shares the relapse/remission pattern of motor-based sequelae or that it is directly impacted by medication. However, withholding treatment in favor of providing extensive education regarding management strategies would not adequately address Faye's current functional language status and the impact it had on her quality of life and ability to return to work. In this particular case, the client, her physicians, family, and the clinician all agreed that SLP intervention was warranted given the acute onset of the impairments, Faye's motivation, and stimulability.

Once the decision to treat was made, an understanding of the source of the impairment was needed to formulate a diagnosis that would later shape the treatment plan. Given the more commonly seen cognitive-linguistic impairments in patients with MS, it was possible that Faye's presentation was resulting from a grossly impaired organizational system impacted by significant fatigue vs. aphasia. To develop a working diagnosis for guiding treatment, standardized assessments including portions from the Western Aphasia Battery (Kertesz, 1982), Boston Diagnostic Aphasia Exam (Goodglass, Kaplan, & Barresi, 2001), and Boston Naming Test (Goodglass, Kaplan, & Weintraub, 2001) were administered to identify patterns of impairment and facilitating strategies. These measures provided a baseline of language abilities and described her status, but did not provide specific information regarding other potentially mitigating factors or contributors.

To look at specific cognitive-linguistic areas both in isolation and as they interacted with each other, the Cognitive Linguistic Quick Test (Helm-Estabrooks, 2001) was used. This provided information regarding attention, memory, visuospatial skills, and executive functions in addition to language skills, with limited expressive language demands. Faye met and surpassed age criteria in all cognitive-linguistic areas with no single target area as an outlier. This was in direct contrast to the results of her aphasia battery, which indicated impairment across all modalities of varying degrees of severity. Given this data, the clinicians felt comfortable developing a diagnosis of aphasia vs. cognitive-linguistic impairment. Following the initial evaluation, Faye's language impairment was described as moderate transcortical motor aphasia.

In this case, the process of developing a differential diagnosis of aphasia was not confounded by visual impairments, dysarthria, or limited attention and/or short-term memory. One should be cautioned that in clients with MS, these sequelae could certainly muddy the diagnostic waters, and subjective observation of performance on standardized measures may prove more beneficial than the objective results when any of these are present.

Another factor in treatment planning for this case was the appropriate dosing. As previously mentioned, Faye and her family were highly motivated to begin treatment and to complete daily home practice activities, both those provided by the therapist and those developed by Faye, her family, and friends. However, one of the obstacles for clients with MS is rapid fatigue and the need for energy conservation. In the "more is more" approach that Faye and her family had adopted, with the extensive time spent in structured activities, was this as likely to result in a positive change as it would with someone with aphasia resulting from stroke? Should both SLP sessions and home practice be limited in favor of energy conservation? Given the positive prognostic indictors for recovery, including Faye's age, time postonset, progress to date, and motivation, coupled with Faye's report that her performance did not deteriorate over time, a schedule of therapy consistent with a client with similar prognostic variables with acute aphasia from gray matter involvement was chosen. It was recommended that Faye attend 2–3 individual SLP sessions per week, with sessions lasting 50 minutes, for an anticipated time frame of approximately 8 weeks.

A final factor in treatment planning was how to prioritize time within each session. Again, given the relapsing and remitting nature of Faye's MS but little understanding of how this impacts aphasia, the clinicians needed to decide how best to use each treatment session—in activities that target remediation of a deficit area, that compensate for a deficit area, or a combination of the two. Faye's preference was for a combination of the two, which she felt would provide her with the best opportunity for a timely, successful return to work by potentially strengthening her efficiency for compensation. The clinicians developed long-term goals over an anticipated 8-week period to address circumlocution, naming in all forms, syntax at the discourse level, and reading comprehension for work-related information. Auditory comprehension and written expression were to be probed and monitored; however, at the onset of treatment Faye felt these areas to be grossly functional for meeting her daily and vocational needs. Verbal expression and reading comprehension were the biggest areas of frustration and the biggest obstacle to returning to activities of daily living.

## Course of Treatment

### SLP Interventions

Therapy began with extensive training of word retrieval strategies. Faye frequently demonstrated anomia in conversation, but did not have an efficient system to facilitate word retrieval. Therapy focused on circumlocution practice and word retrieval exercises, such as work with synonyms and antonyms. Faye quickly initiated the use of compensatory word retrieval strategies such as circumlocution and substitution in conversation, which significantly reduced her frustration. The frequency of Faye's anomic episodes and paraphasias significantly declined, and she was able to correct these errors with greater efficiency. Faye was always anxious for homework, and was provided with regular word retrieval exercises to complete between sessions.

To address Faye's concerns of slowed reading efficiency, the Multiple Oral Re-reading (MOR) approach as described by Beeson & Hillis (2001) was utilized to improve her overall reading speed. The philosophy behind the MOR program is that repeated oral reading will improve the graphemic recognition of written words and improve overall reading speed and efficiency. In the MOR program, Faye was presented with a series of novel, 100-word written passages. Her initial oral reading rate was recorded, and then Faye practiced oral reading of these passages at home until she could achieve her criterion of 100 words per minute (wpm). Faye was highly successful with this program, beginning with an initial oral reading rate of novel passages of less than 50 wpm. Throughout the course of treatment, Faye's initial oral reading rate of novel information improved with each new passage presented. By the end of treatment, Faye was able to achieve an oral reading rate of greater than 90 wpm with novel information.

Throughout the course of therapy, counseling centered on methods for implementation of learned compensatory strategies into home-, work-, and community-based interactions, as well as discussion of energy conservation strategies and resource allocation should Faye experience a change in status with future exacerbations.

## Analysis of Client's Response to Intervention

Faye attended a total of 18 SLP sessions over 12 weeks. Additional scheduled sessions were missed due to a nonrelated illness. Throughout the course of her treatment, Faye's family was very involved in her care. They frequently attended sessions with her, helped her complete homework assignments, and were supportive of her efforts to utilize compensatory word retrieval strategies.

Faye also found ways to enhance her communication opportunities at home, such as returning to her book club. Although reading the lengthy novels and participating in complex discussions were more difficult than before the exacerbation, Faye was able to use her book club as an opportunity to challenge both her verbal expression and her reading skills.

Ultimately Faye was discharged from SLP treatment in June 2007 having reached her long-term goals and feeling equipped to implement both verbal expression and reading comprehension strategies as needed. She planned to return to work on a part-time basis in July. Faye and her family were very satisfied with the improvement that she made throughout the course of treatment. Although it is uncertain if formal SLP treatment was responsible for Faye's improvement, Faye felt that therapy gave her an opportunity to learn compensatory strategies to help her, by her own report, "be a better communicator with aphasia."

## Conclusion and Further Recommendations

The course of therapy and the recovery pattern were consistent with those of a young, educated, motivated woman with acute onset of aphasia from gray matter involvement, despite the fact that there are several prognostic indicators unique to the MS population, which are both positive and negative. The positive indicators include the age of the individual—those with MS are often younger than the cerebrovascular accident population—and use of medications such as steroids to suppress inflammation. The negative prognostic indicators include recovery patterns related to medical stability—the CVA population often demonstrates a linear recovery pattern versus the relapsing, remitting pattern of MS, and rapid access to treatment of aphasia is much more commonly identified in the CVA population. While the mechanism of aphasia in the MS population is not definitively known, this case supports the notion that management of aphasia, when careful differential diagnosis between aphasia and other cognitive-linguistic impairments is established, is not altogether different from management in those with aphasia resulting from stroke or other focal gray matter lesions. However, a careful eye on energy conservation and education in preparation for future exacerbations may be warranted.

## Author Note

The medical information, initial presentation, course of treatment, and outcomes described above are drawn from an actual case; however, the client's name, quotations, and psychosocial details have been changed, as have the specific diagnostic measures used in the initial evaluation.

## References


Achiron, A., Ziv, I., Djaldetti, R., Goldberg, H., Kuritzky, A., & Melamed, E. (1992). Aphasia in multiple sclerosis: Clinical and radiologic correlations. *Neurology, 42,* 2195.

Basso, A. Prognostic factors in aphasia. (1992). *Aphasiology, 6*(4), 337–348.

Beeson, P. M., & Hillis, A. E. (2001). Comprehension and production of written words. In. R. Chapey (Ed.), *Language intervention strategies in adult aphasia* (4th ed., pp. 572–595). Baltimore, MD: Lippincott, Williams & Wilkins.

Devere, T. R., Trotter, J. L., & Cross, A. H. (2000). Acute aphasia in multiple sclerosis. *Archives of Neurology, 57*(8), 1207–1209.

Erdem, H., Stalberg, E., & Calgar, L. (2001). Aphasia in multiple sclerosis. *Upsala Journal of Medical Science 106,* 205–210.

Goodglass, H., Kaplan, E., & Weintraub, S. (2001). *Boston Naming Test* (2nd ed.). Baltimore: Lippincott, Williams & Wilkins.

Goodglass, H., Kaplan, E., & Barresi, B. (2001). *Boston Diagnostic Aphasia Exam* (3rd ed.). Baltimore: Lippincott, Williams & Wilkins.

Greener, J., Enderby, P., & Whurr, R. (1999). Speech and language therapy for aphasia following stroke. *Cochrane Database of Systematic Reviews,* Issue 4, Art. No. CD000425. DOI: 10.1002/14651858.CD000425.

Helm-Estabrooks, N. (2001). *Cognitive Linguistic Quick Test.* San Antonio, TX: The Psychology Corporation.

Jondottir, M., Magnusson, T., & Kjartansson, O. (1998). Pure alexia and word-meaning deafness in a patient with multiple sclerosis. *Archives of Neurology, 55,* 1473–1474.

Kertesz, A. (1982). *Western Aphasia Battery.* New York: Grune & Stratton.

Kidd, D., Barkhof, F., McConnell, R., Algra, P. R., Allen, I. V., & Revesz, T. (1999). Cortical lesions in multiple sclerosis. *Brain, 122*(1), 17–26.

Lacour, A., de Seze, J., Revenco, E., Lebrun, C., Masmoudi, K., Vidry, E., et al. (2004). Acute aphasia in multiple sclerosis: A multicenter study of 22 patients. *Neurology, 62*(6), 974–977.

Pirko, I., Lucchinetti, C., Sriram, S., & Bakshi, R. (2007). Gray matter involvement in multiple sclerosis. *Neurology, 68,* 634–642.

Randolph, J., Arnett, P., & Freske, P. (2004). Metamemory in multiple sclerosis: Exploring affective and executive contributors. *Archives of Clinical Neuropsychology, 19,* 259–279.

Wallin, M., Wilken, A., & Kane, R. (2006). Cognitive dysfunction in multiple sclerosis: Assessment, imaging, and risk factors. *Journal of Rehabilitation Research and Development, 43*(1), 63–72.

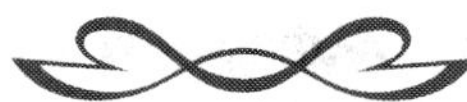



# CASE 43

# Douglas: A Novel Combination Approach to Treating Apraxia of Speech

*Julie A.G. Stierwalt and Joanne P. Lasker*

## Conceptual Knowledge Areas

In order to understand this case, readers should possess a basic understanding of apraxia of speech as an impairment in motor planning, an understanding of basic properties of AAC voice output devices, and a basic understanding of treatment concepts related to drill/practice modeling, feedback, and stimuli selection.

Apraxia of speech (AOS) is a motor speech disorder that results from a disruption of the *motor program* for speech production. For example, when you want to formulate an utterance, first you must select the ideas and the words you want to put together (e.g., "That was a great party last night!"). Once you have formulated what you want to say, the message must be relayed to the speech system with all the sounds in their proper order so the listener can understand the communicative intent. That *message* relayed from the brain, which informs the speech mechanism how to move muscles in order to create words, takes the form of a motor program. Thus, the disruption in apraxia of speech does not occur in formulating language, as it does with aphasia, because individuals with apraxia know what they want to say. Instead, for individuals who have AOS, the disruption comes somewhere between formulating the language and coordinating the structures of the speech mechanism (the diaphragm, the vocal folds, the articulators) to produce speech.

## Description of the Case

The case example provided in this chapter illustrates a new approach to treating apraxia of speech with an individual (Douglas) who suffered from profound AOS. The novel features of this treatment come in the form of combining principles of motor learning (manipulating practice characteristics) and accessing an augmentative and alternative communication (AAC) device for home practice. This approach allowed Douglas, who was initially without speech, to talk functionally with his family and friends using words, phrases, and sentences.

### Background Information and Reason for Referral

At the time of our initial evaluation, Douglas was a 49-year-old right-handed retired sheriff who had experienced a series of 3 strokes 4 years earlier. Immediately following his strokes, Douglas participated in both inpatient and outpatient rehabilitation programs. As part of his rehabilitation plan, a voice-output AAC device using digitized speech recording to store messages was recommended and obtained; however, Douglas never used the device because he felt that it did not meet his needs. The first phase of Douglas's treatment ended 3 years prior to our evaluation. Immediately before our assessment, a brief diagnostic treatment trial with a local speech-language pathologist focused on traditional articulation approaches for apraxia of speech; however, the treatment was terminated when Douglas was still unable to speak. At the end of that treatment trial, the speech-language pathologist referred Douglas to our university clinic for an augmentative and alternative communication (AAC) evaluation.

Before his strokes, Douglas served 20 years in the military and worked as a corrections officer and a sheriff. His educational history included 2 years of college in addition to the training he obtained in the military. Douglas was divorced, had one adult son, and lived with his sister in a town located about 100 miles from the university clinic. Douglas had limited functional use of his right arm and used a cane to walk. Despite his hemiparesis, he drove his own vehicle, used a cell phone, and managed all activities of daily living independently. Douglas was a highly strategic problem-solver. When driving in for his first appointment, he went into the college bookstore, handed his cell phone and the clinician's card to the clerk and indicated that he was lost and needed directions. The clerk called the clinician's number on the card to explain the situation, and Douglas followed the directions to find his way to the appointment.

With regard to lifestyle prior to the series of strokes, Douglas enjoyed fishing, attending church, participating in the fraternal order of Freemasons, shopping, cleaning, and cooking. According to Douglas's sister, he spent the bulk of his time watching TV, shopping, cleaning, cooking, and attending church. His sister reported that Douglas had a desire to communicate with family members, friends, and his pastor. He also wished to be able to communicate on the telephone. When contacted before his evaluation at our clinic, Douglas's sister reported that she hoped we "weren't going to give him one of those talking machines again because Douglas wanted to talk." That statement was not in line with the referral to our clinic for an AAC device by the former clinician, but was an important consideration when selecting treatment options.

## Findings of the Evaluation

### Speech and Language

Because Douglas had an identifiable apraxia of speech, the Praxis subtest of the Western Aphasia Battery (Kertesz, 1982) was administered to determine whether he demonstrated additional forms of apraxia (i.e. limb apraxia or oral apraxia). The subtest assessed his ability to perform and sequence motor movements involving both the upper limbs and facial muscles to voluntary command. Douglas obtained 52 out of 60 possible points (87%) on this subtest. He completed 15 out of 20 tasks (75%) on command and 3 out of 20 tasks by imitation. No limb or oral apraxia was observed.

The results of the Apraxia subtest indicated that Douglas demonstrated a profound AOS without accompanying limb or oral apraxia. Unfortunately, Douglas's expressive speech impairment did not allow for the completion of formal or standardized testing, and we were unable to obtain an Aphasia Quotient from the Western Aphasia Battery (Kertesz, 1982). Specifically, Douglas had a severely restricted repertoire of speech sounds and had difficulty producing even isolated vowel sounds either through imitation or in unison production with the clinician. Informal evaluation revealed that attempts at verbal output were limited to phonation on command and imitation of /ah/ and /oh/. Although it was difficult to determine his language skills due to his limited spoken productions, he was able to communicate successfully using a variety of partner-supported conversation techniques, such as the Written Choice Communication Strategy (Garrett & Lasker, 2005), some handwriting, residual speech sounds, and gestures. When asked to sing along with familiar songs, he was able to imitate melodic line well, but had great difficulty producing any identifiable portion of the words. Throughout the evaluation, Douglas's receptive language skills appeared to be within functional limits for basic conversation.

Because the assessment results confirmed a profound AOS, Douglas was tested for stimulability using the Motor Learning Guided (MLG) approach (Hageman, Simon, Backer, & Burda, 2002). He was presented with 5 index cards containing the words "so," "ah," "no," "mow," and "oh" (targeting vowel sounds "a" and "o"). The vowel "o" was used in 4 of the 5 words because it was the easiest vowel to elicit based on our testing. The clinician provided him with a model of the target and asked him to repeat it. Following the first repetition, Douglas was instructed to wait 4 seconds between repeating the stimulus an additional 3 times. He was instructed to use the intervening pause time to "listen" to his production and change it if necessary to make it sound more like the target. (The MLG approach works to improve clients' awareness of their motor speech system and sound errors.) Douglas produced an approximation of the target for 5 of 15 trials. When the clinician did not provide him with a model (a much more difficult task), Douglas produced approximations on 3 of 15 trials. Many of his productions included delays, articulatory groping, and perseverative errors. However, given his extremely limited output, even an incorrect production was considered a relatively promising prognostic indicator. For example, when Douglas produced "no" instead of the targets "so" or "mow," this demonstrated at least some degree of speech control (ability to execute a motor program). Douglas required cueing and encouragement to "say anything" in order to produce a response for every stimulus card. It was clear that Douglas was, in fact, surprised when he was able to produce any speech at all. Based on the results of this limited trial, we believed it was possible that employing the MLG protocol had the potential to improve aspects of Douglas' speech production.

## Augmentative and Alternative Communication

At the initial evaluation, the voice-output communication device that Douglas owned was a Dynamo (originally made by DynaVox Systems but no longer available), which was funded by his insurance. The Dynamo is a digitized speech communication device, meaning it has no text-to-speech capability. That is, there are no phrases or words contained in the device unless another person previously programmed them into the system. This device was not the optimal choice for Douglas, who had no usable speech and no follow-up support for programming relevant messages into the system. In addition, the Dynamo is geared primarily for "holophrastic" communication, meaning that whole phrases are more readily stored and accessed in the system than words or letters. However, Douglas clearly possessed the ability to formulate and access messages using a variety of letters, words, and phrases. The Dynamo is a dynamic display system, meaning that when Douglas pressed a button, the screen changed to reveal a new set of potential messages. This feature of the Dynamo made sense for a strategic user like Douglas.

During the evaluation, the clinicians presented Douglas with a different voice-output communication device, the DynaMyte (originally made by DynaVox Systems but no longer available). Salient features of this device included the dynamic display, which gives communicators the capability to move from page to page by pressing certain areas on the screen, and the text to speech synthesis. When a user selected different "buttons" on the screen, representing letters, words, and phrases, the speech synthesizer within the device produced a message using a computer-generated voice. Douglas easily navigated to various locations on the screen to access specific messages. For example, when asked which button he would press to find messages related to shopping, he immediately pressed the correct message square linking to the "shopping" page. He clearly understood the concept of navigation and of returning to the "home" page to find other categories of potential messages. When he and his sister heard the machine produce a message using synthesized speech for the first time, it was clear that they were both surprised and impressed by the fact that AAC devices had such capability.

Douglas was also shown the conversation overlay on the DynaMyte, which consisted entirely of whole phrases on buttons arranged according to conversation function, such as greetings, comments, and conversation breakdown repair messages. Douglas was given two hypothetical situations and asked how he would respond. When the clinician presented him with a situation (i.e., "If someone told you you couldn't drive, what would you say to them?") he successfully navigated through the system choosing the representation for "it isn't fair." In another situation, when asked by the clinician what he would say if his niece or nephew drew a picture for him, he responded by choosing the phrase "I love it" from a page of comments.

When asked, through partner-supported conversation strategies, if he liked the synthesized speech-based DynaMyte trialed during the evaluation, Douglas clearly indicated he did.

We suspected that part of his reluctance in using a speech-generating device was related to the fact that he owned an inappropriately prescribed device and received no support or follow-up to help him use it effectively. Given his limited natural speech output, relatively strong reading skills, and strategic communication behaviors, Douglas appeared to be an excellent candidate for voice-output AAC approaches. We began the process of searching for and acquiring a new, more appropriate speech-generating device.

To summarize our evaluation findings, Douglas exhibited profound AOS characterized by his inability to imitate vowel sounds or produce any usable speech. We believed that it was likely that Douglas also had an expressive aphasia, but we were unable to confirm the type or extent due to his speech impairment. Douglas demonstrated strengths in the areas of auditory comprehension (i.e., following verbal commands) and reading comprehension in context (selecting choices presented in Written Choice Conversation by his communication partner). Douglas also possessed adequate skills to use multiple communication strategies, including gesture, limited writing of words, and partner dependent conversation strategies. Douglas's pragmatic behaviors in conversation were good. He appeared to understand requests and his responses were appropriate given his expressive speech constraints. Based on the changes in speech production he achieved using the MLG approach, it appeared that the potential to benefit from a motor learning guided approach was positive. Finally, when provided with an appropriate AAC device, Douglas was able to operate it successfully and was pleased with the benefits that it provided.

## Treatment Options Considered

In making decisions regarding treatment, there are important guidelines to follow, which include selecting a treatment that has the following aspects:

- Has established evidence, or when evidence is not available, is based on sound theory.
- Has shown clinical efficacy through the clinician's experience or through case report.
- Targets behaviors and/or objectives in line with the client's wishes.

With these guidelines in mind, there are several treatments that were considered. Melodic Intonation Therapy (MIT) is a treatment approach used with AOS that has some documented success in the literature. However, that evidence has not been strong and our attempts to probe the technique in our assessment (singing well-known songs such as "Happy Birthday") were not successful in eliciting expression, thus, MIT was not selected for treatment. Traditional approaches such as the Eight-Step Continuum approach had not provided therapeutic benefit in previous treatment with Douglas, therefore they were not selected (Wambaugh, Duffy, McNeil, Robin, & Rogers, 2006). As another option, we considered additional training using AAC, since Douglas appeared more amenable to the concept when provided with an appropriate device. Finally, we decided on a combined approach. Because Douglas *was* able to demonstrate changes in his speech using the MLG approach within the assessment, trial therapy using the technique was warranted. Additionally, while the referral to our university clinic was specifically for an AAC device, Douglas and his sister expressed that they wanted to focus on "speech." Although somewhat new as a technique, MLG is based on sound motor learning theory (Hageman et al., 2002; Schmidt & Wrisberg, 2000), and we have had tremendous success with its application for individuals with acquired and developmental AOS. The second piece of the combination was to utilize AAC as a supplemental practice tool. The combination approach was successful with a similar client we had treated in our clinic. Implementing this approach successfully addressed each of the treatment selection guidelines. There was existing evidence and sound theoretical support, personal clinical experience with the technique, and this technique addressed the client's wish to target speech.

## Course of Treatment

Treatment sessions were conducted in a university clinic once weekly as Douglas drove 100 miles to attend the clinic. The initial portion of every session (during which retention probes were administered) was videotaped and recorded with a lavaliere microphone. In addition to clinic treatment sessions, Douglas practiced the treatment targets at home for 15 minutes a day with the aid of an AAC speech-generating device. These sessions were monitored using a log that was completed weekly. The trained stimuli were programmed into the speech-generating device, with a single target item stored under a single button. When a specific area on the device was selected, the target utterance was "spoken" aloud by the device. For Cycles 1 and 2, Douglas used a small digitized device to practice targets (Dynamo by DynaVox Systems). For Cycles 3 and 4, he used a device with synthesized voice output (Say-it! SAM made by Words+). Douglas reported that he had no strong preference between digitized and synthesized voice output models.

### Stimuli

During each treatment cycle, 20 stimuli were selected for treatment and 20 were designated as untrained. The untrained items were probed approximately every three sessions to determine whether there was a generalization of the treatment effect. We attempted to create lists of trained and untrained stimuli that were similar in terms of length and phonetic structure; however, the primary emphasis was on functionality of the target items. We also took care to create stimuli that were consistent with Douglas's dialect and cultural experiences. The first cycle of stimuli consisted of "real word" CV combinations, including items such as "no," "day," "hi," and "see." Cycle 2 stimulus items included 2-syllable words and phrases such as "amen," "no way," "maybe," "how much," "sweet tea," and "Jesus." In Cycle 3, stimuli included 3–7 syllable words and phrases, including biographical information such as the client's name, medical history, and phone number, and terms Douglas wanted to say in church. These items included: "I had 3 strokes," "paralyzed," "Jerusalem," "arrogance," and "Holy Ghost." Cycle 4 stimuli ranged from 2–5 syllables in length, focusing on phrases that Douglas needed in his daily activities in church, as a member of the Aphasia Group, and using his cell phone, including items such as "How was your weekend?" "seven years ago," "peace be with you," and "I'll call you back."

### Session Procedure

Each MLG treatment session began with random elicitation of the treatment targets as a measure of motor retention. Following the retention task, treatment ensued. The MLG treatment hierarchy, described in Figure 43.1, began with Step 1, in which the clinician modeled a target drawn randomly from a group of 5 of the stimuli, which were printed on index cards. After the model, Douglas attempted an imitation of the target. After that attempt, he produced 3 additional attempts with an imposed delay between each. At the end of the 3 repetitions, the clinician provided the model again with feedback. This process was completed for each of the 5 stimuli. Once the group of 5 stimuli was finished, Step 2 commenced. In Step 2, the process was repeated with the same 5 stimuli presented again in random order, but without the clinician model. This 2-step sequence continued until all 20 items had been completed. At that time, all 20 of the items were addressed once again, elicited in random order.

The unique features of MLG drawn from motor learning theory include the type and schedule of feedback provided and the variable nature of practice (Husak & Reeve, 1979). The feedback clinicians provided was of a "knowledge of results" type, at approximately a 30% schedule. Knowledge of results differs from traditional "knowledge of performance" feedback in which clinicians provide specific instruction on how to change productions (e.g., "Move your tongue between your teeth"). "Knowledge of results" is general information about production accuracy, namely, how close the attempt is to the target item. Feedback consisted of statements such as, "That second try was really good" or "I heard the last part of the target clearly." Knowledge of results encourages the client to self-evaluate his or her productions relying on the auditory and kinesthetic (movement) feedback, rather than the clinician's interpretation. The schedule of feedback is another important consideration. Historically, clinicians have been trained to provide a high schedule of feedback, sometimes as high as 100%. However, delivering feedback at such a high schedule may actually interfere with the client's self-evaluation, which will reduce long-term accuracy (motor learning) (Lee, Magill, & Weeks, 1985).

**The Motor Learning Guided (MLG) Treatment Protocol**

***Environment/Stimuli***

Treatment will take place in a quiet treatment atmosphere as free from distraction as possible. The participant will be instructed to refrain from asking questions during the practice and, more importantly, asked to refrain from talking during the delay interval.

Approximately 20 stimulus items (presented in written form) will be selected for treatment. The stimuli will range from single words to full sentences selected on the basis of their high functionality by the participant or a family member who is well acquainted with the subject and his/her routines. An additional 20 items will be generated and used as untreated items to probe every 3rd–4th session.

**Retention Measure**

Each session will begin with random elicitation of the 20 treated items. These items are scored according to an 11-point rating scale (see Figure 43.2). These ratings demonstrate the extent of motor learning retained from the previous session; thus, they serve as a true index of motor learning. They are uniformly elicited *prior* to the treatment phase of the session in order to eliminate potential practice effects.

***Step 1.*** **The clinician selects a block of 5 stimulus items at random from the group of 20 treated items to be used for Steps 1 and 2. The clinician produces an utterance (participant repeats), waits 4 seconds, and the utterance is elicited from the participant using a written stimulus card.**

Participant attempts utterance without assistance. (No feedback).

Participant produces utterance 3 times with 4-second pause between each attempt.

After the 3 attempts, the clinician will repeat the stimulus and provide *knowledge of results* feedback (general feedback regarding the accuracy of the client's productions).

*(Step 1 continues for a block of 5 stimulus items.)*

***Step 2.*** **Using the same 5 stimulus items as in Step 1, the utterance is elicited from the participant using a written stimulus card in random order.**

Participant attempts utterance without assistance. (No feedback).

Participant produces utterance 3 times with 4-second pause between each attempt.

After the 3 attempts, the clinician will repeat the stimulus and provides knowledge of results feedback.

*(Step 2 continues for a block of 5 stimulus items.)*

***Step 3.*** **Repeat steps 1–2 with another block of 5 stimulus items until completed.**

***Step 4.*** **Upon completion of the 20 treated items, the utterances are randomly elicited from written stimulus cards.**

Participant attempts utterance without assistance. (No feedback).

Participant produces utterance 3 times with 4-second pause between each attempt.

After the 3 attempts, the clinician will repeat the stimulus and provides knowledge of results feedback.

FIGURE 43.1 The Motor Learning Guide Treatment Protocol

Variable practice is another feature incorporated in MLG. It calls for randomizing targets/stimuli during practice. This is in direct contrast to "massed practice" in which a single target is practiced repeatedly for an extended time period. The difference between these practices is a simple one. During massed practice, an individual will retrieve and execute the motor program one time, then hold that program in working memory during the massed repetitions. The variable practice in MLG requires that a client retrieve and execute the motor program for a few repetitions, then move on to another target. Each time these targets are revisited, the motor plan is retrieved. The multiple occurrences provide a greater opportunity for motor learning to occur (Newell & Shapiro, 1976).

| | Retention Measure Rating Scale |
|---|---|
| 11 | Accurate, immediate (may include distortion but maintains immediate intelligibility) |
| 10 | Delayed (greater than 2 seconds) |
| 9 | Delayed (includes silent or audible articulatory groping and/or posturing) |
| 8 | Immediate, acceptable approximation, though not immediately intelligible |
| 7 | Delayed (2+ seconds) acceptable approximation, though not immediately intelligible |
| 6 | Self-correction |
| 5 | Repeat, asks for repetition |
| 4 | Incomplete, similar characteristics but not the target |
| 3 | Error (clearly not the target) |
| 2 | Error plus a delay (2+ seconds) |
| 1 | Perseveration (produces previous response) |

FIGURE 43.2 Retention Measuring Scale

To rate Douglas's performance on the target items at the beginning of the session, clinicians used an 11-point multidimensional scale (with 11 indicating an immediate accurate production and 1 indicating a perseveration). See Figure 43.2 for details of this rating scale. Items were judged to be some degree of "correct" or "intelligible" when ratings were above or equal to a 5 on this scoring system.

### Reliability

Douglas worked with different student clinicians for each of the 4 treatment cycles. The student clinicians transcribed his utterances elicited during the retention measure at the start of each session. They transcribed online and then viewed videotapes to correct any transcription or scoring errors. Discrepancies were resolved by viewing the session recording and consulting with the supervisors. Reliability checks were conducted on a minimum of 30% of all transcripts for each treatment cycle. The overall mean inter-observer agreement for correct productions for all sessions was 88%. Procedural reliability of clinician's adherence to the steps of the MLG protocol was determined for all of the treatment sessions in each cycle and found to be 100%.

## Analysis of Client's Response to Intervention

Figures 43.3, 43.4, 43.5, and 43.6 illustrate the accuracy of production of trained and untrained stimulus items from retention probes conducted in Cycles 1, 2, 3, and 4. In Cycle 1, Douglas did not initially produce any of the treated or untreated stimuli successfully. By the end of the first cycle, accuracy had increased steadily until his productions of treatment targets stabilized at 13 out of 20. Within the first 3 weeks of Cycle 2, 8 out of 20 of the targets were being produced at an intelligible level. At the end of the second cycle, 16 of the 20 targets were produced at an intelligible level. Generalization to untrained items was also seen for 10 of the 20 untreated stimuli that were produced at an intelligible level, although the improvement did not approach the treatment effect demonstrated with target items. At the end of Cycle 3, 14 of the 20 items were produced accurately. Due to the complexity of items in the Cycle 3 treatment set (e.g., "arrogance," "runs a day care") the cycle continued for 2 academic semesters. All treated and untreated stimuli from Cycles 1, 2, and 3 were probed at the end of Cycle 3, and Douglas retained correct production of 46 of 65 targets (71%). When Douglas returned after a summer break to begin Cycle 4, treated and untreated stimuli from Cycle 3 were probed, and Douglas retained correct production of 15 of the trained utterances and 10 of the untrained utterances for a total of 25 of 40 items (63%). Given the fact that Douglas reported that he had not practiced Cycle 3 items over the summer break, it is interesting to

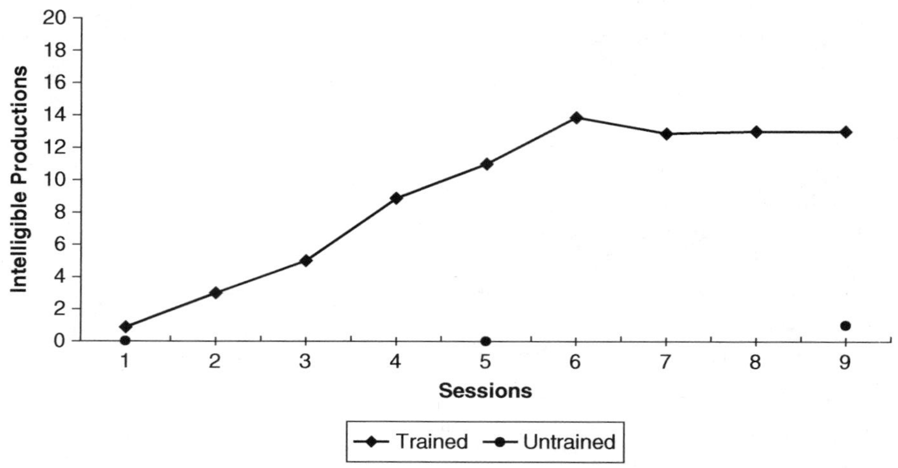


FIGURE 43.3 Number of Intelligible Items (Scores of 5 or Higher) of Trained and Untrained Stimuli in Cycle 1

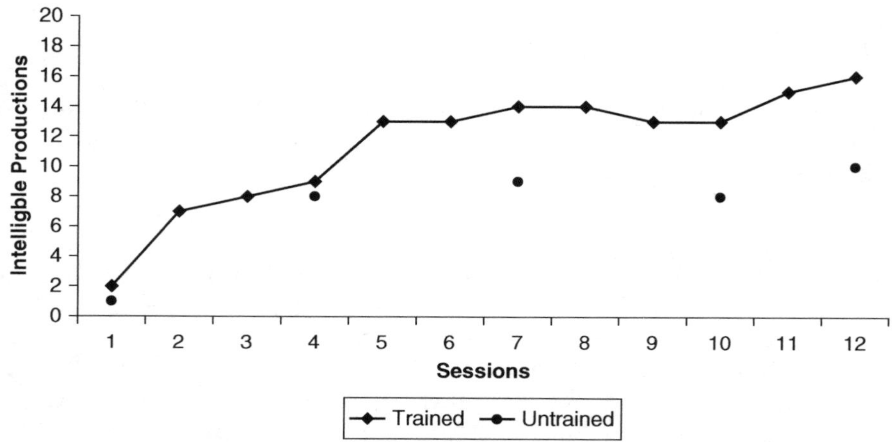


FIGURE 43.4 Number of Intelligible Items (Scores of 5 or Higher) of Trained and Untrained Stimuli in Cycle 2

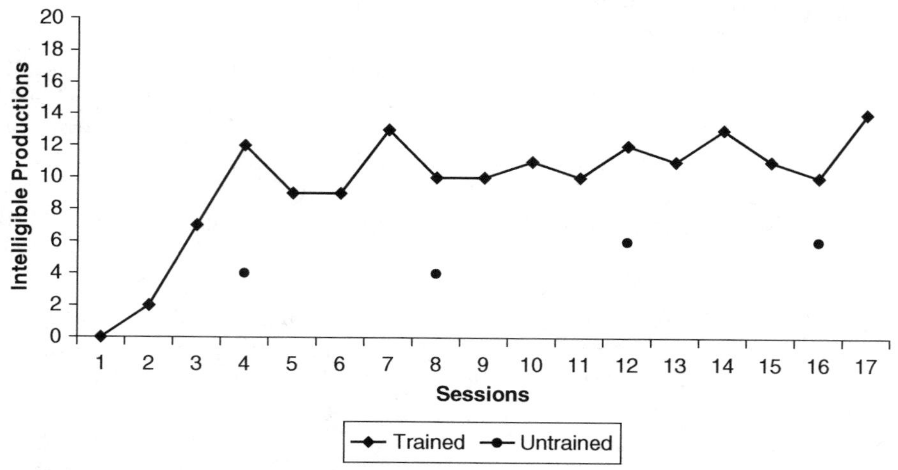


FIGURE 43.5 Number of Intelligible Items (Scores of 5 or Higher) of Trained and Untrained Stimuli in Cycle 3

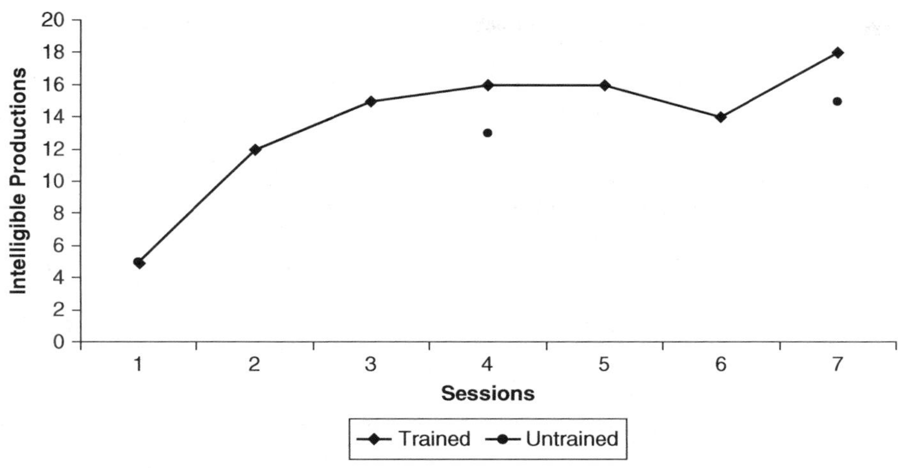


FIGURE 43.6 Number of Intelligible Items (Scores of 5 or Higher) of Trained and Untrained Stimuli in Cycle 4

note that he retained correct production of both trained and untrained items over a period of 4 months without training. Cycle 4 began with both trained and untrained items at a score of 5 correct. By the seventh week of Cycle 4, Douglas produced 18 of 20 trained stimuli and 15 of 20 untrained items correctly.

In addition to changes noted on weekly retention probes, Douglas, his family and other clinicians reported positive changes in Douglas's spoken productions in "real-life" activities. While participating in Cycle 2, Douglas attended a weekly Aphasia Group conducted at a university clinic and began to verbalize during group sessions. He attempted novel and trained words in contexts outside of treatment sessions, as observed by clinicians and through reports from his sister. Douglas continued his participation in Aphasia Group through Cycle 3 with ever-increasing numbers of verbal attempts noted each week. During a particularly engaging group session, Douglas attempted to produce novel 1–3 word utterances at least 40 times. Douglas now speaks during one-to-one conversations with clinicians on a regular basis, usually producing untrained responses. For example, when asked how tall he was, Douglas replied "6–2." He recited his phone number for a clinician when asked and commented on a supervisor's new hairstyle by saying, "your hair." In a recent conversation about Thanksgiving, he independently produced the utterances "fried turkey," "dinner," "fresh," "peanut oil," "throw it away," "nephew," and "Georgia."

## Implications and Hypotheses

Results revealed that a combined treatment approach that utilized the Motor Learning Guided approach (MLG) for apraxia of speech and augmentative and alternative communication (AAC) was effective for this client with long-standing, profound apraxia of speech. The gains Douglas made were particularly notable given his time poststroke (4 years at the start of treatment) and the severity of his impairment (essentially nonverbal). Based on these results, we have noted several interesting features related to this treatment approach:

- While clearly effective for Douglas, this approach was quite effortful, especially at the beginning; he expended both physical and mental effort to complete retention probes. For example, it took a full 60-minute session for Douglas to produce 40 items (all CVs) in Cycle 1 due to persistent groping and restarts.
- As cycles have progressed, Douglas's facility in producing utterances has improved and the time required to produce each utterance has decreased. However, he continues to rely heavily on written input (e.g., concentrating carefully on the written cue card), particularly for untrained stimuli.

- We note that, as utterances have increased in complexity, it has taken Douglas a greater number of weeks to acquire them. For example, he required 17 weeks to reach mastery of trained items in Cycle 3 as compared with 9 weeks in Cycle 1.
- In Cycle 1, minimal change was noted in untrained stimuli as trained stimuli were acquired. In Cycles 2, 3, and 4, untrained items were acquired in conjunction with trained items; however, retention of trained items has always been better than retention of untrained items. This suggests it may take time to "turn on" a motor programming switch, given time postonset and severity of impairment, but once activated, MLG provided a technique that facilitated the relearning of motor programs for speech.
- As Douglas's speech productions outside of clinic settings increased, his agrammatic language became more evident. For example, he left a message on one author's voice-mail to report car trouble, stating his name and the words, "car—no." Now that Douglas has a greater number of words in his spoken repertoire and greater facility with producing untrained words, we believe that the nonfluent aphasia that likely coexists with his apraxia of speech has and will continue to become more apparent. When Douglas first arrived at our clinic, we were unable to detect his aphasia due to his profoundly limited output. When using handwriting or his AAC device to augment his natural speech, Douglas clearly demonstrated difficulty spelling words, retrieving words, and organizing words into sentences.
- At this time, Douglas uses primarily natural speech to communicate, which he augments and supplements with handwriting, gesture, scrolling through names on his cell phone, and accessing prepared messages on his speech-generating device. He best fits the category of a "generative communicator" as defined by the AAC-Aphasia Classification System (Garrett & Lasker, 2005), in that he is highly strategic and uses multiple approaches to formulate novel messages for communication partners.
- Based on our work with Douglas and other clients like him, we have noted characteristics of individuals who appear to benefit most from this unusual treatment approach. Clients who may benefit demonstrate a greater degree of speech impairment (AOS) as compared with a language impairment (aphasia), have adequate auditory comprehension to discriminate accurate from inaccurate productions, are highly motivated to improve speech production, are willing to persevere in using an approach that offers limited short-term benefits and limited clinician feedback, and are able to devote daily practice time to training and at least one weekly session with a clinician for MLG training.

## Author Note

We would like to express our thanks to Douglas (pseudonym). We are grateful for his willingness to share his story and are sincerely impressed by the time, effort, and spirit he exhibits in pursuing his goals. We would also like to thank the following graduate student clinicians, Stephanie Fountain, Min-Jung Kim, Dorian Chen, and Katie Ames, who worked with Douglas and were just as "bowled over" as we have been by his dedication and tremendous progress.

## References

Garrett, K. L. & Lasker, J. P. (2005). AAC for adults with severe aphasia (pp. 467–504). In D. Beukelman & P. Mirenda (Eds.), *Augmentative and Alternative Communication: Supporting Children and Adults with Complex Communication Needs.* Baltimore, MD: Paul H. Brookes.

Hageman, C. F., Simon, P., Backer, B., & Burda, A. N. (2002). *Comparing MIT and motor learning therapy in a nonfluent aphasic speaker.* Symposium conducted at the annual meeting of the American Speech-Language-Hearing Association, Atlanta, GA.

Husak, W. S., & Reeve, T. G. (1979). Novel response production as a function of variability

and amount of practice. *Research Quarterly, 50,* 215–221.
Lee, T. D., Magill, R. A., & Weeks, D. J. (1985). Influence of practice schedule on testing schema theory predictions in adults. *Journal of Motor Behavior, 17*(3), 283–299.
Kertesz, A. (1982). *Western Aphasia Battery (WAB).* New York: Grune & Stratton.
Newell, K. M., & Shapiro, D. C. (1976). Variability of practice and transfer of training: Some evidence toward a schema view of motor learning. *Journal of Motor Behavior, 8*(3), 233–243.
Schmidt, R. A., & Wrisberg, C. A. (2000). *Motor learning and performance* (2nd ed.). Champaign, IL: Human Kinetics.
Wambaugh, J. L., Duffy, J. R., McNeil, M. R., Robin, D. A., & Rogers, M. A. (2006). Treatment guidelines for acquired apraxia of speech: A synthesis and evaluation of the evidence. *Journal of Medical Speech-Language Pathology, 14*(2), xv–xxxiii.

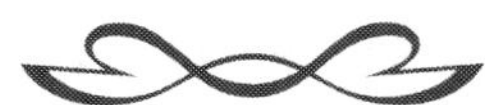

## Articulation

# CASE 44

# Mr. M: Articulation Errors Secondary to Dentures

*Michelle M. Ferketic*

## Conceptual Knowledge Areas

"Although the total U.S. population is expected to increase by 42 percent over the next half century, the number of men and women 65 and older will increase by 126 percent, those 85 and older by 316 percent, and centenarians by 956 percent—nearly 10 times the present number" (U.S. Department of Health and Human Services [USDHHS], 2000, p. 286). Advances in medical and dental care have resulted in more older Americans retaining their teeth, which, therefore, are subject to oral diseases and disorders (Douglass et al. study as cited in USDHHS, 2000). Consequently, there will be an increase in caries, periodontal diseases, and inadequate or absent prostheses (Burt study as cited in USDHHS, 2000).

As people age, the prevalence of medical conditions increases. For example:

- The prevalence of diabetes in the U.S. population of persons age 60 years or older is 10.3 million or 20.9% (Centers for Disease Control [CDC], 2007).
- Approximately one in four adults in the U.S. has hypertension (American Heart Association [AHA], 2004).
- "In 2001, the estimated prevalence of arthritis/chronic joint symptoms among U.S. adults was 33.0% . . . , representing approximately 69.9 million adults" (CDC, 2002).

Medications taken to treat these diseases may contribute to tooth loss secondary to changes in the viscosity of, and/or decrease in, saliva. Changes in pH and dry mouth promote dental decay and negatively influence the oral cavity.

When dental extractions are indicated, complete or partial dentures may be the only option for dental restoration. According to the American Dental Association (ADA, 2007), during the 2005–2006 calendar year, general dentists and prosthodontists performed an estimated 5.5 million complete and 5.5 million partial denture procedures in the United States.

During the past decade, dental implants have become increasingly popular, with an estimated 2 million dental implant procedures performed by active dental private practitioners in the United States (ADA, 2007). Dental implants, a higher cost alternative or supplement to dentures (i.e., dentures supported by implants), are often not covered by dental insurance. For many, especially older individuals and persons with diabetes or heart disease, dental implants are not a viable option. Healing is negatively affected by diabetes, and anticoagulant medications used to treat heart disease reduce clotting.

Ironically, particularly for older individuals, the very health issues that lead to the need for prosthetics often undermine the success these patients experience in adapting to the new oral environment, particularly with regard to the ability to speak and swallow.

Given the large number of denture and dental implant procedures performed in the United States, it is incumbent upon speech-language pathologists to assess the function of dentures for speech and swallowing purposes and to be aware of dental and medical conditions that affect the oral health of individuals and their ability to adjust to dentures.

## Professional Knowledge

1. ***General speech-language pathology evaluation:*** Screening or more in-depth evaluations, as indicated, of the oral mechanism, oral motor, speech articulation, swallowing, cognitive functioning, and language are routine to any speech evaluation. It is important to appreciate the influence of occlusion (i.e., dental and skeletal) on articulatory placement, the effect of maxillary dentures on resonance (Scarsellone, Rochet, and Wolfaardt, 1999), and the role teeth play in the oral preparatory and oral phases of swallowing.
2. ***Assessment of swallowing function:*** Because teeth and saliva play an important role in the oral preparatory and oral phases of swallowing, it is important for the speech-language pathologist to be able to assess this function and to be knowledgeable of factors influencing this function, including sensory feedback and pain. For example, lack of sensory feedback associated with complete dentures and pain during chewing or swallowing may lead to reduced eating or noneating, further compromising health status.
3. ***Assessment and treatment of articulation disorders:*** There is a paucity of information on articulation disorders secondary to dentures. According to Sinescu et al., "not all speech sounds are sensitive to changes of the dental system. The most sensitive sounds which are produced in the oral cavity are /s/, /sh/, /t/, /th/, and they depend on the spoken language" (2008, p. 1206). Displacement of the maxillary incisors to the labial direction was most sensitive in producing speech problems (Ritchie et al. study as cited in Sinescu, 2008; Runte et al., 2001).
4. ***Related matters:*** For many, alterations in physical appearance resulting from dental health issues (e.g., bone deterioration) can have a profound effect on self-image. The clinician needs to be sensitive to this outcome and to the effects social and cultural norms or references (e.g., generation, nationality) can have on the patient's acceptance of dentures and willingness to follow directions or recommendations of the clinician.
5. ***Interdisciplinary management:*** Although many people are fitted with dentures in the United States each year without the benefit of interdisciplinary team management, it is important to be aware of all professionals (dental and other) involved in the patient's treatment. Consider whether there are physicians, psychologists, and/or social workers with whom information should be shared in order to optimize patient care.

6. ***Relevant experiences:*** As with any area of practice, the amount and range of experience a clinician has with a particular client population contributes to his or her ability to successfully assess and treat individual clients. In this particular case, experience with an older group having swallowing and/or articulation disorders as a result of dentures is further enhanced when the clinician has also had experience with individuals within that group who differ in terms of preexisting medical conditions, as well as culture, ethnicity, gender, and race.

# Description of the Case

## Background Information

Mr. R. Michael (hereinafter referred to as Mr. M.), a retired 81-year-old chemist, was referred for a speech evaluation at a university-based medical center by a staff oral surgeon (OS 1) who also had a private practice. His daughter accompanied him to all appointments.

Mr. M. had been widowed 5 years ago. Although he lived alone, 4 of his 6 children lived in close proximity. They, along with a caregiver who visited daily, ensured that Mr. M. received his daily medications and meals. Mr. M. had had 2 years of dental school education following early admission from his undergraduate program.

## Reason for Referral

Mr. M. had a bilateral, symmetric sensorineural hearing loss with a mean pure-tone average of 40 dB in the right ear and 42 dB in the left ear. He had used hearing aids binaurally for the past 4 years. His most recent audiologic evaluation, completed 2 months prior to this assessment, revealed word recognition scores of 86% and 92% respectively for the right and left ear. Middle ear function was normal. Mr. M. reported that while wearing his hearing aids he was able to easily converse in small group situations. Communication was more challenging in crowded venues, which he avoided. He maintained his aids, cleaning and changing batteries as necessary.

Mr. M. reported that his general dentist recommended full mandibular and maxillary dentures and referred him to the oral surgeon on staff. Following an initial oral surgical evaluation, he was referred to the hospital speech clinic because of his concerns regarding the effects of dentures on speech and eating. He also noted that, though he preferred dental implants, his health concerns precluded that option.

His daughter concurred with the reason for referral, but added that the teeth were now affecting his health and medical care. Additionally, until now, Mr. M. had resisted having his teeth extracted because "any teeth are better than dentures."

## Findings of the Evaluation

### Medical and Dental History

Relevant medical history garnered through patient/family interview, referral note, and medical chart included abdominal aortic aneurysm (AAA); severe essential hypertension; chronic myeloid leukemia (CML); osteoarthritis in the knees; Type 2 diabetes; enlarged prostate; depression; and moderate sensorineural hearing loss. With the exception of the AAA, the aforementioned medical conditions were treated with medications: amoxicillin; dutasteride; tamsulosin hydrochloride; bumetanide; warfarin sodium; valsartan; imatinib mesylate; atorvastatin calcium; sertraline hydrochloride; potassium; zolpidem; metformin; tramadol, and timolol maleate ophthalmic solution. Because many of these medications reduce the production of saliva, the speech-language pathologist should screen for any concomitant swallowing difficulties.

An approximate 3.5 cm AAA was diagnosed during a sonogram to assess the effects of imatinib mesylate on the liver. Mr. M. was referred by his oncologist to a vascular surgeon for follow-up. Further evaluation determined that the AAA was over 7 cm in diameter. Surgical repair was recommended and scheduled three weeks later to allow time for the family to obtain preoperative evaluations and to substitute a less potent anticoagulant for the warfarin sodium. Upon medical intake on the day of the surgery, Mr. M. complained that he had an abscessed tooth, which resulted in cancellation of the AAA surgery.

Prior to the diagnosis of the aneurysm, Mr. M. had been referred by his primary dentist for an oral surgery consult because of advanced tooth decay and pain. Additionally, a CT scan of the jaw, ordered because of jaw pain limiting Mr. M.'s ability to open his mouth, was unremarkable. He was evaluated by another oral surgeon (OS 2) with whom his primary dentist had a close working relationship. However, because Mr. M. was a high-risk patient and opposed to dental extractions, OS 2 was reluctant to treat. Consequently, when there was evidence of active dental infections, Mr. M. was treated with antibiotics.

The vascular surgeon postponed AAA surgery until Mr. M. had all infected teeth extracted to reduce the risk of a secondary infection following surgical repair of the aneurysm. Because the OS 2 was reluctant to treat Mr. M., his family identified OS 1, who was associated with the same hospital as his other medical care providers.

Following an examination and review of dental x-rays, OS 1 explained the medical necessity of extracting the teeth and reasons for recommending dentures rather than implants, most notably the history of diabetes and anticoagulant drug therapies. Because Mr. M. had further questions concerning the influence of dentures on his speech and his ability to eat, the oral surgeon referred him for pre- and posttreatment speech and swallowing evaluations, with follow-up 2 months after Mr. M. was fitted with dentures.

## Speech and Swallowing Evaluations

### *Preoperative Evaluation*

- ***Oral Peripheral Exam:*** Consistent with dental findings, inspection of the oral cavity showed extensive dental caries and broken teeth prior to treatment. The patient had a Class I dental occlusion. Evaluation of air emission on nasal and nonnasal sounds was normal. Oral-motor evaluation was within normal limits.
- ***Speech Articulation:*** No articulation errors were noted when using a single-word and sentence screening instrument or during conversation.
- ***Voice:*** Voice quality was within normal limits.
- ***Resonance:*** Perceptual and instrumental assessments of resonance were within normal limits.
- ***Swallowing:*** Despite report and evidence of reduced saliva, Mr. M. had no difficulty swallowing. No swallowing difficulty was present during swallowing screening. It was noted that Mr. M. took small bites of food and sipped water between bites.
- ***Audiology:*** See results of audiologic evaluation done 2 months ago.

### *Postoperative and Fitting Evaluation* (2 Months Following Dentures)

- ***Oral Peripheral Exam:*** Following oral surgical and prosthodontic treatment, with the exception of two mandibular molars (one on either side), all mandibular teeth had been extracted. In the maxilla, all teeth remained, with the exception of the left central and lateral incisors and cuspid. Mr. M. was wearing a complete denture in the mandible and a partial removable denture in the maxilla. A dental class I occlusion was noted. Evaluation of air emission on nasal and nonnasal sounds was normal. The oral-motor evaluation was within normal limits.
- ***Speech Articulation:*** Mr. M. reported that immediately after being fitted with dentures, he had "a lot of difficulty speaking" and his speech initially sounded "slushy." However, more recently his speech had improved, though he noted slushiness was sometimes present and that /s/ sounds were sometimes "whistly." His daughter concurred.
- ***Audiology:*** See most recent evaluation.

Additionally, Mr. M. perceived that when he spoke people looked at his mouth specifically rather than his face, and asked him to repeat himself more often than they had when he did not wear dentures.

With dentures in place, speech was normal with the exception of "whistly" distortions during the production of /s/ and /z/ in all positions of words at the single word level in sentences, and during conversation. Mr. M. produced these sibilants by placing his tongue on the maxillary alveolar ridge. When he produced the sounds by placing his tongue on the mandibular ridge (of the denture), the distortion disappeared. Although changing tongue placement improved articulation, this was not a comfortable placement for Mr. M.

## Treatment Options Considered

### Counseling: Pre- and Postsurgical/Denture Fitting

Prior to surgery, Mr. M. was counseled concerning the role the teeth and tongue have in articulation and the period of adjustment to a "new" oral cavity; how difficult it is to predict the effect of dentures on speech or ability to eat/chew (outcomes are influenced by the extent of the extractions, the type—complete, partial—and fit of dentures); the effects of full plate dentures on sensory feedback; and, if complete maxillary dentures are indicated, their possible effects on resonance.

During the pre-op counseling session, Mr. M. repeatedly commented on the negative influence losing his teeth would have on his appearance; he mimicked a person without teeth talking by pulling his lips over his teeth and smacking them together. In response, the speech-language pathologist reiterated the importance of good oral health and the relationship between oral and general health, as counseled by the oral surgeons. After validating his concerns, the speech-language pathologist stressed that, with well-fitting dentures, his appearance would be enhanced because no decay would be visible.

Following surgical extractions and initial fitting of the dentures, Mr. M. indicated that he had accepted the dentures, but was anxious to improve the quality of his speech and to chew without pain.

## Analysis of Client Response to Intervention and Further Recommendations

1. Mr. M. was to return to his prosthodontist to request that his dentures be adjusted, reducing the space between his maxillary central and lateral incisors, and to determine the best way to secure the mandibular denture. (The results of the evaluation were to be mailed to the prosthodontist.)
2. Following completion of the first recommendation, if speech distortions and chewing difficulty continued, Mr. M. would return to the clinic for a follow-up evaluation and possible treatment.

Rarely does an adult patient present with an isolated speech, language, or swallowing problem. Rather, multiple factors and influences are present and need to be assessed to secure the best possible treatment outcome for any given patient. It is the responsibility of the speech-language pathologist to conduct a thorough history, obtaining medical, dental, and psychosocial information that may directly or indirectly affect the person's communication and swallowing abilities and responsiveness to treatment.

## Author Note

This case is based on a compilation of cases. The author wishes to thank Karen Beverly-Ducker, MA, CCC-A, Michael Kuzmik, DDS, Paula A. Sullivan, MS, CCC-SLP, and Jean C. White, BA for their expert review and helpful comments.

;
.l Association. (2007). *2005–06* ıtal *Services Rendered.* Chicago,

:t Association. (2004). *Heart* *stroke statistics—2004 update.* American Heart Association. ısease Control, National Center .c Disease Prevention and Health Promotion Division of Diabetes Translation. (2007). *National diabetes fact sheet: National estimates on diabetes.* Retrieved April 1, 2010, from http://www.cdc.gov/diabetes/pubs/estimates05.htm.

Centers for Disease Control. (2002). Prevalence of self-reported arthritis or chronic joint symptoms among adults—United States, 2001. *Morbidity and Mortality Weekly Report, 51*(42), 948–950. http://www.cdc.gov/mmwr/preview/mmwrhtml/mm5142a2.htm

Runte, C., Lawerino, M., Dirksen, D., Bollmann, F., Lamprecht-Dinnesen, A., & Seifert, E. (2001, May). The influence of maxillary central incisor position in complete dentures on /s/ sound production. *Journal of Prosthetic Dentistry, 85*(5), 485–495.

Scarsellone, J. M., Rochet, A. P., & Wolfaardt, J. F. (1999). The influence of dentures on nasalance values in speech. *Cleft Palate-Craniofacial Journal, 36*(1), 51–56.

Sinescu, C., Drăgănescu, G. E., Dodenciu, D., Bereteu, L., Negruţiu, M., & Românu, M. (2008). Quantitative parameters which describe speech sound distortions due to inadequate dental mounting. *Physica A: Statistical Mechanics and its Applications, 387,* 1205–1217.

U.S. Department of Health and Human Services. (2000). *Oral health in America: A report of the Surgeon General.* Rockville, MD: U.S. Department of Health and Human Services, National Institute of Dental and Craniofacial Research, National Institutes of Health. http://www.surgeongeneral.gov/library/oralhealth/

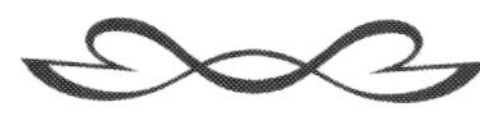

## AUTISM

# CASE 45

# George: An Adult with High-Functioning Autism: Language and Communication Challenges at Work

*Diane L. Williams*

## Conceptual Knowledge Areas

### DSM-IV-TR Diagnostic Criteria for Autism Spectrum Disorders

According to the *Diagnostic and Statistical Manual of Mental Disorders* of the American Psychiatric Association (APA, 2000), to meet the requirements for a diagnosis of autism an individual must have a qualitative impairment in social interaction, a qualitative impairment in verbal and nonverbal language skills and use of communication, and a restricted range of interests and activities that is evident before the age of 3 years.

in order to be diagnosed

## Cognitive Models of Autism Including Complex Information Processing and Theory of Mind

Based on the results from a neuropsychological study of adults with autism, Minshew, Goldstein, and Siegel (1997) proposed the complex information processing (Williams, Goldstein, & Minshew, 2006) model of autism. This conceptualization of autism is derived from models of information processing. According to this model, individuals with autism perform simple information processing tasks across the cognitive domains at or above the level of normal controls but have more difficulty with tasks that require complex processing. "Complex" refers to the processing demands of the task. Large amounts of information, unorganized information, information that requires integration across domains, information that must be processed quickly, information that must be processed parallel to other information, and information that must be processed when the individual is stressed or anxious are all examples of complex processing. Decreasing performance with increasing complexity is not unique to individuals with autism; however, these individuals show deficits at lower levels of complexity than expected relative to age and general ability level. The selective impairments in higher order cognitive functions mean that individuals with autism must accomplish tasks using lower order abilities, resulting in inefficiencies of learning and the oddities of performance associated with autism.

Baron-Cohen (1995) has proposed that a central deficit in autism is the lack of a theory of mind (ToM) or "mindblindness." ToM refers to the understanding that other people have thoughts and the ability to make assumptions about what those thoughts might be. Baron-Cohen suggests that individuals with autism fail to develop a level of ToM that is consistent with their cognitive and language abilities. This deficiency in ToM is thought to explain why individuals with autism have difficulty with reciprocal social interaction even if they develop sophisticated language skills.

## Pragmatic Language (Formation of Gist, Conversational Turn-Taking, Topic Maintenance, Topic Shifting)

Pragmatic language refers to the functional use of language, especially for conversation and discourse. This is an area of language that is particularly affected in individuals with autism even if they are very verbal. For example, when an individual with typical development wants to tell someone else about a personal experience or a movie, the individual forms a gist of the event or the story, telling only the information needed for the other person to understand what happened. Individuals with autism frequently fail to do this. Instead, they tell all the details of the event or story. Individuals with autism may monopolize the conversation and not take turns during conversation, may stay on one topic too long, or jump from topic to topic, making it difficult for listeners to interact with them.

## Generalization

Generalization is the cognitive process by which information learned in response to stimuli in one context is transferred and used in a new context. Individuals with autism are known to have a great deal of difficulty with generalization. This seems to occur because during the learning process the information is strongly connected to both the stimuli that elicit the responses and to the context in which the information is learned.

## Emotion Regulation

Emotion regulation is the ability to control emotional responses so that they are (1) appropriate to the situation, and (2) do not interfere with performance or learning. The ability to regulate emotions is a developmental skill. Older children and adults continue to experience strong emotions but learn self-control so that their responses are measured in consideration of the social situation. Individuals with autism may have pronounced difficulty with emotion regulation even when they have cognitive intelligence that is average or above. They may have age-inappropriate "meltdowns" that interfere with their performance in academic and employment settings.

## Supported Employment

Some individuals with autism require assistance to learn job tasks and/or to learn how to behave appropriately in a work setting from a professional trained to provide this service. Supported employment is employment in an actual work setting but with the assistance of a job coach or counselor who helps the individual learn to perform the tasks essential to successful job performance. The job coach or counselor may break down the steps of the job tasks to make them more explicit and easier for the individual with special needs to learn. The job coach or counselor may also work with the individual on the social skills required to keep the job such as how to interact appropriately with supervisors and fellow employees.

## Vocational Rehabilitation Services

Vocational Rehabilitation Services, commonly known as OVR or the Office of Vocational Rehabilitation Services, is a state-run agency that provides assessment, funding for job training, and assistance with employment for individuals who have special needs but have the potential to work independently. OVR was created by a mandate from the federal government but receives a combination of state and federal funding and is administered at the state level. Individuals who are 18 years old or older who have documented special needs are potentially eligible for services. Eligibility is typically determined following a comprehensive evaluation that includes psychological testing to ascertain general functioning level. OVR works with community educational programs (such as colleges and vocational training programs) and job assistance programs (such as the Work for Life program described in the case of George) to provide for the needs of their clients.

# Description of the Case

George W. was a 26-year-old male diagnosed with autism. He was considered *high functioning* because his Full Scale IQ was above 70. George lived with his parents, Ed and Marjorie W. He had been employed at several part-time jobs in the past. His most recent job was as a stock clerk at a large discount department store. George was laid off from that job about 3 months prior to the evaluation.

## Background Information

### Early Development/Diagnosis

George's parents had been concerned about his development since before he was 3 years of age. He did not talk until he was almost 2.5 years old. When he began to talk, George spoke in full sentences. However, these sentences were primarily imitations of the speech of his mother and father or phrases from television. As a young child, George had some challenging behaviors. He had frequent temper tantrums. Mrs. W. reported that she was never sure what triggered the tantrums. George also spent time turning light switches on and off or opening and closing doors. Mrs. W. said that George would spend hours lining up blocks and toy vehicles. Mr. and Mrs. W. did not have any other children and neither had been around young children very much, so, at the time, they did not think these behaviors were unusual.

From an early age, George had remarkable memory abilities. He could recite children's books word-for-word after only one hearing. In fact, he would become extremely upset if his mother changed even one word of a book when reading it to him. At first, Mr. and Mrs. W. thought George was precocious because he was reading before the age of 4. However, something about his reading struck them as odd. George seemed to get more pleasure from saying the words in the books over and over again to himself than from reading to or with someone.

When George entered preschool, his teacher became concerned that he did not join in with the other children, preferring to play by himself. George spent large amounts of time picking up sand from the sandbox and watching it as it fell slowly from his hand. At other times, he would start squealing and run wildly around the play yard, scaring the other children. He was attracted to anything with a string and would flick the string back and forth while intently examining it. The teacher noticed that, although George seemed to know a lot, he had difficulty answering her questions and she could not engage him in conversation. George preferred to focus on a subject of his own interest; for example, he would talk at length about different types of rocks. He continued to have frequent tantrums.

The teacher suggested that George's parents have him evaluated. George was seen at age 4 years, 8 months at the Child Development Unit of Children's Hospital by a developmental pediatrician, who completed the Childhood Autism Rating Scale (CARS; Schopler, Reichler, DeVellis, & Daly, 1980). Based on the responses of his mother and father, George received a score of 34 (scores less than 30 are not consistent with autism and scores of 36 or greater indicate severe autism). The doctor diagnosed George with autism and referred him for a neuropsychological evaluation. The neuropsychological evaluation indicated that George's overall cognitive functioning was in the low-average range. He was advanced in his ability to decode written words. George had the first of many speech-language evaluations. He received a standard score of 77 in Auditory Comprehension and a standard score of 83 in Verbal Ability on the Preschool Language Scale (PLS; Zimmerman, Steiner, & Pond, 1979). He received a standard score of 103 on the Peabody Picture Vocabulary Test-Revised (PPVT-R; Dunn & Dunn, 1981), which measured his understanding of the meanings of single words. George was referred to his local school district for special education services.

## Elementary School

At the age of 5 years, George was enrolled in a kindergarten program for children with special needs. He received speech therapy once weekly for 50 minutes in a small group with three other special needs children. The therapy focused mainly on following directions and answering questions. As he progressed in school, George continued to be enrolled in a special education classroom and to receive speech therapy once weekly. Beginning in fourth grade, he was mainstreamed into a regular class for music, art, and gym. He was not mainstreamed for academic subjects because he continued to have significant behavioral issues. George would rock his body back and forth and flick papers with his right hand while flapping his left hand. If George had difficulty with a task, he would begin to scream and would sometimes throw himself onto the floor. The teachers thought these behaviors would disrupt the learning of the other children.

## Middle School and High School

By seventh grade, George's parents became concerned that he was not being challenged enough academically. Therefore, at that year's Individualized Education Plan (IEP) meeting, they pressed for mainstreaming in math, science, and social studies. George would continue to receive reading and English in a resource room with other students with challenges to learning. George's behavior problems were reduced, but he continued to have occasional angry outbursts when he became frustrated. Because George's behaviors could be disruptive, a teaching assistant was assigned to the regular education classes that George attended. This general plan continued through high school. As George matured, he managed more of his behaviors in public. He kept a wad of string in his pocket, playing with it only when he thought no one was looking. George's rocking and hand flapping decreased significantly. Emotional outbursts were much less frequent.

George had a comprehensive speech-language evaluation at age 15. The results of the Clinical Evaluation of Language Fundamentals-3 (CELF-3; Semel, Wiig, & Secord, 1995) indicated that George had slight weaknesses in following directions, explaining the relationships between associated words, and formulating sentences when given 3 targeted words. He had relative strengths in vocabulary and syntax. A conversational speech sample revealed that he could hold a conversation on a topic that he initiated for at least 2 minutes. However, George's turns took up significantly more time than those of his conversational partner and he had difficulty with shifting topic. George did not change what he was saying in response to information provided by his communication partner.

Prior to the beginning of his senior year in high school, George was seen for a comprehensive assessment by a psychologist from the local Office of Vocational Rehabilitation Services. The results of that assessment indicated that George had a Verbal IQ of 85, a Performance IQ of 106, and a Full Scale IQ of 95. George was described as being a visual learner, and it was suggested that he go to the local community college to study a visually based field such as computer programming.

George continued to receive speech therapy during high school in a small group once weekly. He practiced social communication skills including conversational turn-taking and social forms such as ordering food in a restaurant and placing phone calls. George graduated from high school at 18 years of age. He finished with a 2.2 (out of 4.0) grade point average. His reading and writing skills were at an eighth-grade level.

### Postsecondary Education

After high school, George enrolled in classes at the community college. He struggled with the coursework. Tutoring was available at a center on campus, but George did not go. He failed to pass his English and history classes and received a grade of D in his math and computer classes. When it was time for the next semester to begin, George refused to attend class and became upset any time his parents mentioned college.

### Work History

Through a friend of the family, his parents helped George get a job at a local pizza restaurant. George worked there 10 hours a week, helping with setup for the dinner shift. He rolled silverware sets into napkins and put paper placemats on the tables. One afternoon, a first-grade class on a field trip was eating at the restaurant. They were in the room that George used to roll the silverware sets. George became increasingly agitated at the noises the children were making. He knocked over the silverware tray and, when he tried to leave the room, was so angry that he pulled the knob off the door. This greatly upset the children, and the manager fired George.

George was unemployed for several months. Then his former resource room teacher called. She had a friend, Mr. D., who was the manager at a local discount department store. Mr. D. was interested in hiring employees with special needs. George began working at the store 15 to 20 hours a week. He stocked the shelves, did daily cleaning (sweeping the aisles, cleaning up spills), and gathered the shopping carts from the parking lot. Mr. D. worked patiently with George until he could perform these tasks proficiently. George worked at the store for 3 years. Then Mr. D. was promoted and moved to a new location. After the new manager came, George began to exhibit more agitation and had occasional outbursts. One day, he could not get a shopping cart to fit in the long line of carts he was gathering from the parking lot. George became angry and pushed the cart really hard, hitting a parked car and causing considerable damage. George was let go from his job.

George sat at home for 3 months while his parents tried to figure out what to do. Mrs. W. finally called the local autism support group and they referred her to the Work for Life program.

## Reasons for the Referral

George is currently a client at Work for Life, an agency that provides evaluations and supported employment services to adults with developmental disabilities. George has had difficulty in his past jobs related to his problems with social communication and emotional regulation. The case manager requested an evaluation of George's language skills to provide suggestions to the support team that would be working with him.

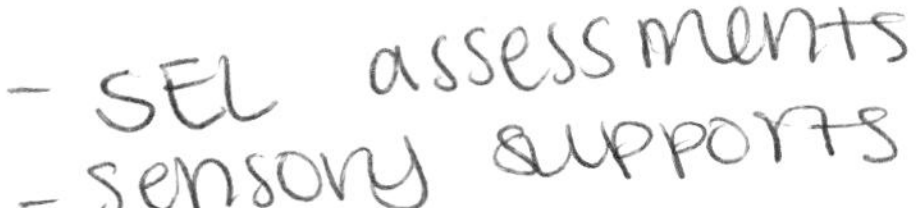

### Proposed Vocational Placement

Following occupational and interest evaluations performed by the support team at Work for Life, and with input from George and his parents, a vocational training plan was developed. It was decided that George needed a work environment that (1) limited his contact with the public to structured interactions, (2) provided supervision by a caring and supportive manager, (3) included tasks in which he had a high degree of interest and knowledge, and (4) allowed him to use skills that he had been successful in using in previous jobs.

Since childhood, George has had a persistent interest in rocks and other areas of geology. He knows the names of all the rocks that are native to the area where he lives and is expert at identifying them and relating relevant facts about the rocks. George reported that one task he enjoyed from his previous job was cleaning and putting stock in order.

George's support team made arrangements for him to get a part-time job at a state park not far from his home. George's duties would include cleaning up and removing trash and clearing overgrown walking trails. He would also help to clean and maintain the displays of geological items and wildlife at the park's education center. The director of the education center was going to work with George on giving short presentations about the rocks and other geological formations that could be found at the state park.

The questions for the speech-language pathologist were: (1) Does George currently have the language/communication skills to be successful in the proposed job placement? (2) If not, what skills would George need to develop? (3) What form of intervention would be most appropriate for the development of these skills?

### Planning the Evaluation

The first decision to be made in planning the evaluation was what form it should take. George had had a number of evaluations throughout his life. He had already been diagnosed with high-functioning autism and had the characteristic language problems associated with that disorder. Therefore, the questions to be answered by an evaluation of George's language skills were more specific. The primary need was to determine whether George had the language and communication skills to be successful in the proposed job placement. In addition, George had significant problems in the *social* use of language and communication or *pragmatic language*, an area that a formal assessment measure might not accurately detect. Therefore, a *functional or ecologically based assessment* appeared to be most appropriate. However, a second consideration was for the evaluation to fulfill the agency requirements of documenting the need for speech and language therapy services. The agency required that all individuals have a formal test measure as the basis for this determination. Therefore, the evaluation needed to include at least one formal measure of language. George's evaluation would be a combination of (1) an ecologically based assessment related to the proposed job placement, and (2) a formal test measure to fulfill the agency requirements of documentation of the need for services.

## Findings of the Evaluation

### Ecologically Based Assessment

An ecologically based assessment is focused on the environments in which the individual needs to communicate to determine the specific demands of those environments. An inventory of the individual's communication skills is also made. The communication demands and the communication skills are then compared to determine what skills need to be developed. The intervention plan targets those skills. Ecological assessments typically include the elements of (1) interviewing parents and other key individuals who can provide information about the demands of the environments and the individual's current skills; and (2) observing the individual in the relevant environments (Elksnin & Elksnin, 2001).

### Interview with the Parents

The parents not only knew George's history, they were also George's primary communication partners. They reported that George did well in interacting with others when he had a clear understanding of what was expected of him. They had successfully taught him a few basic social scripts such as asking people how their days were going. They thought that George would have a hard time telling visitors to the Education Center about the items in the display cases. They were afraid that he would talk about what he was interested in, not what the visitor was interested in. They were concerned that he would talk on and on about an item and that his listeners would become impatient.

### Interview with Past Employer

After securing permission from George, Mr. D., the manager at the department store where George previously worked, was interviewed. He provided information about the challenges George encountered with language and social communication in a work setting. Also, because he had trained George, Mr. D had insight into what learning strategies worked with George. Mr. D. said that whenever George learned a new task, the task needed to be broken down into small, explicit steps. George seemed to remember the steps better if each was given a short verbal description and that verbal description was used repeatedly (First you look at the barcode on the package. Then you find the barcode on the shelf. Then you put the package on the shelf by that barcode.). Mr. D. said that George did better when he worked in an area by himself and did especially well at remembering the order of the tasks to be done during a shift if he was given some choice of how to arrange his schedule.

### Interview with George

George was shown several rock samples and asked to explain the names of the rocks, how they were formed, and what they could be used for. George picked up a piece of granite and talked for 2 minutes without stopping. He did not use the provided organizational structure. When he was asked a question, George answered but then returned to his list of facts about the rock.

### Observations

The SLP accompanied George and his job coach on an initial visit to the state park where he was scheduled to work. While George shadowed one of the park maintenance workers, the speech-language pathologist made observations to determine the communication demands of the environment and what skills George had. These observations indicated that George needed to develop language and communication skills to (1) interact with supervisors and coworkers regarding work assignments and to ask for assistance with unfamiliar tasks, (2) use language to talk himself through unfamiliar tasks, and (3) answer basic informational questions from park visitors.

### Formal Assessments

A challenge in planning a speech-language evaluation for adults with autism is the lack of standardized test instruments to use with this population. Many of the test instruments created for developmental language disorders only provide norms to the age of 21 years. Most of the tests that are available for older adults were constructed for adults with acquired language disorders such as those associated with a traumatic brain injury (TBI) or a cerebral vascular accident (CVA). Therefore, if the use of a standardized test is important, a speech-language pathologist has to decide whether to use an instrument that is slightly out of age range (using the norms for the oldest age group) or whether to restrict choices to the limited number of language areas, such as expressive and receptive vocabulary, for which age-appropriate normed tests are available. In George's case, the Test of Adolescent and Adult Language (TOAL-3; Hammill, Brown, Larsen, & Wiederholt, 1994) was administered. The TOAL-3 has norms to age 24 years, 11 months. George was age 26 years at the time the test

TABLE 45.1 Results of the TOAL-3

| Subtest | Standard Score* | Percentile | Interpretation |
|---|---|---|---|
| Listening/Vocabulary | 7 | 16 | Average |
| Listening/Grammar | 6 | 9 | Below average |
| Speaking/Vocabulary | 9 | 37 | Average |
| Speaking/Grammar | 11 | 63 | Average |
| Reading/Vocabulary | 6 | 9 | Below average |
| Reading/Grammar | 5 | 5 | Below average |
| Writing/Vocabulary | 6 | 9 | Below average |
| Writing/Grammar | 5 | 5 | Below average |

* Scores are based on a mean of 10 and a standard deviation of 3.

was administered. When the scores were reported, it was noted that the norms for the oldest age groups were used. George's performance on this test was as shown in Table 45.1.

Based on a mean of 100 and a standard deviation of 15, George's score of 73 for Receptive Language was below average and his score of 85 for Expressive Language was low average. He had particular weaknesses with reading and writing and in the comprehension of spoken language.

## Treatment Options Considered

### Individual Speech-Language Therapy

In individual sessions George could be explicitly taught about communication interactions with his supervisors, coworkers, and park visitors. He could also be taught scripts to use when teaching park visitors about items displayed in the Education Center.

- ***Advantages:*** George's attention could be focused on the skills that the speech-language pathologist wanted to address without the distractions present in an actual work environment. The cognitive processing load could be more carefully managed in a pull-out session than during teaching that is embedded in the actual work environment. George might be more willing to try skills that he had not mastered if he did not have other people watching him.
- ***Disadvantages:*** Like other individuals with high-functioning autism (HFA), George had difficulty with *generalizing* knowledge learned in one setting to a different one. Even though he performed the desired language/social skill during the pull-out session, George might not generalize this skill to the actual work environment. Social communication cannot be adequately addressed in a session in which the only communication partner is the therapist. Other models of service delivery are more effective for addressing functional outcomes and training of communication partners. Because of these limitations, if used, pull-out services should be directly related to functional outcomes and used on a limited basis for the development of skills that are then quickly translated and established in an actual work environment (ASHA, 2006).

### Social Communication Group

Another option considered for George was group therapy in the form of a social skills group or social "club" (Kilman & Negri-Schoultz, 1987). In this approach, the speech-language pathologist plans each session around preset topics related to social communication challenges. Topics are typically general social problems such as meeting new people, being different, or dealing with stress. The speech-language pathologist may also design the program around topics that relate to the specific needs of the participants. Sessions typically include modeling of appropriate behavior and feedback to the participants about the effectiveness of their communication.

- ***Advantages:*** Interactive behaviors can be targeted because multiple communication partners are available. Under the guidance of the speech-language pathologist, group members can serve as models for one another.
- ***Disadvantages:*** George may spend time on topics that are not directly relevant to him if the needs and skill levels of other participants are different than his own. Other individuals with social communication problems may be inadequate models. George may not generalize what he learns in the social communication group to his work setting.

### Ecological Treatment

Ecological treatment, or treatment within the context where the skills will be used, has been demonstrated to be beneficial for the development of the social communication skills of individuals with autism spectrum disorders (National Research Council, 2001).

- ***Advantages:*** Treatment can focus directly on the skills needed for particular language and social communication tasks. George will not need to generalize the skills learned in one setting to another setting. The skills and strategies will be made explicit to him during the treatment process.
- ***Disadvantages:*** Treatment within the work setting is time-consuming for the professionals involved. The speech-language pathologist would need to travel to the work setting and spend time with George and his communication partners. Different types of tasks require different language and communication demands. Intervention would need to address the skills required for each of these tasks rather than on social communication skills in general. Development of the scripts for George's educational talks might be more difficult within the work setting than during a one-on-one session.

### Peer Modeling

Peer modeling is a strategy that is used as part of an ecological treatment approach. Peer modeling or mediation has been used successfully with children with autism to develop social communication skills (Strain, 2001). George's peers were fellow employees in the work setting. Peers would receive instruction so that they knew what was expected of them and what they were trying to help George do. An example of a strategy that a peer might model is to say aloud what he is thinking while doing the task. George would then use this language to talk himself through the task. This language would help George to structure the task and provide cues so that he could perform independently. Peers could also serve as models for social communication with each other and with park visitors.

- ***Advantages:*** The peers are available to provide guidance on an ongoing basis until the skills become well established. The peers may have an insight into the language needed to do a task that is not obvious to others.
- ***Disadvantages:*** The availability of an appropriate peer model depends on who else is employed at the work setting. These peers may also have limitations in language and social communication, making them inadequate models.

## Course of Treatment

### Training of the Supported Employment Trainer

As he began his new job placement at the state park, George would be assisted by a job coach from Work for Life. This individual would work with him for at least the first 3 months of his placement. Although this individual had a degree in rehabilitation, he might not have experience in working with an individual with HFA in general and in working with George specifically. George's speech-language pathologist would provide preservice and continuing education to this person (American Speech-Language-Hearing Association, 2006). This training would include background information about HFA, the language and social communication challenges encountered by individuals with HFA, and specific information about George's abilities and the skills needed. The speech-language pathologist would work with the job coach to develop the teaching strategies to be used with George as he learned about the environment and duties of his new job.

### Training of the Job Supervisor

The job supervisor was given background information about HFA and specific information about George's abilities. The supervisor received advice on an ongoing basis as particular situations arose. The job coach, SLP, and job supervisor developed a plan to help George use his language to reduce problems with emotional regulation.

### Environmental Adaptations

Visual schedules have been shown to be effective even for high-functioning individuals with autism (Bryan & Gast, 2000). Because George's reading skills were at an eighth-grade level, his schedule could be provided in written form rather than with pictures. George needed to have his weekly and daily work schedules provided in written form. The weekly schedule let him know what days and times he was to report for work. The daily schedule informed him of the specific tasks to do during each work day. When possible, the daily schedule was arranged by time of day so that George knew which tasks to do in a particular time period. George was given the tasks that needed to be completed that day and could choose the order in which they would be addressed (Watanabe & Sturmey, 2003).

### Training of the Client

Skills to be developed with George were language and social communication for work-related interactions with his supervisors, social chit-chat with coworkers, and interactions with park visitors. He needed to learn scripts to structure his work and complete tasks. Peer modeling was used as previously described for language and communication needed when completing tasks and interacting with supervisors and coworkers.

George worked with the speech-language pathologist to develop written scripts for use when explaining the displays in the Education Center. Written scripts have been shown to be an effective teaching strategy to use with individuals with high-functioning autism (Charlop-Christy & Kelso, 2003). During the development of these scripts, George needed to be guided so that he (1) focused on what was the important or salient information that his listeners needed to know, and (2) expressed the information using appropriate pragmatic skills.

To reduce inappropriate behaviors, George was taught socially appropriate ways to communicate frustration. Social stories were developed for this purpose. This technique has been demonstrated to be effective in reducing inappropriate behaviors such as tantrums and aggression in individuals with autism (Kuttler, Myles, & Carson, 1998; Swaggart et al., 1995).

## Analysis of the Client's Response to Treatment

George's response to treatment will not be measured by formal assessment instruments. Rather, his response to treatment will be measured by how successful he is in his job placement. If George performs well and not only is able to retain his job, but becomes a valuable employee, this will indicate that he has the language and social communication skills necessary for that job. However, if George experiences difficulty with completion of his tasks or interactions with his supervisor, coworkers, and/or park visitors, this will suggest that the impact of his difficulties with language and social communication on his job performance need to be further assessed and additional intervention will need to be planned and implemented.

## Further Recommendations

If the job supervisor changes, the new supervisor will need to be trained. The job supervisor needs a consistent person to contact as new challenges arise on the job. George's parents need to remain vigilant for any signs that George is having difficulty at work. These signs might include changes in George's behavior such as increased anxiety as the time to go to work approaches, increases in verbalizations that are not directed to anyone, increase in pacing, sudden outbursts of anger, and other negative behaviors.

## Author Note

George W. is a fictional person who represents a compilation of several adults with autism that the author has worked with during her clinical career.

## References


American Psychiatric Association. (2000). *Diagnostic and statistical manual of mental disorders* (4th ed., text rev.). Washington, DC: Author.

American Speech-Language-Hearing Association. (2006). *Roles and responsibilities of speech-language pathologist in diagnosis, assessment, and treatment of autism spectrum disorders across the life span: Position statement.* Available from http://www.asha.org/docs/html/PS2006-00105.html

Baron-Cohen, S. (1995). *Mindblindness: An essay on autism and theory of mind.* Cambridge, MA: MIT Press.

Bryan, L. C., & Gast, D. L. (2000). Teaching on-task and on-schedule behaviors to higher functioning children with autism via picture activity schedules. *Journal of Autism and Developmental Disorders, 30*, 553–567.

Charlop-Christy, M. H., & Kelso, S. E. (2003). Teaching children with autism conversational speech using a cue card/written script program. *Education and Treatment of Children, 26*, 103–127.

Dunn, L. M., & Dunn, L. M. (1981). *Peabody Picture Vocabulary Test–Revised.* Circle Pines, MN: American Guidance Service.

Elksnin, N., & Elksnin, L. (2001). Adolescents with disabilities: The need for occupational social skills training. *Exceptionality, 9,* 91–105.

Hammill, D. D., Brown, V. L., Larsen, S. C., & Wiederholt, J. L. (1994). *Test of adolescent and adult language* (3rd ed.). Los Angeles, CA: Western Psychological Services.

Kilman, B., & Negri-Schoultz, N. (1987). Developing educational programs for working with students with Kanner's autism. In D. J. Cohen and A. M. Donnellan (Eds.), *Handbook of autism and pervasive developmental disorders* (pp. 440–451). New York: John Wiley & Sons.

Kuttler, S., Myles, B. S., & Carson, J. K. (1998). The use of social stories to reduce precursors to tantrum behavior in a student with autism. *Focus on Autism and Other Developmental Disabilities, 13*, 176–182.

Minshew, N. J., Goldstein, G., & Siegel, D. J. (1997). Neuropsychologic functioning in autism: Profile of a complex information processing disorder. *Journal of the International Neuropsychological Society, 3,* 303–316.

National Research Council. (2001). *Educating children with autism.* Washington, DC: National Academy Press, Committee on Educational Interventions for Children with Autism, Division of Behavioral and Social Sciences and Education.

Schopler, E., Reichler, R. J., DeVellis, R. F., & Daly, K. (1980). Toward objective classification of childhood autism: Childhood Autism Rating Scale (CARS). *Journal of Autism and Developmental Disorders, 10,* 91–103.

Semel, E. M., Wiig, E. H., & Secord W. (1995). *Clinical evaluation of language fundamentals (CELF-3).* San Antonio, TX: Psychological Corporation.

Strain, P. S. (2001). Empirically based social skill intervention: A case for quality-of-life improvement. *Behavioral Disorders, 27*, 30–36.

Swaggart, B. L., Gagnon, E., Bock, S. J., Earles, T. L., Quinn, C., Myles, B. S., et al. (1995). Using social stories to teach social and behavioral skills to children with autism. *Focus on Autistic Behavior*, 10, 1–16.

Watanabe, M., & Sturmey, P. (2003). The effect of choice-making opportunities during activity schedules on task engagement of adults with autism. *Journal of Autism and Developmental Disorders, 33*, 535–538.

Williams, D. L., Goldstein G., Minshew N. J. (2006). Neuropsychologic functioning in children with autism: Further evidence of disordered complex information processing. *Child Neuropsychology, 12,* 279–298.

Zimmerman, I., Steiner, V., & Pond, R. (1979). *Preschool Language Scale-Revised Edition.* Upper Saddle River, NJ: Merrill/Prentice Hall.

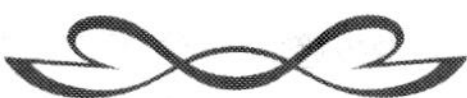



CASE 46

# Dr. JN: An Adult Nonnative Speaker of English: High Proficiency

*Amee P. Shah*

## Conceptual Knowledge Areas

The U.S. Census 2000 report indicates that 28.4 million immigrants now live in the United States, the largest number recorded in the nation's history, and a 43% increase since 1990 (Camarota, 2001). Future projections predict a continuous growth of over 1.2 million each year. With such a large proportion of nonnative speakers in the total population, it is often the case that speech-language pathologists (SLPs) are consulted for intelligibility and accent issues due to foreign (and regional) accents. Recognizing this need, ASHA's 1983 and 1985 position papers have included communication problems related to dialects and accents in the scope of SLP practice. Thus, a majority of graduate programs in the country now address accent modification in the clinical services and academic training of graduate students. Surveys of accredited programs (Schmidt & Sullivan, 2003; Shah, 2005) have revealed several areas of need, including inadequate preparation in accent modification of students, limited coursework focusing on cross-language issues, and a dearth of efficacy-based accent modification clinical practices. Shah (2005) concluded that the absence of normative assessment tools and clinical programs forced clinicians to combine subtests from diverse tests, find and use less-known or obscure tools, and devise their own training procedures. The recent emphasis on evidence-based practice makes it imperative that the area of practice addressing regional dialectal- and foreign-accent-related communication difficulties be considered. Similar to other areas of SLP practice, accent modification needs to be grounded in theory and research, thus fostering an efficacy-based effort. This case presents a high-proficiency client as a model of systematic, evidence-based practice from interview to intervention. Specifically, the ideas and evidence obtained from research conducted in fields such as psychology, sociolinguistics, and speech perception were adapted and applied to various aspects of accent modification practice. Thus, specific areas of clinical practice described include initial case history and interview, assessment as guided by quantitative analyses, and therapy as planned using structured, systematic principles.

### Background Information

The Communicating for Impact program has been especially designed to cater to the highly specialized communication needs of international physicians and scientists at the Cleveland Clinic. Based on experience with a large cohort of such physicians and scientists who had been referred for therapy over the course of the last year, this author was able to design and successfully implement such a program. Specifically, as high-proficiency (or advanced) speakers of English, this particular client group's communication needs are subtle and advanced.[1] Thus, this program consisted of specialized goals and methods to specifically meet the language needs and cognitive styles of such physicians and scientists. In particular, the *goals* addressed advanced skills such as professional vocabulary, language rhythm (suprasegmental features), advanced grammar, and subtle pragmatic differences that may have impeded socialization and acculturation, and thus, indirectly, affected perceived spoken intelligibility. This program helped address these goals in *methods* that would appeal to the cognitive and learning styles of an analytic, knowledgeable, learned, technologically savvy group of professionals. The program used acoustic software that provided audio and visual cues of the clients' speech on computers. The clinician guided the clients to edit and change speech patterns with such audio and visual feedback. Extensive use of clients' recorded samples was used in training, as well as in pre- and posttraining comparisons. The structure of the program was established as more of an equal partnership with the clients, wherein they were consulted and informed at every juncture of the process. Thus, after the initial interview and assessment, they were given a detailed summary of their communication deficits and, together with the clinician, planned therapy priorities. They maintained the diagnostic profile report and referred to it at periodic junctures to monitor their own progress and work on goals at home.

## Description of the Case

### Background Information

Dr. JN, a 38-year-old Asian (Japanese) female anesthesiologist working at the Cleveland Clinic, was referred by her supervisor to the Communicating for Impact program offered by the Office of Diversity at the clinic. The area of primary concern for the referring superior was that Dr. JN was very difficult to understand as she had a strong foreign accent that interfered with her communication with her patients as well as the hospital personnel.

### Reasons for Referral

Based on the Language Background Questionnaire that is part of the Comprehensive Assessment of Accentedness and Intelligibility (CAAI; Shah, 2007), *language history* is as follows. Dr. JN was born and raised in Tokyo, Japan, and spoke Japanese as her primary and native language. In addition, she spoke English and had partial knowledge of French. Her self-rated proficiency in Japanese was "strong" in all language areas including reading, writing, and speaking. She rated her English proficiency as "average" for speaking and "good" for reading and writing, respectively. Her self-rated proficiency for French was "low" in all areas of speaking, reading, and writing. She reported using English and Japanese with nearly equal frequency in the course of her week; English at work and Japanese at home, in her local neighborhood and among friends. She considered Japanese to be her strongest language and continued to prefer using it over English or French. Dr. JN's age of language learning (AOL) for English was 13 years, when she was formally taught English in her middle school in Japan exclusively by Japanese teachers who spoke English with a distinct Japanese accent. Dr. JN's age of arrival (AOA) in the United States was 24 years, and her length of residence (LOR) in the United States was 14 years. Dr. JN came to the United States to pursue her medical degree and completed 8 years of her medical education leading to her present job as an anesthesiologist. Upon arrival she had been enrolled in an English as Second Language (ESL) class through her university; she participated for 1 semester and received English instruction once a week for 2 hours for 16 weeks. Dr. JN's educational history included an M.D. and a postgraduate fellowship in anesthesiology. Her language needs at her work involved spending about 70% of her time conversing in English during active patient care (conversing with patients, their family, the hospital personnel, and colleagues), and about 30% of her time in activities such as giving presentations in conferences or in meetings with colleagues, collaborating on research, reading professional journals, writing journal articles in medical journals, and training residents. Thus, her English language skills were called upon in all areas of communication including speaking, listening, reading, and writing. Her self-reported areas of concern with her communication abilities included primarily needing help with her strong foreign accent to be better understood. She expressed difficulty listening and attempting to understand other speakers of English. Her listening skills were reportedly good in casual conversation and watching television but markedly reduced with unfamiliar work and people. She needed help in acquiring and using more advanced vocabulary skills, especially professional terminology, idiomatic expressions, and slang. Goals involved being able to communicate more intelligibly with patients and colleagues, as well as during her presentations and meetings. She considered her grammar skills to be fairly good in English and did not seek any further direct intervention in speaking and writing.

Her self-perceived communication difficulties included her awareness that, while people appeared to be able to understand the gist of her message and a large number of her sentences, they had frequent trouble understanding single words in her sentences and often asked her to repeat individual words. As part of her awareness and attempts to circumvent her communication challenges, she tried to implement strategies, such as speaking slower, segmenting syllables, and planning the sentence grammar ahead of time as she spoke English. She commented that her communication difficulties had markedly improved after she increasingly attempted to "think in English." No other medical, social, or family history was reported as relevant to the nature of her communication difficulties.

*Note*: Factors such as AOL, AOA, and LOR were part of the interview questions in keeping with the extensive research conducted by James Flege and colleagues (e.g., Flege, 1984) that describes how these variables can affect and shape second language learning and, ultimately, predict success in learning that second language.

## Findings of the Evaluation

After the interview, the Comprehensive Assessment of Accentedness and Intelligibility (CAAI; Shah, 2007) was administered to determine Dr. JN's performance in various aspects of speech, language, and overall communicative abilities in English. The CAAI is *comprehensive* in that it targets a multitude of typical errors that pose communication difficulties for dialect and accented clients. Foreign accentedness and intelligibility issues span speech production, speech perception, and other language areas such as grammar, vocabulary, and nonverbal behavior. It is important to assess the range of area(s) that are implicated and determine which of those specifically interfere with the individual client's communication and integration into mainstream society. Consequently, this test addresses various levels of speech and nonspeech extralinguistic areas. This test distinguishes *articulatory* from *phonological errors* and *segmental errors* of consonants and vowels from *prosodic errors* that span varied lengths of spoken material from syllables and words to sentences and narratives. Auditory and perceptual discrimination abilities are tested in order to make judgments about the underlying causes of accented speakers' production errors, thereby helping to predict goals and target areas for intervention. The test also addresses *language performance* as measured by *grammatical, semantic,* and *pragmatic* differences.

Dr. JN completed 22 sections of the CAAI, which required activities such as reading aloud words, sentences, and/or paragraphs, answering questions, and role playing dialogs. The 22 sections yield numeric data through the scores from each section, which can then be used to make pre- and posttherapy comparisons. In particular, the Diagnostic Profile (see Table 46.1) provided with the Individual Scoring Form helps categorize the scores and enables the examiner to get a quick snapshot of areas of relative difficulty, and thus arrive at the priority order of targeting them in later therapy/training.

The interview and assessment session of the CAAI was audio recorded and later analyzed and scored by two speech-language pathology students to ensure reliability in test scoring and analysis. Results of the analysis are as presented in Table 46.1, which consists of the diagnostic profile

TABLE 46.1 Diagnostic Profile for Dr. JN (from the CAAI)

**Comprehensive Assessment of Accentedness & Intelligibility: Complete Diagnostic Report**

**Amee P. Shah, Ph.D.** **Date:** **Client Name: Dr. J.N.**

| **SECTION TITLE** | **Total possible score** | **90% performance** | **70% performance** | **50% performance** | **Client's Score** |
|---|---|---|---|---|---|
| Degree of difficulty ………………> | | mild difficulty | moderate | strong difficulty | |
| SECTION 1: INTELLIGIBILITY RELATIVE TO ACCENTEDNESS<br>e.g.,"The committee was composed of ten members . . ." | 1 to 5 | 2 | 3 | 4 or more | 2.5 |
| SECTION 2: INTELLIGIBILITY SCORE & RATE OF SPEECH ON NARRATIVE PASSAGE<br>Stimulus: Rainbow Passage | 100% | 90% | 70% | 50% | 89%, normal rate |
| SECTION 3: SENTENCE LEVEL INTONATION<br>"I got promoted!" | 10 | 9 | 7 | 5 | 7 |
| SECTION 4: WORD LEVEL INTONATION<br>e.g.: ("Tuesday comes after Monday.") "Good!" | 4 | 3.6 | 2.8 | 2 | 3 |
| SECTION 5: LEXICAL STRESS IN SINGLE, MULTISYLLABIC WORDS<br>e.g.: "Repellent." | 12 | 10.8 | 8.4 | 6 | 7 |
| SECTION 6: DERIVATIVE STRESS IN MULTISYLLABIC WORDS<br>e.g.: "democracy/democratic" | 24 | 21.6 | 16.8 | 12 | 15 |
| SECTION 7: CONTRASTIVE LEXICAL STRESS<br>e.g.: "I have a birthday present for you."/present | 28 | 25.2 | 19.6 | 14 | 17 |
| SECTION 8: EMPHASIS<br>e.g.: ("Which one was it?") "I made the pumpkin pie." | 12 | 10.8 | 8.4 | 6 | 10 |
| SECTION 9: SENTENCE PHRASING<br>e.g.: "I need milk, eggs, and bread from the market." | 7 | 6.3 | 4.9 | 3.5 | 7 |
| SECTION 10: CONTRASTING SENTECE PAIRS<br>e.g.: "Ben would never leave Woody/would he?" | 10 | 9 | 7 | 5 | 10 |
| SECTION 11: CONSONANTS WORD LIST<br>e.g.: Initial position /p/ in "pan." | 65 | 58.5 | 45.5 | 32.5 | 56 |
| SECTION 12: CONSONANT CLUSTERS WORD LIST<br>e.g.: /r/ blend in "brush." | 59 | 53.1 | 41.3 | 29.5 | 38 |
| SECTION 13a: VOWEL WORD LIST<br>e.g.: /i/ in "meat." | 18 | 16.2 | 12.6 | 9 | 12 |
| SECTION 13b: VOWEL WORD LIST<br>e.g.: /æ/ in "packed." | 22 | 19.8 | 15.4 | 11 | 13 |
| SECTION 14: PHONOLOGICAL PROCESSES | 13 | 11.7 | 9.1 | 6.5 | 4 |
| SECTION 15: AUDITORY DISCRIMINATION | 75 | 67.5 | 52.5 | 37.5 | 53 |
| SECTION 16: PREPOSITIONS<br>e.g.: "I live ____ Ohio." (in) | 20 | 18 | 14 | 10 | 13 |
| SECTION 17: COLLOQUIAL/IDIOMATIC USE OF PREPOSITIONS<br>e.g.: Are we still on __________ tonight? (for) | 8 | 7.2 | 5.6 | 4 | 6 |

TABLE 46.1 *Continued*

| SECTION TITLE | Total possible score | 90% performance | 70% performance | 50% performance | Client's Score |
|---|---|---|---|---|---|
| SECTION 18: CONTRASTING IDIOMATIC PHRASES<br>e.g.: "hold on" vs. "hold out." | 17 | 15.3 | 11.9 | 8.5 | 15 |
| Secondary Cues: sentence fill-in (comprehension of phrases) | secondary score: 8 | 7.2 | 5.6 | 4 | n/a |
| SECTION 19: COMPREHENSION OF IDIOMATIC PHRASES<br>"Don't be upset, he's only pulling your leg." (teasing) | 12 | 10.8 | 8.4 | 6 | 10 |
| SECTION 20: ADVANCED VOCABULARY<br>Defining a word given four choices. | 20 | 18 | 14 | 10 | 13 |
| SECTION 21: CONVERSATIONAL GRAMMAR | | | | | |
| SECTION 22: PRAGMATIC PROBLEMS | | | | | |

for Dr. JN. The table provides a quantitative estimate of the client's accent-severity in each of the 22 sections, as well as an overall estimate of the baseline intelligibility and speaking rate.

### Summary of Assessment Results

Based on the assessment findings, the client was found to typically exhibit mild to moderate degree of difficulty in most areas. As Section 2 in the CAAI indicated, the client's rate of speech was normal and baseline intelligibility was only mildly affected (89%). The client had a distinct moderate accent that did not appear to affect conversational intelligibility (2.5 on a scale of 1–5) and was labeled as a "Mild-Moderate Foreign Accent."

Areas that were judged to be only mildly impaired and relatively low priority for further intervention included suprasegmental aspects such as sentence-level intonation, word emphasis, sentence phrasing, and contrasting sentence phrasing. Areas with moderate degree of impairment and high priority for intervention included word-level stress features (word-level intonation, lexical stress in multisyllabic words, derivative stress, and contrastive lexical stress). In addition, segmental properties were moderately affected and included errors on many consonants (/r/, /ɾ/, /l/, /pʰ/, /tʰ/, /kʰ/, /v/, /θ/, and /ð/), a marked number of clusters (predominantly /r/ blends and /l/ blends), and a variety of vowels (/ɪ/, /æ/, /ʊ/, /a/,/ɚ/, and /ʌ/). Four phonological processes were noted, including final /s/ or /z/ deletion, addition of intrusion schwa, vowel reduction, and deaspiration of initial voiceless consonants.

Auditory discrimination abilities were found to be moderately implicated as well and included confusion between sounds such as (/r/-/l/, /v/-/b/,/θ/-/ð/, /ð/-/d/, /θ/-/t/, /f/-/p/, /f/-/v/, /m/-/n/, /v/-/w/, /ɪ/-/ɛ/, /ɪ/-/e/, /ɔ/-/ʌ/). Other nonspeech aspects of language were affected to a moderate degree and consisted of errors with the colloquial use of prepositions, knowledge of idiomatic expressions, and technical/advanced vocabulary.

## Treatment Options Considered

Therapy goals were identified and an order of priority determined in the overall therapy hierarchy. This goal-setting was done on the basis of the baseline numeric scores and the strength of their deviation from the norm (mild, moderate, or strong), as seen on the diagnostic profile for the client (Table 46.1). Areas that were either moderately or strongly impaired were considered to have the highest priority in treatment.

The following areas were selected, in the order in which they were addressed in therapy:

1. Production and discrimination of consonants
2. Production and discrimination of vowels
3. Phonological processes

4. Word-level stress, including contrastive stress
5. Understanding and appropriate use of prepositions
6. Understanding and appropriate use of everyday idiomatic expressions
7. Everyday conversational skills relevant to client's professional and social settings: addressing all of the preceding goals, with emphasis on overall prosody
8. Presentation skills focusing on technical vocabulary, overall language prosody (intonation, juncture, and pacing), and pragmatics.

In determining the selection of these goals, their priority status, and their respective methods of intervention, several factors were considered along with the immediate results and scores of the assessment battery, including *client preference, experience,* and *need.* Moreover, in keeping with the client's professional needs, the area of improvement in presentation skills was addressed. The selected goals were incorporated in activities involving conversational role-play and making professional presentations (lectures).

The examiner also reviewed well-established knowledge/scientific evidence. For example, Strange and colleagues (Miyawaki et al., 1975; Strange & Dittmann, 1984) have shown how Japanese speakers benefit from training on discrimination and production of /r/-/l/ sound contrasts. Learning accomplished through such training appears to be transferred outside the laboratory situation and maintained for longer periods even after the training is discontinued. As a result of such documented information, /r/-/l/ contrasts were selected for the client. Similarly, Derwing, Munro, and Wiebe (1998) and Derwing & Rossiter (2003) have shown the importance of suprasegmental aspects in the perceived improvement of nonnative speakers' intelligibility. Thus, therapy focused on language prosody skills, including various aspects of lexical stress, and overall sentence intonation through conversational role-plays. Segmentals were addressed before the prosodic goals as the former were relatively few, easier to target, and provided good initial encouragement and reinforcement. After some preliminary practice and improvement with segmentals, prosody aspects were soon introduced in Dr. JN's therapy. Prosody aspects were targeted in a variety of ways, including conversations and presentation skills, and were continued long after segmental goals were discontinued.

The issue of accentedness has been treated here as a category distinct from intelligibility. Munro & Derwing (1995) have shown that the phenomena of perceived accentedness and intelligibility are related, yet distinct. Intelligibility refers to the actual process of decoding the message and is estimated by transcribing each utterance heard by listeners to arrive at the number of words understood. Perceived accentedness, on the other hand, is determined by conducting an accent-rating task on a scale from "no foreign accent" to "strong foreign accent." Although clinical accent-modification and ESL programs are typically geared toward addressing only those speech characteristics that affect intelligibility, these programs should instead test and address perceived accentedness as separate from intelligibility. Indeed, accented speech, even when free of intelligibility concerns, may be stigmatized and pose difficulties to speakers in their personal and professional communication. The CAAI was used to address and separate the methods for arriving at measures of perceived accentedness as distinct from and independent of performance on intelligibility. Sections 1 and 2 in the test help separate these two measures and, consequently, help separate therapy priorities for different clients. Thus, for some clients the goal may be to improve intelligibility, whereas with others, therapy may need to address subtle aspects of speech to minimize the "foreignness."

A third factor considered in therapy was the clinician's *clinical experiences.* Clinical experience revealed intervention on segmentals to be a good starting point in therapy as it gives the client practice with listening to various sounds and identifying subtle differences. Targeting segmentals also allows clients opportunities to vary articulatory maneuvers on individual sounds (as opposed to the length of an entire sentence). Finally, segmentals allow clients to visually *see* the difference in their productions (e.g., on programs where sound waveforms are shown, clients can see the improvement in changing duration, intensity, stress on specific syllables, aspiration for voiceless stops, pause and juncture across syllable and word boundaries, and overall word or sentence contour). A multimodality approach was followed because it was found to yield maximum and relatively fast improvements in therapy. Such an approach involves listening to sounds, producing them and noticing the tactile and kinesthetic differences across articulatory movements, and observing the acoustic properties on a spectrograph or waveform.

The CAAI's individual scoring forms allow recording and comparing baseline and follow-up testing scores side-by-side to track progress as well as show clients their achievements. It is recommended that portions of CAAI be readministered at periodic junctures after a goal in therapy has been addressed for a few sessions. These follow-up scores will ensure a more quantified comparison with baseline scores than their clinician-generated "impressions."

## Course of Treatment

### Session Structure

Therapy consisted of 8 sessions, once a week, for 60 minutes each. The number of sessions was determined by clients' availability in the Communication for Impact program (these physicians were able to devote only 8 hours of time to their communication needs, hence this program had to provide maximum results in the least possible time).

Of the 8 sessions, one was devoted to the initial interview and the comprehensive assessment using CAAI. Two sessions were reserved for consonant-intervention (including auditory discrimination and production), and two more were reserved for vowels. The sessions focusing on segmentals (consonants and vowels) also included 15 minutes of reading paragraphs and producing free-form conversation, wherein prosody-goals were introduced and addressed in tandem with the segmentals. One session was dedicated entirely to introducing and practicing details of suprasegmentals. Two more sessions were availed for "real-life" speaking opportunities, wherein all previously addressed segmental and prosodic goals were addressed together, as relevant.

### Specific Procedures

***Segmentals: Consonants and Vowels*** Consonants were targeted before intervention with vowels. Each session dealing with segmentals involved auditory discrimination exercises first, to allow the client to hear and perceive the differences between the target phoneme in contrast with other phonemes. These minimal pairs were selected from the examples found in the two auditory discrimination subtests in the CAAI. If necessary, additional examples were selected for practice from other accent-modification books (see, for example, Celce-Murcia, Brinton, & Goodwin, 1996; Compton, 1984; Edwards & Strattman, 1996). The clinician would say aloud minimal pairs to provide the client with listening experiences in differentiating various phonemes in these minimal pairs. She was asked to identify these phonemes as "same or different" and write the exact word pairs heard. The clinician provided verbal feedback to point out differences between the sounds if the client failed to identify the difference on her own. Repetitions were provided as necessary until the client began to perceive the difference with at least 80% accuracy.

After this perception-experience, the second half of the session dealt with practice on production of these phonemes. For each target phoneme (consonant or vowel), the production exercises began by showing the client a picture of the typical articulatory position to produce the sound. Concurrently, the clinician demonstrated that movement, asked the client to mimic it, and provided direct instructions to modify the movement, as necessary. For phonemes whose productions were relatively difficult to visualize via pictures and/or clinician's model (e.g., velar and palatal consonants and back vowels), a visual animation software program was used to demonstrate the movement of the articulators on a computer screen. The client was asked to imitate the articulatory movements for each phoneme until the clinician was satisfied that the client realized these gestures correctly on individual sounds. Once the client understood the correct articulatory placement, that target phoneme was introduced in all 3 positions in words of varying syllable length (1-, 2-, and 3- or 4-syllable words). These words were selected from Blockcolsky, Frazer, and Frazer (1979). The client read individual word lists varying in syllable length and monitored the correct production of the articulatory position on the target phoneme. Each list of words was followed by practice with a list of short sentences containing these phonemes. Finally, the client read a paragraph with all target sounds underlined. The client attended to the related articulatory positions, especially as she read the underlined parts. Simultaneously, as the client read these sentences and paragraphs, the prosody goals were introduced and addressed in tandem with the segmentals. The prosody goals involved aspects such as lexical stress, contrastive syllable stress, word emphasis, overall sentence intonation, and pausing at phrase boundaries. Where necessary, the client was instructed and provided appropriate prosodic models for imitation at various junctures.

***Suprasegmental/Prosody*** A session was exclusively dedicated for the prosodic goals. The client's goals involved *word-level stress features* (word-level intonation, lexical stress in multisyllabic words, derivative stress, and contrastive lexical stress). Activities involved reading word-lists with appropriate syllable stress patterns, and where incorrect, repeating after the corrected models provided by the clinician. These word lists were compiled from the corresponding sections of the CAAI as well as from other practice books (such as Celce-Murcia et al., 1996; Compton, 1984; Edwards & Strattman, 1996; Sikorski, 1988; and Stern, 1987). These words varied in syllable length and ranged from 2 to 5 syllables. A wide range of examples was included in these word lists to allow the client to intuit English stress patterns and remap existing stress patterns carried over from the mora-timed Japanese stress patterns. Once the client achieved 80% success rate in her word-level stress productions, she was presented with sentence lists and paragraphs containing the previously used words from the word lists. The client read these sentences and paragraphs as naturally as possible and focused on the appropriate syllable-stress patterns. Where necessary, reinstruction and clinician's models were provided.

***Real-Life Conversational Speaking Opportunities*** The final two sessions of the program were dedicated to bringing together the learning accomplished on the segmental and prosodic goals in the previous sessions and to transferring and generalizing these goals to the client's routine conversational situations. Thus, a secondary goal was to provide specific skills and strategies to enable the client to communicate effectively in her meetings and professional presentations/lectures.

## Analysis of Client's Response to Intervention

At the end of the 8-week program, a determination was made to assess whether the client had made adequate progress and functional improvement to be discharged from therapy, or whether a continuation of therapy was warranted. Three criteria were used to arrive at this decision: (1) pre- and posttherapy scores on the CAAI, (2) intelligibility judgments by neutral listeners, and (3) client's personal response to intervention.

### Pre- and Posttherapy Scores on CAAI

Selected sections of the CAAI were readministered. The client showed marked improvement in most of the targeted areas/sections. Overall intelligibility scores improved from the previous 2.5 to the present 1.5 and baseline passage intelligibility increased from 89% to 97%; these scores indicated a nearly normal range of functioning. Perfect scores were obtained on word-level intonation and contrastive lexical stress; and mild difficulty was noted on lexical stress on multisyllabic words and derivative stress. Consonant production scores improved from 56 to 62 and consonant clusters' scores improved from 38 to 55, indicating normal functioning. Vowel production scores showed mild difficulty, especially with the back vowels. The client demonstrated good use of compensatory strategies and self-cueing in the section of phonological processes, and as a result scores showed a marked improvement from 4 to 10.5 on a scale of 1–13. The nonspeech language areas revealed marked improvement as well. Scores on the two sections of prepositions improved to a normal range, as did use and understanding of idiomatic expressions. Marked progress was seen with vocabulary, and the client's score improved from 13 to 17. Pragmatic issues were noted to improve as the client now made direct eye contact with the speaker and used better sitting posture and vocal loudness to allow projection of voice and its audibility. The client demonstrated better awareness of communication breakdown and immediately responded to listeners' cues. Based on CAAI scores, it was determined that the client had made marked gains in all areas and problems that persisted were of a mild degree. More importantly, she knew and used compensatory strategies and independently self-cued to address communication breakdowns. Thus, based on CAAI scores alone, it appeared that the client did not need further intervention and could be discharged from therapy. However, it was still important to determine whether this improvement was apparent to neutral listeners, and also whether the client was satisfied with her current communication status.

### Intelligibility Judgments by Neutral Listeners

Audio recordings made of the client reading sections 1 and 2 (sentences and the Rainbow Passage, Fairbanks, 1998) were presented individually to three neutral listeners for judgment. They were undergraduate students at Cleveland State University and received partial credit in their class for participating in this task. These listeners had no prior listening training or familiarity with the client's speech or voice. Individual scores were computed from each listener and interrater reliability of their scores yielded a high 96% correlation. An average of their scores was 2 in section 1, and 92% in section 1, thus matching the CAAI scores reported above very closely (1.5 and 97%, respectively). It appeared that neutral, untrained listeners' judgments corresponded well with the trained speech-language pathologist's estimation of the client's functional improvement.

## Further Recommendations

It was important to ascertain whether the client felt there were any areas that were not addressed and to determine whether she had any additional concerns that would prevent her from demonstrating gains and/or independently using speech strategies in real-life situations. Thus, in the course of debriefing and discussing the follow-up scores on the CAAI, the clinician probed for her opinion about her performance. Pre- and posttherapy audio recordings were also played to the client for an objective comparison. This discussion revealed that the client was very pleased with the outcome of therapy. She reported that the scores confirmed her own intuitions and self-assessment of progress. She noted feeling more comfortable and confident in her communication with patients and during professional presentations. Her concerns were about how to ensure that she would retain what she had accomplished. To address this concern, some long-term maintenance skills and strategies were provided. She was given samples of the audio recording files from her baseline and final sessions. Specific issues in her baseline recording were identified and strategies to articulate those consonants, vowels, or prosodic patterns were reviewed. The client recorded these detailed instructions and where necessary included examples and drawings of articulators showing the incorrect and correct postures of sound production. Additional examples of sentences and paragraphs were provided for take-home practice and review. She was asked to continue practicing the sounds and their pronunciation daily on her own as well as in conversations with others. Finally, a 6-month follow-up visit was scheduled to monitor and review her status and maintenance of the progress achieved at present.

## Author Note

This report is based on a real case; some of the background details of the case, including the client's name, have been altered in order to preserve anonymity. The research and therapy treatment were conducted with the appropriate permissions from Cleveland State University's

Institutional Review Board and the Cleveland Clinic Foundation's Office of Diversity. All necessary permissions to present the data and the case findings have been sought and obtained from the client and the collaborating colleagues and institutions.

## Acknowledgments

This research was supported in part by the Faculty Research Development Grant awarded to the author from Cleveland State University. Assistance of the personnel and students in the Speech Acoustics and Perception Laboratory is greatly appreciated. The author appreciates the support and resources provided by the director, Dr. Deborah Plummer, and various staff members of the Office of Diversity at Cleveland Clinic Foundation.

## Endnote

1. In contrast, skills, goals, and methods that apply to low-English-proficiency clients are addressed in the following case.

## References

Blockcolsky, V. D., Frazer, D. H., & Frazer, J. M. (1979). *40,000 selected words.* San Antonio, TX: Communication Skill Builders.

Camarota, S. A. (2001). *Immigrants in the United States—2000: A snapshot of America's foreign-born population.* Washington, DC: Center for Immigration Studies.

Celce-Murcia, M., Brinton, D., & Goodwin, J. (1996). *Teaching pronunciation: A reference for teachers of English to speakers of other languages.* Cambridge, MA: Cambridge University Press.

Compton, A. (1984). *Pronouncing English as a second language.* San Francisco: Institute of Language and Phonology.

Derwing, T. M., Munro, M. J., & Wiebe, G. (1998). Evidence in a favor of a broad framework for pronunciation instruction. *Language Learning, 48*(3), 393–410.

Derwing, T. M., & Rossiter, M. J. (2003). The effects of pronunciation instruction on the accuracy, fluency, and complexity of L2 accented speech. *Applied Language Learning, 13*(1), 1–17.

Edwards, H. T., & Strattman, K. H. (1996). *Accent modification manual: Materials and activities.* San Francisco: Singular.

Fairbanks, G. (1998). *Voice and articulation drillbook.* New York: Addison Wesley Educational.

Flege, J. E. (1984). The detection of French accent by American listeners. *Journal of the Acoustical Society of America, 76,* 692–707.

Flege, J. E., & Fletcher, K. L. (1995). Talker and listener effects on degree of perceived foreign accent. *Journal of the Acoustical Society of America, 91,* 370–389.

Flege, J. E., Munro, M. J., & Mackay, I. R. A. (1995). Factors affecting strength of perceived foreign accent in second language. *Journal of the Acoustical Society of America, 97,* 3125–3134.

Miyawaki, K., Strange, W., Verbrugge, R., Liberman, A. M., Jenkins, J. J., & Fujimura, O. (1975). An effect of linguistic experience: The discrimination of [r] and [l] by native speakers of Japanese and English. *Perception & Psychophysics, 18,* 331–40.

Munro, M. J., & Derwing, T. M. (1995). Foreign accent, comprehensibility and intelligibility in the speech of second language learners. *Language Learning, 45*(1), 73–97.

Schmidt, A. M., & Sullivan, S. (2003). Clinical training in foreign accent modification: A national survey. *Contemporary Issues in Communication Science and Disorders, 30,* 127–135.

Shah, A. (2005). *Accent modification: Is it efficacy-based? Results from a nationwide survey.* Paper presented at the Annual Conference of the American Speech and Hearing Association (ASHA), San Diego, CA. Abstract in *ASHA Leader, 10*(11), 86, 513.

Shah, A. P. (2007). *Comprehensive Assessment of Accentedness and Intelligibility (CAAI).* Self-published assessment battery. For further information, e-mail Amee P. Shah, Ph.D., at a.shah101@csuohio.edu.

Sikorski, L. (1988). *Mastering the intonation patterns of American English.* Santa Ana, CA: LDS and Associates.

Stern, D. (1987). *The sound and style of American English: A course in foreign accent reduction.* Los Angeles: Dialect Accent Specialists.

Strange, W., & Dittmann, S. (1984). Effects of discrimination training on the perception of /r-l/ by Japanese adults learning English. *Perception & Psychophysics, 36,* 131–45.

# CASE 47

# Ms. PW: An Adult Nonnative Speaker of English: Low Proficiency

*Amee P. Shah*

## Conceptual Knowledge Areas

This case offers a profile of a low-English-proficiency client to contrast and supplement the information in the previous case on a high-English-proficiency client. Together, these cases provide speech-language pathology students and professionals with evidence-based models to attempt systematic assessment and treatment for clients with regional and foreign accents. Accent modification is a relatively recent area of practice in the discipline of speech-language pathology, and thus lacks a sufficiently robust research base to inform its clinical practice. These cases are intended to introduce clinicians to a relevant literature base, available assessment tools and methods, and variables to consider in treatment as related to accent-modification therapy in contrasting scenarios (low- and high-proficiency speakers of English). It is suggested that the previous case be read first for additional details that are relevant to this case as well, but not repeated here to prevent redundancy.

The present case was undertaken in the course of an ongoing research project in the Speech Acoustics and Perception Laboratory at Cleveland State University. International students on the CSU campus were recruited to participate in a pilot program to help them with speech and language difficulties related to their foreign accents. This training study was geared toward relatively low-proficiency speakers of English, newly arrived in the United States, who were struggling to navigate the classroom and to acculturate and adapt to their new country.

As low-proficiency (or introductory) speakers of English, this specific client group's communication needs are in contrast to the subtle and advanced skills reported in the previous case. Communication issues in a low-proficiency subgroup would typically involve markedly low intelligibility; wide-ranging differences in the production of consonants, vowels, and consonant clusters; marked carryover of phonological patterns from the native language; and limited experience perceiving the second-language sound contrasts. An overall difficulty with the second language is also predicted, including issues such as limited vocabulary, limited fluency, and presence of large number of grammatical errors. Furthermore, due to limited acculturation, knowledge of idiomatic expressions, colloquialisms, and pragmatic awareness of the mainstream culture tends to be rather limited.

## Description of the Case

### Background Information and Reason for Referral

Ms. PW, a 21-year-old female, presented with a moderate-strong foreign accent characterized by difficulties in the production of Standard American English phonemes common to native Russian speakers. A graduate student in engineering at Cleveland State University, she was concerned that her dialect would interfere with her ability to obtain gainful employment. She was referred to the Speech Acoustics and Perception Laboratory by her psychology class instructor, who noticed PW's marked difficulty in understanding what other people were saying to her and her inability to make herself understood. The initial interview revealed that PW had moved to the United States at the age of 19 years (AOA = 19 yrs.) and had lived in the United States for 2 years (LOR = 2 yrs.). She began learning English at age 10 years (AOL = 10 yrs.) in her home country.[1] She never received any ESL or accent-modification training. She was a bilingual speaker, with Russian as her first and dominant language and English as the second language. She rated her English as medium-proficiency in speaking and writing modalities but strong in reading. She had brief experiences as a cashier in a Subway sandwich franchise and was a parking attendant on campus. She reported severe difficulty with pronunciation relative to her listening skills, vocabulary issues, and writing skills. The latter were reported to be mildly affected and grammar issues were reported to be moderately affected.

## Findings of the Evaluation

The Comprehensive Assessment of Accentedness and Intelligibility (CAAI; Shah, 2007) was administered to determine performance in various aspects of speech, language, and overall communicative abilities in English. Please refer to the previous case for details and an overview of CAAI, including the test design rationale, purpose, and structure. To briefly review, the CAAI consists of 22 sections including intelligibility, consonant and vowel production, phonological processes, auditory discrimination, prosody and contrastive stress, emphasis, prepositions, idiomatic phrases, grammar, vocabulary, and pragmatics. The 22 sections yield numeric data in the form of individual section scores, which can be used to make pre- and posttherapy performance comparisons. The resulting diagnostic profile for PW summarizing the scores, patterns, and severity of disruption to communication is provided in Table 47.1.

### Summary of Assessment Results

Based on the assessment findings (see Table 47.1), the client exhibited a moderate to strong degree of difficulty in most areas. As section 2 in the CAAI indicated, the client's rate of speech was normal but her baseline intelligibility was strongly reduced (44%). The client was found to have a "Strong Foreign Accent" as her accent markedly affected conversational intelligibility.

Areas with moderate-strong degree of impairment, and in turn, those considered high priority for intervention, included segmental errors, namely, errors with the following consonants (/r/, /ɾ/, /w/, /v/, /s/, /z/, /θ/, /ð/, /ŋ/, /p$^h$/, /t$^h$/, /k$^h$/) and a variety of vowels (/ɪ/, /i/, /æ/, /o/, /ɔ/, /ʊ/, /a/,/ɚ/, /ə/, and /ʌ/). The phonological processes noted included deaspiration of initial voiceless stops, devoicing of final fricative (/s/ for /z/), and tense-lax vowel confusion. Auditory discrimination abilities were found to be markedly implicated as well and included confusion between sounds such as a/ɛ, i/e, ɚ/r, v/w, e/ɛ, s/θ, z/g, ʃ/s, ɔ/ʌ, æ/ɛ, d/t, a/ʊ, ŋ/n, ɪ/e, aʊ/æ, a/o, a/ʌ, o/ɔ.

Among suprasegmental features that appeared to be moderately impaired were lexical stress in multisyllabic words, derivative stress, and contrastive stress; these were targeted next in the hierarchy. Suprasegmental features that were relatively spared and did not require further intervention at this point included word emphasis, sentence phrasing, and contrasting sentence pairs. Other nonspeech aspects of language were markedly affected and needed to be addressed as well, although they played less of a role on perceived intelligibility and accentedness and were thought not as high a priority. These included prepositions, advanced vocabulary, understanding and use of idiomatic phrases and colloquialisms, and certain pragmatic features of conversation.

TABLE 47.1 Diagnostic Profile for Ms. PW (from the CAAI)

**Comprehensive Assessment of Accentedness & Intelligibility: Complete Diagnostic Report**

**Amee P. Shah, Ph.D.** **Date:** **Client Name: Ms. PW**

| SECTION TITLE | Total possible score | 90% performance | 70% performance | 50% performance | Client's Score |
|---|---|---|---|---|---|
| Degree of difficulty ·······················> | | mild difficulty | moderate | strong difficulty | |
| SECTION 1: INTELLIGIBILITY RELATIVE TO ACCENTEDNESS<br>e.g.,"The committee was composed of ten members . . ." | 1 to 5 | 2 | 3 | 4 or more | 4.08 |
| SECTION 2: INTELLIGIBILITY SCORE & RATE OF SPEECH ON NARRATIVE PASSAGE<br>Stimulus: Rainbow Passage | 100% | 90% | 70% | 50% | 44%, normal rate |
| SECTION 3: SENTENCE LEVEL INTONATION<br>"I got promoted!" | 10 | 9 | 7 | 5 | 9 |
| SECTION 4: WORD LEVEL INTONATION<br>e.g.: ("Tuesday comes after Monday.") "Good!" | 4 | 3.6 | 2.8 | 2 | 4 |
| SECTION 5: LEXICAL STRESS IN SINGLE, MULTISYLLABIC WORDS<br>e.g.: "Repellent." | 12 | 10.8 | 8.4 | 6 | 8 |
| SECTION 6: DERIVATIVE STRESS IN MULTISYLLABIC WORDS<br>e.g.: "democracy/democratic" | 24 | 21.6 | 16.8 | 12 | 19 |
| SECTION 7: CONTRASTIVE LEXICAL STRESS<br>e.g.: "I have a birthday present for you."/present | 28 | 25.2 | 19.6 | 14 | 19 |
| SECTION 8: EMPHASIS<br>e.g.: ("Which one was it?") "I made the pumpkin pie." | 12 | 10.8 | 8.4 | 6 | 10 |
| SECTION 9: SENTENCE PHRASING<br>e.g.: "I need milk, eggs, and bread from the market." | 7 | 6.3 | 4.9 | 3.5 | 7 |
| SECTION 10: CONTRASTING SENTECE PAIRS<br>e.g.: "Ben would never leave Woody/would he?" | 10 | 9 | 7 | 5 | 9 |
| SECTION 11: CONSONANTS WORD LIST<br>e.g.: Initial position /p/ in "pan." | 65 | 58.5 | 45.5 | 32.5 | 35 |
| SECTION 12: CONSONANT CLUSTERS WORD LIST<br>e.g.: /r/ blend in "brush." | 59 | 53.1 | 41.3 | 29.5 | 32 |
| SECTION 13a: VOWEL WORD LIST<br>e.g.: /i/ in "meat." | 18 | 16.2 | 12.6 | 9 | 13 |
| SECTION 13b: VOWEL WORD LIST<br>e.g.: /æ/ in "packed." | 22 | 19.8 | 15.4 | 11 | 16 |
| SECTION 14: PHONOLOGICAL PROCESSES | 13 | 11.7 | 9.1 | 6.5 | 8 |
| SECTION 15: AUDITORY DISCRIMINATION | 75 | 67.5 | 52.5 | 37.5 | 42 |
| SECTION 16: PREPOSITIONS<br>e.g.: "I live ____ Ohio." (in) | 20 | 18 | 14 | 10 | 15 |
| SECTION 17: COLLOQUIAL/IDIOMATIC USE OF PREPOSITIONS<br>e.g.: Are we still on ___________ tonight? (for) | 8 | 7.2 | 5.6 | 4 | 1 |

*(continued)*

TABLE 47.1 *Continued*

| SECTION TITLE | Total possible score | 90% performance | 70% performance | 50% performance | Client's Score |
|---|---|---|---|---|---|
| SECTION 18: CONTRASTING IDIOMATIC PHRASES<br>e.g.: "hold on" vs. "hold out." | 17 | 15.3 | 11.9 | 8.5 | 8 |
| Secondary Cues: sentence fill-in (comprehension of phrases) | secondary score: 8 | 7.2 | 5.6 | 4 | n/a |
| SECTION 19: COMPREHENSION OF IDIOMATIC PHRASES.<br>"Don't be upset, he's only pulling your leg." (teasing) | 12 | 10.8 | 8.4 | 6 | 3 |
| SECTION 20: ADVANCED VOCABULARY<br>Defining a word given four choices. | 20 | 18 | 14 | 10 | 2 |
| SECTION 21: CONVERSATIONAL GRAMMAR | | | | | |
| SECTION 22: PRAGMATIC PROBLEMS | | | | | |

## Treatment Options Considered

The following areas were selected and are included in the order in which they were addressed:

1. Production/auditory discrimination of consonants
2. Production/auditory discrimination of vowels
3. Phonological processes
4. Word-level stress properties (lexical stress, contrastive stress, and derivative stress)
5. Everyday conversational skills

As mentioned in the previous case, important factors in selecting the goals and their importance were the *client's preference, experience,* and *need.* In contrast to the high-proficiency client in Case 46, the present client was relatively new to the country and not very proficient in English. Limited English skills precluded working on any of the advanced language skills targeted with the previous client. Instead, the emphasis was on speech pronunciation abilities, and in particular, those that would directly influence intelligibility and the strength of accent. Thus, the majority of the treatment sessions focused on segmentals, including consonant and vowel discrimination practice, articulation drills, and coarticulation of these sounds in narratives and conversations.

## Course of Treatment

### Session Structure

Therapy consisted of 12 once weekly sessions of 1.5 hours each. The number of sessions was determined by the client's availability (once a week), and session duration was determined by the severity of the client's communication needs (moderate-severe).

### Goals and Specific Procedures[2]

***Long-Term Goal*** PW will use Standard American English (SAE) patterns and speech sounds with 80% accuracy in two 10-minute conversational speech samples as measured by analysis of the speech samples.

***Short-Term Goal 1*** PW will discriminate sound-pairs (consonants or vowels) with 80% accuracy while listening to the clinician read from a list of minimal pairs of words.

- Client will discriminate contrasting vowels /i/, /ɪ/, /ɛ/ at the word level with 80% accuracy while listening to the clinician read from a list.
- Client will discriminate contrasting consonants /r/ and /l/ at word level with 80% accuracy while listening to the clinician read from a list.
- Client will discriminate contrasting consonants /v/ and /w/ at word level with 80% accuracy while listening to the clinician read from a list.

***Short-Term Goal 2*** PW will use SAE to produce the following consonant sounds in all positions of words with 80% accuracy:

- Client will correctly produce aspiration on word-initial voiceless consonants /$p^h$/, /$t^h$/, and /$k^h$/.
- Client will correctly produce /r/ in all positions of words using SAE with 80% accuracy.
- Client will correctly produce contrasting consonants /r/ and /l/ at word level while reading from word lists with 80% accuracy.
- Client will correctly produce /s/ in all positions of words using SAE with 80% accuracy.
- Client will produce /z/ in all positions of words using SAE with 80% accuracy.
- Client will produce /v/ and /w/ contrasts at word level while reading from word lists with 80% accuracy.

***Short-Term Goal 3*** PW will use SAE to produce vowel sounds in all positions of words with 80% accuracy.

- Client will correctly produce /ʌ/ in all positions of words using SAE with 80% accuracy.
- Client will correctly produce /a/ in all positions of words using SAE with 80% accuracy.
- Client will correctly produce /o/ in all positions of words using SAE with 80% accuracy.
- Client will produce contrasting vowels /ɪ/ and /i/ at word level while reading from word lists with 80% accuracy.

***Short-Term Goal 4*** PW will correctly use SAE stress and intonation patterns in conversational speech with 80% accuracy.

- Client will produce correct syllable stress in multisyllable words at both word and sentence level while reading from word lists and passages with 80% accuracy.
- Client will use SAE stress patterns when asking a question with 80% accuracy.
- Client will use SAE stress patterns when answering a question with 80% accuracy.
- Client will use SAE intonational patterns in scripted conversation with 80% accuracy following clinician's model.

## Specific Procedures

***Segmentals: Consonants and Vowels*** Intervention began with work on consonants, including: /r/, /w/, v/, /s/, /z/, /$p^h$/, /$t^h$/, /$k^h$/). Vowels including /ɪ/, /i/, /o/, /a/ and /ʌ/ were then addressed. Initially, auditory discrimination exercises were conducted using examples from the CAAI and other word samples from accent-modification books. The clinician read minimal pairs of words with target sound contrasts and the client had to indicate which of the two words represented a given target sound. The exercise was varied on other days to require the client to say "same" or "different" in response to hearing these minimal pairs with either the same sounds (e.g., "rate-rate") or different sounds (e.g., "rate-late"). Word-identification exercises required the client to write the string of words that the clinician read aloud.

These listening exercises were conducted before addressing production errors. Consonants were targeted before vowels in production exercises. For each target sound goal, the activity started by showing the client a picture of the articulatory position for that sound. Next, the clinician demonstrated and asked the client to mimic the correct posture and movement for that sound, and provided direct instructions to modify the movement, as necessary. Once the client had learned the correct posture and movement for a sound in isolation, words containing that sound were presented to the client to be read aloud. These lists of words were taken from the book of 40,000 words by Blockcolsky, Frazer, and Frazer (1979). Words were selected so that each target sound occurred in word-initial, medial, and final positions, as well as in words increasing in syllable length, that is, 2-, and 3-, and 4- or 5-syllable words. The client practiced producing these various word positions and word lengths. In tandem, the client practiced to contrast the target sound with others in minimal pairs. For example, while working on /p/, words with /f/ and /b/ were also presented for practice. Once 80% of mastery was accomplished with these word-level sound productions, the client was led through practice with sentences containing these sounds. All sounds were practiced in the two consonant-dedicated sessions. Finally, the client was asked to read a paragraph wherein all the sounds targeted thus far were underlined and to pay attention to the related articulatory positions while reading the underlined parts.

***Suprasegmental/Prosody*** The client's prosody goals involved *word-level stress features* (lexical stress in multisyllabic words, derivative stress, and contrastive lexical stress). Activities involved reading word lists with contrastive lexical stress (e.g., OBject vs. obJECT) and varying degrees of lexical stress over words with increasing syllable length (one to five syllables). Once the client achieved 80% success rate in word-level stress productions, she was presented with sentence lists and paragraphs containing previously used words. The client read these sentences and paragraphs as naturally as possible and focused on the appropriate syllable-stress patterns. In addition to reading word lists and sentences, the client engaged in role-plays with scripted conversations to produce stress and sentence intonation patterns that matched appropriate contexts such as asking questions, answering factual questions, exclaiming, conveying sadness, and so on. The sentences represented a variety of pitch contours reflecting a wide range of pragmatic contexts. Where necessary, reinstruction and clinicians' models were provided.

## Analysis of Client's Response to Intervention

At the end of the semester, a follow-up evaluation was conducted to determine the client's progress and gauge whether to continue therapy. Progress was noted as follows. The client discriminated contrasting vowels /i/, /ɪ/, and /ɛ/ at the word level with 60% accuracy while listening to the clinician read from a list. She discriminated contrasting sounds /r/ and /l/ with 90% accuracy at word level. She produced voiceless consonants with marked improvement, /$p^h$/ and /$t^h$/ with 90% accuracy, and /$k^h$/ with 85% accuracy in all positions. She produced /r/ with 65% accuracy in all positions of words using SAE, /s/ in all positions with 70% accuracy, and /z/ in all positions with 60% accuracy. In the vowel category, she produced /ʌ/ in all positions of words with 75% accuracy, /a/ in all positions of words with 80% accuracy, and /o/ in all positions of words with 80% accuracy. She used SAE stress patterns when asking a question with 80% accuracy, SAE stress patterns when answering a question with 80% accuracy, and SAE intonation patterns in scripted conversation with 80% accuracy.

A debriefing discussion was conducted with the client to elicit her response to intervention, check her evaluation of her progress, and to understand her expectations. She reported noticing marked improvement in her ability to perceive the differences in the sound patterns in English as they differ from her native language, Russian. Moreover, she reported being better able to self-correct her production errors when they occurred in conversations by reminding herself of their correct articulatory position and specific oral movements. She learned when to slow down and repeat, when to paraphrase, when to enunciate carefully, and when to speed up her utterances in order to sound more natural. She reported maximum success with producing and monitoring the production of the voiceless consonants, /$p^h$/, /$t^h$/, and /$k^h$/. She expressed continued difficulties in producing vowels and a few consonant clusters.

## Further Recommendations

In light of these evaluation findings and the client's self-report, it was concluded that the client had benefited from speech therapy and shown marked progress, and that therapy needed to be continued further in the course of the next semester. The client had fewer errors and communication issues, but needed increased practice with gains made and future ones expected. Thus, it was determined that the client would be seen 3 times a week (instead of 2 times weekly as before) for 30-minute (instead of 1.5 hour) sessions. The client was provided with strategies and assignments for the winter break to maintain the progress and learning achieved thus far. These assignments included copies of materials involving words, sentences, and paragraphs with highlighted sounds, all of them targeting the specific consonant and vowel targets addressed. In addition, the client was given conversational assignments wherein she was supposed to role-play situations with her teenage daughter at home to mimic interactions with various people in her everyday situations and audio-record these situations (e.g., discussing a product in a store with a sales clerk, discussing a simple banking transaction with a bank teller, placing an order over the telephone). She analyzed these recordings and identified features in which she had incorporated the new strategies learned in therapy, as well as those features which she failed to do so. Finally, she was asked to practice pronouncing the individual words that she identified as errors from this analysis and to bring recordings to the therapy sessions.

## Author Note

This report is based on a real case; some of the background details of the case, including the client's name, have been altered to preserve anonymity. The research and therapy treatment were conducted with the appropriate permissions from Cleveland State University's Institutional Review Board, and from the Speech and Hearing Clinic at Cleveland State University. All necessary permissions to present the data and the case findings have been sought and obtained from the client and the collaborating colleagues and institutions.

## Acknowledgments

This research was supported in part by a Faculty Research Development Grant awarded to the author from Cleveland State University. Assistance of the personnel and students in the Speech Acoustics and Perception class and the Speech and Hearing Clinic is greatly appreciated.

## Endnotes

1. For information regarding the terms AOA, AOL, and LOR, please refer to the case history information in the previous case.
2. Please note that the format of this section is different from that of the previous case. The clients seen in the Speech Acoustics and Perception lab are treated in keeping with the structure of the speech and hearing clinic. Thus, long- and short-term goals, procedures, and report-writing reflects those followed in the clinic. This structure is different from that specially designed for the high-proficiency clients seen in the Communication for Impact program described in the previous case.

## References

Blockcolsky, V. D., Frazer, D. H., & Frazer, J. M. (1979). *40,000 selected words.* San Antonio, TX: Communication Skill Builders.

Shah, A. P. (2007). *Comprehensive Assessment of Accentedness and Intelligibility (CAAI).* Self-published assessment battery. For further information, e-mail Amee P. Shah, Ph.D., at a.shah101@csuohio.edu.

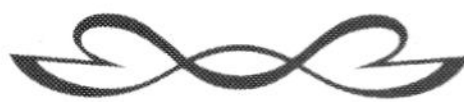



# CASE 48

# Mr. K: An Adult with Dementia of the Alzheimer Type: Screening, Assessment, and Cognitive-Linguistic Interventions

*Nidhi Mahendra*

## Conceptual Knowledge Areas

### What Is Dementia?

Grabowski and Damasio (2004) define dementia as a syndrome characterized by acquired and persistent impairment of multiple cognitive domains that is severe enough to impair competence in daily living, occupation, and social interaction. Affected cognitive domains include memory, language, attention, executive function, and visuospatial abilities. Importantly, cognitive impairments in these domains occur in the absence of delirium, which is an acute but reversible state of confusion associated with temporary impairments of attention, perception, and cognition.

### Characteristics of Dementia of the Alzheimer Type

Dementia can be reversible (e.g., when resulting from depression or nutritional deficiencies) or irreversible (e.g., when resulting from Alzheimer's disease or other neurological diseases) and can be caused by multiple diseases and health conditions. Alzheimer's disease (AD) is the most common cause of irreversible dementia in adults over the age of 65 years. It accounts for approximately 50% of clinical diagnoses of dementia. Other causes of dementia include vascular dementia (VaD), frontotemporal dementia (FTD), and subcortical dementias (e.g., when associated with Huntington's disease or progressive supranuclear palsy). Memory impairment, specifically episodic memory decline, is the earliest appearing symptom of AD (Bayles, 1991). The presence of pervasive memory impairments is required for a clinical diagnosis of dementia.

### Episodic Memory Impairments in Dementia of the Alzheimer Type

Episodic memory, one component of the declarative system of human long-term memory (see Mahendra & Apple, 2007 for a comprehensive review of human memory systems), refers to the ability to consciously recollect events and episodes, with specific information about the time/space constraints in which these events occurred. Episodic memory allows us to quickly learn new information and is highly vulnerable to the effects of aging and dementia, especially Alzheimer's disease. Assessment tasks that involve episodic immediate and delayed recall of new information (e.g., a short story, word list) are most sensitive to distinguishing age-associated episodic memory changes from those associated with neurodegenerative disorders like AD. Working memory and semantic memory are also affected in AD, the former being affected much earlier in the disease process than the latter. Such memory impairments also negatively impact linguistic communication because of the inextricable link between memory and language as related aspects of cognition.

### Linguistic Communication Impairments in Dementia of the Alzheimer Type

The aforementioned impairments in multiple cognitive domains result in persons with AD manifesting linguistic communication impairments. The earliest noted linguistic communication impairments include anomia and discourse-based impairments. The discourse of persons with AD is characterized by lack of coherence, repetitiousness, tangentiality, inability to maintain a topic during conversation, and reduced content. The ability to express ideas verbally and in writing deteriorates as the severity of dementia increases. A decline in receptive language abilities is also dependent on the integrity of attention, working memory, and episodic memory, all of which deteriorate in dementia. Interestingly, phonological and syntactic processing abilities remain relatively preserved until more advanced stages of the disease.

### Spaced Retrieval Training (SRT)

Spaced retrieval training (SRT) is a type of shaping procedure applied to memory training that is increasingly being used to teach new information or skills to persons with dementia (see Hopper et al., 2005 for a recent review of evidence for using SRT with dementia patients). This technique entails presenting new information or demonstrating a new motor procedure to a person with dementia and requiring successful immediate recall (or recall and demonstration of a procedure) followed by successful recall over gradually increasing time intervals until a client can recall that information for everyday tasks. Time intervals following successful recall are doubled, whereas intervals following failure to recall are halved. For example, clients with mild to moderate dementia were successfully trained to recall faces and names of persons as long as 3 months after stopping spaced retrieval training (Mahendra, Apple, & Reed, 2008). Similarly, a clinician can train a client to perform a compensatory strategy or a safety maneuver during therapy using spaced retrieval training.

### Semantic Feature Analysis (SFA)

Semantic feature analysis (SFA) is an elaborate, systematic cueing technique whereby a client has to produce words or exemplars semantically related to a target item. For example, if the target word is "fork," the cues might be questions targeting use of the item (eating), its physical attributes (metal/plastic, three prongs, etc.), the semantic category to which it belongs (flatware), and generating other items that are associated with "fork" (e.g., knife, spoon, plate, napkin). The intent of producing semantically related exemplars is to facilitate access to semantic memory. It is thought that repeated practice activating conceptual information related to a target increases the likelihood that this target can be accessed and named more easily. Researchers have documented that SFA improves confrontation naming performance in persons with aphasia for treated picture stimuli, and that enhanced performance generalizes to untreated pictures (Boyle, 2004; Boyle & Coelho, 1995; Coelho, McHugh, & Boyle, 2000).

## Description of the Case

This case profiles the cognitive and communicative functioning of a client with dementia of the Alzheimer type and details the implementation and outcomes of spaced retrieval training (SRT) and semantic feature analysis (SFA) with this client. The screening, assessment, and interventions reported here were conducted under the aegis of a clinical research program administered at a continuum-of-care facility where Mr. K resided. The spaced retrieval training described was conducted using a laptop computer.

## Background Information

Mr. K was an 81-year-old, monolingual, biracial (Caucasian and Latino) male who lived in the assisted living section of a continuum-of-care facility in the San Francisco Bay Area in California for 7 years. He was referred to the aging and dementia research team by the social services director and the director of nursing (DON) at the facility where he lived.

Mr. K had an eighth-grade education and had served in the U.S. Navy for 8 years, following which he ran a small business buying and selling automobile spare parts. Owing to the success of his small business, Mr. K and his wife were comfortably well off in their lifetime and reported their socioeconomic status as "upper-middle-class." Mr. K was born and raised in Mesa, Arizona and had lived in Arizona, Seattle, Hawaii, and California over the past 30 years, spending the most time in Hawaii. Mr. K's medical history was significant for diabetes, hypertension (well controlled), bilateral sensorineural hearing loss, and a history of surgery on both knees. One year prior to this referral, Mr. K had been diagnosed with probable Alzheimer's disease by an interdisciplinary team comprised of his primary care physician, a neurologist, a neuropsychologist, and the facility nursing staff. For the past year, he had been taking Aricept, an acetylcholinesterase inhibitor, to slow down the cognitive decline resulting from AD. Mr. K was a tall, well-nourished, friendly, and rather talkative gentleman who often told jokes and occasionally made pragmatically inappropriate comments during conversation. Mr. K was not very insightful about changes in his cognitive functioning and talked openly about being very upset about not being allowed to drive his car following the diagnosis of AD. There was no reported positive family history for Alzheimer's dementia or other non-Alzheimer's dementia.

## Reasons for the Referral

Mr. K was initially referred for consultation about his declining cognitive status. Specifically, his wife was concerned about his progressively declining memory, increased agitation over trivial matters, and recent behavior of making uninhibited, inappropriate comments to their friends during conversation. Mrs. K also was concerned about him routinely forgetting to take his walker and subsequently having falls. She reported that he would leave their apartment, be gone for several hours, and return without being able to state where he had been or what he had been doing. When she questioned him about his whereabouts, he would counter, "Have I been gone that long? That's impossible." She had spoken with the social services director and the director of nursing about the possibility of conducting an evaluation and wanted advice about whether it was time to leave their assisted living apartment and transition to the dementia unit (a locked unit with higher level of care) within this same continuum-of-care facility.

## Findings of the Evaluation

The consultation began with a short, 30-minute screening (see Table 48.1 for a time-ordered agenda of screening activities) with a plan to use the results of the screening to determine the subsequent need for a comprehensive assessment and/or intervention. This was explained to Mr. K and his wife; she provided her consent for the initial screening and Mr. K gave his verbal assent to participate. During the screening, the clinician reviewed Mr. K's medical chart, spoke with nursing staff, and administered the Mini Mental State Exam (Folstein, Folstein, & McHugh, 1975), the Geriatric Depression Scale-Short Form (Sheikh & Yesavage, 1986), and pure-tone audiometric hearing screening.

### Initial Screening and Related Findings

***Medical Chart Review*** In addition to confirming the active medical diagnoses reported earlier, from reviewing Mr. K's medical chart, the clinician noted that he recently had two atraumatic falls, both of which resulted because he had forgotten to take his walker. Mr. K had been

TABLE 48.1 Time-Ordered Plan for Screening Activities

| Activity | Time Allotted | Rationale |
|---|---|---|
| Brief Chart Review | <5 minutes | To ensure no relevant medical information about Mr. K had been overlooked |
| Conversation with Nursing Staff | <5 minutes | To obtain information about staff concerns and perceptions about Mr. K |
| Mini Mental State Exam | 10 minutes | To obtain a rough estimate of Mr. K's dementia severity and his possible candidacy for skilled interventions |
| Geriatric Depression Scale (Short Form) | 5 minutes | To rule out depression as an alternative explanation for Mr. K's declining cognitive performance |
| Otoscopy, Pure-Tone Audiometric Hearing Screening, Word Recognition Testing | 10 minutes | To obtain information about Mr. K's hearing ability |

briefly hospitalized for three days three weeks prior for a urinary tract infection (UTI) that had been successfully treated with antibiotics and since resolved. From the chart notes, it appeared that his cognitive abilities might have deteriorated further since this UTI.

***Brief Conversation with Nursing Staff*** The staff described Mr. K as getting confused easily with verbal directions and having difficulty clearly stating what he needed. He routinely forgot detailed conversations with the staff about events and would get upset about them not helping him with tasks that they had earlier helped him to complete.

***Mini Mental State Exam (MMSE)*** The MMSE is an 11-item, 30-point brief cognitive status assessment that documents performance on items pertaining to orientation, registration, attention and calculation, verbal episodic memory, and language (naming, repetition, reading, writing, following a command). Mr. K scored 17 out of 30. Given his age (81 years) and confirmed eighth-grade education, the expected normative MMSE score would be 25 (Crum, Anthony, Bassett, & Folstein, 1993). Thus, his MMSE score of 17 indicated below expected cognitive functioning and definite cognitive impairment of mild to moderate severity.

***Geriatric Depression Scale–Short Form (GDS)*** The GDS-Short Form consists of 15 questions that require a yes or no response (for example, "Do you have more problems with memory than most people?" "Is it wonderful to be alive now?"). Depending on the client's answers, a score out of 15 is generated and scores of 5 or greater require referral to a physician to address the possibility of clinical depression. Mr. K scored 1 out of 15, indicating that he was not depressed at the time of this screening.

***Otoscopy, Pure-Tone Audiometric Screening, and Word Recognition Testing*** Mr. K's wife revealed that he had been prescribed and fitted with bilateral in-the-ear (ITE) hearing aids by an audiologist four years ago. He had received no subsequent audiological assessment and data from his last assessment were not available for review. Given this situation and because it was important to have some objective data about his current hearing abilities, otoscopy was conducted followed by pure-tone audiometric hearing screening. Mr. K complained that he did not like his hearing aids and preferred not to wear them. Otoscopy revealed no gross abnormalities, discharge, or impacted cerumen in either ear. Mr. K did not pass a pure-tone audiometric hearing screening developed for geriatric listeners at 35 dB HL at 500 Hz, 1 kHz, and 2 kHz in either ear. He also did not pass a pure-tone screening at 45 dB HL at 4 kHz, 6 kHz, and 8 kHz in the right and left ears. The clinician had to maintain a reasonably loud conversational volume, and then Mr. K was able to follow most directions when seated in a quiet room facing the clinician. His word recognition was tested by having him repeat a phonemically balanced word list spoken by the clinician at her normal conversational volume. He was able to repeat 9 out of 20 words accurately. During the screening, Mr. K's wife was observed to often be uncomfortably loud (perhaps compensating for Mr. K not wearing his hearing aids) and occasionally condescending in how she communicated and interacted with him.

### Comprehensive Evaluation

Based on the aforementioned results of the screening, it was determined that Mr. K should have a comprehensive evaluation to obtain more information about dementia severity and his profile of spared and impaired cognitive abilities. Further, initial information obtained about Mr. K and his level of functioning during the screening and observations based on interacting with him revealed that he would likely be a good candidate for implementing direct interventions. It was noteworthy that incidental observations of his spouse and of communicative exchanges between Mr. K and his wife suggested that indirect intervention would be very appropriate for Mrs. K and select nursing staff with the goal of enhancing Mr. K's cognitive and communicative functioning and Mrs. K's and his quality of life.

The central hypothesis was that Mr. K presented with mild to moderate dementia. A comprehensive evaluation would be conducted with the following goals:

- Obtain an objective index of the severity of his cognitive and communicative functioning.
- Identify Mr. K's most significant cognitive and communicative impairments.
- Identify select spared abilities that could be capitalized upon during therapy.
- Test Mr. K's responsiveness to multiple possible intervention options and document their initial feasibility.

A comprehensive evaluation is the foundation of developing an efficacious therapy plan. It reveals a client's spared and impaired abilities (Tomoeda, 2001) and is an invaluable opportunity to further determine if the client is a good candidate for specific evidence-based therapeutic interventions. It is noteworthy that Medicare intermediaries look for evidence in a clinician's evaluation documentation that a client with dementia has restorative potential or has demonstrated some ability to benefit from skilled therapy before reimbursing a claim for therapy services provided. From this perspective of demonstrating a client's ability to participate in and benefit from an intervention, a comprehensive evaluation must include *dynamic assessment* as described by Gutiérrez-Clellen and Peña (2001). Dynamic assessment, an alternative to traditional standardized assessments, refers to an approach in which a clinician invests time during an evaluation to identify skills that a client possesses and to obtain evidence of a client's learning potential. Such assessments are process-oriented and emphasize the learning process with a goal to identify what conditions optimally facilitate client performance (e.g., test-teach-retest methods, response modeling, simplified instructions, increased processing time, supportive cues, or environmental modification). Dynamic assessment is routinely used by speech-language pathologists (SLPs) during stimulability testing for clients with articulation disorders or when testing what language stimulation strategies (parallel talk, expansion, etc.) facilitate improved language production in children. Dynamic assessment is rarely used during evaluation with adult clients who have dementia.

A 75-minute comprehensive evaluation was planned to build on information obtained during the screening. The evaluation comprised a brief client interview, the Dementia Rating Scale (DRS-2; Mattis, Jurica, & Leitten, 1982), select subtests of the Arizona Battery for Communication Disorders of Dementia (ABCD; Bayles and Tomoeda, 1993), and a dynamic assessment of Mr. K's candidacy to participate in spaced retrieval training (SRT; Brush & Camp, 2000) and semantic feature analysis (SFA; Boyle, 2004; Boyle & Coelho, 1995). Table 48.2 provides a time-ordered agenda for this comprehensive evaluation including time allotted for each activity and a rationale for its inclusion (see Mahendra and Apple, 2007 for a list of other assessment options and rationale for their consideration). Given that Mr. K was unwilling to wear his hearing aids and the need for the clinician to

TABLE 48.2 Time-Ordered Plan for Assessment Activities

| Activity | Time Allotted | Rationale |
|---|---|---|
| Client Interview | 10 minutes | To obtain information on client perceptions and motivation to participate in intervention |
| Mattis Dementia Rating Scale (DRS-2) | 30 minutes | To better quantify dementia severity, correct scores for age and education level; and to use an assessment measure that has alternate forms for future assessment |
| Subtests of the Arizona Battery for Communication Disorders of Dementia<br>- Immediate and Delayed Story Recall<br>- Confrontation Naming<br>- Concept Definition<br>- Object Description | 20 minutes | To obtain information about staff and family perceptions/concerns |
| Dynamic Assessment for Use of Spaced Retrieval Training | 5 minutes | To determine if spaced retrieval training would be an appropriate intervention for Mr. K |
| Dynamic Assessment for Use of Semantic Feature Analysis | 5 minutes | To determine if semantic feature analysis would be an appropriate intervention for Mr. K |

maintain a loud conversational volume throughout testing, an assistive listening device (ALD) was introduced. He responded very well to the ALD and agreed to keep it on during the entire evaluation.

## Results of Comprehensive Assessment

***Interview Findings and Observations*** On the day of the evaluation, Mr. K did not remember that he was to come to the clinic for an evaluation. He had to be escorted to the clinic area by a certified nursing aide (CNA). He walked into the assessment room with his walker and was well groomed and alert. As he entered the therapy room, he paused and unbuttoned his shirt down to his waist, stating, "I am ready for action." He seated himself and made no attempt to button up his shirt for several minutes until directly asked to do so by the clinician. His behavior was appropriate for the remainder of this session. During the interview, Mr. K was asked a few questions about his perceived areas of difficulty, his interests and things that he missed being able to do, and his willingness to participate in therapy with the clinician. Mr. K responded by describing his frustration with instances in which he could not recall the name of a friend or his granddaughter, Kirsten, or when he could not name an item he could visualize clearly. He also stated that he wanted to resume using his laptop computer but felt too frustrated with it lately. He stated that he missed driving, that he was very bored at the facility, and that the activities that were being recommended to him did not keep him engaged. He reported that his wife talked to him as if he was stupid and this made him angry.

***Dementia Rating Scale (DRS-2)*** The Dementia Rating Scale-2 (DRS-2) is the second and extensively revised edition of the original Dementia Rating Scale (DRS). The DRS-2 is a widely used, brief, comprehensive neuropsychological measure of cognitive status in adults with degenerative cortical impairments that also can be used to monitor changes in cognitive status over time. It consists of 36 tasks that yield information about 5 subscales—Attention, Initiation/Perseveration, Construction, Conceptualization, and Memory. Mr. K's total raw score on the DRS-2 was 104 (out of a possible 144 points), which falls below the first percentile when compared to an age- and education-matched cohort for Mr. K. In other words, less than 1% of healthy elders receive this total score on the DRS-2. A detailed profile revealed mildly impaired performance on the Attention and Conceptualization subscales with moderately impaired performance on the Initiation/Perseveration, Construction, and Memory subscales.

***Arizona Battery for Communication Disorders of Dementia (ABCD)*** The ABCD is a comprehensive assessment and screening tool for use with persons who have dementia. It was standardized on persons with Alzheimer's disease and Parkinson's disease as well as young and older healthy adults without cognitive impairments. The ABCD assists clinicians in differential diagnosis, monitoring change over time, developing therapy goals, and discharge planning. It contains 14 subtests that may be administered individually and together provide information on 5 constructs—linguistic expression, linguistic comprehension, verbal episodic memory, visuospatial construction, and mental status.

The clinician already had information on Mr. K's medical diagnosis of probable Alzheimer's disease, his mental status (based on the MMSE), and his overall dementia severity (based on results of the DRS-2). Therefore, instead of administering the entire ABCD, the clinician chose to do a nonstandardized assessment using 4 subtests of the ABCD, including the story retelling (immediate and delayed retelling), confrontation naming, object description, and concept definition subtests. The intent was to obtain more information about his verbal episodic memory, semantic memory, naming, and oral discourse abilities.

### Dynamic Assessment to Determine Candidacy for Spaced Retrieval Training (SRT)

The clinician adapted a published screening protocol for SRT (Brush & Camp, 2000) to evaluate Mr. K's candidacy for this therapy technique. This involved having Mr. K recall discrete information about the clinician (her place of work) over 1- and 2-minute short delays and over a longer delay of 5 minutes. Mr. K demonstrated successful recall, indicating that he was a good candidate for this intervention.

### Dynamic Assessment to Determine Candidacy for Semantic Feature Analysis (SFA)

The clinician chose to implement SFA with Mr. K based on three considerations. First, he had notably impaired confrontation naming (naming pictures on the ABCD, naming real objects on the DRS-2) and generative naming (a.k.a. verbal or category fluency). Next, whereas his naming abilities were rather impaired, he was much better at describing common objects and defining concepts (on the ABCD Object Description and Concept Definition subtests). Third, SFA therapy has a strong evidence base (Boyle, 2004; Boyle & Coelho, 1995; Coelho, McHugh, & Boyle, 2000) and has been successfully used to facilitate the confrontation naming performance of persons with aphasia. Although SFA has not been implemented with persons who have dementia, it was felt that this rationale was strong. Dynamic assessment was used to confirm that SFA would be a useful therapeutic technique for him. Five items were selected that Mr. K had not been able to name on confrontation naming, and methods detailed by Boyle (2004) were applied to test the utility of SFA. The clinician presented these 5 items to Mr. K, asking him to name them, and then asked Mr. K to produce words that were related to the picture or semantically associated. To elicit this information about semantic features, Mr. K was either questioned or provided with sentence stems to complete. He was given the following 3 cues for each item:

1. What category does this item belong to? (Goal: To elicit information about superordinate category)
2. This item is used for ________ (Goal: To elicit information about the use of the item)
3. What does this item look like? (Goal: To elicit information about the item's physical attributes)

Following 2 learning trials, Mr. K was able to answer 1–2 questions for each of the 5 selected items, indicating that he would be able to benefit from a simplified version of SFA to compensate for his word-finding difficulties.

## Treatment Options Considered

Based on Mr. K's performance on screening and assessment measures, his episodic memory impairments and word retrieval deficits were identified as the primary targets of intervention. Secondary goals of intervention were to address caregiver communication patterns and to provide Mr. K with some personally relevant and cognitively stimulating activities in which he could successfully participate. Thus, the clinician implemented spaced retrieval training (SRT) and semantic feature analysis (SFA) directly with Mr. K and conducted caregiver education and training on effective communication patterns with Mrs. K and the CNAs. The rationale for selecting SRT was based on the extensive evidence supporting its successful use with persons with dementia (Hopper et al., 2005) and Mr. K's success with participating in SRT during dynamic assessment. Finally, it was thought that SRT could be used effectively to address Mr. K's failure to remember to take his walker and to train a compensatory strategy of describing an object or item that he could not name.

SFA was chosen because this therapeutic technique is well detailed in the literature on treating anomia (see Boyle, 2004 for a detailed description of SFA), and the described methodology in published studies allowed us to replicate this with Mr. K. Also, our client had relatively well-preserved semantic memory and responded fairly well to a trial implementation of SFA during dynamic assessment. Therefore, the clinician decided to use SFA to facilitate Mr. K's successful naming of 30 everyday objects that he was not able to name consistently at baseline testing. To address Mrs. K's communication with her husband, two 45-minute sessions were devoted to educating her about the effects of AD on communication and cognition, and to instruct her about effective communicative strategies that she should use with Mr. K. Our clinical hypotheses were that:

1. Spaced retrieval training (SRT) would be beneficial in teaching Mr. K to remember:
   a. To take his walker with him every time he left his apartment
   b. To learn a compensatory strategy of describing the attributes of an object to help him with his word retrieval impairments
2. Semantic feature analysis (SFA) would be beneficial in directly improving Mr. K's word retrieval abilities by enhancing his ability to describe characteristics of everyday items that he could not name.
3. Caregiver training would help his wife modify her communication patterns to be most effective for Mr. K.

## Course of Treatment

Mr. K was seen for a total of 12 50-minute sessions, 3 times a week, focusing on the above goals.

### Spaced Retrieval Training (SRT)

SRT was used to sequentially train two procedures. Procedure 1 was trained by asking Mr. K the question, "Mr. K, what do you need to take with you each time you leave your apartment?" Mr. K was to answer, "I'll take my walker with me." Initially, this question was presented verbally by the clinician and simultaneously appeared in writing on a laptop screen to provide a multimodal input. One minute later, if Mr. K did not recall the answer to the question, the clinician provided the answer verbally and in writing on the computer screen and had him repeat it. Then the question was subsequently re-presented 1 minute later (with no increase in time interval). If after the initial 1 minute he successfully recalled the information, he was asked the target question 2 minutes later (doubling the previous 1 minute interval). Thus, each time he correctly recalled the answer, the next interval before testing recall was doubled. Using this expanded rehearsal and shaping procedure, Mr. K was trained to successfully recall the answer to the target question over gradually increasing time intervals of 1, 2, 4, 8, 16, and 32 minutes. After Mr. K successfully recalled this information over 32 minutes over 2 consecutive sessions, therapy sessions were conducted in his apartment. Sessions included a daily actual probe of this procedure when he was ready to leave the apartment by asking him the target question in the everyday context for which it was trained. Mr. K maintained successful recall over the remainder of therapy. To maintain recall, environmental cues were placed to help him remember to take his walker via a wristband that he wore, which contained the reminder "Don't forget your walker" and a laminated card posted on the inside of his apartment door.

After this first procedure had been trained up to a 32-minute interval, it was probed weekly until the end of therapy. Mr. K maintained his recall of this first target information. Subsequently, SRT was used to teach Mr. K a second procedure in response to the question "What will you do if you cannot think of the name of an object?" Mr. K had to answer "I will describe the object." This compensatory strategy was trained using SRT, whereas the ability to systematically describe a target object in detail was trained using semantic feature analysis (SFA). One of the advantages of SRT is that it can be nested within other therapy goals for a client. For instance, if a client is recalling information over a 16-minute interstimulus interval, the clinician can address other therapy goals during that interval. The clinician implemented SFA during interstimulus intervals that were 8 minutes or longer in duration. For time intervals shorter than 8 minutes, Mr. K was engaged in casual conversation.

### Semantic Feature Analysis

SFA was implemented for approximately 20–25 minutes of each of Mr. K's 12 sessions, and was nested within spaced retrieval training. Target items for SFA training were selected based on analysis of Mr. K's naming performance during testing with the DRS-2 and the ABCD. Incidental data on naming performance was also gathered about reported and observed naming difficulties that Mr. K experienced. Additional baseline testing was conducted during the first few therapy sessions using naming subtests from the DRS-2 and the ABCD as well as the Snodgrass and Vanderwart (1980) black-and-white line drawings to identify object names for training. Thus, a core vocabulary of 30 common and highly functional items was identified for SFA training. Figure 48.1 contains a list of the words that Mr. K could not name on multiple baseline sessions that he was trained to name and describe using SFA.

Multiple stimuli were similarly presented in 5-word blocks with data collected regarding the number of sessions in which a particular item was treated using SFA. Each item was targeted in 8–10 sessions. The schematic in Figure 48.2 illustrates a typical therapy session with Mr. K in which both SRT and SFA were implemented. Once a target response could be recalled over 8 minutes during spaced retrieval training, SFA was implemented during the interstimulus intervals exceeding 8 minutes.

### Caregiver and CNA Training

Caregiver training was conducted with Mrs. K in the first two sessions of therapy. This helped keep the first two sessions short for Mr. K and allowed the clinician to monitor the effects of caregiver training over the next several weeks. One live inservice workshop was conducted by the clinician for CNAs and nurses on effective communication strategies for residents with dementia. This inservice was videotaped and available as a permanent resource for other CNAs and registered nurses who were not able to attend on the day that the workshop was conducted. Mrs. K was provided a published brochure titled *Communication: Best Ways to Interact with the Person with Dementia* (Alzheimer's Association, 2005) and the contents of the brochure were discussed with her and explained. The clinician also showed Mrs. K a 21-minute videotape titled *Dealing with Alzheimer's Disease: A Common Sense Approach to Communication*

FIGURE 48.1 List of 30 Items Targeted Using SFA

**Meals/Food Items (12):** Oatmeal, Fork, Straw, Napkin, Steak, Chicken, Cottage Cheese, Pears, Grapes, Peas, Splenda (sugar substitute), Microwave

**Toiletries (6):** Mouthwash, Floss, Towel, Comb, Deodorant, Toothpaste

**Clothing and Personal Items (5):** Vest, Robe, Wristwatch, Slippers, Sunglasses

**Items Pertaining to Hobbies (6):** Cards, Calendar, Computer, DVD Player, Camera, Remote (for TV)

**People's Names (1):** Kirsten* (granddaughter)

* *Note:* Names of people have not been typically trained using SFA. The clinicians chose to implement SFA for Mr. K's granddaughter's name given the high personal relevance of this target for this client. Questions and sentence stems used in SFA were modified for training this name. The cues used were exactly as those in the section describing dynamic assessment using SFA.

EXAMPLE: Target—Toothpaste

1. What category does toothpaste belong to? (Toiletries)
2. You use toothpaste for __________ (cleaning your teeth)

What does it look like? (Soft, pasty, often white or blue in color, comes in a tube)

(Ramsey Foundation, 1990). The contents of this video were debriefed with Mrs. K and specific techniques (using short, simple sentences; rephrasing and repeating; avoiding metaphors; providing tangible stimuli during conversation using written cues, photos, or objects) were demonstrated to her. After the first two sessions that included direct training with Mrs. K, she was asked to return demonstrations of these techniques as she interacted with Mr. K in 5 of the next 10 sessions.

## Analysis of the Client's Response to Intervention

By the end of 12 sessions, Mr. K was able to recall both responses trained during SRT spontaneously over multiple weeks. His ability to remember to take his walker with him improved

FIGURE 48.2 Typical Therapy Session with Mr. K

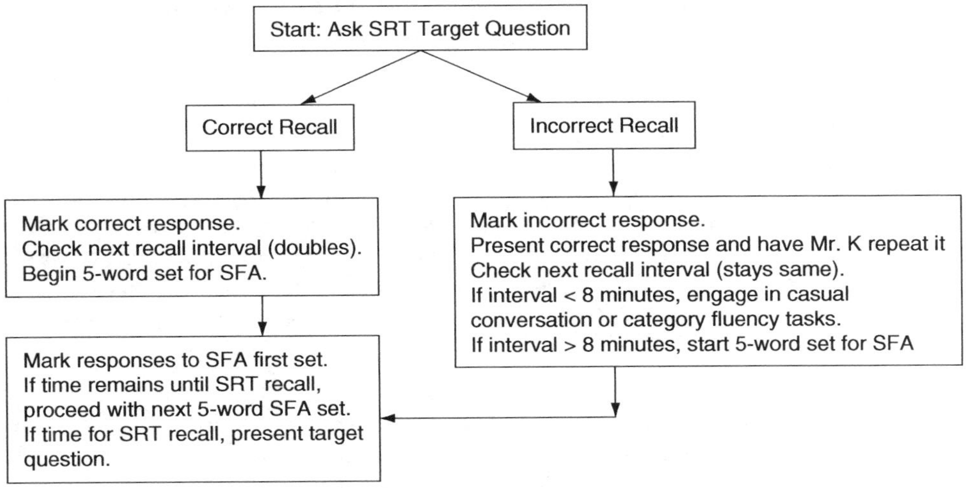

Start: Ask SRT Target Question

Correct Recall

Incorrect Recall

Mark correct response.
Check next recall interval (doubles).
Begin 5-word set for SFA.

Mark incorrect response.
Present correct response and have Mr. K repeat it
Check next recall interval (stays same).
If interval < 8 minutes, engage in casual conversation or category fluency tasks.
If interval > 8 minutes, start 5-word set for SFA

Mark responses to SFA first set.
If time remains until SRT recall, proceed with next 5-word SFA set.
If time for SRT recall, present target question.

dramatically from 20% of situations tracked by the clinician, the CNAs, and his spouse to 90%. His spouse and the CNAs were instructed to provide the same target question that had been used during therapy to continue to help him maintain his recall. Over the 4 weeks that Mr. K was enrolled in therapy, he did not have a single fall. With the help of the CNAs, data were tracked for 2 months after he stopped therapy and he still had not had any subsequent falls, largely because of his improved ability to remember to take his walker with him.

Regarding SFA, a posttreatment naming assessment of the 30 items selected for training was conducted with Mr. K. He correctly named 21 of 30 items spontaneously; for the remaining 9 items, he spontaneously described 6 out of 9 items using 1–2 trained object attributes. For the remaining 3 items, he had to be reminded of this compensatory strategy of describing objects by asking the target question, "Mr. K, what will you do if you cannot think of the name of an object?" He most often used functional attributes of objects and less often used physical attributes or superordinate category descriptors. His posttreatment naming performance is strong evidence that SFA resulted in improved lexical access. Further, when he could not retrieve an object label, he benefited from the SFA cueing and the spaced retrieval training by using a compensatory strategy of describing objects so listeners could determine what he was attempting to say.

Regarding caregiver training, Mrs. K was inconsistent in using the trained communicative strategies when she interacted with Mr. K. Multiple 5-minute verbal exchanges were observed during five sessions subsequent to her training. In three of these sessions, she used strategies appropriately. In the other two sessions, she displayed verbal frustration ("I give up," "I don't know how to explain to you"), inconsistent use of strategies, raising her voice and talking very fast, and choosing to end a conversation before Mr. K had a chance to respond. The clinician pointed out these observations to her while reinforcing her positive changes in communicative behavior, and counseled her to maintain the strategies that she had learned and about the importance of persisting in improving her communication with Mr. K. Given that Mrs. K felt very responsible for Mr. K, she also was counseled about caregiver burden and was encouraged to see the social services director for respite care arrangements so that she could pursue her own hobbies and outings without worrying about Mr. K.

## Further Recommendations

Speech-language pathologists are uniquely positioned to make significant contributions to the care of older adults with dementia by utilizing knowledge and skills and intervening for cognitive, communicative, and swallowing impairments. However, we must achieve a fundamental attitudinal shift if we indeed want to make a difference to our clients with dementia. We cannot stand back and not use our knowledge and skills to intervene for fear that claims for therapeutic services may be denied. Nor can we hesitate to request the number of sessions that will be needed to achieve outcomes, or to ask for additional therapy time if the client's performance and response to therapy necessitate this. Indeed, if we implement methodologically sound therapy approaches after dynamically assessing client candidacy for these approaches, we demonstrate to third-party payers that our clinical decision making is sound for recommending specific skilled services. Further, if we organize therapy sessions to deliver the most "bang for the buck" and collect meaningful data on client and/or caregiver performance that reveal positive changes in functioning, we can be successful in providing much-needed services to our clients with dementia. Finally, it is imperative that there be a tight link between our comprehensive evaluation and subsequent recommendations for intervention. This link is best achieved through compelling and clear documentation as well as organized data collection during therapy. If services we have provided are questioned or scrutinized, we must be able to stand by our clinical decisions and have the data to support our practice.

## Author Note

Preparation of this paper was supported by an Everyday Technology for Alzheimer Care (ETAC) research grant awarded to the author by the Alzheimer's Association. This case is based on a compilation of assessment and intervention outcomes of two actual clients with dementia. Approval from the California State University East Bay IRB was obtained for the original intervention study in which these clients participated. Informed consent by proxy was obtained from caregivers of both participants as well as verbal assent from the participants themselves.

## References


Alzheimer's Association. (2005). *Communication: Best ways to interact with the person with dementia* (12-page brochure). Retrieved November 24, 2008 from http://www.alz.org/national/documents/brochure_communication.pdf

Bayles, K. A. (1991). Alzheimer's disease symptoms: Prevalence and order of appearance. *Journal of Applied Gerontology*, 10(4), 419–430.

Bayles, K. A., & Tomoeda, C. K. (1993). *The Arizona Battery for Communication Disorders of Dementia*. Tucson, AZ: Canyonlands Publishing.

Brush, J. A., & Camp, C. J. (2000). *Spaced retrieval: A therapy technique for improving memory.* Available at http://www.nss-nrs.com (Northern Speech Services, Inc. and National Rehabilitation Services).

Boyle, M. (2004). Semantic feature analysis treatment for anomia in two fluent aphasia syndromes. *American Journal of Speech Language Pathology, 13*(3), 236–249.

Boyle, M., & Coelho, C. (1995). Application of semantic feature analysis as a treatment for aphasia dysnomia. *American Journal of Speech Language Pathology, 4,* 94–98.

Coelho, C., McHugh, R., & Boyle, M. (2000). Semantic feature analysis as a treatment for aphasic dysnomia: A replication. *Aphasiology, 14*(2), 133–142.

Crum, R. M., Anthony, J. C., Bassett, S. S., & Folstein, M. F. (1993). Population-based norms for the Mini-Mental State Examination by age and education level. *Journal of the American Medical Association, 269*(18), 2386–2391.

Folstein, M. F., Folstein, S. E., & McHugh, P. R. (1975). Mini-Mental State: A practical method for grading the cognitive state of patients for the clinician. *Journal of Psychiatric Research, 12,* 189–198.

Grabowski, T. J., & Damasio, A. R. (2004). Definition, clinical features, and neuroanatomical basis of dementia. In M. Esiri, V. Lee, & J. Trojanowski (Eds.), *Neuropathology of dementia* (2nd ed., pp. 1–10). Cambridge, UK: Cambridge University Press.

Gutiérrez-Clellen, V. F. & Peña, E. (2001). Dynamic assessment of diverse children: A tutorial. *Language, Speech, and Hearing Services in Schools, 332,* 212–224.

Hopper, T., Mahendra, N., Kim, E., Azuma, T., Bayles, K., Cleary, S., et al. (2005). Evidence-based practice recommendations for working with individuals with dementia: Spaced retrieval training. *Journal of Medical Speech Language Pathology, 13,* xxvii–xxxiv.

Mahendra, N., & Apple, A. (2007, November 27). Human memory systems: A framework for understanding dementia. *The ASHA Leader, 12*(16), 8–11.

Mahendra, N., Apple, A., & Reed, D. (2008). *Computer-assisted training of face-name associations in persons with dementia.* Poster presented at the 2008 meeting of the International Neuropsychological Society, Waikoloa, Hawaii.

Mattis, S., Jurica, P., & Leitten, C. (1982) *Dementia Rating Scale (DRS-2).* Lutz, FL: Psychological Assessment Resources.

Ramsey Foundation. (1990). *Dealing with Alzheimer's disease: A common sense approach to communication* (21-minute videotape). St. Paul, MN: Ramsey Foundation.

Sheikh, J. I., & Yesavage, J. A. (1986). Geriatric Depression Scale (GDS): Recent evidence and development of a shorter version. *Clinical Gerontologist, 5*(1–2), 165-173.

Snodgrass, J. G., & Vanderwart, M. (1980). A standardized set of 260 pictures: Norms for name agreement, image agreement, familiarity and visual complexity. *Journal of Experimental Psychology (Human Learning), 6*(2), 174–215.

Tomoeda, C. K. (2001). Comprehensive assessment for dementia: A necessity for differential diagnosis and management. *Seminars in Speech and Language, 22*(4), 275–289.

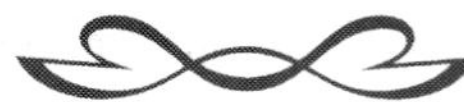



# CASE 49

# Jessica: Treatment of Stuttering for an Adult

*Sue O'Brian, Mark Onslow, Ross G. Menzies, and Tamsen St Clare*

## Conceptual Knowledge Areas

Stuttering is a speech motor disorder that begins in early childhood. In adulthood, the incidence is around 1% with a male to female ratio of 4:1. Adults who stutter may find normal communication extremely difficult, and in severe cases their rate of transfer of information can be reduced by up to half that of nonstuttering speakers. They may also avoid speaking for much of their day-to-day lives. Stuttering can cause low self-esteem, social maladjustment, and failure to attain educational and occupational potential (Craig & Calver 1991; Hayhow, Cray, & Enderby 2002; Klein & Hood, 2004; Klompas & Ross, 2004). Anxiety is a common clinical symptom associated with stuttering, with half of those seeking clinical help warranting a comorbid psychiatric diagnosis of social phobia (Menzies et al., 2008; Stein, Baird, & Walker, 1996).

Social phobia, or social anxiety disorder, is one of the commonly diagnosed anxiety disorders. It involves a morbid and debilitating expectation of negative evaluation by others in social situations, with the expectation of being humiliated and embarrassed. The response of those affected is disproportionate to the reality of the threat, and in severe cases involves high levels of avoidance and social isolation.

Cognitive behavior therapy (CBT) is widely considered the most efficacious treatment for anxiety. Five meta-analytic reviews (Chambless & Hope, 1996; Fedoroff & Taylor, 2001; Feske & Chambless, 1995; Gould, Buckminster, Pollack, Otto, & Yap, 1997; Taylor, 1996) have summarized studies evaluating cognitive and behavioral therapies for social anxiety. All have reached a similar conclusion: that behavior therapy and CBT are consistently more efficacious than wait-list conditions. Taylor (1996) concluded that CBT is superior to placebo and various control conditions. CBT has been found to be significantly more efficacious in reducing social anxiety than both pharmacologic interventions (Clark et al., 2003) and alternate forms of psychotherapy (for example, Heimberg, Salzman, Holt, & Blendell, 1993).

Cognitive behavior therapy has been associated with excellent maintenance of gains following treatment. Heimberg and colleagues (1993) found that patients receiving CBT maintained their gains at five-year follow-up, and remained significantly less symptomatic than those who had received the control intervention of education and supportive counseling.

## Description of the Case

### Background Information

Jessica presented at the Australian Stuttering Research Centre as a pleasant, somewhat reserved, articulate young woman of 29 years at the time of assessment. She was single and lived alone, having recently moved from South Africa to Sydney. She had no immediate family support and a very small circle of friends. She had initially trained as a librarian but soon after beginning treatment, she began work with a publisher of educational texts.

Jessica said she had had difficulty with her speech for as long as she could remember. Although it had been a consistent problem for her throughout her primary school years, it was only during adolescence that she identified her problem as stuttering. Her family never discussed the issue with her and she had always been too embarrassed to bring it up with them. Jessica was unaware of any other family members who stuttered but had never felt able to ask about its existence in her extended family.

Jessica's stuttering had remained mild but persistent throughout her years at school and university. She had never sought treatment, although she had tried many techniques herself to overcome the problem. She had practiced reading out loud when nobody was listening. She had tried to slow down her speech rate when experiencing difficulty, and she reported scanning ahead when talking and substituting other words for those on which she anticipated stuttering. However, she reported that none of these techniques had any impact on her stuttering.

### Findings of the Evaluation

A speech sample in conversation with the clinician at the first clinic visit revealed 3.4 percent syllables stuttered (%SS) and a clinician severity rating (SR) of 4 on a 9-point scale (1 = no stuttering, 9 = extremely severe stuttering; O'Brian, Packman, & Onslow, 2004). Repeated movements, usually several incomplete syllable repetitions, characterized Jessica's stuttering and very occasional short fixed postures. Jessica's self-reported stuttering SRs in five situations representative of her daily life confirmed typical severity ratings of between 3 and 4. These findings are presented in Table 49.1.

Jessica's speech history also revealed several cognitive and behavioral indicators of speech anxiety. First, she had never sought advice about nor discussed her stuttering with anyone, including family members and friends, despite experiencing considerable long-term concern about her speech. She reported being tormented by embarrassment and feelings of inadequacy all her life because she sounded different from her peers. She felt that her stuttering had significantly affected her social relationships as well as her occupational potential, because she avoided many speech-related situations. She felt continually frustrated by using word avoidance strategies, because this meant that she was unable to express herself precisely. Her presentation to the clinic at 29 years of age was significant, because it was the first time she had ever acknowledged her stuttering to another person.

During the assessment, Jessica showed symptoms of speech-related anxiety, which were considered to be in excess of those expected in the context of a quite mild stuttering problem. It was acknowledged that Jessica might have difficulty applying speech techniques in everyday social settings and that consequently her speech outcomes might be compromised by her anxiety.

During her treatment (see "Description of Course of Treatment") Jessica was assessed by a clinical psychologist (the third author). The clinical psychologist conducted a comprehensive clinical interview to determine the specific nature of Jessica's anxiety and to assess for comorbid psychiatric disorders. Jessica reported the following specific anxiety symptoms in the three domains of anxiety.

*Cognitive* symptoms included acute embarrassment when she stuttered and high levels of anticipatory anxiety when thinking about speaking situations. Reported beliefs about stuttering included: "People will notice that I stutter," "I won't be able to say what I want to say," "People will think I'm incompetent because I stutter," and "People will evaluate me negatively because I stutter." She also expressed concern that other people would discover not only that she stuttered, but also that she became anxious about speaking. *Behavioral* symptoms reported were marked avoidance of the following speaking situations: the telephone, formal work meetings, and telephone answering machines. She also reported using word avoidance. Physiological symptoms reported were blushing, dry throat, sweaty hands, nausea, and stomach distress.

Jessica met Stein, Baird, and Walker's (1996) modified diagnostic criteria for social phobia. She also reported having been diagnosed with irritable bowel syndrome (IBS). This is common in anxious people and stress is thought to exacerbate the symptoms. Her IBS symptoms included intermittent stomach bloating, decreased appetite, and abdominal pain. Jessica did not meet criteria for any other psychiatric diagnoses.

In addition to the clinical interview, Jessica completed a battery of psychometric measures to assess social anxiety. The measures chosen were the Fear of Negative Evaluation (FNE) Scale, the Social Avoidance and Distress (SAD) Scale, and the Social Phobia and Anxiety Inventory (SPAI). Results from these measures are summarized in Table 49.2 and show that Jessica scored significantly above the mean on the three measures. This confirmed that she was suffering from high levels of social anxiety despite having mild stuttering.

## Reason for Referral

In summary, Jessica presented as an intelligent 29-year-old woman with mild stuttering, which was complicated by significant speech-related anxiety. Her stated aim in seeking therapy at the time of assessment was to eliminate or at least reduce her stuttering.

## Treatment Options Considered

Onslow, Jones, O'Brian, Menzies, and Packman (2008) argue that a reasonably liberal definition of a clinical trial is a prospective study involving speech measures beyond the clinic with at least 3 months follow-up. Using that definition, there have been 20 speech pathology clinical trials published of five treatment categories for adults who stutter (> 17 years of age).

By far the best evidence for control of stuttering in this age group is for speech restructuring techniques, with 13 trials published that meet the Onslow et al. criteria (Block, Onslow, Packman, Gray, & Dacakis, 2005; Boberg, 1981; Boberg & Kully, 1994; Harrison, Onslow, Andrews, Packman, & Webber, 1998; Howie, Tanner, & Andrews, 1981; Ingham & Andrews, 1973; Langevin & Boberg, 1993; Langevin & Boberg, 1996; O'Brian, Onslow, Cream, & Packman, 2003; O'Brian, Packman, & Onslow, 2008; Onslow, O'Brian, Packman, & Rousseau, 2004; Onslow, Costa, Andrews, Harrison, & Packman, 1996; Perkins, Rudas, Johnson, Michael, & Curlee, 1974). These treatments control stuttering by changing aspects of speech production, such as reduced rate, prolonged vowels, "soft" articulatory contacts, and "gentle" vowel onsets (Packman, Onslow, & Menzies, 2000). However, despite short-term benefits from these treatments, posttreatment relapse is common. In addition, posttreatment speech with these treatments often feels unnatural to the speaker, takes effort to maintain, and may sound unnatural to the listener.

An alternative treatment technique, for which there are three clinical trials according to the definition of Onslow et al. (2008), is time-out (Hewat, O'Brian, Onslow, & Packman, 2001; Hewat, Onslow, O'Brian, & Packman, 2006; James, 1981). Time-out is a verbal response contingent procedure that involves a person pausing for a short period contingent on stuttering. It may be imposed by the clinician or by the client, or some combination of the two. Clinical trials of this procedure have demonstrated up to 80% reduction in stuttering in some clients in as few as 6–8 treatment hours. Another advantage of this procedure is that clients do not have to learn to use a new speech pattern. There has been one clinical trial showing positive results when time-out is combined with speech restructuring (James, Ricciardelli, Rogers, & Hunter, 1989).

According to the Onslow et al. criteria, there has been one clinical trial of the regulated breathing method (Saint-Laurent & Ladouceur, 1987) and one trial of the machine-based modification of phonation intervals procedure (Ingham et al. 2001). In the former case, the treatment was not thought to be adequately operationalized for use. The Ingham et al. trial was preliminary and the equipment not yet available. Additionally, there are many reports of drug treatments for stuttering, particularly using Haloperidol, Risperidone, and Olanzapine. These interventions were not considered because of the limitations of their evidence base (Bothe, Davidow, Bramlett, Franic, & Ingham, 2006).

Menzies et al. (2008) reported a clinical trial of CBT for adults who stutter, based on the procedures of McColl, Onslow, Packman, & Menzies (2001). Participants in the Menzies et al. trial were treated with a CBT package specifically developed to target speech-related anxiety. Results suggested that the addition of CBT to standard speech restructuring procedures for adults may lead to improved outcomes. In this study, patients receiving CBT for anxiety as an adjunct to speech restructuring experienced less general anxiety, were less avoidant, and engaged in more everyday speaking tasks than subjects who received speech restructuring alone.

## Course of Treatment

Referral to a clinical psychologist for treatment (the third author) was considered at the start of treatment. However, since stuttered speech was Jessica's primary complaint, a trial of speech treatment was offered first. Referral to a clinical psychologist could follow later if required.

The clinician tried self-imposed time-out (SITO) as a first treatment option for Jessica for the following reasons:

1. She had no previous successful or unsuccessful stuttering treatment to take into consideration.
2. Her stuttering was quite mild and therefore might not need the continued effort and focus involved in using a speech restructuring technique.
3. She had a fear of "sounding different" that may have made her feel uncomfortable using any speech restructuring technique.
4. SITO involves a shorter period of clinical time than speech restructuring techniques.
5. Speech restructuring could be introduced if a trial of SITO was unsuccessful.

A stable baseline was first established for Jessica's stuttering in the clinic, and then several 2-minute monologues using clinician-imposed time-out were trialed. Jessica's stuttering did not decrease at all in response to this technique. A further period of 2-minute monologues, this time using SITO, showed Jessica's stuttering to be unresponsive to the SITO technique, although she was able to use it very well. She identified accurately all instances of stuttering and timed herself out for several seconds; however, her stuttering rate did not reduce sufficiently during preliminary trials for the technique to be considered viable. Therefore, the clinician decided to introduce speech restructuring treatment. The Camperdown Program (O'Brian, Cream, Onslow & Packman, 2000, 2001; O'Brian et al., 2003; O'Brian, Packman, & Onslow, 2008) was the treatment model chosen because the evidence at the time suggested that it was the simplest and least time-consuming delivery model for speech restructuring. Materials for this program, including the exemplar video, can be downloaded from the website of the Australian Stuttering Research Centre (O'Brian, Onslow, Packman, & Cream, 2008).

### Description of Course of Treatment

The Camperdown Program consists of four stages: (1) teaching of the treatment components, (2) within-clinic control of stuttering, (3) generalization of stutter-free speech into everyday speaking situations, and (4) maintenance. It can be implemented in group or individual sessions and in weekly or intensive format. A telehealth version of this treatment is known to be efficacious in two clinical trials available (Carey, O'Brian, Onslow, Block, & Jones, 2008; O'Brian et al., 2008); however, the face-to-face version (O'Brian et al., 2003) was chosen.

Jessica attended weekly 1-hour sessions for Stage 1 of the program. She easily learned to use the speech pattern as demonstrated in the video exemplar, although she commented that she did not like the sound or the feel of the speech pattern and was initially somewhat uncomfortable and embarrassed using it even in the clinic. She had no difficulty learning to use the 9-point severity and naturalness scales.

She attended a group day with two other people for Stage 2 of the program as it was thought that she might benefit from exposure to and support from other adults who stuttered. At the completion of this day, she was able to use natural-sounding, stutter-free speech consistently within the clinic.

Stage 3 of the program was again implemented in weekly individual sessions. The focus of these problem-solving sessions was to establish appropriate speech practice routines, initially with familiar and supportive partners, and general consolidation of the speech restructuring technique in everyday situations. Practice routines were difficult for Jessica because she had not told anyone that she was attending treatment, had never spoken to her friends or family about her stuttering, and still was uncomfortable to do so. Therefore, she had no one with whom she could overtly practice her speech. Arrangements were therefore made for her to practice over the telephone with another client who had attended the group day with her, and with a clinic reception staff member. She was also encouraged to begin to use her speech technique in various everyday situations and to collect severity and naturalness ratings of her speech in these situations.

After a few sessions, Jessica returned to South Africa for a month to attend a family wedding. During this time, she did no speech practice and did not attempt to use speech restructuring to control her stuttering in any situation. When her mother decided to return to Australia with her for a holiday, Jessica felt compelled to tell her about the stuttering treatment program. Her mother was critical and unsupportive of her decision to attend therapy and, in particular, her use of a speech technique.

After a few clinic sessions, Jessica's self-reports of stuttering severity beyond the clinic differed little from those reported before treatment. She could be consistently stutter-free and natural-sounding, with Speech Naturalness scores of 1–2, while talking to the clinician, the clinic reception staff member, the other members of her initial group, and her mother. However, Jessica was reluctant to attempt to use her speech technique to control her stuttering in everyday situations. She was only comfortable using the speech pattern to control her stuttering with people with whom she had discussed her problem, which involved a limited group, particularly as her mother had now returned home.

In summary, despite being able to use speech restructuring to control her stuttering at a Speech Naturalness of 2, and listening to recordings of this speech and agreeing that it sounded quite normal, Jessica was unwilling to use it in everyday situations. She remained concerned about other people's reactions to both her stuttering and her use of the speech technique. Jessica's speech-related anxiety had not decreased as a result of her speech treatment, and it was prohibiting her from making further progress with her speech treatment.

Consequently, a referral was made for Jessica to be assessed by a clinical psychologist. At the time of referral to the clinical psychologist (see "Findings of the Evaluation," above) Jessica had attended approximately 16 hours of speech therapy: 3 initial teaching hours, 7 group hours, and 6 problem-solving hours.

Given that Jessica met diagnostic criteria for social phobia, was motivated to overcome her anxiety, and did not exhibit any comorbid diagnoses thought to interfere with response to treatment, she was considered an ideal candidate for CBT. Her CBT program was based on the package developed by McColl and colleagues (2001), with modifications to reflect current best practice in the treatment of social anxiety. The individual CBT components are outlined in the following paragraphs.

***Education*** Jessica was provided with information on the following topics: (1) the relationship between anxiety and speech performance, (2) the nature of anxiety, (3) the cognitive-behavioral model of anxiety acquisition and maintenance, and (4) cognitive-behavioral interventions for anxiety. Detailed information was presented and Jessica's own experiences were discussed.

***Cognitive Restructuring*** Jessica was taught to identify and change her dysfunctional beliefs about stuttering using the following steps.

1. Jessica was taught that there are many possible ways to interpret a specific situation. This was achieved with a series of "thinking exercises" in which she was required to generate several alternative interpretations for an ambiguous hypothetical situation.
2. Jessica learned to identify the thoughts that led her to feel anxious in speaking situations. She was asked to analyze the various components of her anxiety response by writing the following information in a diary each time she became aware of anxiety symptoms: date and time, situation, feelings, perceived threat, and behavior.
3. Jessica learned to challenge her thoughts by analyzing how realistic and helpful they were. She was asked to explore the evidence for and against her unhelpful thoughts. She was then asked to consider other ways in which that same situation could have been interpreted and to generate more adaptive thoughts and beliefs about the social situations she entered.
4. As is typical of social anxiety, Jessica's primary fear was of negative evaluation by others. She tended to overestimate both the likelihood and "badness" or cost of negative evaluation. Cognitive therapy was aimed at helping Jessica learn to analyze the real probability and cost of such evaluation by others, and repeatedly to challenge her automatic interpretations by generating more realistic and helpful alternatives.

***Behavioral Experiments*** Behavioral experiments are another method of producing cognitive change. They involve testing beliefs and interpretations with direct experiments. Initially, Jessica was convinced that her stuttering was obvious to others and that the likelihood that others would notice it increased as she became more anxious. She was also convinced that as she became anxious she would show other signs of physiological arousal such as blushing and sweating, and that others would notice them. She was convinced that once others knew of her stuttering, or once they noticed her blushing and sweating, they would judge her as being incompetent.

Jessica was encouraged to test these beliefs rather than accepting them as true without supporting evidence. One task involved her speaking to a large group and videotaping her presentation. She then analyzed the video and compared her predicted speech and appearance with her actual speech and appearance. She discovered that she did not stutter as much as expected and that there were no obvious signs of physiological arousal. A second task involved her telling several close friends that she had a stutter and comparing their reactions to her predictions. Interestingly, her best friend had not realized that Jessica stuttered, despite having known her for more than 20 years. Once Jessica collected evidence from these behavioral experiments, she was encouraged to use it in her cognitive restructuring exercises to further facilitate cognitive change.

***Attentional Training*** Many socially anxious people have difficulty focusing on the task in which they are engaged, such as the speech they are giving or the content of the conversation they are having. This is because their attention is focused on how they are being perceived by others. Jessica described having a mental image of herself stuttering, blushing, and sweating when talking to others, and that this preoccupied her to such an extent that she could not focus on the content of conversations. In order to overcome this, Jessica was taught an attentional training exercise, which she was asked to practice twice each day.

The attentional training component involved two tasks. First, Jessica was encouraged to strengthen her attentional ability with meditation exercises. In this task, she learned to focus on alternative cognitive targets by counting her breaths rather than focusing on intrusive thoughts. The second task involved intentionally changing the focus of her attention when in anxiety-provoking speaking situations.

The above components were delivered across 10 weekly 1-hour sessions. Jessica was then reassessed to determine treatment response. Jessica made significant improvements in her social anxiety. She described being less anxious when speaking in formal work meetings and said that she no longer avoided participating in them. She was no longer concerned that others might see her blush or sweat and was markedly less concerned about other people noticing her stutter. She had reduced her use of e-mail and was making many more telephone calls

TABLE 49.1 Jessica's Pretreatment and Posttreatment Scores and Population Means for Social Anxiety Measures

| Measure | Jessica Pretreatment | Jessica Posttreatment | Nonanxious control subjects |
|---|---|---|---|
| FNE | 27 | 16* | 13.97[a] |
| SADS | 18 | 10* | 11.2[a] |
| SPAI Difference Score | 98 | 62* | 32.7[b] |

* $p < 0.05$

[a] Watson & Friend, 1969

[b] Turner, Beidel, & Dancu, 1986

TABLE 49.2 Pretreatment and Posttreatment Percent Syllables Stuttered (%SS) and Severity Ratings (SR) for Jessica

| | Pretreatment | Posttreatment |
|---|---|---|
| Within clinic (%SS) | 3.4 | 0 |
| Within clinic (SR) | 4 | 1 |
| Talking to family (SR) | 3 | 1 |
| Social—friends (SR) | 4 | 2 |
| Telephone (SR) | 4 | 2 |
| Work—talking to clients (SR) | 4 | 2 |
| Work—seminar presentations (SR) | 4 | 2 |

SRs are measured on a 9-point scale where 1 = no stuttering and 9 = extremely severe stuttering.

to customers. She was actively confronting difficult words rather than avoiding them. Posttreatment scores on psychometric measures reflected this reported reduction in anxiety. Posttreatment questionnaire scores are presented in Table 49.1. This shows that Jessica had significantly reduced her scores on all three measures following CBT.

## Analysis of Client's Response to Intervention and Further Recommendations

After completing the CBT program Jessica attended several further sessions with the speech-language pathologist (SLP) before moving into a performance-contingent maintenance program. During these sessions, strategies were discussed for using her speech technique when needed to control her stuttering in everyday speaking situations. Her maintenance sessions, some of which occurred by telephone, were spaced as she took control of her stuttering management. Clinical measures collected before and after treatment are presented in Table 49.2.

## Author Note

This case was based on a real client. Names, places, and some details of treatment were changed to preserve anonymity.

## References

Block, S., Onslow, M., Packman, A., Gray, B., & Dacakis, G. (2005). Treatment of chronic stuttering: Outcome from a student training clinic. *International Journal of Language and Communication Disorders, 40,* 455–466.

Boberg, E. (1981). Maintenance of fluency: An experimental program. In E. Boberg (Ed.), *Maintenance of fluency* (pp. 71–111). New York: Elsevier.

Boberg, E., & Kully, D. (1994). Long-term results of an intensive treatment program for adults and adolescents who stutter. *Journal of Speech and Hearing Research, 37,* 1050–1059.

Bothe, A. K., Davidow, J. H., Bramlett, R. E., Franic, D. M., & Ingham, R. J. (2006). Stuttering treatment research 1970–2005: II. Systematic review incorporating trial quality assessment of pharmacological approaches. *American Journal of Speech-Language Pathology, 15,* 342–352.

Carey, B., O'Brian, S., Onslow, M., Block, S., & Jones, M. (2008). A randomised controlled non-inferiority trial of a telehealth treatment for chronic stuttering: The Camperdown Program. *Manuscript submitted for publication.*

Chambless, D. L., & Hope, D. A. (1996). Cognitive approaches to the psychopathology and treatment of social phobia. In P. M. Salkovskis (Ed.), *Frontiers of cognitive therapy* (pp. 345–382). New York: Guilford Press.

Clark, D. M., Ehlers, A., McManus, F., Hackmann, A., Fennell, M., Campbell, H., et al. (2003). Cognitive therapy versus Fluoxetine in generalized social phobia: A randomized placebo-controlled trial. *Journal of Consulting and Clinical Psychology, 71,* 1058–1067.

Craig, A. R., & Calver, P. (1991). Following up on treated stutterers: Studies of perceptions of fluency and job status. *Journal of Speech & Hearing Research, 34,* 279–284.

Federoff, I. C., & Taylor, S. (2001). Psychological and pharmacological treatments of social phobia: A meta-analysis. *Journal of Clinical Psychopharmacology, 21,* 311–324.

Feske, U., & Chambless, D. L. (1995). Cognitive-behavioral versus exposure only treatment for social phobia: A meta-analysis. *Behavior Therapy, 26,* 695–720.

Gould, R. A., Buckminster, S., Pollack, M. H., Otto, M. W., & Yap, L. (1997). Cognitive-behavioral and pharmacological treatment for social phobia: A meta-analysis. *Clinical Psychological Science Practice, 4,* 291–306.

Harrison, E. Onslow, M. Andrews, C., Packman, A., & Webber, M. (1998). Control of stuttering with prolonged speech: Development of a one-day instatement program. In A. Cordes & R. J. Ingham (Eds.), *Treatment efficacy in stuttering.* San Diego, CA: Singular.

Hayhow, R., Cray, A. M., & Enderby, P. (2002). Stammering and therapy views of people who stammer. *Journal of Fluency Disorders, 27,* 1–16.

Heimberg, R. G. (2002). Cognitive behavioral therapy for social anxiety disorder: Current status and future directions. *Biological Psychiatry, 51,* 101–108.

Heimberg, R. G., Salzman, D. G., Holt, C. S., & Blendell, K. A. (1993). Cognitive-behavioral group treatment for social phobia: Effectiveness at 5-year follow-up. *Cognitive Therapy and Research, 14,* 1–23.

Hewat, S., O'Brian, S., Onslow, M., & Packman, A. (2001). Control of chronic stuttering with self-imposed time-out: Preliminary outcome data. *Asia Pacific Journal of Speech, Language, and Hearing, 6,* 97–102.

Hewat, S., Onslow, M., O'Brian, S., & Packman, A. (2006). A phase II clinical trial of self-imposed time-out treatment for stuttering in adults and adolescents. *Disability and Rehabilitation, 28,* 33–42.

Howie, P., Tanner, S., & Andrews, G. (1981). Short- and long-term outcome in an intensive treatment program for adult stutterers. *Journal of Speech and Hearing Disorders, 46,* 104–109.

Ingham, R., & Andrews, G. (1973). An analysis of a token economy in stuttering therapy. *Journal of Applied Behavior Analysis, 6,* 219–229.

Ingham, R. J., Kilgo, M., Costello Ingham, J., Moglia, R., Belknap, H., & Sanchez, T. (2001). Evaluation of a stuttering treatment based on reduction of short phonation intervals. *Journal of Speech, Language, and Hearing Research, 44,* 1–16.

James, J. (1981). Behavioural self-control of stuttering using time-out from speaking. *Journal of Applied Behavior Analysis, 14,* 25–37.

James, J. E., Ricciardelli, L. A., Rogers, P., & Hunter, C. E. (1989). A preliminary analysis of the ameliorative effects of time-out from speaking on stuttering. *Journal of Speech and Hearing Research, 32,* 604–610.

Klein, J. F., & Hood, S. B. (2004).The impact of stuttering on employment opportunities and job performance. *Journal of Fluency Disorders, 29,* 255–273.

Klompas, M., & Ross, E. (2004). Life experiences of people who stutter, and the perceived impact of stuttering on quality of life: Personal accounts of South African individuals. *Journal of Fluency Disorders, 29,* 275–305.

Langevin, M., & Boberg, E. (1993). Results of an intensive stuttering therapy program. *Journal of Speech-Language Pathology and Audiology, 17,* 158–166.

Langevin, M., & Boberg, E. (1996). Results of intensive stuttering therapy with adults who clutter and stutter. *Journal of Fluency Disorders, 21,* 315–327.

McColl, T., Onslow, M., Packman, A., & Menzies, R. G. (2001). A cognitive behavioural intervention for social anxiety in adults who stutter. *Proceedings of the 2001 Speech Pathology Australia National Conference,* 93–98.

Menzies, R., O'Brian, S., Onslow, M., Packman, A., St Clare, T., & Block, S. (2008). An experimental clinical trial of a cognitive behavior therapy package for chronic stuttering. *Journal of Speech, Language, and Hearing Research, 51,* 1451–1464.

O'Brian, S., Cream, A., Onslow, M., & Packman, A. (2000). Prolonged speech: An experimental attempt to solve some nagging problems. *Proceedings of the 2000 Speech Pathology Australia National Conference*, Sydney, Australia.

O'Brian, S., Cream, A., Onslow, M., & Packman, A. (2001). A replicable, nonprogrammed, instrument-free method for the control of stuttering with prolonged-speech. *Asia Pacific Journal of Speech, Language, and Hearing, 6,* 91–96.

O'Brian, S., Onslow, M., Cream, A., & Packman, A. (2003). The Camperdown Program: Outcomes of a new prolonged-speech treatment model. *Journal of Speech, Language, and Hearing Research*, 46, 933–946.

O'Brian, S., Onslow, M., Packman, A., & Cream, A. (2008). Camperdown Program Treatment Manual. Retrieved October 24, 2008, from The University of Sydney, Australian Stuttering Research Centre Web site: http://sydney.edu.au/health_sciences/asrc/health_professionals/asrc_download.shtml

O'Brian, S., Packman, A., & Onslow, M. (2004). Self-rating of stuttering severity as a clinical tool. *American Journal of Speech-Language Pathology, 13,* 219–226.

O'Brian, S., Packman, A., & Onslow, M. (2008). Telehealth delivery of the Camperdown Program for adults who stutter. *Journal of Speech, Language, and Hearing Research, 51,* 184–195.

Onslow, M., Costa, L., Andrews, C., Harrison, E., & Packman, A. (1996). Speech outcomes of a prolonged-speech treatment for stuttering. *Journal of Speech and Hearing Research, 39,* 734–49.

Onslow, M., Jones, M., O'Brian, S., Menzies, R., & Packman, A. (2008). Biostatistics for clinicians: Defining, evaluating, and identifying clinical trials of stuttering treatments. *American Journal of Speech-Language Pathology*, 17, 401–415.

Onslow, M., O'Brian, S., Packman, A., & Rousseau I. (2004). Long-term follow-up of speech outcomes for a prolonged-speech treatment for stuttering: The effects of paradox on stuttering treatment research. In A. K. Bothe (Ed.), *Evidence-based treatment of stuttering: Empirical issues and clinical implications.* Mahwah, NJ: Lawrence Erlbaum Associates.

Packman, A., Onslow, M., & Menzies, R. (2000). Novel speech patterns and the control of stuttering. *Disability and Rehabilitation, 22,* 65–79.

Perkins, W., Rudas, J., Johnson, L., Michael, W., & Curlee, R. (1974). Replacement of stuttering with normal speech: III. Clinical effectiveness. *Journal of Speech and Hearing Disorders, 39,* 416–428.

Saint Laurent, L., & Ladouceur, R. (1987). Massed versus distributed application of the regulated-breathing method for stutterers and its long-term effect. *Behaviour Therapy, 18,* 38–50.

Stein, M. B., Baird, A., & Walker, J. R. (1996). Social phobia in adults with stuttering. *American Journal of Psychiatry, 153,* 278–280.

Taylor, S. (1996). Meta-analysis of cognitive-behavioral treatments for social phobia. *Journal of Behavior Therapy and Experimental Psychiatry, 27,* 1–9.

Turner, S. M., Beidel, D. C., & Dancu, C. V. (1986). *SPAI: Social Phobia and Anxiety Inventory.* New York: Multi-Health Systems.

Watson, D., & Friend, R. (1969). Measurement of social-evaluative anxiety. *Journal of Consulting and Clinical Psychology, 33,* 448–457.

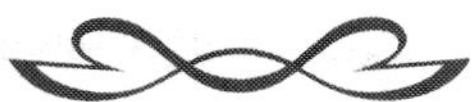



# CASE 50

# Joel: Management of a Patient with Advanced Head and Neck Cancer

*Roxann Diez Gross*

## Conceptual Knowledge Areas

To work successfully with patients that are being treated for head and neck cancer, the speech-language pathologist (SLP) must have an understanding of normal oral, laryngeal, and pharyngeal anatomy and function. Competency in evaluating and treating adult speech intelligibility disorders and dysphagia is required. The clinician must also be familiar with a variety of swallowing exercises, postural strategies, and swallowing maneuvers. Examples of swallowing exercises and maneuvers that are often used for this patient population are the effortful swallow, Mendelsohn maneuver, Shaker exercise, super-supraglottic swallow, and tongue hold maneuver. The effortful swallow increases the strength of all swallowing muscles by requiring patients to repeatedly swallow as hard and long as they can. The Mendelsohn maneuver improves the strength of the muscles that elevate the larynx by teaching the patient to maintain laryngeal elevation for several seconds when swallowing. The Shaker exercise increases the opening of the upper esophageal sphincter and is completed by lying on the back and raising the head to the chest while keeping the shoulders down. The super-supraglottic swallow increases airway protection and assures correct breathing-swallowing coordination by teaching the patient to breathe in and close the vocal folds, bear down, and then swallow. The tongue hold maneuver improves the anterior motion of the posterior pharyngeal wall. It is completed by protruding the tongue and holding it between the teeth while swallowing. Positional strategies alter bolus (food or drink) flow from the mouth and into the esophagus. For example, turning the head to a weak side diverts the bolus to the stronger side. Tucking the chin to the chest can have a variety of effects on the swallow, from preventing premature spillage from the back of the mouth to narrowing the laryngeal vestibule.

Clinicians should also have basic knowledge of the different surgical procedures that are used to excise tumors and the potential effects on speech and swallowing. Additionally, familiarity with the imaging techniques and fundamental terminology that physicians use in relation to the medical management of these patients is beneficial. Strong counseling skills are necessary because these patients are often upset about their diagnoses and have little knowledge about speech and swallowing function. Furthermore, many patients are now aware of the painful side effects involved in cancer treatment and are understandably anxious about the effects of any pending surgical procedures or chemotherapy drugs.

Small tumors of the oral tongue and true vocal folds can be treated with surgical procedures that do not often impair speech or swallowing function; however, large tumors require wide excisions and can profoundly impair communication and swallowing.

Treatment that preserves organs is rapidly becoming the primary method to destroy tumors in the larynx and oropharynx; however, the function of these organs can decline as a result of this form of management. Currently, the main organ preservation treatment for oropharyngeal and laryngeal tumors is the combination of chemotherapy and radiation therapy. The main purpose for the chemotherapy is to increase the effects of the radiation. Chemotherapy drugs are continually being evaluated and clinicians should be familiar with the names of the drugs and aware of the potential side effects. New methods that limit radiation exposure to surrounding tissues are also continually in development. The SLP should recognize the terminology used to describe the different modalities that deliver radiation as well as the effects of radiation on the surrounding tissues. Basic understanding of diagnostic imaging and tumor staging is also beneficial and can assist in determining the size and location of the tumor when postulating the potential effects on speech and swallowing in light of the various treatments. Observational and interview experience in providing emotional support is crucial, because patients are often very fearful and seek assurance from the medical community. Speech-language pathologists should be sensitive to the patient's fears and anxiety in relation to a diagnosis as grave as cancer and should provide emotional support without exceeding the scope of practice (such as by implying that a cure is certain or uncertain).

## Description of the Case

### Background Information and Reasons for Referral

Joel was a 48-year-old male, nonsmoker, nondrinker, with no significant past medical history. He had a college education and was employed full-time as an accountant. His family history included a father who died of heart disease and a mother who died of colon cancer. His sister had diabetes and a remote history of stroke. He initially presented to his primary care physician with a persistent "sore throat" of four weeks duration. Two courses of antibiotics were not effective in relieving his symptoms. A dental exam found the need for a root canal, which was performed in hopes of providing relief, yet the pain did not subside. In fact, Joel began to develop increased pain upon swallowing (rated by the patient as 6 on a scale of 10), and he began to experience a new onset of intermittent ear pain.

Joel was then referred by his primary care physician to an otolaryngologist who, based upon the recent medical history, completed a thorough head and neck assessment. During the examination, the physician palpated a firm base of tongue mass. A transnasal endoscopic examination was then performed by the doctor. The mucosal surface of the nasopharynx and soft palate were normal in appearance. When the flexible scope was advanced into the oropharynx, a large, irregular base of tongue mass was clearly visible. Upon continued visual inspection, the tumor did not appear to involve laryngeal structures or the pyriform sinuses. A small portion of the mass was excised and sent to pathology. A more in-depth imaging procedure called positron emission tomography (PET) and computerized tomography (CT) or a PET CT scan was ordered.

### Findings of the Evaluation

Joel's case was discussed by the head and neck cancer team at the weekly multidisciplinary conference. The team discussed treatment options and weighed the effects of surgery alone vs. surgery with radiation vs. organ preservation treatment to determine which treatment would provide the maximum potential to cure the disease while limiting the impact on Joel's post-treatment quality of life. The biopsy results confirmed the presence of squamous cell carcinoma. PET CT scan images showed strong uptake of the radiopharmaceutical and increased metabolic activity in the tongue base and bilaterally in the neck. Measurements of the size of the tumor and nodes were made so that the tumor could be staged. The 2.5 x 2.4 cm mass in the base of the tongue extended up to the right palatine tonsil and down to the pediole of the epiglottis. Several lymph nodes within the neck also showed increased activity. None of the nodes were greater than 6 cm. The biopsy was also positive for human papilloma virus (HPV). The possibility that the tumor was a result of HPV was discussed (Gallegos-Hernandez et al., 2007). The tumor was staged as T2, N2C, M0, indicating stage IV head and neck cancer (Patel & Shah, 2005).

## Treatment Options Considered

The risks and benefits of surgical, radiation, and combined treatment modalities were discussed by the medical team. Treatment options included a wide surgical excision of the base of the tongue and selected neck dissection to remove the cancerous nodes and surrounding nodes. The removal of a tumor that large with so much lingual tissue would most likely result in permanent and severe pharyngeal dysphagia as well as articulatory impairment from reduced range of motion of the tongue. In addition, Joel would still require radiation and could develop other unwanted effects. For these reasons, team members agreed that a combination of chemotherapy and radiation (CRT) was the best option for successful treatment and functional outcome. Chemotherapy treatment options were (1) neoadjuvant or induction chemotherapy, which is chemotherapy given prior to radiation therapy, and (2) adjuvant chemotherapy, where the chemotherapy drug(s) are given concomitantly with radiation therapy (chemoradiotherapy).

The radiation was to be given in a "fractionated fashion," meaning that a total dose would be given in fractions over a period of time. Additional options for radiation therapy were (1) conventional external beam radiation, and (2) intensity-modulated radiation therapy (IMRT), a more advanced form of radiotherapy that uses a computer-controlled method to deliver a more precise radiation dose to tumors that invade deeply into tissue.

The effects of the CRT on swallowing can vary, but the probability is that patients are at risk to develop some degree of speech and/or swallowing impairment during and after treatment (Nguyen, Sallah, Karlsson, & Antoine, 2002). Consequently, referral to speech-language pathology was made. The team decided that Joel should be followed and periodically assessed by the dietitian throughout the course of treatment to assist with nutritional counseling as necessary.

The primary reason for the initial referral was to enable the SLP to instruct Joel in the appropriate swallowing exercises prior to the start of his cancer treatment (Carroll et al., 2008; Rosenthal, Lewin, & Eisbruch, 2006), to take a baseline quality of life (QOL) measurement and a baseline evaluation of swallowing function, and to provide counseling in relation to preservation of speech precision and swallowing function during CRT. Joel and his wife came to the outpatient speech-language pathology clinic three days after he received his final diagnosis from the otolaryngologist and following a meeting with the radiation oncologist and medical oncologist. He stated that he was to receive one dose of chemotherapy prior to the initiation of radiation therapy (induction chemotherapy), followed by adjuvant chemotherapy and radiation therapy over the course of 7 weeks. Because of the tumor characteristics, he would receive intensity-modulated radiation therapy (IMRT), which can deliver high doses of radiation with reduced exposure to surrounding and uninvolved tissues such as the parotid gland, mandible, and spinal cord. Joel stated that he was eager to begin CRT so that the cancer would not progress, but he was also anxious about both the short- and long-term side effects of the treatment.

## Course of Treatment

Joel had a large tumor that appeared to have a negative effect on swallowing function primarily by causing pain; however, there was a very real possibility that the tumor could alter or partially obstruct bolus flow. Perceptually, his speech intelligibility was within normal limits at this time. When questioned further, he revealed that he had lost 10 pounds in the past 4 weeks. His taste sensation was unchanged (normal) at the time of the initial visit. Although he was evaluated endoscopically by a physician, a swallowing assessment had not been completed.

The large tumor would likely obstruct the view should a fiber-optic endoscopic evaluation of swallowing take place (FEES); therefore a videofluoroscopic evaluation of swallowing or modified barium swallow study was planned. Because pre-CRT treatment swallowing exercises have been shown to improve swallowing outcomes (Carroll et al., 2008; Kulbersh et al., 2006), Joel would be instructed in a series of exercises during the first visit. Also, counseling was necessary in relation to the need to continue to swallow despite the onset of odynophagia (painful swallowing), dysgeusia (altered taste sensation), and hypogeusia (low taste sensation).

During the first visit, Joel was instructed in prophylactic range of motion exercises (ROM) for tongue and mandible to prevent loss of motion from scarring and synechia (adhesions) that can result from high doses of radiation that are intensified further by the chemotherapy. Both he and his wife were counseled on the importance of continuing to swallow throughout the course of CRT even if he could only swallow water. They stated that they had received the same suggestion from the radiation oncologist. It was also recommended that, should he develop the side effect of painful mucositis (inflammation and ulceration of the oral and pharyngeal mucosa), he should take the prescribed pain medicine rather than stop eating and/or drinking. Because CRT would alter taste sensation and cause eating to be unpleasant, he was given guidance to change his expectation of food and drink from "pleasure" to "medicine," or to think of himself as an athlete in training in which food is consumed for a purpose (i.e., build muscle). Joel, his wife, and the SLP were hopeful that he could continue to obtain adequate nutrition and hydration by mouth and avoid the necessity of having a feeding tube placed into his stomach.

Joel was then instructed in a series of strengthening exercises such as effortful swallow, Mendelsohn, and tongue-hold maneuver. He was unable to perform them with sufficient effort at the time because of pain and tumor size. He was able to perform the Shaker exercise and agreed to do at least 3 repetitions every other day. He was instructed to make the lingual and mandibular ROM exercises part of his morning and evening grooming routine, such as face washing and teeth brushing, and to use the mirror for visual feedback. It was explained that the purpose of the ROM exercises was not to increase motion, but to maintain the current function, particularly lingual motion for speech and swallowing. These twice daily exercises were to continue for the rest of his life (adding that, hopefully, he will be doing the ROM exercises for many years). It was explained that the effects of the radiation would continue long after the radiation therapy had ended and that some of the tissue changes would be permanent. The MD Anderson Dysphagia Inventory (MDADI) was also administered for the purpose of obtaining a baseline quality of life measurement (Chen et al., 2001). This scale has been shown to be valid and reliable for use in patients with head and neck cancer. The scale runs from 0 (extremely low functioning) to 100 (high functioning). The results showed that, overall, Joel felt that his quality of life (QOL) was high with a global score of 100/100, emotional score of 96/100, and functional score of 92/100. He gave the lowest rating to his physical status with a score of 87.5/100.

A baseline videofluoroscopic swallowing study or modified barium swallow was completed while Joel sat in lateral view and swallowed a variety of standardized viscosities from thin liquid to pudding and a solid. The evaluation showed that the oral phase was within normal limits as indicated by complete and controlled mastication, anterior to posterior movement of each entire bolus, no posterior oral cavity loss, and no oral residue. There was good velar seal and a prompt pharyngeal response. The large base of tongue tumor was easily visible in the lateral view and altered, but did not obstruct bolus flow. Pharyngeal transit was within functional limits with hyoid elevation to the level of the mandible; laryngeal elevation was within normal limits for both height and duration of elevation; the posterior pharyngeal wall moved well; and the upper esophageal sphincter opening was adequate for bolus passage. There was no pharyngeal residue or aspiration observed during the evaluation. It was recommended that he continue with his current diet and food selections including thin liquids.

As stated previously, CRT side effects can include mucositis (painful inflammation and ulceration of the tongue and mucous membranes), making it too painful to eat by mouth, and/or hypogeusia (reduced taste ability) and/or dysgeusia (distortion of taste), which make it difficult and undesirable to eat. Joel began CRT the next week with chemotherapy to be given at the beginning, middle, and end of 7 weeks of radiation. He was scheduled to return to the clinic in 3 weeks or sooner if he noticed a decline in swallowing function indicated by symptoms such as coughing during meals and/or a sensation of food sticking.

After approximately 3 weeks into his cancer treatment, Joel developed painful oropharyngeal mucositis and voluntarily switched to very soft and then smooth puree as tolerated. He continued to drink thin liquids. He lost his sense of taste and had a very poor appetite. He was reminded to try to change his expectation of food and to consider only the nutritional aspects as well as the importance of trying to continue to swallow, even if it was only water. He was not able to overcome the barriers to oral intake that had developed and lost greater than 10% of his body weight. At that point the dietitian recommended the placement of a percutaneous endoscopic gastrostomy (PEG) tube so that nonoral nutrition and hydration could be given. Joel's preference was to be relieved of the burden of eating by mouth and he had the PEG placed. During the next session, he and his wife were again advised as to the importance of continuing to swallow even if only small sips of water were taken. He was encouraged to continue to complete the daily ROM activities and Shaker exercise.

Two weeks after the CRT was completed, Joel's pain had resolved; however, he refused to eat because he felt that it was unsafe to do so. He continued drinking water because his salivary glands were affected by the CRT, and he developed severe mouth dryness, called xerostomia. He stated that all other liquids tasted bitter and, although he did attempt to take small amounts of food on occasion, he was unable to consume anything because he "couldn't swallow" and "everything tasted like paper." Because CRT patients' perceptions of their swallowing ability is not always consistent with their function, and having nothing by mouth for as little as 2 weeks is associated with a poorer outcome (Gillespie, Brodsky, Day, Lee, & Martin-Harris, 2004), a second videofluoroscopic swallowing evaluation was scheduled. Additionally, it was felt that a fluoroscopic examination of swallowing would make it possible to identify the pathophysiology that might have resulted from the CRT so that a treatment plan specific to the patient could be designed. Also, compensatory and positional strategies could be explored, if indicated.

At this point, Joel's swallowing ability was likely functional, but anxiety and perhaps altered sensation were, in part, preventing him from eating by mouth. In addition, dysgeusia, or significantly altered taste sensation, had a significant negative impact on his desire for food. Radiation-induced xerostomia was another major complaint that often causes patients to perceive greater swallowing difficulty than may actually be present (Logemann et al., 2003).

The videofluoroscopic evaluation was completed in lateral and anterior-posterior views using the same standardized amounts and viscosities as the baseline exam. It was found that the oral phase had remained unchanged from the baseline examination. The large base of tongue tumor was no longer visible. Reduced base of tongue retraction was identified by the lack of normal posterior motion and failure to contact the posterior pharyngeal wall. Laryngeal elevation was also reduced as indicated by reduced superior motion from approximately 1½ vertebral bodies on the first exam to less than 1 cervical body. The anterior motion of the posterior pharyngeal wall was mildly diminished when compared to the baseline evaluation. Epiglottic inversion was not observed on any swallow, a finding that further supported the reduced range of motion of the base of tongue and laryngeal elevation. These changes combined to result in moderate residue in the valleculae (cavity approximately 50% full) with puree and soft solid (cookie), plus mild bilateral residue in the pyriform sinuses (bases only contained residue) with puree and solid. No material given was observed to enter the laryngeal vestibule or subglottis. A liquid wash was found to be an effective method to clear all residue. A deep chin tuck narrowed the pharyngeal space and altered biomechanics sufficiently to improve pharyngeal transit and prevent residue in the pharyngeal spaces. A soft diet with thin liquids was recommended. Based upon this assessment and Joel's concerns for swallowing safety, the video of the swallowing study was reviewed with him and his wife so that it could serve as a teaching tool. After a brief orientation to the swallowing structures and review of basic swallowing function, both stated that they were assured that the material he consumed had not entered his airway. They were also able to determine the effectiveness of the compensatory strategies, since this was observed directly. The patient stated that he was motivated to work toward having the feeding tube removed.

In a therapy session that followed, Joel was instructed to resume oral intake gradually using chin tuck and/or a liquid wash to manage pharyngeal residue. To assist with anxiety related to swallowing safety, the clinician gave him smooth purees and liquids during the treatment session and allowed him to practice the chin tuck and liquid wash. Because his pain had resolved, Joel and the clinician both felt that he was able to begin an exercise program. Therefore, based upon the pathophysiology observed fluoroscopically, the following therapeutic exercise program was established: To increase base of tongue retraction, the effortful swallow and super-supraglottic swallow were to be the primary exercises. To improve laryngeal elevation, the Mendelsohn maneuver was instructed using submental EMG biofeedback for instruction. In addition, he was to continue to perform the Shaker head lift exercise. To increase anterior motion of the posterior pharyngeal wall, the tongue hold maneuver was instructed. The exercises were to be completed independently at home in sets of 20, every other day. He was asked to return in 1 week, so that it could be assured that he was performing the exercises correctly. The results of the fluoroscopic swallowing study and the recommendation to gradually resume oral intake were sent to the dietician, so that she could manage the gradual transition from nonoral to oral feedings without compromising nutritional status.

Upon his return, Joel demonstrated that he could perform each exercise accurately. He had not been able to reach 20 repetitions, but was gradually increasing the intensity of his home program. Because he demonstrated independence with his exercises, he was not scheduled to be seen again for 1 month. Clinician contact information was provided along with written instructions. During this time period, it was expected that he would have begun to transition off the PEG feedings and resume oral intake to meet at least 50% of his nutritional and hydration needs. A fiber-optic endoscopic examination of swallowing function (FEES) was to be performed upon his return. FEES was selected for the reevaluation because the absence of residue in the valleculae and pyriform sinuses would indicate improved functioning and benefit from therapy without additional exposure to radiation. FEES was also indicated because there had been no oral phase swallowing impairment, and an endoscopic swallowing examination could easily be performed in the office.

After 1 month, Joel returned to the clinic. He stated that he had maintained his weight and possibly gained a pound or two. A quick weight check confirmed a 2-pound weight gain. He stated (and his wife confirmed) that he had been completing his swallowing exercises on a consistent basis with improved motivation since subsidence of his pain and reduced anxiety. In addition, he stated that he felt more confident about his ability to swallow safely since viewing his swallowing function under fluoroscopy. In spite of the expected trepidation in relation to having a nasoendoscope passed, he was eager for the examination because he expected to see significant improvement. Although it is out of the scope of practice of the SLP to evaluate or comment on tumors and masses, and Joel was informed of this, he and his wife were anxious to visually inspect the base of his tongue.

The FEES was completed using a range of viscosities that had contrast color added to assist with visualization. Joel's head was in neutral position. Preswallowing observations showed slight swelling of the arytenoid cartilages and a smoothed appearance of the pharyngeal mucosa, both of which are indicative of dryness and radiation changes. The presence of obvious tumor was not appreciated and the tongue base appeared to be normal in size. There was no pooling of secretions. The true vocal folds adducted well. Premature spillage was not observed with any consistency. Postswallowing observations showed minimal, diffuse residue throughout the pharynx with pudding consistency only. An effortful swallow eliminated the residue. No contrast color of any of the materials given was observed within the laryngeal vestibule or subglottis. The impressions were that Joel no longer required a chin tuck or liquid wash because pharyngeal transit was much improved. The recommendations were to continue with a soft diet and thin liquids. It was also recommended that he continue to work with the dietitian until he was able to obtain all nutrition and hydration by mouth. The physician and dietitian were then to decide when to remove the PEG tube.

## Analysis of Client's Response to Intervention

At this time, Joel was asked to take the MDADI once again so that his quality of life in relation to eating and drinking could be reassessed. His post-CRT global score was 60 (down from 100), the emotional subscale was 80 (down from 96), the physical component score was 70.5 (down from 87.5), and the functional score was 96 (increased from 92). The lower scores likely reflected his lack of taste, dryness, and other postradiation changes. The importance of continuing to complete twice daily lingual and mandibular range of motion exercises to prevent scar tissue formation that can negatively affect speech and swallowing was reinforced, and Joel was discharged.

## Author Note

The case is highly typical of patients who undergo organ preservation treatment of head and neck cancer; however, many personal details are fictional.

## References


Carroll, W. R., Locher, J. L., Canon, C. L., Bohannon, I. A., McColloch, N. L., & Magnuson, J. S. (2008). Pretreatment swallowing exercises improve swallow function after chemoradiation. *Laryngoscope, 118*(1), 39–43.

Chen, A. Y., Frankowski, R., Bishop-Leone, J., Hebert, T., Leyk, S., Lewin, J., et al. (2001). The development and validation of a dysphagia-specific quality-of-life questionnaire for patients with head and neck cancer: The M. D. Anderson dysphagia inventory. *Archives of Otolaryngology—Head & Neck Surgery, 127*(7), 870–876.

Gallegos-Hernandez, J. F., Paredes-Hernandez, E., Flores-Diaz, R., Minauro-Munoz, G., Apresa-Garcia, T., & Hernandez-Hernandez, D. M. (2007). [Human papillomavirus: Association with head and neck cancer]. *Cirugia y cirujanos. 75*(3), 151–155.

Gillespie, M. B., Brodsky, M. B., Day, T. A., Lee, F. S., & Martin-Harris, B. (2004). Swallowing-related quality of life after head and neck cancer treatment. *Laryngoscope, 114*(8), 1362–1367.

Kulbersh, B. D., Rosenthal, E. L., McGrew, B. M., Duncan, R. D., McColloch, N. L., Carroll, W. R., et al. (2006). Pretreatment, preoperative swallowing exercises may improve dysphagia quality of life. *Laryngoscope, 116*(6), 883–886.

Logemann, J. A., Pauloski, B. R., Rademaker, A. W., Lazarus, C. L., Mittal, B., Gaziano, J., et al. (2003). Xerostomia: 12-month changes in saliva production and its relationship to perception and performance of swallow function, oral intake, and diet after chemoradiation. *Head & Neck, 25*(6), 432–437.

Nguyen, N. P., Sallah, S., Karlsson, U., & Antoine, J. E. (2002). Combined chemotherapy and radiation therapy for head and neck malignancies: Quality of life issues. *Cancer, 94*(4), 1131–1141.

Patel, S. G., & Shah, J. P. (2005). TNM staging of cancers of the head and neck: Striving for uniformity among diversity. *CA: A Cancer Journal for Clinicians, 55*(4), 242-258; quiz 261–242, 264.

Rosenthal, D. I., Lewin, J. S., & Eisbruch, A. (2006). Prevention and treatment of dysphagia and aspiration after chemoradiation for head and neck cancer. *Journal of Clinical Oncology, 24*(17), 2636–2643.

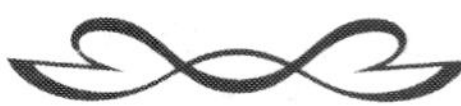



# CASE 51

# Bob: Adult Audiologic Rehabilitation: The Case of the Difficult Patient

*Jill E. Preminger and Jonathon P. Whitton*

## Conceptual Knowledge Areas

We present the case of a patient referred to as Bob and explore the concept of the "difficult patient." Some of the clinicians who have worked with Bob found him to be demanding and "difficult to treat." Bob exhausted multiple audiologic rehabilitation tools (i.e., hearing aids, FM systems, group audiologic rehabilitation classes, and cochlear implantation). His case provides a unique perspective on the effectiveness of audiologic rehabilitation.

Bob first came to a private pay audiology practice in 2000. He presented with a moderate precipitously sloping to profound sensorineural hearing loss (see Figure 51.1). Essentially, Bob had little functional hearing above 1,500 Hz. His subjective experience related to this hearing loss was reflected on a questionnaire completed prior to his appointment. Bob's responses on the questionnaire indicated that he heard poorly in all listening situations. Bob

FIGURE 51.1 Audiogram from 2000

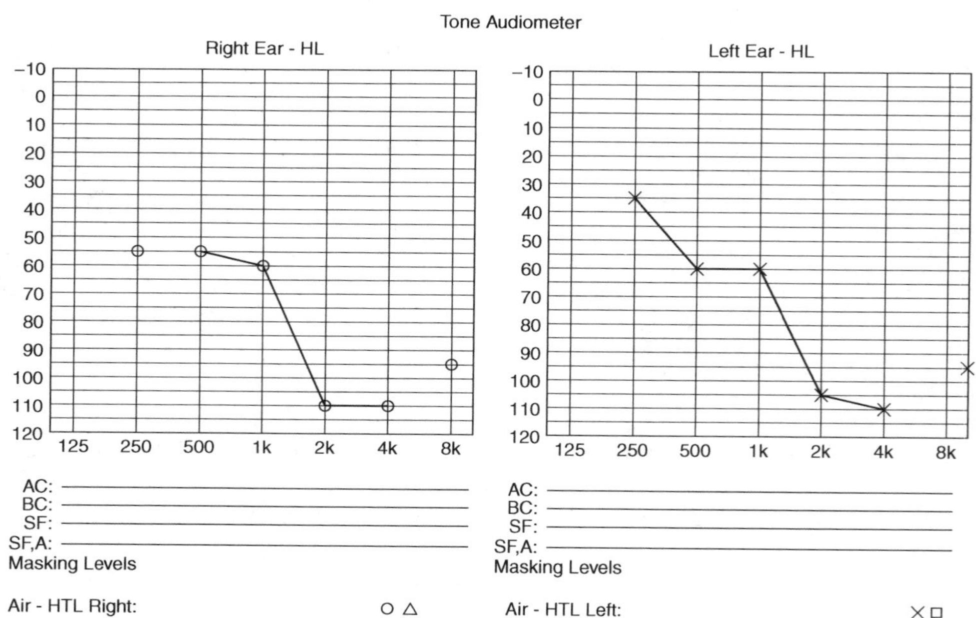

TABLE 51.1 A Summary of Bob's Visits to the Practice

| Year | 2000 | 2001 | 2002 | 2003 | 2004 | 2005 | 2006 | 2007 |
|---|---|---|---|---|---|---|---|---|
| **Services** | HAE = 1 | HAF = 1<br>PROG = 3<br>CHECK = 1<br>IN = 1 | PROG = 1<br>OUT = 1 | PROG = 1<br>CHECK = 1<br>IN = 1 | HAE = 1<br>HAF = 1<br>PROG = 3<br>CHECK = 1<br>ADP = 1<br>ADR = 1<br>IN = 3<br>OUT = 7 | PROG = 1<br>OUT = 2 | IN = 2<br>OUT = 5 | OUT = 1 |

HAE = hearing aid evaluation; HAF = hearing aid fitting, PROG = patient request for hearing aid reprogramming, CHECK = hearing aid check/cleaning, ADP = assistive device purchase, ADR = assistive device return, IN = hearing aid in office repair, OUT = out of office repair

was an experienced hearing aid user, but he came to the practice with hopes that the clinicians might be able to help him "hear" better.

During the 8 years that Bob was in the care of the practice, the audiologists came to know him well; see Table 51.1 for a listing of all visits during this period. He was fitted with hearing aids twice and seen for programming adjustments to his hearing aids 9 times. He purchased and subsequently returned an FM system and later inquired about purchasing one again. During a 3-year period, his hearing aids were sent out for repair 14 times. Bob was frustrated with the constant hearing aid repairs and adjustments; he was especially frustrated with his poor communication abilities even while wearing his hearing aids. Bob's audiologists were also troubled by these same issues.

During clinical rotations students likely hear stories about "difficult" patients. Practicing clinicians may describe a difficult patient as an individual who makes unreasonable demands, or one whose outcomes are poorer than would be expected based on his or her physical condition. It is not clear that this was the case with Bob. However, before addressing the question of whether Bob was a difficult patient, we will describe the audiologic rehabilitation process and how it related to Bob's treatment. First, we review the process of audiologic rehabilitation; then we examine these rehabilitation principles through the lens of Bob's case, describing his experiences with hearing aid use, FM use, group audiologic rehabilitation, and cochlear implantation. Finally, we explore the concept of "the difficult patient" and whether Bob fit that concept.

## What Is Audiologic Rehabilitation?

There is confusion among students and professionals about the definition of *audiologic rehabilitation*. Some professionals view audiologic rehabilitation quite narrowly and consider it to be services ancillary to the provision of hearing aids, cochlear implants, and/or assistive listening devices. These ancillary services might include speechreading training, auditory training, and group audiologic rehabilitation. However, we prefer to take a broader view. According to Tye-Murray (2004), audiologic rehabilitation is "intervention aimed at minimizing and alleviating the communication difficulties associated with hearing loss" (p. 2). With this broad definition it becomes clear that audiologic rehabilitation includes many services; please see Table 51.2 for a list of potential adult audiologic rehabilitation services.

To determine which audiologic rehabilitation services are most appropriate for a particular patient, the audiologist should consider both the communication difficulties imposed by hearing loss as well as the psychosocial ramifications of the hearing loss. The psychosocial aspects of hearing loss are multidimensional and have been well described in the literature (Hetu, 1996; Hogan, 2001; Trychin, 2002). Trychin (2002) has classified reactions to hearing loss in terms of emotional, cognitive, interpersonal, behavioral, and physical responses. See Figure 51.2 for an interpretation of these reactions described by Preminger (2007).

TABLE 51.2 Possible Adult Audiologic Rehabilitation Services

| Device Specific | Individual | Group |
|---|---|---|
| • Hearing aid (or cochlear implant) programming and fitting<br>• Hearing aid (or cochlear implant) orientation<br>• Hearing aid (or cochlear implant) checks and counseling<br>• Assistive listening device selection and coaching | • Speechreading training (office-based, or home-based via computer)<br>• Auditory training (office-based, or home-based via computer)<br>• Informational counseling | • Communication strategies training<br>• Psychosocial support activities<br>• Speechreading and auditory training<br>• Informational counseling |

Research has consistently demonstrated that hearing aids can alleviate the psychological, social, and emotional effects of hearing loss (Chisolm et al., 2007a). However, in many cases residual hearing-loss-related participation restrictions and activity limitations remain. This can occur in an individual with a particularly severe hearing loss or in an individual who is having difficulty adjusting to and/or accepting hearing loss. In these cases it can be difficult for the audiologist to determine the appropriate course of treatment; self assessment scales can be used in order to tease out a particular patient's needs.

## Self-Assessment Scales

Hearing-loss-specific quality of life scales measure the degree to which patients' hearing loss or hearing aids affect their self-perception of daily functioning and well-being and provide a systematic measure of the success of treatment and/or the need for further treatment (Chisolm et al., 2007a). Appropriate scales can also be useful in determining the type of audiologic rehabilitation treatment that would be most beneficial. For example, a hearing aid benefit scale such as the Abbreviated Profile of Hearing Aid Benefit (Cox & Alexander, 1995) is useful for determining whether a hearing aid fitting is successful. If it is not, results on the scale could suggest whether assistive listening technologies would be a useful addition. A scale such as the Communication Strategies Scale for Older Adults (Kaplan, Bally, Brandt, Busacco, & Pray, 1997) measures whether a patient uses communication strategies successfully. Those who do not may benefit from an individual or group audiologic rehabilitation program that focuses on communication strategy training. A hearing-loss-related quality of life scale such as the Hearing Handicap Inventory (for the Elderly or for Adults; Newman, Weinstein, Jacobson, & Hug, 1990; Ventry & Weinstein, 1982) is useful to determine whether an individual has effectively dealt with the emotional reactions and interpersonal reactions to hearing loss. Those who have not effectively dealt with these reactions could benefit from

FIGURE 51.2 Psychosocial Reactions to Hearing Loss

1. Emotional reactions: This dimension refers to the stigma of hearing loss and may include shame, guilt, anxiety, anger, frustration, embarrassment, and depression.
2. Cognitive reactions: These reactions may include inattentiveness, difficulty in concentration, low self-esteem, or low self-confidence. This may also include increased effort required for comprehension in difficult listening situations.
3. Interpersonal reactions: These responses may include bluffing, social withdrawal, dominating conversations, and a loss of intimacy in relationship(s).
4. Behavioral reactions: These reactions may include a limitation of activities or self-isolation.
5. Physical reactions: These include health issues that can be caused or exacerbated by hearing loss, such as fatigue, muscle tension, headaches, stomach problems, and sleep problems.

participation in a group audiologic rehabilitation program that focuses on the psychosocial aspects of hearing loss.

The preceding discussion of audiologic rehabilitation and self-assessment scales demonstrates how treatment should occur under ideal conditions. In a busy clinic, the professional may not always adhere to best practices. Important data may go uncollected and useful treatment options may be ignored.

## Description of the Case

### Background Information and Reason for Referral

#### Hearing Aid Use

Bob was treated by the practice for 8 years. During that time he had two primary problems with his hearing aids: physical problems and unresolved hearing-loss-related participation restrictions and activity limitations. When Bob became a patient in the practice, the audiologists switched him from in-the-ear-style hearing aids to behind-the-ear-style hearing aids to provide him with increased gain. The clinician was unaware that this would create a problem. Bob was an avid gardener with a history of skin cancer. As a result, he used large amounts of sunscreen on a frequent basis. Merely 1 month after he was fitted with his new hearing aids, the right hearing aid casing cracked. Over the course of 3 years, his hearing aid casing cracked 9 different times. The clinicians eventually discovered (through conversations with a representative from the hearing aid manufacturer) that the cracking was likely caused from contact with Bob's sunscreen. Despite the use of hearing aid coatings and sweatbands, this problem never resolved satisfactorily.

### Findings of the Evaluation

If Bob's problems were restricted to the cracked casing of his hearing aids, the clinicians would have been glad to repair them every few months. However, despite wearing two hearing aids, Bob continued to experience significant communicative difficulties. This is evident by his frequent returns for hearing aid adjustments (nine times shown in Table 51.1). These adjustments are referred to as "tweaking" by some audiologists. Bob's requests for tweaking were sometimes contradictory (he asked for increased gain at one visit and requested reduced gain at the next visit). It is not clear if tweaking actually improves speech understanding or just "appeases" the patient. Cunningham, Williams, and Goldsmith (2001) compared the success of 2 groups of hearing aid patients in response to tweaking. For one group, the clinicians responded to all of the patients' requests for tweaking by making appropriate electroacoustic adjustments to the hearing aids. For the other group, the clinicians made no adjustments to the hearing aids and instead counseled the patients when they requested such changes. Cunningham and colleagues found that there were no differences in level of benefit, measured subjectively and objectively, between the groups.

### Treatment Options Considered

Rather than "tweak" Bob's hearing aids, the clinicians might have attempted to determine why Bob was so dissatisfied with his hearing aids and whether additional assessment and/or treatment was warranted. The reasons for Bob's limited hearing aid benefit can begin to be understood by examining Figure 51.3 showing the "aided speech maps" for the left and right ear following Bob's first hearing aid fitting in 2001. These graphs are basically an audiogram flipped upside down. The $y$-axis of the graphs show sound pressure level (the intensity of the sound), and the $x$-axis of the graphs show the frequencies of the sounds. The Xs and Os connected by straight lines represent Bob's left ear and right ear hearing thresholds. The shaded region above the thresholds represents the target area for the audiologist to place the speech sounds that are presented through Bob's hearing aids. If the audiologist can adjust the hearing

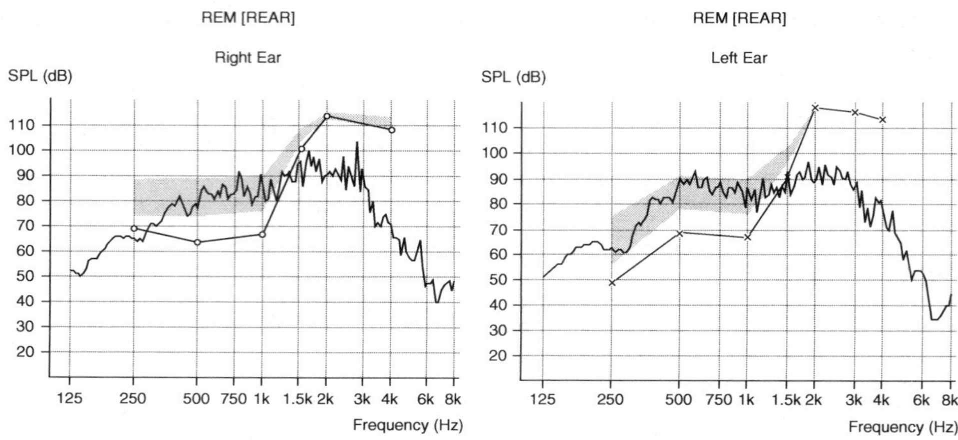


FIGURE 51.3 Live Speech Maps in 2001

aids to amplify sounds of different frequencies to reach the target (shaded) area, then all of the speech signal will be audible. Finally, the squiggly lines represent the speech sounds that were presented to Bob. As a result of Bob's profound hearing loss above 1,500 Hz, the audiologist was unable to provide any functional amplification in those frequencies. (The squiggly lines fell below the shaded area above 1,500 Hz in each ear.) Basically, Bob was unaidable in the mid to high frequencies.

Another way to look at the success of the hearing aid fitting is to consider the articulation index (AI). The articulation index is a method to calculate the audibility of speech for a particular individual (American National Standards Institute, 1969; Pavlovic, 1989). Without hearing aids Bob has an AI of approximately .02 for each ear. That is, if someone were to speak to him at a normal level, only 2% of the speech signal would be audible. The speech maps in Figure 51.3 demonstrate that when Bob wore his hearing aids his AI improved to 23%. While this may seem to represent poor hearing aid performance, with an articulation index of .23, it is expected that he would be able to understand about 50% of sentences presented to him in quiet listening situations (American National Standards Institute, 1969). That is not bad considering Bob's significant hearing loss, but not good enough considering his communication demands. Despite their best efforts, the clinicians could never improve Bob's audibility to 100%. Unfortunately, Bob never understood this, as will be discussed later.

Notwithstanding careful hearing aid fitting and multiple reprogramming, Bob had unmet needs. The staff knew this because he kept coming back to the practice, but they were unable to determine the exact nature of his concerns because a standardized hearing-loss-related quality of life scale was never used. As a result, it was unclear if his unmet needs were emotionally related, interpersonally related, or so on (see Figure 51.2). If this information had been gathered, it might have expedited his audiologic rehabilitation plan. Despite this, Bob's audiologists did try a number of additional audiologic rehabilitation strategies.

## FM Use

Bob's audiologists knew that his audibility would never reach 100% and tried to explain this. With reduced audibility, most adults can follow conversations due to the redundancy and predictability of speech. Even with only 30% of the signal audible, patients can typically repeat sentences with high accuracy (American National Standards Institute, 1969). Bob could do this under ideal "quiet" listening situations. But when the environment became noisy and masked (covered up) some of the speech signal, speech understanding became impossible. A way of combating this problem is through FM use.

FM systems overcome the difficulty encountered in challenging listening environments (i.e., background noise, distance, and reverberation) by delivering the target acoustic signal (speaker's voice) directly to the listener's ear. This is accomplished through the use of a remote microphone (a microphone used by the talker) that transmits sound directly to the hearing aid through some type of FM receiver. The result of FM use is a favorable signal to noise ratio, ranging from 15–25 dB (for a review, see Chisolm, Noe, McArdle, & Abrams, 2007b). Despite the advantages in communication abilities provided through the use of an FM system, many patients do not choose to try or to keep an FM system. Although FM systems typically work well, they involve a great deal of "technology." The patient must learn when and how to use this system and must feel comfortable handing the remote microphone to an individual talker. One solution to this problem is FM coaching. The successful use of FM systems requires additional counseling, instruction, and coaching over several visits rather than the one-time explanation that many patients receive before beginning FM use. Chisolm et al. (2007b) examined the effectiveness of FM coaching and found that benefits were seen over a 6-month period of FM use and coaching as measured by multiple outcome scales and FM retention. However, the authors concluded that the additional cost associated with the purchase of an FM system on top of the high cost of hearing aids may create a barrier to FM acceptance.

The FM system that Bob initially purchased was offered at a discounted rate of $2,285 (in 2004), still a significant investment to make over and above the purchase of hearing aids. Bob's willingness to undertake such a purchase revealed his desire to improve his communicative abilities. Nevertheless, Bob later returned the entire system for credit. Would Bob have continued to use the FM device if he had been provided with FM coaching? Bob reported satisfaction with the device to his clinician and later (in 2006) inquired about purchasing another FM system. These behaviors seem to indicate that Bob recognized some benefit from using the device. FM coaching might have optimized this benefit and allowed Bob to accept the FM system.

## Course of Treatment

### Group Audiologic Rehabilitation Classes

During Bob's 6th year of treatment in the practice, a research study was initiated at the university evaluating the efficacy of audiologic rehabilitation (AR) programs. Bob was invited to participate and attended a 6-hour, 6-week program. Each week a group of 7 experienced hearing aid users discussed the problems and feelings associated with their hearing loss. In addition, they were given informational lectures about hearing loss, hearing aids, assistive devices, and communication strategies. Prior to beginning the study, Bob completed the Hearing Handicap Inventory (HHI; Ventry & Weinstein, 1982). This is a 25-item hearing-loss-related quality of life scale that measures social and emotional responses to hearing loss. A score near 0 indicates no hearing-loss-related difficulties, while a score near 100 suggests severe hearing-loss-related participation restrictions and activity limitations.

Table 51.3 shows all of Bob's HHI scores. Prior to participating in the group program, Bob scored 86. Despite his hearing aid use, Bob reported significant social and emotional reactions to his hearing loss. Hetu (1996) developed a framework for understanding the psychosocial effects of hearing loss. According to this author, most individuals consider their hearing loss to be a "stigma," defined as a discredited or discreditable attribute. In other words, a stigma is the shame or disgrace associated with something that is regarded as socially unacceptable. As a result of a perceived stigma of hearing loss, individuals may isolate themselves, avoid social interactions, and/or bluff their way through communication breakdowns. These behaviors and feelings can result in a change of one's social identity and an enduring sense of social uncertainty (Hetu, 1996; Hogan, 2001). Participation in group audiologic rehabilitation programs is one way to deal with feelings related to the loss of social identity associated with hearing loss (Hetu, 1996). As a result, hearing loss is seen as typical rather than deviant. Participation in a supportive group reinstates the feeling of belonging (Hetu, 1996).

Audiologic rehabilitation groups can focus exclusively on the needs of individuals with hearing loss or they can provide information and training for individuals with hearing loss as well as their significant others (Getty & Hetu, 1991; Preminger, 2003). Groups that include

TABLE 51.3 Hearing Handicap Inventory Scale Scores

| | HHI (Emotional) | HHI (Social) | HHI (Total) |
|---|---|---|---|
| 1. Prior to group AR class participation (2005) | 42 | 44 | 86 |
| 2. Postgroup AR class participation (2005) | 26 | 32 | 58 |
| 3. Six months after group AR class participation (2006) | 38 | 44 | 82 |
| 4. Prior to cochlear implantation (2007) | 36 | 46 | 82 |
| 5. Two and a half months post–cochlear implant stimulation (2008) | 26 | 34 | 60 |

significant others may include training specifically designed for them, such as, "Only speak to the person with hearing loss when you are in the same room and when he or she can see your face," and clear speech training (Schum, 1996).

After participating in the 6-week group program for people with hearing loss, Bob's HHI score dropped to 58, a significant improvement (Weinstein, Spitzer, & Ventry, 1986). Bob also reported to the group leader that for the first time, he understood why he was having so much difficulty understanding, even with his hearing aids. He told the group leader: "I have come to realize I have no miracle coming that will improve my hearing. I feel I have the best type of hearing aid for me. I have always felt like my audiologists did not know how to program them, and now I realize the poor guy has nothing to work with. I have been told this several times, but I guess I never believed it until you explained it so well."

In 2006 Bob told the audiologist who led his group class that for the first time he understood his hearing loss. Yet in 2000 and in 2004 previous audiologists had discussed the same information with Bob at his hearing aid evaluation and at his subsequent hearing aid counseling sessions. Unfortunately, this is a common occurrence. Research indicates that patients remember only about 50% of what is told to them at their office visits (Margolis, 2004). Perhaps patient retention of information could improve with the use of written materials, CDs, and DVDs.

## Cochlear Implant Use

While Bob benefited from the group audiologic rehabilitation program, this benefit was brief. Six months after completing the program his HHI score increased to 82, a significant hearing handicap. Bob's audiologists recommended that he consider a cochlear implant. Why wasn't Bob referred for a cochlear implant earlier? Bob's pure-tone audiogram and lack of perceived benefit from hearing aids made him a potential cochlear implant candidate when he first began treatment in the practice in 2001. Bob could have been recommended for a cochlear implant evaluation in 2001 when he purchased a new set of hearing aids, or in 2004 when he purchased another set of hearing aids. However, the audiologist might not have recognized Bob was a cochlear implant candidate at those times. When the U.S. Food and Drug Administration first approved cochlear implants for adults in 1985, only adults with hearing losses greater than 100 dB HL and no discernible communication benefit from hearing aids were considered candidates (Zwolan, 2007). According to these old guidelines, Bob was not a candidate for a cochlear implant. Candidacy has changed over time as cochlear implants have improved and benefits from cochlear implantation have increased. Between 1998 and 2001 candidacy for the three major cochlear implant companies changed to moderate to profound hearing loss in the low frequencies and profound hearing loss in the middle to high speech frequencies (pure-tone average at. 5, 1 and 2 kHz of 70 dB HL or greater) with limited benefit from amplification, as defined by open set sentence recognition scores of 50% correct or less in the ear to be implanted and 60% or less in the best aided condition (Food and Drug Administration, 2008). Bob's audiologist was either not aware of the change in candidacy or simply did not think about Bob as a cochlear implant candidate since he was already viewed as a hearing aid user. In addition, Bob had quite a bit of "aid-able" hearing in the lower frequencies, which might have prevented his audiologists from viewing him as a cochlear implant candidate. Bob received a cochlear implant in 2007. Two and a half months after activation of the implant he scored a total of 60 on the HHI, a significant decrease of 22 points compared to his pre-implantation score. It is likely that his benefit from the cochlear implant will continue to improve, as adult cochlear implant patients typically see slow improvements in performance over time (Valimaa, Maatta, Lopponen, & Sorri, 2002a, 2002b). There is a growing body of evidence that adult cochlear implant users can benefit from auditory training, which can speed the rehabilitation process and may improve peak performance (Fu & Galvin, 2007). Unfortunately, many facilities do not offer auditory training for adult cochlear implant users.

## Analysis of Client's Response to Intervention

### Is Bob a Difficult Patient?

Hahn and colleagues have described 3 characteristics of "difficult" patients: (1) patient psychopathology, (2) abrasive interpersonal style, and (3) multiple physical symptoms (Hahn, Thompson, Will, Stern, & Budner, 1994; Hahn et al., 1996; Hahn, 2001). These characteristics combine in a variety of ways that foster negative feelings in the clinician, such as frustration and dislike (Wasan, Wooton, & Jamison, 2005). Based on informal reports from audiologists who participated in this patient's care, Bob was considered a "difficult" patient. There have been no reports of psychopathology in Bob's case; however, all the audiologists indicated that Bob had an abrasive interpersonal style and certainly presented with significant communicative impairment and self-perceived participation restrictions.

According to Hahn, the term *difficult patient* is really a misnomer as the "difficulty" is experienced by the clinician; therefore, the clinician's characteristics also influence the level of difficulty (Hahn et al., 1996, Hahn, 2001). Part of the frustration involved in treating a difficult patient is generated by the clinician's perceived inability to successfully diagnose and/or treat the patient. Bob's abrasive personality, significant activity limitations, and participation restrictions, as well as the frustration his case had generated for the clinicians involved in his care, would classify him as a difficult patient. However, three clinician-related variables also could have contributed to clinician-experienced difficulty in Bob's case. First, the clinicians never measured Bob's perception of his activity limitations or participation restrictions. Second, the clinicians never documented Bob's expectations for rehabilitation. Therefore, Bob's expectations and prognosis were never clear. A patient's expectations can be assessed through administration of questionnaires such as the Hearing Demand, Ability and Need Profile (Palmer & Mormer, 1997). This questionnaire allows the patient to establish goals for treatment and then document expectations in meeting those goals. The audiologist can modify the patient's goals based on professional expertise. Unreasonable goals for rehabilitation can dramatically confound rehabilitation outcomes. Many patients expect hearing aids to "fix" their hearing, just as glasses "fix" vision. These patients do not understand the complexity of hearing loss, including outer versus inner hair cell damage, loss of compressive qualities within the cochlea, and changes to the central auditory nervous system (Hardie & Shepherd, 1999; Moore, 2007; Oxenham & Bacon, 2003). Bob's unrealistic expectations might account for the multiple requests for "tweaking" made throughout his time in the practice and his lack of satisfaction with amplification. Finally, the clinicians treating Bob might not have been providing him with the most appropriate treatment tools. Bob's pure-tone audiogram, lack of perceived benefit from hearing aids, challenging auditory environment, and motivation to achieve better communication made him a potential cochlear implant candidate when he first arrived for rehabilitation in 2000.

## Further Recommendations

Although Bob's clinician still reports that he has an abrasive personality, his communicative needs are being met more appropriately by his current treatment plan (i.e., bimodal cochlear implant and hearing aid use). The efficacy of the treatment plan is evidenced by the reduction in his hearing loss participation restrictions and activity limitations as reported on the Hearing Handicap Inventory. It is argued that a significant portion of the "difficulty" associated with Bob's case can be attributed to inadequate verification of treatment efficacy, delay in provision of best treatment options, and Bob's poor communicative abilities coupled with high communicative demands. Bob's rehabilitative progress will continue to be monitored through validated self-assessment measures, and as cochlear implant technology advances, he might benefit from bilateral implantation in the future. In the meantime an auditory training program may help Bob adjust to and benefit from his cochlear implant, and both Bob and his spouse may benefit if she attends an audiologic rehabilitation program designed for significant others of people with hearing loss.

## Author Note

The case described is an actual case; no modifications to the case data have been made. The authors would like to thank the many audiologists who worked with this patient and who provided thorough documentation of their work. This case report was acknowledged by the Human Studies Protection Program at the University of Louisville; this case was not considered human subjects research and was not reviewed.

## References

American National Standards Institute. (1969). American National Standard methods for the calculation of the articulation index. ANSI S3.5–1969. New York: ANSI. Ref Type: Generic.

Chisolm, T. H., Johnson, C. E., Danhauer, J. L., Portz, L. J. P., Abrams, H. B., Lesner, S., et al. (2007a). A systematic review of health-related quality of life and hearing aids: Final report of the American Academy of Audiology task force on the health-related quality of life benefits of amplification in adults. *Journal of the American Academy of Audiology, 18,* 151–183.

Chisolm, T. H., Noe, C. M., McArdle, R., & Abrams, H. B. (2007b). Evidence for the use of hearing assistive technology by adults: The role of the FM system. *Trends in Amplification, 11,* 73–89.

Cox, R. M., & Alexander, G. C. (1995). The Abbreviated Profile of Hearing Aid Benefit (APHAB). *Ear and Hearing, 16,* 176–186.

Cunningham, D. R., Williams, K. J., & Goldsmith, L. J. (2001). Effects of providing and withholding postfitting fine-tuning adjustments on outcome measures in novice hearing aid users: A pilot study. *American Journal of Audiology, 10,* 13–23.

Food and Drug Administration. (2008). *Devices @ FDA.* Food and Drug Administration [Online].

Fu, Q. J., & Galvin, J. J., III. (2007). Perceptual learning and auditory training in cochlear implant recipients. *Trends in Amplification, 11,* 193–205.

Getty, L., & Hetu, R. (1991). Development of a rehabilitation program for people affected with occupational hearing loss. 2. Results from group intervention with 48 workers and their spouses. *Audiology, 30,* 317–329.

Hahn, S. R. (2001). Physical symptoms and physician-experienced difficulty in the physician-patient relationship. *Annals of Internal Medicine, 134,* 904.

Hahn, S. R., Kroenke, K., Spitzer, R. I., Brody, D., Williams, J. B., Linzer, M., et al. (1996). The difficult patient: Prevalence, psychopathology, and functional impairment. *Journal of General Internal Medicine,* 1–8.

Hahn, S. R., Thompson, K. S., Will, T. A., Stern, V., & Budner, N. S. (1994). The difficult doctor-patient relationship: Somatization, personality and psychopathology. *Journal of Clinical Epidemiology, 47,* 647–657.

Hardie, N. A., & Shepherd, R. K. (1999). Sensorineural hearing loss during development: morphological and physiological response of the cochlea and auditory brainstem. *Hearing Research, 128,* 147–165.

Hetu, R. (1996). The stigma attached to hearing impairment. *Scandinavian Audiology, 25,* 12–24.

Hogan, A. (2001). *Hearing rehabilitation for deafened adults: A psychosocial approach.* London, England: Whurr.

Kaplan, H., Bally, S., Brandt, F., Busacco, D., & Pray, J. (1997). Communication Scale for Older Adults (CSOA). *Journal of the American Academy of Audiology. 8*(3), 203–217.

Margolis, R. H. (2004). Page ten: What do your patients remember? *The Hearing Journal, 57,* 10–17.

Moore, B. C. J. (2007). *Cochlear hearing loss* (2nd ed.). West Sussex, England: John Wiley & Sons.

Newman, C. W., Weinstein, B. E., Jacobson, G. P., & Hug, G. A. (1990). The Hearing Handicap Inventory for Adults: Psychometric adequacy and audiometric correlates. *Ear and Hearing, 11,* 430–433.

Oxenham, A. J., & Bacon, S. P. (2003). Cochlear compression: Perceptual measures and implications for normal and impaired hearing. *Ear and Hearing, 24,* 352–366.

Palmer, C. V., & Mormer, E. (1997). A systematic program for hearing aid orientation and adjustment. *Hearing Review, 1,* 45.

Pavlovic, C. V. (1989). Speech spectrum considerations and speech intelligibility predictions in hearing aid evaluations. *Journal of Speech and Hearing Disorders, 54,* 3–8.

Preminger, J. E. (2003). Should significant others be encouraged to join adult group audiologic rehabilitation classes? *Journal of the American Academy of Audiology, 14,* 545–555.

Preminger, J. E. (2007). Issues associated with the measurement of psychosocial benefits of group audiologic rehabilitation programs. *Trends in Amplification, 11,* 113–124.

Schum, D. J. (1996). Intelligibility of clear and conversational speech of young and elderly talkers. *Journal of the American Academy of Audiology, 7,* 212–218.

Trychin, S. (2002). *Guidelines for providing mental health services to people who are hard of hearing* (Rep. No. ED466082). University of California, San Diego.

Tye-Murray, N. (2004). *Foundations of aural rehabilitation: Children, adults, and their family members* (2nd ed.). Clifton Park, NY: Delmar Learning.

Valimaa, T., Maatta, T., Lopponen, H., & Sorri, M. (2002a). Phoneme recognition and confusions with multichannel cochlear implants: Consonants. *Journal of Speech, Language, and Hearing Research, 45,* 1055–1069.

Valimaa, T., Maatta, T., Lopponen, H., & Sorri, M. (2002b). Phoneme recognition and confusions with multichannel cochlear implants: Vowels. *Journal of Speech, Language, and Hearing Research, 45,* 1039–1054.

Ventry, I. M., & Weinstein, B. E. (1982). The hearing handicap inventory for the elderly: A new tool. *Ear and Hearing, 3,* 128–134.

Wasan, A. D., Wooton, J., & Jamison, R. N. (2005). Dealing with difficult patients in your pain practice. *Regulatory Anesthesia and Pain Medicine, 30,* 184–192.

Weinstein, B. E., Spitzer, J. B., & Ventry, I. M. (1986). Test-retest reliability of the Hearing Handicap Inventory for the Elderly. *Ear and Hearing, 7,* 295–299.

Zwolan, T. (2007). Selection of cochlear implant candidates. In S. Waltzman & J. T. Roland (Eds.), *Cochlear implants* (2nd ed., pp. 57–68). New York: Thieme Medical Publishers.

# CASE 52

# Claude: Evaluation and Management of Vestibular Problems and Tinnitus Following Head Trauma

*Richard A. Roberts*

## Conceptual Knowledge Areas

### Benign Paroxysmal Positional Vertigo (BPPV)

This vestibular disorder is the number one peripheral cause of spinning dizziness (vertigo; Roberts & Gans, 2008). It is common in most age groups and becomes more prevalent as we get older. BPPV is caused by displacement of the crystalline otoliths from the utricle of the vestibular labyrinth into the semicircular canals, which do not have such structures in a normal state. Common causes of BPPV include the normal aging process, head trauma, ear surgery, ear infection, and so on. Movement of the otoliths within the semicircular canal causes an inappropriate response to changes in head position leading to intense vertigo and nystagmus (eye movement) in the plane of the affected canal. BPPV also has a negative influence on balance and can contribute to falls, particularly in older patients. Approximately 90% of the time the posterior semicircular canal becomes affected by the displaced otoliths given its inferior location relative to the utricle. The modified Dix-Hallpike maneuver is used to identify BPPV. To complete this test, the patient is seated on an examination table with the clinician positioned behind. The patient is then gradually lowered until lying flat on the exam table with the clinician seated behind in a position to observe the eyes of the patient. The clinician is supporting the head and neck of the patient during this maneuver. A positive response includes a subjective report of vertigo along with a transient rotary-type nystagmus. This disorder does not respond to medication, although there are surgical interventions that are successful. Most agree that repositioning maneuvers, which consist of moving the head and body of the patient through a set protocol, are able to deposit the otoliths back to the utricle with complete resolution of symptoms in 1–2 repositioning treatments 80–96% of the time (Roberts & Gans, 2008).

## Uncompensated Peripheral Vestibulopathy

This terminology describes the status of the balance system following insult to one or both of the vestibular structures. This insult may be secondary to disorders such as labyrinthitis, vestibular neuritis, Meniere's disease, and so forth, and can follow head trauma, which may lead to labyrinthine concussion. When one or both of the vestibular structures become damaged, there is often a functional alteration in the two main reflex pathways, which rely on vestibular information to a great extent: the vestibulo-ocular reflex (VOR) and the vestibulospinal reflex (VSR). The VOR pathway is in large part responsible for maintenance of gaze on a visual target during head movement. Correspondingly, damage to the vestibular structure(s) may lead to blurred vision with head movement (Roberts & Gans, 2007). Reportedly, visual acuity may degrade from 20/20 with no head movement to 20/200 with head movement, which can be debilitating for the patient. The VSR pathway connects the vestibular structures to antigravity muscles, and is key to maintenance of postural stability. Patients with disruption of VSR may notice difficulty maintaining balance during ambulation, particularly in poorly lit environments with an uneven walking surface.

Patients with uncompensated peripheral vestibulopathy often experience significant reduction of symptoms through vestibular rehabilitation therapy (VRT; Shepard, Telian, Smith-Wheelock, & Raj, 1993). The goal of VRT is not to "fix" the peripheral vestibulopathy but to get the VOR and VSR pathways to utilize information from unaffected vestibular structures, as well as other resources such as visual and somatosensory input (Whitney & Rossi, 2000). In this way, the balance system recalibrates to the altered set of inputs. This is accomplished through an individualized VRT program incorporating specific exercises to target *adaptation* to the altered vestibular information, *habituation* to head and body movements that lead to unpleasant symptoms (i.e., nausea, fatigue), and *substitution* of other resources to supplement vestibular information. Following successful VRT, a patient may be said to have compensated to the peripheral vestibulopathy.

## Tinnitus

Perception of sound(s) in the ears or head without an acoustic/vibratory source is tinnitus. Types of tinnitus include ringing, roaring, whistling, buzzing, humming, crickets, pulsing, and so on. There are many causes of tinnitus, such as buildup of ear wax (cerumen), temporomandibular joint problems, head and neck trauma, certain medications (including aspirin), and thyroid problems (Henry et al., 2005). By far, hearing loss is the most common cause of tinnitus. It is estimated that 90% of patients with cochlear-based sensorineural hearing loss report the presence of tinnitus. Damage to the hair cell structures in the cochlea by excessive noise, ototoxic medications, and the normal aging process are often implicated as causes of tinnitus. For many patients with tinnitus, there is little effect on quality of life. Other patients with tinnitus find it extremely troubling and potentially debilitating with difficulty concentrating, relaxing, and sleeping (Henry et al., 2005).

Given the relationship between hearing loss and tinnitus, it is fortunate that many patients report a decrease in their tinnitus when fitted with hearing aid amplification (Henry, Dennis, & Schechter, 2005). The hearing aids reduce stress from communication difficulties related to the hearing loss and also increase the perception of other sounds in the environment of the patient. The patient is less likely to focus on the tinnitus in this situation. Likewise, many patients with tinnitus report a decrease in perception of their tinnitus when they maintain an acoustically rich environment. Other forms of tinnitus intervention include masking devices, tinnitus retraining therapy, and biofeedback (Henry, Schechter, et al., 2005; Henry, Dennis, et al., 2005). Often, appropriate counseling about the causes of tinnitus by a trained audiologist or physician will reduce the impact of tinnitus on the patient's quality of life.

## Description of the Case

### Background Information

Claude was a 71-year-old male with onset of symptoms following a motor vehicle accident (MVA) during which a head trauma occurred. Immediately postimpact, the patient developed constant vertigo with nausea and emesis that gradually improved over 3 days. There was no change in hearing status or tinnitus reported at the time of hospital admission. He was placed on medication to suppress his symptoms. A CAT scan was unremarkable. His symptoms improved to brief episodes of vertigo with slight nausea. The patient was tapered off the medication and discharged after 5 days.

### Reasons for the Referral and Findings of the Evaluation

Claude reported two types of dizziness. One was described as "a strange sensation of dizziness that was not quite spinning" and which was provoked by head movement. He felt best when he was lying still in bed. Claude reported experiencing very intense but brief vertigo when lying down or turning over in bed. In between the episodes of vertigo, he reported imbalance worse with ambulation in the dark and outside his home. He noted having to touch the walls inside his home and other objects such as furniture to steady himself during ambulation. Claude also reported that his "eyes do not keep up with his head." He noticed difficulty reading the newspaper, which was always an activity he enjoyed prior to onset of the current symptoms. He noticed that his constant ringing tinnitus, which was present prior to the MVA, was more troubling since his discharge from the hospital and was causing him some difficulty falling asleep at night.

Claude was referred for comprehensive vestibular and equilibrium evaluation to rule out a peripheral vestibular involvement contributing to his symptoms. Audiometric evaluation revealed a bilateral, symmetric mild to moderately severe sensorineural hearing loss. Otoacoustic emissions and immittance results were in agreement with audiometric data. Tinnitus was matched to a 3 kHz tone with 20 dB sensation level. Claude reported that the tinnitus seemed momentarily softer following a presentation of 60 seconds of 3 kHz narrow band noise. He stated that his tinnitus immediately became more noticeable when he entered the sound-treated suite. Subjective assessment with the Tinnitus Handicap Inventory (THI) was 73 (Newman, Jacobson, & Spitzer, 1996).

The vertebrobasilar artery screening test (VAST; Roberts & Gans, 2008) revealed a slight transient dizziness with hyperextension of the neck and rotation of the head to the right. Results to the left were unremarkable. Postural stability testing revealed a vestibular pattern with a right turn on the Fukuda stepping test and a fall on dynamic surface with eyes closed. This is consistent with functional impairment of the VSR as the patient could not remain standing without visual information, though vestibular information should have been available.

During the Fukuda stepping test, Claude was asked to march in place for about 30 steps with eyes closed. The fact that he turned instead of staying in one place is remarkable. Dynamic visual acuity testing revealed a degradation from 82% correct with no head movement to 42% with horizontal volitional head movement and 60% with vertical volitional head movement. These results are consistent with functional impairment of the VOR (Roberts & Gans, 2007). Greater difficulty with horizontal compared to vertical is also a common finding with VOR dysfunction.

Vestibular evoked myogenic potentials (VEMP) revealed normal P13–N23 waveforms with stimulation to both ears. Saccule and inferior vestibular nerve function is required for normal VEMP responses. Random saccade, smooth pursuit, and optokinetic results were unremarkable, which is consistent with intact oculomotor function. Gaze testing was unremarkable, but high-frequency headshake elicited a transient left beating nystagmus. Claude also reported a subjective increase in his dizziness, though not to the point of vertigo. Modified Dix-Hallpike positioning to the right provoked an intense sensation of vertigo and upbeating torsional nystagmus consistent with right posterior semicircular canal BPPV (Roberts & Gans, 2008). Results to the left were negative. Static positional testing was unremarkable. Caloric testing produced a 50% right unilateral weakness. Directional preponderance and fixation suppression index were within normal limits. Subjective assessment with the Dizziness Handicap Inventory (DHI) was 85 (Jacobson & Newman, 1990).

### Key Findings

- Right posterior semicircular canal BPPV (from head trauma)
  - Supported by: positive modified Hallpike
- Partial peripheral vestibulopathy affecting the right labyrinth (labyrinthine concussion due to head trauma)
  - Supported by: Provokable left beating nystagmus, right unilateral weakness in presence of normal VEMP
- Functional VOR and VSR deficits related to vestibulopathy and possibly contributed to by BPPV
- Bilateral sensorineural hearing loss
- Dizziness Handicap Inventory (DHI) = 85 points, classified as severe with activity limitation and participation restriction
- Tinnitus Handicap Inventory (THI) = 73 points, also consistent with a severe perception of handicap (McCombe et al., 2001)

## Treatment Options Considered

### Benign Paroxysmal Positional Vertigo

Medications are not typically successful in treating BPPV. There are surgical options (singular neurectomy and semicircular canal occlusion), but these are quite involved and are usually reserved for patients who do not respond to repositioning maneuvers. Clearly, the literature indicates that repositioning the displaced otoliths into the utricle is the most efficient intervention that provides immediate relief of symptoms in 80–96% of patients (Roberts & Gans, 2008). Brandt-Daroff exercises have been reported to be successful but usually require 9–14 days of patients working on their own to disperse the otoconia. This is not a good choice for treatment given that most of the other repositioning techniques provide an immediate positive response. The canalith repositioning maneuver initially described by Epley is a good choice for many patients. In the current case, Claude had a positive VAST. Although that response may be related to the presence of BPPV on the right, the clinician cannot be certain. The CRM requires the patient to be in a state of hyperextension for an extended time and would certainly be contraindicated in the current case in view of the positive VAST (Roberts & Gans, 2008). The Semont Liberatory Maneuver (SLM) or Gans Repositioning Maneuver (GRM; Roberts, Gans, & Montaudo, 2006) are both excellent alternatives to the CRM as both methods avoid the neck hyperextension associated with the CRM, but have the same efficacy. For this case, a GRM was chosen but the SLM could have been used quite easily.

### Uncompensated Peripheral Vestibulopathy

Overall, the results of the current case indicated a unilateral right peripheral vestibulopathy for which the patient is uncompensated. Although some patients will compensate to the peripheral vestibulopathy over time, the literature indicates that an individualized program of VRT allows the patient to realize a faster functional recovery (Whitney & Rossi, 2000). Patients who are highly motivated with predominantly a disruption of VOR are often candidates for a self-directed program of VRT. The audiologist or physical therapist would work with the patient in a single session to teach the appropriate form for the various exercises. The clinician then follows the patient by phone until an appointment to determine the outcomes.

In other cases, and especially with VOR and VSR deficits, a clinician-directed program is more appropriate with either an audiologist or a physical therapist. As the level of VSR dysfunction increases and if there are additional comorbid factors such as peripheral neuropathy, artificial knee or hip, and so on, a physical therapist (PT) would likely be the best choice. Since there was an obvious functional impact on VSR (supported by postural stability findings and patient symptoms), it was decided that the patient should be referred for a clinician-directed program with a PT.

### Tinnitus

In view of the complexity of this case in terms of the dizziness and imbalance along with tinnitus, it was not felt that more time-intensive tinnitus interventions such as tinnitus retraining therapy (TRT), biofeedback, and so forth were appropriate. Claude was a candidate for hearing aid amplification based on the bilateral sensorineural hearing loss. It was decided to fit the hearing loss of the patient as an initial plan and keep other tinnitus intervention options open if there was not an appropriate level of improvement following successful use of hearing aid amplification. The hearing aid amplification was expected to reduce communication stress by allowing him to hear sounds important for speech intelligibility (Henry, Schechter, et al., 2005). It was anticipated that VRT would diminish any stress associated with Claude's dizziness and imbalance. Decreasing the overall stress in his life, it was hoped, would produce a concomitant decrease in perception of the tinnitus.

## Course of Treatment

Claude was immediately treated for the BPPV using a GRM, which was well tolerated. After two successive treatment maneuvers, he no longer exhibited symptoms of BPPV when placed in the provoking position, which is indicative of a successful treatment maneuver. He was scheduled to return in 1 week for follow-up to treatment of the BPPV to ensure treatment efficacy.

Vestibular retraining therapy (VRT) was initiated with a local physical therapist 1 week after treatment for BPPV. The therapy was scheduled for twice weekly 45-minute sessions. Claude was provided with supplemental VRT exercises to complete at home. Therapy incorporated adaptation and habituation techniques for home and clinic use. Substitution strategies were used mainly with the clinician in a controlled situation and focused more on the patient's balance. Claude became frustrated during the first week of VRT because the therapeutic exercises provoked his symptoms quite a bit. This is expected with VRT and all patients should be warned that this may occur, but they should be encouraged to continue with the program (Shepard et al., 1993). Encouragement by the audiologist and physical therapist helped the patient continue with VRT for the remaining 3 weeks, during which he noted significant subjective improvement. Claude admitted that he was not diligent about his home VRT exercises initially, but performed them faithfully after he started noticing improvement during the second week.

Claude was fitted with appropriate hearing aid amplification at the start of his VRT. He became frustrated and felt that "nothing was working." It was decided to wait until he noted improvement in the symptoms of dizziness and imbalance and then refit the hearing aid amplification. In the third week of VRT, Claude noted that his tinnitus was less troubling. At that point, the hearing aid amplification was refitted. He felt that he was receiving excellent benefit from the amplification and decided to keep the instruments at the end of his trial period. The tinnitus was only noticeable intermittently by the end of the trial period.

## Analysis of Client's Response to Intervention

On his follow-up to treatment of the BPPV, Claude indicated that he was no longer experiencing any vertigo. He did note that the dizziness with head movement was still present, but he was quite pleased with the immediate resolution of the vertigo. He was checked with side-lying and there was no BPPV response. Rechecking of his VAST was initially positive and then was also negative, suggesting that the initial responses were likely related to the BPPV in the right ear. Claude was then checked using a modified Hallpike position since there was no issue with vertebrobasilar insufficiency. This was also negative. He was placed in left and right lateral positions to ensure that no otoconial debris migrated into the adjacent right horizontal canal and this was negative. Claude was considered clear of the BPPV.

As mentioned above, Claude reported some initial frustration with VRT. This was due, in part, to the immediate success he realized with the treatment for BPPV. It was explained that VRT takes longer and requires more effort on the part of the patient. He continually used a rating scale from 0 (no dizziness) to 5 (extreme dizziness) to report his subjective impressions of each exercise. During the first week, most of the VRT elicited reports of "4" and "5." This gradually declined until the fourth week when the reports were mainly of "0" and "1." Claude reported little to no dizziness with head movement and also noted significantly improved balance. Posttherapy DHI was assessed by the patient and was a "4," suggesting no activity limitation or restriction of participation. Claude returned to the audiologist for follow-up assessment. His SOP was normal with no fall on dynamic surface with eyes closed. This result indicated functional recovery of the VSR. His DVA scores were 76% and 72% for horizontal and vertical volitional head movement, respectively. This result indicated functional recovery of the VOR. In addition, no provocable nystagmus was recorded during headshake testing using video-oculography. This is also consistent with intact VOR function. All results suggested that Claude was compensated to the peripheral vestibulopathy.

Tinnitus intervention via hearing aid amplification was initially postponed to allow the patient time to see the positive effects of BPPV treatment and get over the initial symptoms provoked during VRT. Claude noticed a decrease in his tinnitus symptoms after the BPPV was resolved and after he began to have some positive gains in VRT. This continued with successful fitting of hearing aid amplification, and a postfitting THI was 24. This is consistent with a mild impact with tinnitus easily masked by environmental sounds and easily forgotten during activity (McCombe et al., 2001). This is a significant improvement over the initial THI score.

## Further Recommendations

Over 5 months this patient was able to achieve (1) complete resolution of BPPV, (2) significant functional and subjective improvement in dizziness and imbalance symptoms associated with uncompensated peripheral vestibulopathy, and (3) significant improvement in subjective perception of tinnitus through appropriate fitting of hearing aid amplification.

Upon release from treatment, Claude was advised that recurrence rates for BPPV range from 5–30%, barring a precipitating event such as head trauma or inner ear infection. He was to contact the audiologist immediately with any recurrence of positional vertigo.

Outcome studies indicated the patient compensated to the peripheral vestibulopathy. It was explained that some patients experience a "relapse" of symptoms occasionally with extreme fatigue or acute illness. He was to begin his home program of VRT immediately after onset of these symptoms. If the symptoms persisted, he was to contact the audiologist for further evaluation.

It is quite possible that reducing the stress associated with the dizziness and imbalance as well as any hearing-loss-related communication stress helped to decrease this patient's perception of his tinnitus. Claude will continue to wear his hearing aid amplification and was instructed to maintain an acoustically rich environment. It was emphasized that this is especially important when he is in quieter situations, such as trying to go to sleep at night. The use of environmental noise machines was discussed and Claude will consider these if needed. At this time, there is no reason to pursue ear-level tinnitus maskers and/or tinnitus retraining therapy.

## Author Note

The patient described in this case is fictional but based on a composite of real cases evaluated and managed by the author.

## References


Henry, J. A., Dennis, K. C., & Schechter, M. A. (2005). General review of tinnitus: Prevalence, mechanisms, effects, and management. *Journal of Speech, Language, and Hearing Research*, *48*, 1–32.

Henry, J. A., Schechter, M. A., Loovis, C., Zaugg, T. L., Kaelin, C., & Montero, M. (2005). Clinical management of tinnitus using a "progressive intervention" approach. *Journal of Rehabilitation Research and Development*, *42*(4, Suppl. 2), 95–116.

Jacobson, G., & Newman, C. (1990). The development of the dizziness handicap inventory. *Archives of Otolaryngology—Head and Neck Surgery, 116*, 424–427.

McCombe, A., Bagueley, D., Coles, R., McKenna, L., McKinney, C., & Windle-Taylor, P. (2001). Guidelines for the grading of tinnitus severity: The results of a working group commissioned by the British Association of Otolaryngologists, Head and Neck Surgeons, 1999. *Clinical Otolaryngology, 26,* 388–393.

Newman, C., Jacobson, G., & Spitzer, J. (1996). Development of the tinnitus handicap inventory. *Archives of Otolaryngology—Head and Neck Surgery, 122,* 143–148.

Roberts, R., & Gans, R. (2007). Comparison of horizontal and vertical dynamic visual acuity in patients with vestibular dysfunction and non-vestibular dizziness. *Journal of the American Academy of Audiology, 18,* 236–244.

Roberts, R., & Gans, R. (2008). Non-medical management of positional vertigo. In G. Jacobson & N. Shephard (Eds.), *Balance function assessment and management* (pp. 447–468). San Diego, CA: Plural Publishing.

Roberts, R., Gans, R., & Montaudo, R. (2006). Efficacy of a new treatment for posterior canal benign paroxysmal positional vertigo. *Journal of the American Academy of Audiology, 17,* 598–604.

Shepard, N., Telian, S., Smith-Wheelock, M., & Raj, A. (1993). Vestibular and balance rehabilitation therapy. *Annals of Otology, Rhinology, & Laryngology, 102,* 198–205.

Whitney, S., & Rossi, M. (2000). Efficacy of vestibular rehabilitation. *Otolaryngology Clinics of North America, 33,* 659–672.

# CASE 53

# Ella: Sudden Idiopathic SNHL: Autoimmune Inner Ear Disease

*Laurie Wells*

## Conceptual Knowledge Areas

### Sudden Sensorineural Hearing Loss (SSHL)

Sudden sensorineural hearing loss (SSHL) presents complex emotional and physical challenges for the patient as well as unique diagnostic and treatment challenges for audiologists and other medical professionals. As the name implies, the onset of the hearing loss occurs over a short period of time, typically within 3 days or less. The degree of change is generally defined as a 30 dB or greater decrease in hearing thresholds at three adjacent audiometric frequencies and is sensorineural in nature. SSHL accounts for 1% of all cases of sensorineural hearing loss (Hughes, Freedman, Haberkamp, & Guay, 1996). Of the approximately 15,000 cases of sudden hearing loss reported around the world each year, about 4,000 occur in the United States (Hughes et al., 1996). The reported incidence of SSHL is approximately 5–20 cases in every 100,000 people (Byl, 1984).

### Idiopathic Sudden Sensorineural Hearing Loss (ISSHL)

Only about 10% of SSHL cases ever receive a formal diagnosis. Those without a known etiology are termed *idiopathic* SSHL. It is estimated that 60–65% of ISSHL cases recover spontaneously, without medical intervention, within the first 14 days after onset (Mattox & Simmons, 1977). This characteristic further complicates the ability of researchers to judge treatment effectiveness. Most SSHL prevalence studies do not distinguish between idiopathic or known etiology.

SSHL appears to affect women and men in equal numbers and there is no right or left ear preference. It occurs at nearly any age with few reported pediatric cases (Argup, 2008), and is most common in those who are middle-aged, 50–60 years (Bly, 1984). SSHL is often accompanied by tinnitus and vestibular symptoms (Wynne et al., 2001). It is estimated that vertigo accompanies hearing loss in 40% of SSHL cases (Mattox & Simmons, 1977). Possible causes of SSHL can be broadly classified into six categories: (1) viral infections, (2) compromised immune system, (3) vascular disease/disorder limiting the blood supply to the inner ear, (4) neurologic disorders, (5) neoplastic lesions, and (6) inner ear trauma such as disruptions of the membranous system within the cochlea. Diagnosis of hearing loss requires physical examination, detailed medical history, comprehensive audiological assessment, and laboratory studies including hematologic, urinalysis, serologic, and immunologic studies (Muller, Vrabec, & Quinn, 2001). Timing of intervention is critical in terms of hearing recovery. The opportunity for reversal of the hearing loss improves if treatment is received within the first 1 to 2 weeks of onset (Sing, 2006).

### Immune System in the Inner Ear

It was long thought that the inner ear was not capable of housing immune activity because the blood-labyrinth barrier, which separates the labyrinth from circulation, was presumed to separate the inner ear from cellular and humoral activity. However, in 1958 Dr. E. Lenhardt speculated that the inner ear could be affected by anticochlear antibodies in a group of patients with bilateral sudden sensorineural hearing loss (Bovo, Aimoni, & Martini, 2006). Many studies followed in an attempt to define the role of the immune system in the inner ear. Since the early 1980s studies have shown immune activity within the cochlea. It appears that the enolymphatic sac plays a key role. Damage to the delicate inner ear structures can occur secondary to the inflammatory process of immune activity, but also from the autoimmune reactions of the immune system response (Stroudt & Vrabec, 2000).

## Autoimmune Inner Ear Disease (AIED)

In 1979, Dr. Brian McCabe introduced the term *autoimmune hearing loss* and described the first cohort of 18 patients exhibiting similar clinical characteristics, whose symptoms did not fit into an existing disease classification. McCabe described a disease manifested as sensorineural hearing loss, which is bilateral, asymmetrical, and advances over a period of weeks or months, rather than in hours, days, or years, and which responds favorably to treatments traditionally used for autoimmune disease. The argument for a separate designation as autoimmune inner ear disease (AIED) was largely due to the potential for treatment, unlike the other causes of sensorineural hearing losses (McCabe, 1979). Many studies have been conducted to determine the exact relationship of the immune system to the audiovestibular system and, although much has been discovered, there is still no known cause for the disorder. Because the pathophysiology of the immune system in the inner ear has not been directly linked, another term for the disease process has been introduced: *immune-mediated ear disease*.

Although incidence figures are inexact, AIED is considered a rare disease making up less than 1% of all cases of hearing loss or dizziness (Bovo et al., 2006). AIED appears to affect more women (65%) than men (35%) and is most apt to occur in middle age (Hughes et al., 1996). There may be a genetic component to acquiring AIED. AIED can be a localized event, but in 15–30% of patients, there is an underlying systemic autoimmune disorder (systemic lupus, Cogan's syndrome, rheumatoid arthritis, etc.; Bovo et al., 2006).

The hallmark indicator for AIED is the progressive sensorineural hearing loss, which advances too quickly to be age-related hearing loss and too slowly to be classified as SSHL. It is often fluctuating and may originate in one ear first, followed several months later by symptoms in the other ear (79% of patients have bilateral hearing loss). Nearly 50% of patients also experience vestibular symptoms, which range in severity from general imbalance to violent, episodic vertigo. Tinnitus and fullness of the ears occurs in nearly 25–50% of cases (Bovo et al., 2006). Typically, the otologic physical examination of the patient is normal with no visible sign of disease to the outer or middle ear. Because they share similar symptoms, it is difficult to differentiate between AIED and Meniere's disease (MD). There is some evidence that MD may have an underlying autoimmune etiology, and one proposed subcategory of AIED is immune-mediated Meniere's disease (Harris & Keithley, 2003).

### Laboratory Testing for AIED

There is no specific diagnostic test available to definitively identify AIED. Diagnosis is achieved with a combination of clinical manifestation of hearing loss and vestibular symptoms, a detailed medical history, the response to immunosuppressant drugs, and evidence of immune activity in the blood. In a detailed comparison of patients with progressive hearing loss, Hirose, Wener, and Duckert (1999) recommended using either erythrocyte sedimentation rate (ESR) or C-reactive protein (CRP) and Western blot hsp-70 to investigate immune activity in the blood.

***Sedimentation Rate (Erythrocyte Sedimentation Rate or ESR)*** ESR or "sed-rate" is a measure of inflammatory or immune activity in the body. When erythrocytes, or red blood cells, are placed in a test tube, they settle to the bottom, creating sediment, while leaving the clear blood serum above it. The sed-rate is the distance in millimeters from the top that the layer of red blood cells falls within a given time, typically 1 hour. An elevated sed-rate indicates the presence of particular proteins generated during the inflammation process. The proteins cause the red blood cells to clump together and fall more quickly. Thus, the higher the sed-rate, the greater the degree of inflammation. Using a Westegren method, normal sed-rate for males is 0–15 millimeters per hour and for females, 0–20 millimeters per hour.

***C-Reactive Protein (CRP)*** CRP is a specific protein that, with increased presence in the blood, indicates immune activity. It is a marker of inflammation but also is theorized to have a protective mechanism against autoimmune disease (Szalai, 2004).

***Western Blot Analysis*** Western blot analysis is a technique used to identify the presence of a specific antibody in the serum. Specifically, a positive test for an antibody to an antigen of the molecular weight 68 kDA was considered evidence of AIED. Later studies suggest this antigen was actually heat shock protein 70 (hsp 70); however, this conclusion has since been disproved (Bovo et al., 2006). Presence of the antibody was also thought to predict a favorable response to steroids (Moscicki, San Martin, Quintero, Rauch, Nadol, & Bloch, 1994); however, the value of the Western blot analysis is now in question, since as many as 50–60% of patients who do respond favorably to steroid treatments are Western blot–negative (Bovo et al., 2006).

## Treatment for AIED

Successful treatment of AIED involves both medical and audiological management. It is important for both to be coordinated to maximize outcomes.

***Medical Treatment*** There is little consensus regarding the treatment regimens for AIED due to limited research, the relatively few cases seen, and the high number of hearing losses that spontaneously recover. Many cases of sudden hearing loss may be either ignored or discovered only as a secondary finding when investigating a different complaint. Unfortunate delays in identifying SSHL and/or AIED diminish the chances for treatment and potential recovery. Sudden hearing loss should be considered a medical emergency and warrants immediate attention. Steroid therapy is the typical treatment for SSHL and AIED, although the exact mechanism of steroid interaction with cochlear function is not well understood. The type of steroid, the length of treatment, and the delivery mechanism are all variables. A classic regimen is the administration of oral prednisone of up to 1 mg/kg for up to 1 month, with a tapered dosage to diminish use over the next 2-week period. Alternatives to steroids are methotrexate and cyclophosphamide (Cytoxan), but these medications have serious side effects and must be monitored closely (Sargent, 2002).

***Aural Rehabilitation*** CROS and BiCROS hearing aids are designed for people with unilateral hearing loss, to the extent that the poorer ear cannot benefit from traditional amplification (Hayes, 2006). Patients with relatively normal hearing in the "good" ear and no aidable hearing in the "poor" ear can benefit from the technology of contralateral routing of signal (CROS). A CROS aid is used to direct sound received on the patient's poor hearing side and transmit it to the better hearing side. This is done by placing a microphone on the poor ear, which receives the signal and transmits it to a receiver worn on the good ear. The patient hears the sound from the poor ear through the receiver on the good ear, while hearing sound from the good side naturally through the open ear canal. This can be accomplished either by hard-wiring the transmitter and receiver together with a wire worn behind the head, or wirelessly by frequency modulated transmission.

The BiCROS aid was developed for patients who also need amplification on the good ear due to reduced hearing acuity. The BiCROS differs from the CROS in that the good ear is fitted with a hearing aid, which receives the transmitted sound from the poor ear, but also functions as a stand-alone device for the better hearing ear.

CROS and BiCROS hearing aids allow users to hear sound they might otherwise miss from the poor ear. This gives awareness of sound and also some idea about location of the sound source. However, not all unilateral hearing loss patients will accept the aided configuration, because the sound crossed over to the good ear may interfere with processing natural sound in the better hearing ear and may prove confusing as to directionality of sound.

## Description of the Case

"Suddenly, I realized I couldn't hear anything from my right ear," she recalled. This dramatic discovery triggered a long journey: medical intervention, audiological rehabilitation, and an emotional struggle that continues today, nearly 25 years later. This case illustrates a classic sudden hearing loss of unknown etiology including the evolution of the disease, the number of specialists involved, and the emotional struggle of the patient and her family as they all learn to cope with the hearing and balance disorder. Information for this case presentation has been compiled from medical record review and personal interview with the patient.

### Background Information

Rev. Ella Star is a 75-year-old woman. An only child, she learned to entertain herself by reading, writing, and imaginative play. Her father was a high school principal and her mother a piano teacher in rural Kansas. Rev. Star grew up in a small town and loved summertime, when she lived with her grandparents on their farm. Perhaps it was these early experiences that allowed her to better cope with her eventual audiovestibular disability.

### Reason for the Referral

#### Onset of the Hearing and Balance Disorder

Rev. Star graduated from college with a bachelor's degree in music education. She married her husband in 1957 and settled in Iowa where they raised their son and daughter. She supplemented the family income by teaching piano lessons, substitute teaching in the elementary schools, freelance writing, and as an apprentice in the local string instrument repair shop. She is Caucasian, a nonsmoker, and does not drink alcohol. Rev. Star was physically active: walked, exercised regularly, and coached her daughter's church basketball team. After the youngest child left home for college, Rev. Star pursued her own dream: She enrolled in seminary in 1980 and in 1983, at the age of 50 years, was ordained a United Methodist minister. Her new career allowed her to study, write, teach, and counsel people of all ages.

In 1984, Rev. Star underwent a hysterectomy due to a fibroid tumor. As she recalls, some time during her 5-day hospitalization she developed "chirping sounds, like crickets" in the right ear. Approximately 6 weeks later, she consulted a local ear, nose, and throat physician to investigate the tinnitus complaint. An audiology evaluation was conducted and Rev. Star was surprised to learn that she had a "50% hearing loss" in the right ear. Until then, she had no awareness of a hearing problem. Neither medical intervention nor rehabilitation was prescribed by the ear, nose, and throat physician (Dr. 1), who told her she might have Meniere's disease, for which no treatment was recommended. She coped with the tinnitus by learning to "tune out" the sound much as she did as a child when she learned to ignore the sounds of her mother's piano students.

Approximately 1 year later, in July 1985, Rev. Star and her husband were vacationing. During the outbound flight, Rev. Star conversed with her fellow passenger seated to her right. Oddly, after the plane landed, she could no longer hear what the gentleman was saying to her. As they deplaned, Mr. Star noted that Rev. Star was also having difficulty negotiating the ramp. He had to hold her hand to steady her as he guided her through the airport. When they greeted their friends outside the airport, Rev. Star remembered apologizing because she couldn't hear anything from the right ear. No one paid much attention, and she eventually returned to her hotel room to be alone. Assuming that her hearing would return, she didn't consider it to be an emergency and vacation plans were unaltered.

Ironically, one of Rev. Star's parishioners had a daughter who had recently graduated with a master's degree in audiology. When learning of Rev. Star's condition, the parishioner volunteered to call her daughter for advice. The young audiologist contacted a colleague, who quickly arranged an appointment with an otologist at a national medical facility. Three weeks later, Mr. and Rev. Star drove out of state for the consultation.

## Findings of the Evaluation

The otologist (Dr. 2) found nothing remarkable on the physical examination. However, a detailed medical history evoked some additional information including a previous vertiginous attack approximately 2 years prior. His handwritten chart notes follow:

> 51 y.o. w.f. Pastor United Methodist Church who first noted a fullness and rushing sound like fluid in R ear 3 years ago. This eventually resolved. She developed sudden onset of vertigo and nausea ~ 2 years ago lasting < 24 h but followed by ~ 8 weeks of unsteadiness. This was followed by mild positional vertigo which to some extent persists. More tinnitus and decreased hearing became apparent in January 1984 – this fluctuated some in the past year and a half – most recent outside audiogram 2/11/1985 shows 50+dB loss & 36% discrimination. No vertiginous episodes. Audio today – ō R. Now had fluctuation in L ear after flying ~ 1 month ago. No pain.

A diagnostic audiology evaluation on August 22, 1985, revealed a mild degree, sloping sensorineural hearing loss in the left ear with excellent word recognition at 40 dB SL. There was no response to air or bone conduction stimuli in the right ear. Stenger was negative. Immitance findings showed Type A tympanograms in both ears. Contralateral and ipsilateral acoustic reflex thresholds were absent when stimulating the right ear, and present at expected levels when stimulating the left ear. Acoustic reflex decay was negative at 500 and 2,000 in the left ear.

Electronystagmography also conducted on August 22, revealed no spontaneous nystagmus observed in any of the positions tested. Cold and warm water caloric stimulation revealed a unilateral weakness on the right: 0% response in the right ear and 100% in the left ear (nystagmus was suppressed with eyes open). Ice water caloric stimulation to right ear revealed 3.7 degrees/second left beating nystagmus. Findings were consistent with right peripheral deficit.

Dr. 2 noted that the condition "may be hydrops but unusual scenario." He ordered a computed tomography (CT) scan, which was negative with no evidence of lesion. He suggested a repeat audiological evaluation in 1 year and a hearing aid evaluation for a CROS aid. It was speculated that the right ear hearing loss was the result of a viral infection, which would be unlikely to affect the hearing in the left ear.

In December that same year, Rev. Star experienced increased difficulty communicating on the telephone. Terrified that she was losing hearing in her left ear, she immediately made an appointment with her local ear, nose, and throat physician, Dr. 1. After reviewing the results of a new audiogram, Dr. 1 told her that he "didn't see much difference since the last visit." Astonished and angered, Rev. Star responded: "I've lost all of the hearing and balance in my right ear. Now I'm starting to lose the hearing in my left ear, and you don't see the difference?" Dr. 1 left the room and called Dr. 2., the otologist who had seen her in August. After discussing her case, it was agreed to refer her to another otologist, Dr. 3, who had expertise in autoimmune inner ear disease (AIED). An appointment was scheduled within 2 weeks.

### Diagnosis: AIED

When she asked Dr. 3 how one arrives at a diagnosis of autoimmune inner ear disease, he replied: "By ruling out every other known disease." The process of elimination was well underway and a pattern was beginning to emerge. By looking at Rev. Star's total health history, rather than at the audiovestibular mechanism as an isolated system, seemingly unrelated symptoms became connected. A review of salient points follows:

- In college, Rev. Star had episodes of canker sores in her mouth, throat, and bronchial tubes. Later episodes included lesions in the throat and mouth that responded to prednisone treatments.
- Rev. Star's mother had a long history of Meniere's disease and wore hearing aids in both ears.
- During a routine physical done in her early 40s, a blood test revealed an extremely high erythrocyte sedimentation rate (ESR). Her internal medicine physician told her at the time that she could expect to develop rheumatoid arthritis in the future.
- In approximately 1982 she experienced aural fullness and a rushing sound in the right ear, which spontaneously resolved.
- In 1983 she experienced vertigo so severe that she was hospitalized overnight. She was treated with medication for 3 months and had lingering unsteadiness.
- In 1984 she experienced tinnitus in the right ear while hospitalized for a hysterectomy. That summer she noticed that she couldn't keep her balance when riding her bicycle and was unable to make turns when riding. When ascending and descending the steps in her home, she found herself reaching for the banister to make the turn at the bottom of the stairwell.
- In May 1984 she was diagnosed with sensorineural hearing loss in the right ear.
- Later that year she developed severe episcleritis in both eyes. She was treated by her internal medicine physician with monthly steroid injections, which alleviated the symptoms.
- She frequently experienced shortness of breath, which she attributed to being out of shape, although she was physically active. She described "huffing and puffing" when walking a short distance uphill. She was easily fatigued in spite of being weight appropriate.
- In July 1985 she lost all hearing and balance function in the right ear and had mild hearing loss in the left ear. In December 1985 hearing in the left ear decreased.
- In December 1985 her ESR was 93 mm/hr (abnormal).

For Rev. Star, the AIED diagnosis was based on her medical history, which included other autoimmune conditions: canker sores, episcleritis (inflammation of the connective tissue between the conjunctiva and the sclera), and unspecified lung condition causing shortness of breath. The acquisition of the hearing loss fit the time course of AIED, namely, sensorineural hearing loss in one ear, occurring over weeks or months, followed by fluctuating hearing loss in the opposite ear. The hearing loss was preceded by aural fullness, tinnitus, and vertigo. She had at least a 10-year history of high ESRs. In the subsequent years after the initial diagnosis, her CRP has been abnormally high. In 1999, during an episode of reduced hearing, Rev. Star tested negative for the Western blot 69 kDA, even though she did respond favorably to the steroid treatment.

## Course of Treatments

In 1985, Dr. 3 prescribed aggressive treatment to stop the progression of hearing loss in the left ear. Rev. Star underwent 2 weeks of chemotherapy with intravenous injection of cyclophosphamide (Cytoxan): 30 minutes/day, followed by 3 months of oral prednisone and immunosuppresants. Cytoxan has been used for treating rheumatoid arthritis, multiple sclerosis, and leukemias. After the conclusion of the treatment, Rev. Star had a mild, sloping to moderate degree sensorineural hearing loss in the left ear. Word recognition was excellent in quiet. She became extremely ill from the side effects of the powerful drug; however, Rev. Star credited this treatment with preserving the hearing in the left ear.

Rev. Star's subsequent health care involved a team of subspecialty physicians under the supervision of a rheumatologist for her continued physical ailments. She continued to exhibit ulcerations in the throat, soft palate, and mouth; dyspnea upon exertion; and episcleritis, scleral thinning, and arthritis. In November 1986 she was diagnosed as possibly having

Wegener's granulomatosis. This, and also Behcet's disease, were subsequently ruled out after a nasal septum biopsy. Pulmonary function testing and an open lung biopsy led to diagnoses of pulmonary hypertension with possible thromboembolic component. Her symptoms are managed by medication: anticoagulant, immunosuppressants, and tapered doses of both oral and topical prednisone for the reoccurring bouts of episcleritis. Because of past Cytoxan treatment, she was monitored for hematuria (blood in urine). Due to long-term steroid treatment a medication was given to counteract the effect of calcium malabsorption.

From the time of the initial AIED diagnosis (December 1985) until December 2008, Rev. Star has experienced multiple reoccurrences of left ear hearing fluctuations. There were approximately four episodes/year between 1986 and 1988, which reduced in frequency to two episodes/year until 2006. There was one reoccurrence in 2007 and one in 2008. Each episode was treated with high doses of oral prednisone in tapered regimen. The most recent course prescribed was 60 mg/day for 2 weeks, followed by 1 day each at 40 mg/day, 30 mg/day, 20 mg/day, and 10 mg/day. Additional diagnostic tests were conducted over the years, including in 1998 "ENG Tullio and neurocom pressure" tests, which were negative in both ears.

Audiology evaluations are conducted throughout the treatment to monitor hearing change. Typically, there is a 10–25 dB drop in the low–mid-frequency thresholds. Usually, one to two days after beginning the prednisone treatment, Rev. Star noticed a marked subjective improvement in hearing. Objectively, her hearing thresholds showed a return to her baseline levels at the end of the steroid therapy; however, over the course of 23 years, there was some permanent decrease of about 15–20 dB across all test frequencies. Interestingly, word recognition remained excellent at a comfortable listening level in a quiet environment. Refer to Figure 53.1 for audiogram results from 1985 to 2008.

## Living with Hearing and Balance Loss

Because communication is so integral to human interaction, the effects of hearing loss extend to all relationships. Adjusting to a loss of hearing and balance function has implications for both career and family life.

### At Work

According to Rev. Star, being a good pastor was "more about listening than it is about preaching." Several listening situations are encountered, from one-on-one counseling sessions to large social gatherings, with all types of meetings in between. She needed to hear children

FIGURE 53.1 Air Conduction Thresholds for Three Audiograms: 1985, After Initial Onset of Total Right Hearing Loss; 1990; and Most Current, 2008

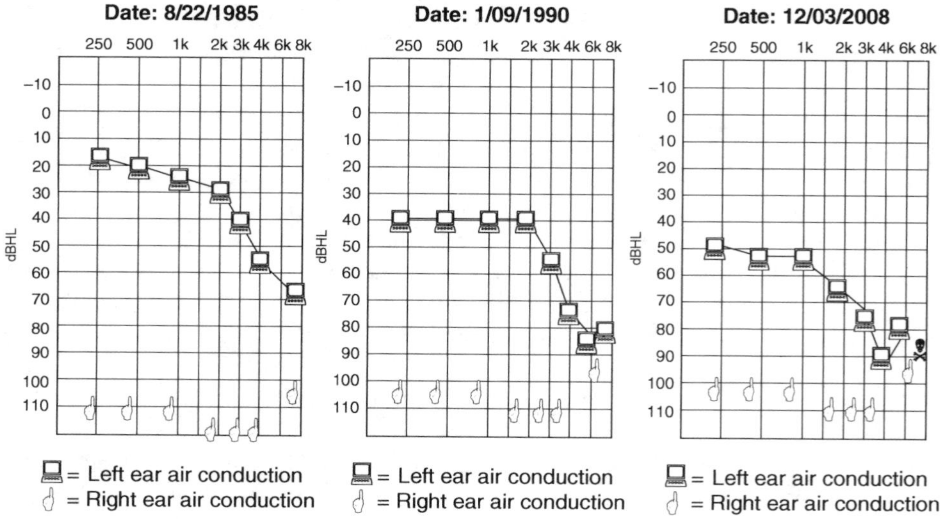

Date: 8/22/1985 | Date: 1/09/1990 | Date: 12/03/2008

= Left ear air conduction
= Right ear air conduction

when teaching Sunday school, elderly people in nursing homes, and sick patients in hospitals. There were weddings, funerals, and multiple worship services to officiate weekly. She was integrally involved in composing, rehearsing, and performing music in her ministry. The repercussions of not responding appropriately in conversation or worse, failing to respond at all, could be severe. Parishioners tend to take it personally when the pastor doesn't acknowledge them. While there were humorous situations caused by misunderstanding words, there were more serious instances of parishioners with hurt feelings from being "ignored" and accusations of purposeful neglect. She desperately needed to hear well and decided she must be open and honest about her hearing loss with her congregation. To maximize sound reception, Rev. Star was fitted with a wireless behind-the-ear BiCROS hearing aid. Having a transmitter on the right side allowed her to know when someone on her right side was speaking; however, she still struggled with sound localization and with understanding speech in a noisy environment, such as the fellowship hour after a church service. As her hearing and other health conditions worsened, she eventually applied for and received medical disability many years before she would have voluntarily retired.

### At Home

Mr. Star, a loving and devoted husband, had to face the reality of his wife's disabilities. He battled his own impatience with having to repeat himself, the frustration of watching his normally astute wife misunderstand conversations, and he grieved lost intimacy and easy laughter. To be effective, communication had to be purposeful and calculated, rather than spontaneous and unconscious. Simple accommodations included rearranging the furniture in the living room so that Mr. Star's chair was on Rev. Star's left side. More difficult accommodations included controlling anger and exasperation in his voice when saying things the second or third time. There were countless medical appointments and the constant worry that some day, the left ear will suddenly drop permanently, making natural communication all but impossible.

The Stars' son and daughter were both grown and away from home when the symptoms of the disease began. At first, there was denial regarding the severity and permanency of the disorder. Like most people, they were unfamiliar with the complications hearing loss adds to conversations and family activities. As the hearing loss fluctuations occurred, their daughter noticed that the quality of Rev. Star's voice changed when her hearing loss increased. This became an important indicator to identify the need for intervention. Both children have become very supportive of their parents through the years. Their daughter researched options for amplified telephones and encouraged Rev. Star to request assistive listening devices at the theater.

Hearing loss changed many of Rev. Star's daily activities. Although she was able to continue playing piano, she eventually withdrew from singing in the choir and from participating in other musical groups. Listening to recorded music at home became less pleasurable, and she stopped listening to music as a pastime. She still enjoyed attending live music events and she and Mr. Star held season tickets to the symphony.

### Coping Strategies

Accepting Rev. Star's new identity as "disabled" came with many changes. The Stars got a puppy and trained her to bark when the phone and doorbell rang. Rev. Star learned that she had to see where she was walking to compensate for the lack of balance. She began to carry a flashlight with her to illuminate the pathway whenever it was dark. Her physical activity changed since something as simple as ducking to avoid a Frisbee could result in a fall. Often, she steadied herself by holding on to another person as she walked, making her feel older than her true age. She stopped swimming and boating to avoid the danger of disorientation while under water. The side effects of large doses of prednisone caused extreme weight gains and mood swings. She constantly apologized for getting things wrong and sensed the negative reactions of others when she did not hear accurately. As painful as it was to give up her ministry, she could no longer trust her hearing ability. She was unable to answer questions with certainty or assume that what she heard was correct. When asked recently what it was like to have a hearing loss, Rev. Star said, "The most insulting part for me is that I am an educated, intelligent, woman. Yet when I make a mistake in a conversation, people look at me as if I am *stupid*."

The combination of the general health disorders and the effort involved to listen made it easier to retreat into her hobbies. Being on immunosuppressant medication makes one more susceptible to any infection and the patient is advised to avoid crowds of people and germ-rich environments. While the autoimmune disease kept her away from many social gatherings, she enjoyed being alone to write, sew, and create jewelry. When she stopped working, she discontinued using the BiCROS-style hearing aid. Over the years she used in-the-ear aids and now used a monaural digital behind-the-ear–style hearing aid with FM compatibility on her left ear. Her positive attitude toward overcoming her limitations contributed to an eagerness to teach others about hearing loss, balance disorders, and autoimmune disease. Rev. Star intended to donate her temporal bones to research and has registered with the National Temporal Bone, Hearing, and Balance Pathology Resource Registry.

## Analysis of Client's Response to Intervention

Key to understanding this case is the difficulty with regard to diagnosing SSHL. Rev. Star experienced the importance of consulting physicians and audiologists who were current with the latest research and connected with their professional peers. The diagnosis of AIED occurred in 1985, just six years after the hallmark study proposing the definition of AIED was published. It took three different physicians, three different audiologists, and over one year of elapsed time to arrive at a diagnosis. There are several relevant observations in reviewing the facts of this case study:

- The technological advancements in the past 25 years have yielded new understandings of how the ear functions and new diagnostic tools have been developed. Still, the primary diagnostic information for AIED are the clinical manifestations, supplemented by medical history and laboratory studies. Today, the audiologist can play a larger role in the diagnosis of AIED by providing a comprehensive assessment strategy and collaborating with other medical professionals.
  - Current audiology test batteries might include:
    - Pure-tone air and bone conduction audiometry
    - Stenger
    - Speech audiometry
    - Multifrequency tympanometry
    - Contra and ipsilaterally stimulated acoustic reflexes
    - Acoustic reflex decay
    - Otoacoustic emissions
    - Electrophysiological tests including early, middle, late evoked potentials
    - Electrocochleography
    - Electronystagmography/videonystamography
    - Posturography
    - Rotary chair testing
  - Hearing aid evaluation and appropriate aural rehabilitation
  - Tinnitus assessment and treatment
  - Vestibular rehabilitation
- The disease process began several years before the diagnosis was made. A culmination of episodes and comprehensive medical history intake was needed to identify the pattern of the audiovestibular disorder and connect the seemingly unrelated symptoms. According to Rev. Star's report, Dr. 1 did not advise any further investigation nor rehabilitation for her symptoms in 1984. There is still risk today that a diagnosis of AIED will be overlooked because there is not one definitive diagnostic test (Bovo et al., 2006).
- The diagnostic process involved ruling out several known disease patterns, including vestibular schwannoma, Meniere's disease, viral infection, and vascular disorder.

- The effectiveness and necessity of Cytoxan chemotherapy is questionable. Though the patient attributes this treatment with stopping the progression of the left ear hearing loss, there is no way of knowing how the outcome would differ with a different treatment approach. The side effects of Cytoxan are unpleasant to the patient and have potential long-term serious effects. For Rev. Star, there was no recovery of hearing thresholds after the Cytoxan treatment. Subsequent record review by another physician indicated the treatment was "to no avail."
- Although early in the disease process Rev. Star experienced vertigo severe enough to be hospitalized, she apparently did not see an ear, nose, and throat specialist nor an audiologist at the time. The primary care physician, emergency room physician, otologist, and audiologist should be in collaboration when patients exhibit audiovestibular dysfunction.
- Unilateral hearing loss has unique behavioral effects: difficulty localizing sound, increased difficulty hearing in background noise, and lack of awareness of activity on the impaired side. CROS or BiCROS hearing aids offer some benefit for some, but not all patients.
- Fluctuation in the hearing levels in the left ear pose challenges for treatment and rehabilitation management.
  - The patient must be quick to recognize a subtle change in hearing to obtain medical/pharmacological treatment as quickly as possible.
  - The hearing aid must be adaptable to compensate for swings in hearing acuity.
  - The spouse and family must learn to accept variations in the patient's ability to communicate and respond to sound.
- Professionals often focus on the effects of hearing loss, yet overlook the complications caused by loss of balance function.
- After the initial diagnosis and treatment, a multidisciplinary approach to medical management is important. Rev. Star had numerous subspecialty physicians all under the supervision of her rheumatologist. She relied heavily on her audiologist to communicate test results with the otologist and manage her hearing aid status. An audiologist has the opportunity to become an advocate for the hearing impaired patient and may also be a resource for the patient when filing a disability claim for hearing loss.

The process of acquiring and adjusting to AIED challenged Rev. Star physically, emotionally, and spiritually. Her family strived to be supportive and understanding. They became keenly aware of the value of good hearing and the fragility of health. Regardless of the hardship, Rev. Star was determined to hear and to be heard no matter how much effort it took. She knew that although the disease changed her, she was still the vital, intelligent, and strong woman she was before the disease.

## Author Note

Many of the facts in this case were drawn from medical records and personal patient interview, used with permission from the patient. However, some descriptive and identifying information, as well as location references, have been fabricated to preserve anonymity. Any resemblance to actual people or places should be assumed to be accidental. Note that all instances of sudden sensorineural hearing loss and autoimmune disease are different and should be treated on a case-by-case basis. This case study is not to be used as a treatment protocol.

## References


Argup, C. (2008). Immune-mediated audiovestibular disorders in the paediatric population: A review. *International Journal of Audiology, 47*(9), 560–565.

Bovo, R., Aimoni, C., & Martini, A. (2006). Immune-mediated inner ear disease. *Acta Oto-Laryngologica, 126,* 1012–1021.

Byl, F. M., Jr. (1984). Sudden hearing loss: Eight years' experience and suggested prognostic table. *Laryngoscope, 94*(5, Pt. 1), 647–61.

Harris, J., & Keithley, E. (2003). Autoimmune inner ear disease. In J. Snow Jr. & J. Ballenger (Eds.), *Ballenger's otorhinolaryngology head and neck surgery* (16th ed., pp. 396–407). Ontario: BC Decker.

Hayes, D. (2006). A practical guide to CROS/BiCROS fittings. Retrieved from Audiology Online: http://www.audiologyonline.com/articles/article_detail.asp?wc=1&article_id=1632

Hirose, K., Wener, M. H., & Duckert, L. G. (1999). Utility of laboratory testing in autoimmune inner ear disease. *Laryngoscope, 109,* 1749–1754.

Hughes, G., Freedman, M., Haberkamp, T., & Guay, M. (1996). Sudden sensorineural hearing loss. *Otolaryngologic Clinics of North America, 29*(3), 393–405.

Mattox, D., & Simmons, F. (1977). Natural history of sudden sensorineural hearing loss. *Annals of Otology, Rhinology & Laryngology, 86,* 463–80.

McCabe, B. (1979). Autoimmune sensorineural hearing loss. *Annals of Otology, Rhinology, and Laryngology, 88*(5), 585–589.

Moscicki, R. A., San Martin, J. E., Quintero, C. H., Rauch, S.D., Nadol, J.B. Jr., & Bloch, K. J. (1994). Serum antibody to inner ear proteins in patients with progressive hearing loss. Correlation with disease activity and response to corticosteroid treatment. *Journal of the American Medical Association, 272*(8), 611–616.

Muller, C., Vrabec, J., & Quinn, F. (2001). Sudden sensorineural hearing loss. Grand Rounds Presentation, UTMB, Dept. of Otolaryngology. Retrieved from: http://www.utmb.edu/otoref/Grnds/SuddenHearingLoss-010613/SSNHL.htm

Sargent, E.W. (2002). Autoimmune inner ear diseases: Autoimmune disease with audiovestibular involvement. Retrieved from Audiology Online: http://www.audiologyonline.com/articles/article_detail.asp?article_id=364

Sing, T. (2006). Prognostic indicators in idiopathic sudden sensorineural hearing loss in a Malaysian hospital. *The Internet Journal of Otorhinolaryngology, 5*(2). Retrieved from: http://www.ispub.com/journal/the_internet_journal_of_otorhinolaryngology/volume_5_number_2_21/article/prognostic_indicators_in_idiopathic_sudden_sensorineural_hearing_loss_in_a_malaysian_hospital.html

Stroudt, R., & Vrabec, J. (2000). Autoimmune inner ear disease. Grand Rounds Presentation, UTMB, Dept. of Otolaryngology. Retrieved from: http://www.utmb.edu/otoref/grnds/Autoimmune-Ear-200001/Autoimmune-Inner-Ear.doc

Szalai, A. (2004). C-reactive protein and autoimmune disease: Facts and conjectures. *Clinical & Developmental Immunology, 11*(3/4), 221–226.

Wynne, M., Diefendorf, A., & Fritsch, M. (2001, December 26). Sudden Hearing Loss. *The ASHA Leader.* Retrieved from: http://www.asha.org/Publications/leader/2001/011226/sudden_hearing_loss.htm

# CASE 54

# Jack: Noise-Induced Hearing Loss: A Work-Related Investigation

*Deanna K. Meinke*

## Conceptual Knowledge

### Noise-Induced Hearing Loss

The relationship between loud sound and hearing loss is well documented. Historically, the phrase *noise-induced hearing loss* (NIHL) has been the nomenclature used to label sensorineural hearing loss caused by hazardous sound levels. More recently, "noise induced" is being replaced by a broader term, *sound induced,* to include loud sound sources not typically characterized as "noisy" or "undesirable." Sound, if it is loud enough, has the potential to cause hearing loss, regardless of how it is perceived by the individual. For instance, the roar of a motorcycle engine, which is thrilling to one person but exacerbating to another, poses a potentially hazardous sound exposure to both listeners. For the purposes of this case report, the terminology NIHL will be utilized to maintain consistency with references to the disorder in the literature and clinical reports.

Hazardous sound exposure has the potential to damage delicate hair cells and other structures in the auditory system (Henderson, Bielfefeld, Harris, & Hu, 2006; Henderson, Bielfefeld, Hue, & Nicotera, 2007). This results in hearing loss most evident at the frequencies of 3, 4, or 6 kHz, at least in the early stages. When plotted on an audiogram, this characteristic dip in the hearing threshold data is commonly referred to as a "noise-notch" and is first evident during the decade 10–19 years old (see Figure 54.1). Gradual onset NIHL may not be subjectively apparent to an individual until it worsens to a greater degree of loss and spreads to adjacent audiometric test frequencies due to continued unprotected exposures. The presence of a "noise notch" in combination with a history of unprotected noise exposure usually distinguishes NIHL from other causes of hearing loss. NIHL diagnosis is confounded by the presence of age-related hearing loss in later decades (60+ years), since the "notch" configuration erodes into a sloping configuration as illustrated in Figure 54.1 for the 70+ decades. Consequently, ongoing periodic monitoring records that include .5, 1, 2, 3, 4, 6, and 8 kHz are critical for regulatory compliance and the determination of work-related NIHL.

## Temporary vs. Permanent Threshold Shift

Hazardous sound exposure can cause both temporary and permanent damage to the auditory system depending on the sound level and duration of sound exposure(s). Audiometric monitoring is used to detect changes in hearing, which may be either short-term noise-induced temporary threshold shift (NITTS) or long-term noise-induced permanent threshold shift (NIPTS). Both ongoing and instantaneous hazardous sound exposures have the potential to cause NIPTS. In the case of acoustic trauma, hearing loss occurs instantaneously after noise exposure and is immediately evident to the affected individual. Specifically, hearing a firearm shot (Humes, Joellenbeck, & Durch, 2005), a vehicle airbag deployment (Yaremchuk, 2001), or an explosion (Van Campen, Dennis, Hanlin, King, & Velderman, 1999) are reported to cause NIPTS. In the occupational setting, long-term unprotected exposure to hazardous levels of noise leads to NIPTS.

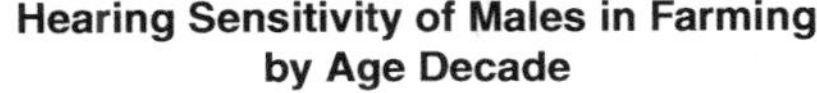

Hearing Sensitivity of Males in Farming
by Age Decade


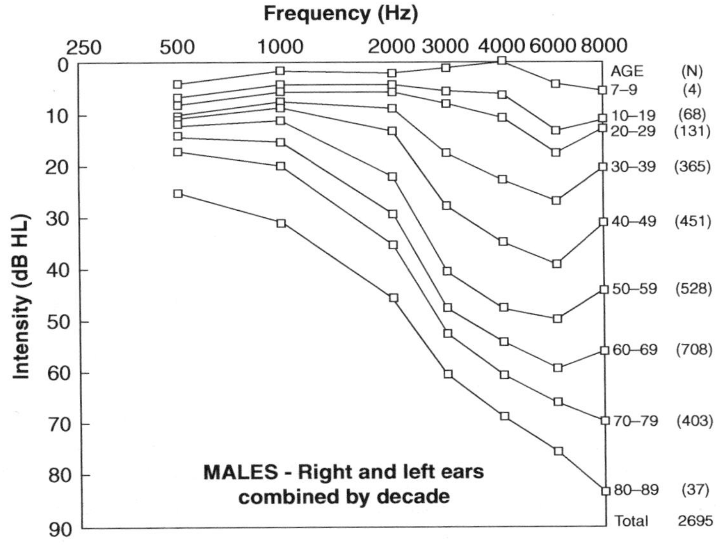


FIGURE 54.1 Averaged Audiometric Threshold Values Plotted by Age Decade for U.S. Males Engaged in Farming

* Note the changes in the notched configuration beginning at 6 kHz for those age 10–19 years.

*Source:* Reprinted with permission from ADVANCE Newsmagazines; Lankford, Zurales, Garrett & Delorier. 10-Year Study of Agricultural Workers. *Advance for Audiologists,* 4, #5, pp. 34, 36–37, 2002.

### Significant Threshold Shift

The audiometric monitoring component of occupational hearing loss prevention programs defines a significant threshold shift (STS) as an average change in hearing of 10 dB or more for the test frequencies of 2,000, 3,000, and 4,000 Hz in either ear. Baseline testing is required to be performed on individuals who have not been exposed to noise within the previous 14 hours to avoid the effects of NITTS on baseline testing references. If an STS occurs and is confirmed on subsequent tests, then the baseline reference is revised to a new reference for determining future significant changes in hearing.

### Occupational Noise-Induced Hearing Loss

NIHL is among the top three most common occupational illnesses. Approximately 10 million persons in the United States (Jackson & Duffy, 1998) and 25–30 million in Europe (Quaranta, Sallustio, & Quaranta, 2001) have permanent hearing loss from long-term continuous noise exposure or acoustic trauma. The National Institute for Occupational Safety and Health (NIOSH; 2004) noted a 26% increase in hearing loss between 1971 and 1990 for 18–44-year-olds. The most commonly recognized "at-risk" occupations include agriculture (farming, forestry, commercial fishing), mining, construction, manufacturing, utilities, transportation (aircraft, railroad, and marine), service personnel (firefighters, emergency medical technicians, surgeons), musicians, and military. Employers are required to report the specifics of any work-related hearing loss on the Occupational Safety and Health Administration (OSHA) 300 log per the requirements of 29 CFR 1904.10 (2002). Hager (2006) summarized the U.S. Bureau of Labor Statistics data relative to the OSHA injury and illness recordable hearing loss statistics for 2004 and reported that 11% of all OSHA recordable occupational injuries were due to hearing loss.

### Prevalence

Audiologists are routinely involved in the evaluation, diagnosis, and treatment of patients with NIHL and tinnitus. Patients with hearing loss and/or tinnitus resulting from noise exposure are pervasive in the ontological clinical population. Dobie (1993) estimates that approximately 20% of patients may attribute at least a part of their hearing loss to noise exposure. Godlee (1992) estimates that 4.5% of the general population has NIHL, as compared to 35–51% of the occupationally noise-exposed population. Estimates of the prevalence of tinnitus in noise-exposed workers range from 10–58% (Axelsson, 1995; Coles, Smith, & Davis, 1990; Cooper, 1994). Workers' compensation is given for tinnitus as well as hearing loss in some jurisdictions (Dobie & Megerson, 2000). Tinnitus is also implicated as an early warning indicator of NIHL (Griest and Bishop, 1998). It is important for clinicians to consider tinnitus history and status when evaluating patients with NIHL and when managing programs for the prevention of NIHL.

### Preventive Approaches

Audiologists have numerous opportunities to interface with patients exposed to hazardous sound levels. Four models incorporating preventative approaches for practicing audiology are the (1) regulatory model, (2) educational model, (3) medical treatment model, and (4) preventative medicine model (Meinke & Stephenson, 2007). A regulatory model relates to the audiologist's role in hearing loss prevention programs mandated by the Occupational Safety and Health Administration (OSHA), the Mine Safety and Health Administration (MSHA), and the Federal Railroad Administration (FRA). The following case study illustrates the regulatory role of the audiologist.

## Description of the Case

Adults are known to be at risk for progressive sensorineural hearing loss if unprotected from hazardous sound exposures over a lifetime. Early detection and intervention is critical for the prevention of noise-induced hearing loss whether due to occupational or avocational sources. In the absence of preventive action, hearing loss may occur and accrue to a disabling degree. Employees who are hearing-impaired are likely to seek workers' compensation for the disabling condition if they believe the employer is responsible for the noise levels that may have damaged their hearing. This case illustrates that a professional team-based approach, combined with critical investigation and diagnostics facilitates individual considerations for workers' compensation claim determinations and settlements. More importantly, it demonstrates that when opportunities for early intervention are missed, additional hearing loss ensues and may be costly to the employer and/or insurer as well as to the employee.

## Background Information

This case of Jack, a worker with NIHL, describes the history, audiometric data, noise exposure profile, and interventions provided by a team of health and safety professionals. There were missed opportunities for the prevention of NIHL in Jack and the reader is encouraged to identify these stages and implement a more proactive, preventive medicine approach in his or her own practice. Note that this case occurred in Colorado so allowances should be made for variations in workers' compensation laws in different states. It is imperative that clinicians be familiar with the workers' compensation statutes and requirements in their geographical region(s). Additionally, this case was uncontested and ultimately was processed through the state workers' compensation insurer for settlement. The employer was obligated under OSHA CFR 29 1910.95 (1983) for hearing loss prevention and OSHA 29 CFR 1904.10 (2002) for occupational injury and illness reporting requirements.

### Relevant Facts

Jack, a 58-year-old male, was first evaluated for the workers' compensation claim in January 2003 and the claim was settled in November 2003. There was no evidence of functional hearing loss and he did not require special testing to rule out malingering. The involved health and safety professionals and their affiliations included the following:

- Industrial hygienist (IH); employer affiliated
- Occupational health nurse (OHN); employer affiliated
- Occupational physician (OPhys); consultant to employer
- Occupational audiologist (OAud); consultant to employer and occupational physician
- Otolaryngologist (ENT); private practice provider
- Clinical audiologist (CAud); private practice provider, affiliated with ENT
- Patient (WRK); employed as a maintenance worker by the employer

## Patient-Reported History Information

The initial case history may be the most important adjunct to the audiologist's test battery, and it often requires more than one effort to complete since information has to be gathered not only from the patient and referring physician, but also from the worksite. A comprehensive history provides direction and confidence for future clinical decisions and reporting. It also serves as a check for consistency between histories given to the occupational health nurse, the physicians, and the audiologists at different times. An example of the complete case history taken for WRK (Jack) via a patient interview (March 2003), is summarized in the following paragraphs. All relevant topics are included for reference.

### General Medical History

Jack was negative for diabetes, kidney disease, thyroid disease, autoimmune disease, neurological disorders/disease, seizure disorders, high blood pressure, circulatory system disorders, stroke, cancer/tumors, metabolic disorders, head injury/unconsciousness, meningitis, and scarlet fever. There was a positive history of childhood mumps and measles. He had a long history of tobacco smoking.

## Otologic Medical History

Jack had negative otologic history for ear pain, drainage, fullness, and discomfort. There were no reports of facial numbness/paralysis, head injuries, ear surgeries, cerumen impactions, or dizziness/vertigo. There were no reports of allergies or sinus/cold symptoms affecting his hearing in the past. He denied taking any ototoxic medications (quinines, -myacins, or long-term high-level aspirin regimens) or knowingly being exposed to chemicals/solvents. There was a negative history for familial hearing loss. Jack reported gradual onset of bilateral hearing loss and noted that he had had problems communicating for the past several years. The loss was not subjectively asymmetrical and did not seem to fluctuate. He also reported bilateral mild tinnitus and described it as primarily "annoying in quiet." He had not been previously evaluated by an ENT or audiologist as part of his personal health care and had never worn hearing aids. He stated that his hearing was checked intermittently at work in the past and that the results were "abnormal, but nothing was done about it."

## Communication History

Jack reported minimal problems understanding speech in quiet or communicating in the course of performing his job duties. He indicated difficulty understanding speech in noisy listening environments, in meetings, on the telephone, and while transcribing voice messages. Warning signals and safety hazard communications were audible and supplemented by a pager. His family complained about his ability to hear at home and during social activities.

## Work-Related Environmental Noise Exposure and Hearing Protector Use History

Jack reported no school/vocational, voluntary work, or second job noise exposure. His work related history is as follows:

- 1967–1969: Served in the United States Air Force with intermittent noise exposure from jet engine props; occasional earmuff use when exposed.
- 1969–1971: Assembled vehicles with some noise exposure reported. No hearing protection was used.
- 1971–1972:[1] Worked a variety of different jobs (building construction and maintenance) in a large manufacturing plant with variable noise exposures; no hearing protection was used.
- 1973: Drove a truck for manufacturer; no hearing protection was used.
- 1973–1993: Worked in mechanical equipment rooms and provided maintenance services to the plant. No hearing protection was used in the early employment years. Earmuffs were required for specific tasks in the later employment years, with hearing protector use "some of the time."
- 1994–2003: Worked in a different mechanical division. Hearing protection was required in the work area, especially while grinding, welding, and using jackhammers. Jack reported faithful use of a foam moldable earplug on a cord during the past few years.

Jack was asked, "What do you think caused your hearing loss?" He answered that between 1989 and 1996 he was required to use a jackhammer and a hammer chisel to remove brittle tile epoxy and cut cement from the plant flooring. He stated that this was very difficult and time-consuming work. He reportedly worked on his hands and knees chiseling the floor for extended periods of time. He noted that earmuffs were the only style of hearing protection offered to employees at that time. Jack had to wear a face-shield to keep tile pieces from flying into his face. The earmuffs were not compatible with the face-shield and consequently hearing protection was not worn. He stated, "I had to make a choice, my ears or my eyes, and I chose my eyes." Reportedly, earplug-style hearing protectors were not available to the workers until 1995. (Note: Jack reportedly had been advised that since "earmuffs are better than earplugs," the employer did not offer both styles to the workforce).

### Nonoccupational Noise Exposure and Hearing Protector Use History

- Firearms: Lifelong exposures as a hunter and target shooter. Jack reported that he is right-handed and shoots right-handed. Frequency of firearm use was reported as once a year while hunting big game. Hearing protection was not used when hunting. Earmuffs were used for target shooting since the 1990s.
- Power tools: Operated household power tools including lawnmowers, weed eaters, construction power tools (saws, sanders, etc.) with occasional use of earmuffs at home reported for "loud tasks."
- Chainsaw: Occasional use of chainsaw for firewood cutting. Earmuffs were used.
- Farm equipment: Grew up on a farm and returned to the family farm to help during planting and harvesting seasons. No hearing protection was used.

### Supplemental Occupational Physician History and Exam Information (March 2003)

- Jack reported routine use of ibuprofen for headaches.
- Jack smoked 1 package of cigarettes per day for about 30 years; he was tobacco-free for the past 4 years, but he began smoking again this year.
- Jack did not do woodworking or sheet metal work or have other noisy hobbies besides hunting.
- Jack enjoyed calf roping and arrowhead hunting as hobbies.
- On physical exams, ear canals were clear of wax impactions and otoscopy was normal bilaterally. No cervical adenopathy was evident and his throat was clear.

### Employer-Reported History Information

The industrial hygienist (IH) and occupational health nurse (OHN) provided information in March 2003 after review and summary of noise surveillance and employer medical records.

### Occupational Noise Exposure

Personal noise dosimetry measurements were not obtained on Jack during the course of employment. Area sound-level measurements were not completely available for most of Jack's employment period. Only a few potentially hazardous exposures were reported:

- 1994–1996: Mechanical room area sound-level measurement reported as 83–92 dBA. Hearing protection was required for these work areas.
- 1996–1998: Area sound-level measurements for various shops and mechanical rooms ranged between 74–100 dBA. Hearing protection was required when operating certain pieces of equipment such as metal hammers, hand-held air motor grinders, welding grinders, band saws, metal spinner, metal shearer, metal saw, and metal hole-punch.
- 1998–2003: No noise exposure records were available. Employee frequented and maintained mechanical rooms with boilers, chillers, and large industrial building fans.

### Hearing Protection Device (HPD) Records

Hearing protection became available at the plant in the middle 1980s. At the time the history was provided, the IH reported that Jack was utilizing a foam expandable earplug with a noise reduction rating (NRR) of 33 dBC. There were no records pertaining to compliance with hearing protection policies available from the employer. The 1995 IH report indicated that the worker should have been enrolled in the OSHA-mandated hearing loss prevention program and should have received annual audiometric exams and hearing conservation training. (Note: For unknown reasons, Jack was never formally enrolled in the hearing loss prevention program and annual audiometric monitoring exams and training were not provided.)

TABLE 54.1 Left Ear Audiometric Threshold Summary

| Date | 500 Hz (dBHL) | 1,000 Hz (dBHL) | 2,000 Hz (dBHL) | 3,000 Hz (dBHL) | 4,000 Hz (dBHL) | 6,000 Hz (dBHL) | 8,000 Hz (dBHL) | STS** Status |
|---|---|---|---|---|---|---|---|---|
| Jan. 1971 | 10 | 10 | 15 | 15 | 35 | 20 | NT* | Original Baseline Exam |
| Sept. 1979 | 15 | 10 | 20 | 40 | 55 | 40 | 30 | Initial STS evident |
| March 1984 | 10 | 05 | 30 | 60 | 65 | 65 | 45 | Second STS evident |
| February 2003 | 20 | 30 | 55 | 80 | 75 | 70 | 50 | Worsening trend |
| March 2003 Diagnostic Evaluation | 10 | 20 | 55 | 65 | 75 | 75 | 55 | Improved trend from Feb. 2003 |

* NT = not tested.

** STS: ≥10 dB average change from baseline at 2,000, 3,000, and 4,000 Hz after application of age corrections permitted by OSHA 29 CFR 1910.95.

## Audiometric Records

Jack's hearing had been monitored sporadically while employed. The initial baseline exam was obtained 2 days prior to the hire date. The baseline exam was essentially normal for both ears with the exception of a slight loss at 4,000 Hz in the left ear. Subsequent audiograms were obtained in September 1979 and March 1984. No other onsite hearing testing was completed until his workers' compensation claim was filed in February 2003. Threshold comparisons indicated a progressive high-frequency hearing loss for both ears on all exams subsequent to the first (baseline) exam. The absolute thresholds and standard threshold shift (STS) status is summarized in Tables 54.1 and 54.2. Note that the employer used existing audiograms as the baseline test for OSHA 29 CFR 1910.95 compliance purposes after 1983. Under OSHA CFR 1910.95, the employer had the option to perform 30-day STS retests; however, none were completed for Jack.

## STS Status

Retrospective analysis of the audiometric test data revealed STSs were present in both of Jack's ears in 1984 and again in 2003. Note that the STSs would have met the OSHA criteria

TABLE 54.2 Right Ear Audiometric Threshold Summary

| Date | 500 Hz (dBHL) | 1,000 Hz (dBHL) | 2,000 Hz (dBHL) | 3,000 Hz (dBHL) | 4,000 Hz (dBHL) | 6,000 Hz (dBHL) | 8,000 Hz (dBHL) | STS** Status |
|---|---|---|---|---|---|---|---|---|
| Jan. 1971 | 10 | 00 | 00 | 10 | 00 | 25 | NT | Baseline Exam |
| Sept. 1979 | 10 | 05 | 15 | 25 | 35 | 15 | 00 | Initial STS evident |
| March 1984 | 05 | 15 | 35 | 35 | 40 | 35 | 20 | Second STS evident |
| February 2003 | 15 | 45 | 60 | 70 | 65 | 65 | 45 | Third STS evident |
| March 2003 Diagnostic Evaluation | 15 | 40 | 55 | 65 | 65 | 65 | 45 | Third STS confirmed |

* NT = not tested.

** STS: ≥10 dB average change from baseline at 2,000, 3,000, and 4,000 Hz after application of age corrections permitted by OSHA 29 CFR 1910.95.

for recording on the injury and illness log in 1984 and again in 2003 if they had been detected at the time of the testing and if a work-related component had been identified. There was no evidence of any audiometric follow-up, medical evaluation, or intervention at any time despite these decreases in hearing. Seemingly, the audiometric technician filed the test results in Jack's medical file at the conclusion of the test without professional review or guidance.

Age corrections were applied to the calculation of STS in Jack's case as it was the standard procedure utilized by the employer for OSHA 29 CFR 1910.95 compliance. STSs were evident with or without the application of age correction. The National Institute of Occupational Safety and Health (NIOSH) does not advocate correction for presbycusis for STS purposes (NIOSH, 1998, pp 59–60):

> NIOSH does not recommend that age correction be applied to an individual's audiogram for significant threshold shift calculations. Although many people experience some decrease in hearing sensitivity with age, some do not. It is not possible to know who will and who will not have an age-related hearing loss. Thus, applying age corrections to a person's hearing thresholds for calculation of significant threshold shift will overestimate the expected hearing loss for some and underestimate it for others, because the median hearing loss attributable to presbycusis for a given age group will not be generalizable to that experienced by an individual in that age group.

(Note: The OSHA age correction procedure is available at www.osha.gov/pls/oshaweb/owadisp.show_document?p_id=9741&p_table=STANDARDS and the OSHA occupational hearing loss recording and reporting criteria reference is available at www.osha.gov/pls/oshaweb/owadisp.show_document?p_table=STANDARDS&p_id=9641.)

## Audiological Evaluation

Jack was referred to the occupational audiologist by the occupational physician for a complete diagnostic exam for workers' compensation purposes in March 2003. The evaluation was scheduled when he had been away from noise for 48 hours. The absolute thresholds are reported in Tables 54.1 and 54.2. The report stated:

> *Right Ear:* Normal hearing progressing to a severe high-frequency sensorineural hearing loss with partial recovery at 8,000 Hz. Speech reception threshold was 30 dBHL and word recognition score was 80% when stimuli were presented at 60 dBHL. Type A tympanogram and normal compensated static acoustic admittance. Contralateral and ipsilateral acoustic reflexes were present at expected sensation levels for 500, 1,000, and 2,000 Hz and absent at 4,000 Hz. The presence of an STS is confirmed as compared to the original 1971 baseline after age correction. The total age-corrected average shift is 39.33 dB. The hearing loss meets current OSHA 300 log injury and illness reporting requirements (the presence of STS and average hearing thresholds at 2,000, 3,000 and 4,000 Hz greater than or equal to 25 dBHL). Distortion product otoacoustic emissions presented at 65/55 dB SPL were absent for 1,000–6,000 Hz.
>
> *Left Ear:* Normal hearing progressing to a severe high-frequency sensorineural hearing loss with partial recovery at 8,000 Hz. Speech reception threshold was 20 dBHL and word recognition score was 80% when stimuli presented at 50 dBHL. Type A tympanogram and normal compensated static acoustic admittance. Contralateral and ipsilateral acoustic reflexes were present at expected sensation levels for 500, 1,000, and 2,000 Hz and absent at 4,000 Hz. The presence of an STS is confirmed as compared to the original 1971 baseline after age correction. The total age-corrected average shift is 29.33 dB. The hearing loss meets current OSHA 300 log requirements (the presence of an STS and average hearing thresholds at 2,000, 3,000, and 4,000 Hz greater than or equal to 25 dBHL). Distortion product otoacoustic emissions presented at 65/55 dB SPL were marginally present at 1,000 Hz (4 dB SNR) and absent for 2,000–6,000 Hz.

A graphic representation of the progressive hearing loss over the 32 years is provided in Figure 54.2.

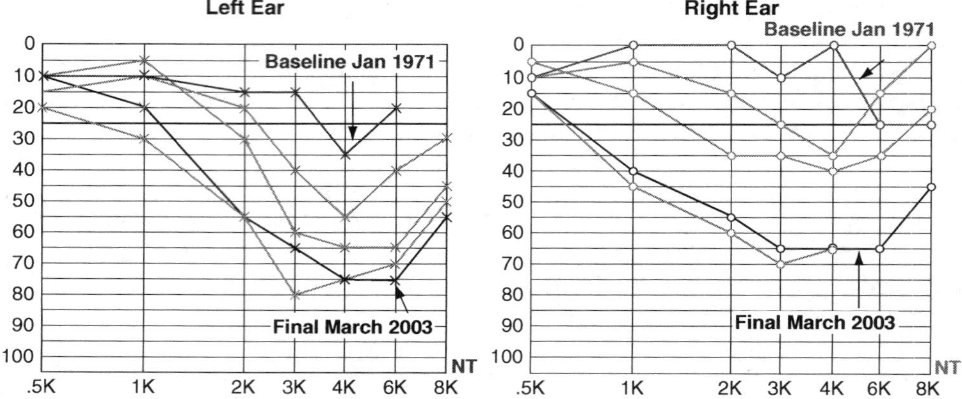


FIGURE 54.2 Serial Audiograms from Baseline in 1971 (gray) Progressing to Final Audiogram in March 2003 (black).

* NT is "not tested" on baseline audiogram.

## Impairment Rating

Colorado uses the American Academy of Otolaryngology (AAO) 1979 impairment rating formula for workers' compensation determinations. The formula is:

- Monaural: [(Average threshold at 500, 1,000, 2,000, and 3,000 Hz) – 25 dB] 1.5%
- Binaural: 5:1 better ear weighting

The subtraction of 25 dB is to account for "normal hearing" and is considered the "low fence." An online impairment calculator is available at: http://www.occupationalhearingloss.com/master_calculator.htm

Jack's AAO-1979 impairment rating at the time of the diagnostic evaluation in March 2003 was 28.1% for the right ear and 18.8% for the left ear. Binaural impairment was 20.3%. A disparity exists between the degree of hearing loss and the impairment rating values for NIHL due to the high-frequency nature of the disorder. This disparity is not as great in other jurisdictions in which high frequencies are included in the impairment formula, such as in Oregon, which includes threshold values for 500, 1,000, 2,000, 3,000, 4,000, and 6,000 Hz (Dobie & Megerson, 2000).

## Hearing Protection Assessment

During scheduling of the evaluation, Jack was asked to bring his current hearing protection with him to the appointment. He used foam expandable earplugs with an NRR of 33 dBC. He was asked to insert his earplugs and the relative fit was assessed both visually and by gently tugging on the earplug cord to check for resistance. Jack subjectively reported an occlusion effect especially when vocalizing. Upon removal, the earplugs were evenly compressed and reflected the contours of the canal. No creases or twisting that might impair the attenuation provided were observed. Hearing thresholds were measured in sound-field using warbled tones first with open ear canals and second with the binaural earplugs inserted by Jack. Attenuation for the least protected ear was 15 dB at 250 and 500 Hz, 25 dB at 1,000 Hz, 30 dB attenuation at 2,000–3,000 Hz, and 40 dB for 4,000–8,000 Hz.

## Work-Relatedness

The determination of work-relatedness is facilitated by addressing a series of questions relative to this employee:

1. Is there a hearing loss? Yes.
2. Is the hearing loss consistent with NIHL? Yes.
3. Was Jack exposed to noise at work? Yes.

4. Did he consistently wear HPDs at work? No.
5. Was he exposed to noise away from work? Yes.
6. Did he consistently wear HPDs for off-the-job noise exposures? No.
7. Did the HPDs have sufficient attenuation for workplace noise exposure? Probably.
8. Was the hearing protector fit adequate and did it provide effective attenuation? Yes.

Related to question 8, individual ear hearing protector fit-testing equipment is now available and audiologists are encouraged to incorporate these ear-specific attenuation measures into their clinical assessment of NIHL. It is widely recognized that the laboratory measured noise NRR overestimates the actual attenuation achieved during field use (Berger, 2000). Individual attenuation measures will serve to quantify the actual field benefit and afford opportunities to improve hearing protector fit and use compliance.

Upon review of these questions it is evident that Jack had unprotected hazardous noise exposure at work and also during nonoccupational activities. The Colorado workers' compensation system relies upon medical opinion for the determination of workers' compensation and does not require apportionment of the impairment between occupational and nonoccupational noise-induced hearing loss nor for the contributions of aging. In some states, such as Iowa, the apportionment procedure is specified and relies upon the International Standards Organization (ISO) 1999 guidelines (ISO, 1990). Also, there is no separate compensation for tinnitus in Colorado at this time.

### Summary Impression

Jack presented with bilateral sensorineural hearing loss. His audiometric configuration and timeline were consistent with progressive NIHL. There was no suspicion of functional hearing loss.

### Recommendations by OAud

1. Refer to an otolaryngologist or otologist for medical evaluation of progressive sensorineural hearing loss, medical determination of work-relatedness, and medical clearance for amplification.
2. Refer to an audiologist for a hearing aid consultation.
3. Continue use of hearing protection for all noise exposures at or above 85 dBA at work and home.
4. Use electronic hearing protection for firearm noise exposures.
5. Monitor hearing loss via annual audiometry.
6. Obtain personal noise dosimetry for current job and HPD requirements.
7. Verify OSHA 29 CFR 1910.95 requirements for hearing loss prevention program after noise dosimetry completed. Recommend an STS follow-up including retraining and refitting of hearing protection.
8. Enroll in workplace hearing conservation program if noise-exposed at or above 85 dBA time-weighted average work.
9. Consider submitting a request for employer accommodations for assistive listening device(s) for meetings and difficult on-the job communication settings.

## ENT Evaluation

An ENT evaluation was conducted in April 2003. The ENT completed a comprehensive physical exam and diagnostic workup. No additional otologic history was provided; however, Jack's general health history indicated surgeries on his hand, shoulder, and stomach. Laboratory testing consisting of CBC, sedrate, TSH, T4, and FTA-ABS was conducted to rule out other systemic causes of sensorineural hearing loss. No radiographic studies were conducted. The tympanic membranes were normal as well as the ear canals. The remainder of the head and neck exam was normal except for smoker's pharyngitis. A repeat audiogram was conducted by the ENT affiliated clinical audiologist and was consistent with the previously reported audiometric evaluation.

### ENT Diagnostic Impression

Jack's diagnosis was a bilateral sensorineural hearing loss secondary to noise exposure. The greatest losses seemed to coincide with the period of unprotected noise injury during Jack's jackhammer work activities. It was felt that the contribution of nonoccupational noise exposure was minimal and if any, might account for 5% of the total injury. Ninety-five percent of the loss was attributed to workplace noise exposure. (Note: Colorado does not require apportionment for workers' compensation purposes, but does require a medical opinion that the hearing loss is work-related. Hence, the ENT provided an indication that the majority of the hearing loss was felt to be attributed to work-related noise exposure.)

### ENT and Clinical Audiologist Recommendations

1. Bilateral digital hearing aids
2. Periodic audiological monitoring
3. Continued use of hearing protection for all noise exposures
4. Lifetime replacement of hearing aids on an approximately 4–6-year cycle

## Final Disposition

### Amplification

Binaural digital hearing aids were dispensed 4 months after the workers' compensation claim was filed. Jack reported excellent subjective benefit and acceptance. He reported using the hearing aids full-time and especially noted the improved ability to hear his granddaughter better. The employee reportedly removed his hearing aids at work and continued to use foam earplugs. He declined the need for assistive listening devices at work and felt his hearing aids sufficed during meetings and other group situations.

### Medical Treatment

No specific medical treatment was advised. The occupational physician (OPhys) completed the final impairment rating and concurred with the ENT's diagnosis. Medical follow-up was advised on an as-needed basis in the future.

### Audiological Monitoring

This will be pursued on an annual basis either through the employer or the worker's personal audiologist.

### Workers' Compensation Claim

Confirmed work-related noise-induced hearing loss, bilaterally. Jack's final impairment rating was consistent with the previously reported impairment percentages. He received a $12,000 financial settlement and negotiated a lifetime provision for bilateral hearing aids, batteries, repairs, and audiological/medical care related to his hearing loss. It is worth noting that financial settlements vary greatly from state to state. Colorado is among the states providing the lowest monetary compensation for hearing loss (Dobie & Megerson, 2000). Compensation is based on a percentage of a lump sum payment set by the workers' state compensation board. In addition, settlements can be negotiated to include the lifetime amplification needs of the worker, an important consideration given the limitations of monetary settlements, which may not be adequate for long-term hearing health care provision.

## Summary

Jack's case illustrates the unique situations and multiple missed opportunities for intervention and prevention of permanent hearing loss. Each individual deserves the dedicated attention and efforts of a team of professionals to prevent NIHL.

## Author Note

The case presented is adapted from a real case with identifying features, absolute timelines, and noncritical components altered to provide anonymity. It is also worth noting that this is a unique case presentation and as such cannot be interpreted as applicable to all individuals presenting with NIHL. Work-related determinations are to be made on a case-by-case basis.

## Endnote

1. Work history from 1971–2003 was for the same employer.

## References


American Academy of Otolaryngology. (1979). Committee on Hearing and Equilibrium and the American Council of Otolaryngology Committee on the medical aspects of noise: Guide for the evaluation of hearing handicap. *Journal of the American Medical Association, 241*(19), 2055–2059.

Axelsson, A. (1995). Tinnitus epidemiology. In G. Reich & J. Vernon (Eds.), *Proceedings of the fifth international tinnitus seminar* (pp. 249–254). Portland, OR: The American Tinnitus Association.

Berger, E. H. (2000). Hearing protection devices. In E. H. Berger, L. H., Royster, J. D. Royster, D. D. Driscoll, & M. Layne (Eds.), *The noise manual* (pp. 379–454). Fairfax, VA: American Industrial Hygiene Association.

Coles, R., Smith, P., & Davis, A. (1990). The relationship between noise-induced hearing loss and tinnitus and its management. In *New advances in noise research. Part I* (pp. 87–112). Stockholm: Swedish Council for Building Research.

Cooper, J. C. J. (1994). Tinnitus, subjective hearing loss and well-being. Health and Nutrition Examination Survey of 1971–75: Part II. *Journal of the American Academy of Audiology, 5*, 37–43.

Dobie, R. A. (1993). *Medical-legal evaluation of hearing loss.* New York: Van Nostrand Reinhold.

Dobie, R. A., & Megerson, S. C. (2000). Workers' compensation. In E. H. Berger, L. H. Royster, J. D. Royster, D. D. Driscoll, & M. Layne (Eds.), *The noise manual* (pp. 689–710). Fairfax, VA: American Industrial Hygiene Association.

Godlee, F. (1992). Noise: Breaking the silence. *British Medical Journal, 304*(6819), 110–113.

Griest, S. E., & Bishop, P. M. (1998). Tinnitus as an early indicator of permanent hearing loss: A 15 year longitudinal study of noise exposed workers. *American Association Occupational Health Nurses Journal, 46*, 325–329.

Hager, L. (2006). *Recordable hearing loss in the United States 2004.* Paper presented at the 31st Annual Conference of the National Hearing Conservation Association, Tampa, FL.

Henderson, D., Bielfefeld, E. C., Harris, K. C., & Hu, B. H. (2006). The role of oxidative stress in noise-induced hearing loss. *Ear & Hearing, 27*(1), 1–19.

Henderson, D., Bielfefeld, E. C., Hu, B. H., & Nicotera, T. (2007). Cellular mechanisms of noise-induced hearing loss. In K. C. M Campbell, (Ed.), *Pharmacology and ototoxicity for audiologists* (pp. 216–229). New York: Thomson Delmar Learning.

Humes, L. E., Joellenbeck, L. M., & Durch, J. S. (2005). *Noise and military service: Implications for hearing loss and tinnitus.* Washington, DC: National Academies Press.

ISO 1999. (1990). Acoustics—Determination of occupational noise exposure and estimation of noise-induced hearing impairment. Retrieved from http://www.iso.org/iso/catalogue_detail.htm?csnumber=6759

Jackson, L. D., & Duffy, B. K. (1998). *Health communication research: A guide to developments and directions.* Westport, CT: Greenwood Publishing Group.

Meinke, D. K., & Stephenson, M. R. (2007). Noise induced hearing loss: Models for prevention. In R. S. Ackley, T. N. Decker, & C. J. Limb (Eds.), *An essential guide to hearing and balance disorders* (pp. 287–323). Mahwah, NJ: Lawrence Erlbaum Associates.

NIOSH. (1998). *Revised criteria for a recommended standard: Occupational noise exposure* (NIOSH Publication No. 98–126). Cincinnati, OH: NIOSH.

NIOSH. (2004). *Worker health chartbook 2004* (DHHS Publication No. 2004–146). Cincinnati, OH: NIOSH.

OSHA. (1983). 29 CFR 1910.95, *Occupational noise exposure.* Washington, DC: U.S. Department of Labor, Occupational Safety and Health Administration. Fed. Reg. Vol. 48, pp. 9738–9744.

OSHA. (2002). 29 CFR 1904.10, *Occupational injury and illness recording and reporting requirements.* Washington, DC: U.S. Department of Labor, Occupational Safety and Health Administration. Fed. Reg. Vol. 67, No. 242, pp. 77165–77170.

Quaranta, A., Sallustio, V., & Quaranta, N. (2001). Noise induced hearing loss: Summary and perspectives. In D. Henderson, D. Prasher, R. Kopke, R. J. Salvi, & R. P. Hamernik (Eds.), *Noise induced hearing loss: Basic mechanisms, prevention and control* (pp. 539–557). London: Noise Research Network Publications.

Van Campen, L. E., Dennis, J. M., Hanlin, R. C., King, S. B., & Velderman, A. M. (1999). One-year audiologic monitoring of individuals exposed to the 1995 Oklahoma City bombing. *Journal of the American Academy of Audiology, 10*(5), 231–247.

Yaremchuk, K. (2001). Otologic injuries from airbag deployment. *Otolaryngology—Head and Neck Surgery, 125*(3), 13–134.

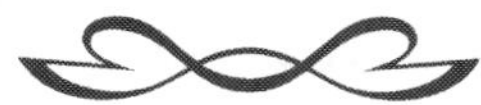

## LARYNGECTOMY

# CASE 55

# Mr. S: Successful Voice Restoration Following Total Laryngectomy with TEP

*Jodelle Deem and Ellen Hagerman*

## Conceptual Knowledge Areas

For a basic understanding of the concepts in this case study the reader should have had a course in basic anatomy and physiology of the speech and hearing mechanism with a specific focus on respiratory, laryngeal, and articulatory anatomy. In-depth understanding of the case will be facilitated if the reader has had at least an introductory course in disorders of voice and/or an introductory course in alaryngeal speech. An introduction to basic medical and surgical terminology would be beneficial as well. Specific knowledge in laryngeal, head, and neck cancer would be very helpful but is not necessary.

## Description of the Case

### Background Information and Reason for Referral

Mr. S, an active 63-year-old, was first seen by the otolaryngology and speech-language pathology staff when he came to the clinic in 2002 with a complaint of persistent hoarseness. He was accompanied by his wife who had been by his side and supportive throughout the years of medical uncertainty. Mr. S had been a 2-pack-per-day smoker for almost 40 years and in his initial appointment he expressed his fears about a possible cancer diagnosis. He was an equine auctioneer and was quite dependent upon his voice for his preferred livelihood. Mr. S loved his work and was very goal-directed in his quest to get his voice problems cleared up. At the time of the initial appointment in the fall of 2002, Mr. S demonstrated a hoarse or rough voice quality with an indirect laryngeal visualization revealing a smooth mass on the right true vocal cord with intact mucosa overlying it. It was decided that Mr. S should have a direct laryngoscopy in the operating room with microlaser removal of the mass on the right true vocal cord. During the surgical procedure, a portion of the lesion on the right true vocal cord was excised and sent to pathology for biopsy. Biopsy results of the section removed from the right vocal cord revealed squamous cell mucosal hyperplasia, keratosis, and chronic inflammation, but no evidence of carcinoma. *Keratosis of the larynx* refers to laryngeal lesions that are characterized by abnormal growth of the laryngeal epithelium. Abnormal epithelial development may occur in response to (1) laryngeal trauma, especially cigarette smoking and other forms of vocal hyperfunction, or (2) protracted cases of chronic laryngitis. The terms *leukoplakia, hyperkeratosis*, and *keratosis* are used to refer to these lesions. The major concern with these lesions is that some of them have been associated with laryngeal carcinoma (Deem & Miller, 2000).

Over the course of the next 2 years, Mr. S underwent no less than 4 separate laryngoscopy and microlaser procedures to explore his chronic hoarseness, as well as multiple CT scans. He underwent multiple $CO_2$ laser surgeries to remove the recurrent swelling on his right true vocal cord. He also was on a typical regimen of antireflux medications and steroids during that 2-year period in an attempt to resolve his dysphonia or voice problems.

## Findings of the Evaluation

### Laryngeal Cancer Diagnosis and Tumor Staging

In January 2004, Mr. S once again came to his otolaryngologist, this time with a complaint of dyspnea, or difficulty breathing, in addition to his chronic hoarseness. Once again he was taken to surgery for a biopsy of the recurrent mass on his vocal folds. This time the biopsy revealed invasive squamous cell carcinoma, a cancerous lesion, on the right vocal fold. The tumor was diagnosed as $T_4N_0M_0$ in the traditional tumor staging system, indicating that the tumor itself was substantial in size but that there was no apparent involvement of regional lymph nodes and no metastasis to distant sites (National Cancer Institute, 2008). In the tumor staging system, T stands for tumor and is usually followed by a subscript number from 0 through 4, or by the letters i and s. $T_0$ means that no tumor was found; $T_{is}$ means tumor in situ, the earliest identifiable tumor; and $T_1$–$T_4$ indicates the range of tumor sizes, with $T_4$ being the largest and $T_1$ the smallest. The N stands for nodes or lymph nodes. It is assigned numbers from 0 through 3, depending on the presence or absence of tumor cells in lymph nodes in the region around the primary site. The final letter of the staging system is M, which stands for metastasis. The M is assigned numbers 1 or 0, depending on the presence or absence of metastasis of the tumor cells to distance sites (Benninger & Grywalski, 1998).

## Treatment Options Considered

Based upon the biopsy results of squamous cell carcinoma, Mr. S was scheduled for a total laryngectomy and possible neck dissection the following week. Prior to the procedure he was seen by a speech-language pathologist (SLP) for preoperative counseling. In the preoperative counseling session he was introduced to a very competent postlaryngectomy esophageal speaker, and he was informed of methods of speaking that would be available to him following his laryngectomy. These include (1) speech with an electrolarynx, (2) esophageal speech, and (3) tracheoesophageal puncture (TEP). He also received instructions on how to use an electrolarynx with an oral adapter, which would be provided to him immediately after his surgery.

## Course of Treatment

### Surgical Procedures and Therapy—Total Laryngectomy

Mr. S was seen for a total laryngectomy with modified left and right neck dissection and total thyroidectomy in January 2004. There was substantial presence of the tumor in both vocal cords. The tumor appeared to originate in the right true vocal cord, but it had crossed the midline at the anterior commissure and had invaded the tissue of the left true cord as well.

There was also some subglottic invasion (below the vocal folds) of the tumor but little supraglottic invasion (above the vocal folds).

In a total laryngectomy, the entire cartilaginous larynx, (including all of its intrinsic muscles and membranes), the hyoid bone, and perhaps the upper two or three rings of the trachea are removed. The trachea is then tilted forward and attached to the external neck region just above the notch of the sternum. This external opening, through which the patient must breathe forever, is called a *stoma* or *tracheostoma*. For those patients in whom the cancer has spread to the neck and cervical lymph nodes, a surgical procedure called a *neck dissection* may be performed on the right, left, or both sides of the neck. During such a procedure, the following structures are typically removed: the sternocleidomastoid muscle, omohyoid muscle, internal jugular vein, spinal accessory nerve (CN XI), and submaxillary salivary gland (Deem & Miller, 2000). Mr. S did have a neck dissection, and his thyroid gland was removed, because of the extent of the invasion of the tumor.

## Mr. S's Postsurgical Voice Recovery and Radiation Treatment

Mr. S recovered well from his surgery and was discharged to his home to begin his recovery and rehabilitation. Voice rehabilitation in patients who have a total laryngectomy can be achieved by (1) esophageal speech, (2) electrolarynx, or (3) TEP with voice prosthesis. In the week following surgery Mr. S began follow-up appointments with otolaryngology and speech pathology. In his early appointments after surgery the speech-language pathologist focused on helping Mr. S to develop intelligible, functional electrolarynx speech. Patients are offered an electrolarynx with an oral "straw" adapter immediately after their total laryngectomy because the electrolarynx usually provides the fastest route back to functional communication. The oral straw adapter is used because the patient's neck is simply too sore for several weeks following laryngectomy to use a traditional neck-held electrolarynx. In his early therapy sessions following surgery, Mr. S used an electric larynx with the plastic straw-like oral adapter and no attempt was made to remove the oral adapter to try neck placement due to soreness in his neck.

As Mr. S began his postsurgery voice rehabilitation, he also began a 6-week series of 2 times per day radiation therapy treatments to his neck. Postsurgical radiation is typical following total laryngectomy for patients with $T_4$ tumors. When Mr. S was asked about radiation he often talked about how much he hated the treatments and how they "just about burned him up." The speech-language pathologists have seen patients who are left with tight, thin, almost leather-like skin on their neck following radiation therapy. Mr. S's otolaryngologists described the skin on his neck as "woody" following radiation. Radiation can negatively affect taste buds, skin, and saliva. Mr. S's skin remained tight and leathery due to the radiation, which had a profound impact on his success with the electrolarynx as his clinicians began to have him try neck placement. Two to three weeks postsurgery, and as his soreness began to decrease, Mr. S used both oral placement with the straw adapter and began trying neck placement.

A neck-held electric larynx works well when it is applied to a spot on the neck that has soft, pliable vibratory properties. The key to good electric larynx speech is to be able to find that perfect "spot" on the neck that vibrates well when the electric larynx is placed against it. Because of the radiation changes in his neck, Mr. S had virtually no spot on his neck that would vibrate well to produce good sound. As previously stated, Mr. S was an auctioneer in the equine industry. The electric larynx did not appear to be an acceptable alternative for him. As the weeks progressed Mr. S became increasingly resistant to the electric larynx. Mr. S's wife made several calls during that time in which she stated that Mr. S was not able to use his electric larynx, that she could not understand him, and that he was very frustrated with it.

Therapy continued on a weekly basis and Mr. S practiced with both neck placement and oral placement during each session. Activities in therapy focused on good articulation with the electric larynx and rate control for intelligibility, but Mr. S was not making progress, was not intelligible, and was not practicing at home. The electric larynx was not meeting Mr. S's communication needs and was definitely not taking him on a path to return to his profession in equine sales. The most difficult part of this period following surgery and radiation was watching the changes in Mr. S as a person. He was becoming noticeably discouraged, frustrated, and angry. Esophageal speech was introduced as an option. Mr. S expressed concern about his ability to learn the procedure because he had been impatient as he tried to learn the electrolarynx. It was agreed that learning esophageal speech might be challenging. He had already been introduced to a skilled esophageal speaker, but he told the clinicians that he did not want to try esophageal speech. He was also informed about TEP voice but was not interested in this alternative either. At 4 months postlaryngectomy the clinicians consulted with Mr. S, his wife, and his surgeon, and all agreed that it was time to try a secondary TEP procedure. Subsequently, Mr. S underwent a secondary procedure under general anesthesia to place a TE fistula for TE voice restoration.

### Tracheoesophageal Puncture and Voice Restoration

Since it first became available in the 1980s, TE voice restoration has been an excellent alternative for voice restoration. The TEP voice restoration procedure was developed by Singer and Blom (1980) and is a solution to many of the problems experienced with other surgical voice restoration procedures. With this approach a small silicone voice prosthesis is inserted into a surgically created, midline, tracheoesophageal fistula, and the patient uses pulmonary air that is conducted from the trachea to the esophagus for voice production. The TEP surgery is a relatively simple endoscopic procedure that can be performed at the time of primary laryngectomy, or later under general anesthesia as a secondary procedure. The major advantage of TE voice restoration is that patients use pulmonary or lung air as their power source for speech production, rather than the limited air supply available in esophageal speech. A second important advantage of the TEP voice restoration procedure is that the surgical procedure can be performed on most patients, including those who have been irradiated heavily. A third advantage of the TEP procedure is that it is reversible because the patient's fistula tends to close within a matter of hours if it is not maintained by the presence of the voice prosthesis or a catheter. A fourth advantage of TEP is that this procedure and the design of the various voice prostheses have effectively eliminated the problems of aspiration and the difficulties in swallowing that have consistently plagued the various tracheoesophageal shunt procedures (Deem & Miller, 2000).

Patients are considered to be good candidates for TEP if they meet several important criteria. A primary requirement is that the patient must have enough manual dexterity to remove, clean, and reinsert the small prosthesis into the TE fistula. Therefore, a patient with arthritis or poor vision may not be a good candidate. The patient must have a tracheostoma that is large enough for the prosthesis to be inserted into, with a diameter of no less than 2.0 cm. A speech-language pathologist who is familiar with TEP procedures should be easily accessible to the patient. If radiation therapy is performed, 6 to 12 weeks should pass before the TEP is done to allow the effects of radiation to subside. Patients should be motivated to attempt TEP voice restoration, and they should be psychologically stable (Case, 1996).

The speech-language pathologist's procedure for inserting TE devices is theoretically similar. However, the clinician must follow instructions exactly for each device to permit the patient to develop optimal voice (E. Hagerman, personal communication, 2008; Deem & Miller, 2000).

1. Every procedure should begin with the use of surgical gloves and universal precautions (Centers for Disease Control, 1988) to prevent the spread of contamination between the speech-language pathologist and the patient.
2. The catheter, placed at the time of the surgical procedure, is removed and a dilator is used to dilate the patient's tracheostoma up to the appropriate size for the selected prosthesis (e.g., 22 Fr. dilator for a 20 Fr. Blom-Singer Indwelling device).
3. The sizer that is included with the kit is pushed carefully into the tracheoesophageal puncture and slightly downward. The sizer is then pulled back, gently allowing the

flange on the sizer to stop on the posterior side of the tracheoesophageal wall. The mark or size number visible on the anterior side of the tracheoesphageal wall is noted. The sizer is adjusted to make sure it is sitting in the proper location and then released. The size that can be read on the anterior side of the tracheoesophageal wall is the size that the patient should use.

4. Using the Blom-Singer Indwelling Low Pressure Voice Prosthesis starter kit, the appropriate size valve (after sizing) is placed onto the loading device that comes with the kit.
5. The valve is pulled slowly through the loading device so that the flange on the prosthesis folds up into the loading device.
6. A gel cap (included in the starter kit) is placed over the outside of the loading device.
7. The push rod (included in the starter kit) is placed gently onto the loading device and the prosthesis is pushed into the gel cap.
8. The tracheoesophageal valve is removed from the push rod.
9. The voice prosthesis (valve) is placed onto the inserter (included in the starter kit) and the flange is attached to the security hook of the inserter.
10. The prosthesis is lubricated lightly, using a very small amount of surgilube.
11. In a continuous motion, the dilator is removed from the tracheostoma and the prosthesis is inserted into the tracheostoma.
12. The gel cap (which has been placed on the valve and is now inserted into the tracheostoma) takes approximately 3 minutes to dissolve. During this time the patient is instructed to begin swallowing gently. After 2 to 3 minutes, the patient should be instructed to drink a little warm water to help dissolve the remainder of the gel cap.
13. The valve is turned manually with the inserter device still on. The valve should turn freely in the patient's neck without any twisting of the attached flange.
14. The flange is removed from the security hook. The patient is instructed to occlude the tracheostoma with a thumb to produce voice. The patient should attempt to sustain vowels first, then count, then recite, and so on and should be encouraged to practice daily. The patient is given a sip of water and the valve is checked for leakage. If all appears well, the security flange is cut and discarded. If the prosthesis is properly in place, the patient should have intelligible conversational speech. Patience should be encouraged while learning to use the prosthesis.
15. To determine whether the valve is properly in place and opened, the patient should be taken to radiology by the speech-language pathologist to see if the circular radiopaque ring is visible on X-ray.
16. The patient should be educated in the use of Nystatin Oral Suspension to prevent fungal growth on the voice prosthesis. One teaspoon of Nystatin should be swished in the oral cavity 2 times per day for at least 5 minutes to reduce the buildup of candida yeast on the prosthesis, which can shorten prosthesis life and cause leakage. Fewer than 5 minutes is thought to be ineffective (Blom, 1996). If the patient is interested in a one-way, hands-free tracheostoma valve, instructions in its application should be given at this time. The one-way or hands-free valve option allows patients to talk while doing other tasks with their hands. This option is particularly useful for patients whose work requires use of both hands. A humidifilter is available to be added to the Blom-Singer hands-free valve. The filter permits incoming air to be warmed, filtered, and moistened (InHealth, 2008).

## Mr. S's Experience with Tracheoesophageal Voice Restoration

To say that the TEP made a difference in Mr. S's life would do injustice to the term "understatement." Mr. S consulted with the speech-language pathologists regarding placement of his TE prosthesis within 3 weeks of his TE fistula surgery. In the visit the SLPs placed an InHealth Blom-Singer® indwelling voice prosthesis (InHealth, 2008). InHealth prostheses are used in this clinic because experience has shown that the similar Provox prostheses are initially more expensive and are sometimes more difficult to fit, depending on the location of the patient's TE fistula. After placing the prosthesis, Mr. S was encouraged to thumb occlude the prosthesis opening and he was instantly able to voice with good volume. By the time he left the therapy session on that day, Mr. S was speaking in phrases with good intelligibility and good speech volume. The SLPs could actually see Mr. S's mood brighten.

Mr. S's progress following placement of his TEP was remarkable. In the first month of his new "TEP voice" he used his thumb to occlude the prosthesis to speak. As he became more comfortable with the device and his speech improved, he tried a hands-free valve with his TEP. After proper fitting, a flexible diaphragm rests in an open position and may be adjusted by rotating the diaphragm for relaxed, quiet breathing, or routine physical activity. During speech, a slight increase in exhalation causes the diaphragm to close and divert air through the prosthesis to provide air for voicing. At the completion of speech, the diaphragm automatically reopens as exhalation pressure decreases (InHealth, 2008).

Mr. S did not have great success with the hands-free valve. Although the literature suggests that it takes very little pressure to close the hands-free diaphragm for speech, that was not Mr. S's experience. He felt that it took too much effort to close the hands-free valve and that his speech rate and rhythm were adversely affected by it. As an alternative to the hands-free valve, an ATOS Provox HME (heat moisture exchange) system was placed on Mr. S's TEP. The Provox HME System is a disposable device that comes fully assembled with a 20-day supply. The patient puts on a new device each day and discards the previous unit. The HME is a two-piece unit that consists of an HME cassette or speech button and an adhesive housing. There is a foam filter for heat and moisture exchange with an antimicrobial agent to inhibit bacterial growth on the filter. The speech button makes thumb occlusion easy for speech production.

The heat moisture exchange system has worked very well for Mr. S. Although the manufacturer recommends changing the filter on the heat moisture exchange system on a daily basis, Mr. S occasionally needed to change his twice per day, especially if he was working around horses, because the filter in his HME system became black after a half day of work. An HME system is costly. A box of 20 filters is $50, and 20 housings for his HME system is also $50. Some insurers will cover part of the cost of the HME systems, but the only way to know with certainty whether the HME will be covered by insurance is to contact the insurance company to review the coverage and reimbursement procedures each time one is ordered or recommended (Acton, 2004). Importantly, these products are generally considered medically necessary for pulmonary health. In spite of this cost, Mr. S was quite satisfied with the HME system and did not use any other type of stoma cover or bib to protect his airway. The HME system was all he needed.

### Primary versus Secondary Tracheoesophageal Puncture

Mr. S's surgeon chose not to perform a TEP procedure at the time of his total laryngectomy, although the surgeon did perform a cricopharyngeal myotomy (to relieve potential spasm of the cricopharyngeus muscle) at the time of the total laryngectomy to help assure that the voice restoration (primary or secondary) would be successful. Surgeons vary in their approach to the TEP procedure. Some surgeons prefer doing the relatively simple endoscopic procedure at the time of the primary laryngectomy. Others wait for several months and then perform a second (or "secondary") TE procedure under general anesthesia in the postlaryngectomized patient. Mr. S's surgeon preferred secondary TEP procedures.

The issue of primary versus secondary TEP has been investigated. Boscolo-Rizzo, Zanetti, Carpene, and DaMosto (2008) expressed a preference for primary TEP procedures, stating that primary and secondary TEP with indwelling voice prosthesis are equally safe and effective procedures and that primary TEP should be preferred to avoid a second surgery and allow early voice restoration with positive psychological impact. Chone, Gripp, Spina, and Crespo (2005) also reported a preference for primary TEP because patient success rate with TEP was similar on outcome measures regardless of whether the patient's TEP was primary or secondary.

In the clinicians' experience, patients seem to do better with secondary TEP procedures rather than with primary procedures. Although the success rate appears to be similar for the primary and secondary procedures, preference for a secondary TEP procedure is based, experientially, upon "process" in addition to outcomes. Clinical experience suggests that primary

TEP can be a less desirable alternative for many patients who are stressed by so much change in the very short period of time after their laryngectomy. These are some of the issues seen in primary TEP patients:

1. Primary TEP patients express feelings of being overwhelmed because they already have so much to deal with surrounding loss of voice and tracheostoma care. The presence of a TE fistula at the time of primary surgery seems to be an additional burden. Many patients express confusion and concern about the presence of the second "hole" or TE fistula. Primary TE patients cannot have their speaking valve fitted for at least 2 weeks while they are healing, so they have an extra tube sutured in place on their neck to keep the TE fistula open. Patients may express confusion about the extra tube and ask what they are supposed to do with it.
2. Many times, even at 2 weeks postlaryngectomy, patients are still sore from surgery and congested with mucous secretions. That makes it difficult for them to occlude the stoma to speak and to keep a primary TE prosthesis clean and open.
3. Patients who have radiation may have changes in the tissue of the neck, which can impact the shape and size of the TE fistula, causing it to stretch or migrate and requiring a surgical revision. These clinicians have seen primary TE fistulas migrate as much as half an inch because of tissue changes following radiation. TEP patients also have to have their prosthesis resized at least three times in the first months following laryngectomy. If the patient is having radiation treatment as well, this can further complicate resizing.
4. Some patients do not like TEP. A patient who waits for a secondary TEP has the opportunity to explore other options before having TEP surgery. This gives the patient a real chance to try both electrolarynx speech and esophageal speech. If the patient does not want to try TEP, then unnecessary fistula surgery will have been avoided.
5. Some primary TEP patients simply do not like the TEP. If it is not properly used or cared for, there is the possibility for leakage around or through the prosthesis. The clinicians have had several patients with primary TEP who would not use it. Some of those patients had tissue breakdown following radiation and their necks became too sore to thumb occlude the TE fistula. Some of those patients became depressed and decided that they would never be able to talk.
6. Finally, in the SLPs' experience, primary TEP is the "best" type of voice restoration. Bastian and Muzaffar (2001) stated that TEP is the preferred method of voice restoration. Yet many patients are quite happy with their esophageal voice or electrolarynx speech. This is an important issue of patient choice and empowerment. There are three methods of voice restoration following total laryngectomy. Patients should be introduced to all three and be allowed to choose what works best for them. There are excellent esophageal speakers and electrolarynx users who are quite satisfied with these choices of communication.

## Analysis of Client's Response to Intervention

Mr. S was satisfied with his TEP voice restoration and returned to an active life traveling and conducting sales in the equine industry. His secondary TEP was the key to his ability to return to his former lifestyle. It is possible that Mr. S would have been successful with a primary TEP as well; however, because of the difficulties he experienced following surgery and radiation treatments, it is believed that the timing of a secondary TEP was perfect for Mr. S because he was well enough to focus only on the TEP and move forward with his life and a new voice.

## Author Note

Mr. S was a real patient seen at University of Kentucky's Ear, Nose, & Throat, Speech & Hearing outpatient clinic. Permission was obtained from the client prior to development of this manuscript. Mr. S continues to function very well with his TEP to this day and has successfully returned to his work in equine sales.

## References


Acton, L. (2004). *Heat moisture exchange: Laryngectomy issues and answers.* Retrieved March 21, 2008, from Speech Pathology.com: http://www.speechpathology.com/articles/article_detail.asp?article_id=224

Bastian, R., & Muzaffar, K. (2001). Endoscopic laser cricopharyngeal myotomy to salvage tracheoesophageal voice after total laryngectomy. *Archives of Otolaryngology, Head and Neck Surgery, 127,* 691–693.

Benninger, M., & Grywalski, C. (1998). Rehabilitation of the head and neck cancer patient. In A. Johnson & B. Jacobson (Eds.), *Medical speech-language pathology: A practitioner's guide.* New York: Thieme Medical.

Blom, E. D. (1996). Tracheoesophageal speech. *Seminars in Speech and Language, 16*(3), 191–203.

Boscolo-Rizzo, P., Zanetti, F., Carpene, S., & DaMosto, M. (2008, January). Long-term results with tracheoesophageal voice prosthesis: Primary versus secondary TEP. *European Archives of Otorhinolaryngology, 265*(1), 73–77.

Case, J. (1996). *Clinical management of voice disorders* (3rd ed.). Austin, TX: PRO-ED.

Centers for Disease Control. (1988). Perspectives in disease prevention and health promotion. Atlanta, GA: Author.

Chone, C., Gripp, F., Spina, A., & Crespo, A. (2005). Primary versus secondary tracheoesophageal puncture for speech rehabilitation in total laryngectomy: Long-term results with indwelling voice prosthesis. *Otolaryngology-Head and Neck Surgery, 133*(1), 89–94.

Deem, J., & Miller, L. (2000). *Manual of voice therapy* (2nd ed., pp. 261–294). Austin, TX: PRO-ED.

InHealth (2008). *Blom-Singer voice prostheses.* Retrieved March 21, 2008, from InHealth Technologies: http://www.inhealth.com/featuredprdvppage1new.htm

National Cancer Institute. (2008). *Staging: Questions and answers.* Retrieved April 2, 2008, from National Institutes of Health: National Cancer Institute: http://www.cancer.gov/cancertopics/factsheet/detection/staging

Singer, M. I., & Blom, E. D. (1980). An endoscopic technique for restoration of voice after laryngectomy. *Annals of Otology, Rhinology, and Laryngology, 89,* 529.


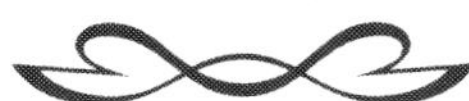

## SWALLOWING

# CASE 56

# Janelle: Diagnosis and Management of Adult Dysphagia


*Christina A. Baumgartner*


## Conceptual Knowledge Areas

### Assessment of Dysphagia

Dysphagia, or impaired swallowing, can be defined as difficulty transferring a bolus from the mouth to the stomach. The swallowing impairment may occur in any or all of the three stages of swallowing: oral, pharyngeal, and esophageal. Both oropharyngeal dysphagia and esophageal dysphagia impact a person's overall health and nutrition. Dysphagia resulting in aspiration may lead to an aspiration pneumonia. Another common consequence of dysphagia is the inability to meet nutritional needs orally. The speech-language pathologist (SLP) is the professional who determines whether a patient has dysphagia.

### Differential Diagnosis of Dysphagia

To manage dysphagia appropriately, it is necessary to determine the location (oral, pharyngeal, and/or esophageal) and cause(s) of the dysphagia. Some dysphagias can be managed therapeutically through changes in diet and liquids, through the use of swallowing compensatory techniques, or through therapy. Other dysphagias require medical management such as surgery or medications.

## Ethical Considerations in Management of Dysphagia

For patients who have a poor prognosis or who are at the end of life, managing dysphagia requires the consideration of medical status, patient preferences, quality of life, and contextual features such as family preferences, social and cultural influences, and legal and financial issues (Sharp & Genesen, 1996). Recommendations change based on each patient's situation, prognosis, and personal wishes. A recommendation of nothing by mouth and nonoral nutrition might be appropriate for someone who is 55 years old, was relatively healthy, suffered an acute stroke, and is now significantly aspirating food and drink due to an oropharyngeal dysphagia. Based on what is known about general recovery patterns from stroke (Jorgensen et al., 1995), this person is likely to improve. Therefore, an aggressive recommendation to provide the patient with nonoral nutrition only to reduce the risk of aspiration pneumonia and provide adequate nourishment and hydration may be made. The focus of dysphagia management in this case is on rehabilitating this patient's swallow function. However, if the patient is an 89-year-old nursing home resident with end-stage Alzheimer's disease, whose only pleasure in life was eating, but aspirated everything he ate and drank, the recommendation might not be as aggressive. Instead, more conservative management focusing on quality of life might be more appropriate. In this case, after discussing evaluation findings with the patient's family and medical team, it may be decided that the patient should continue to eat and drink despite the high risk of developing an aspiration pneumonia, and dysphagia management would focus on facilitation. The goal would be to provide the patient with the safest feeding techniques and compensatory strategies that led to the least amount of aspiration.

# Description of the Case

## Background Information and Reason for Referral

On April 17, Janelle, a 69-year-old female, was admitted to the hospital with complaints of a 1-week history of lethargy, shortness of breath, and poor appetite without significant weight loss. Relevant medical background revealed recent diagnosis of acute myelogenous leukemia (AML), esophageal cancer, and reflux. Janelle began chemoradiation therapy 21 days before she was admitted to the hospital. Janelle was a retired elementary school teacher who had been living independently with her husband of 40 years. She had two adult daughters who live in the area.

Physical examination by the internal medicine physician revealed reduced breath sounds bilaterally with poor inspiratory effort. Cranial nerve examination was normal. Chest x-ray showed progressive right upper lobe and right lower lobe infiltrates. Janelle was diagnosed with pneumonia and was to continue chemotherapy in the hospital and be treated for pneumonia.

Two hours after dinner that first evening in the hospital, Janelle's nurse entered her room and observed that she was minimally responsive. Janelle did not respond to her name and exhibited difficulty breathing. An emergency call was placed to the physicians. Janelle was intubated and transferred to the intensive care unit (ICU). The pulmonology service physician, a specialist in the diagnosis and management of lung disease, was consulted and determined that Janelle was in acute respiratory failure (ARF).

Janelle remained in the ICU for 9 days. She was intubated and sedated for 7 of those days and received medications and hydration through an IV. Janelle was extubated on day 8. She was diagnosed with mucositis at that time. Mucositis, a common side effect of chemotherapy, results in painful inflammation and ulceration of digestive tract mucous membranes (Rosenthal, Lewin, & Eisbruch, 2006). Oral mucositis can result in difficulty talking, eating, and swallowing due to pain from oral sores or ulcers. Some medications used to treat mucositis, such as Lidocaine, are anesthetics that can produce reduced oral and pharyngeal sensation.

## Findings of the Evaluation

On the eighth day of Janelle's ICU stay, the speech-language pathologist was consulted to determine whether Janelle could safely initiate oral intake after extubation. A clinical, bedside swallow evaluation was completed that morning. An oral mechanism examination revealed many atypical findings. Her oral cavity appeared red and inflamed. Overall mild, bilateral labial weakness and reduced range of motion (ROM) was exhibited during protrusion and retraction. Lingual range of motion (ROM) was mildly reduced upon protrusion, retraction, elevation, and lateralization. Lingual strength was also mildly reduced. Buccal tension was grossly WFL and Janelle was able to impound air. Velopharyngeal function was WFL. Phonation was mildly breathy and hypophonic postextubation. Janelle exhibited difficulty initiating visceral swallows due to oral sores and dryness. The overall, mild generalized weakness and reduced ROM exhibited during the oral mechanism examination could be explained by a combination of any or all of the following factors: general debilitation from the cancer diagnosis, xerostomia, fibrosis, and neuromuscular damage due to chemoradiation (Kulbersh et al., 2006), oral pain caused by the mucositis (Rosenthal et al., 2006), and recent prolonged intubation (Colice, Stuckel, & Dain, 1989).

Oral swallow stage at bedside appeared to be mildly impaired. Anterior loss of thin liquids by cup occurred, possibly due to labial weakness and/or reduced sensation. Bolus formation and control of nectar-thick liquids and pureed solids were grossly WFL. Janelle requested to defer soft solid trials due to oral cavity soreness. Bolus transit times were adequate. Swallow responses were timely with adequate laryngeal elevation. However, delayed throat clearing and wet vocal quality were exhibited following swallows of thin liquids indicating possible penetration and/or aspiration of the boluses. Pharyngeal stage dysphagia was suspected. A videofluoroscopic swallow study was recommended to further assess pharyngeal swallow function and to rule out aspiration. Janelle continued to receive nutrition intravenously through total parenteral nutrition (TPN) and remained NPO (nothing by mouth).

A videofluoroscopic swallow study was completed the following day. The patient sat at 90 degrees and lateral and anterior-to-posterior (A-P) views were taken. Swallow function was assessed with thin liquids by teaspoon and cup sip trials, nectar-thick liquid consistency by teaspoon and cup sip trials, pureed consistency, and solids (cracker). Oral swallow stage was moderately impaired, characterized by early spillover of thin liquids into the pyriform sinuses before the swallows. It was suspected that reduced lingual ROM due to oral pain from mucositis, as well as iatrogenic reduction of oral and pharyngeal sensitivity from the medication used to treat the mucositis, may have led to reduced bolus control. Improved bolus control with decreased premature spillage over base of tongue occurred with nectar-thick liquids and pureed consistency. The more viscous consistencies likely resulted in increased sensation. Janelle was unable to masticate a cracker due to oral pain from the mucositis and expectorated that trial.

Pharyngeal swallow stage was moderately impaired and characterized by reduced posterior lingual retraction and absent epiglottic inversion, resulting in consistent, trace penetration during swallows of thin liquids and after swallows from vallecular residue. Reflexive coughing did not clear the penetrated residue, and it was subsequently aspirated. The

Rosenbek 8-point Penetration-Aspiration Scale score was 7 (Rosenbek, Robbins, Roecker, Coyle, & Wood, 1996). Chin down posture was attempted to assess if widening the vallecular space would reduce the amount of residue, and, hence, the potential of penetration and aspiration after the swallows. A chin tuck reduced the amount of vallecular residue, but was inconsistently successful in eliminating the penetration events. Marked amounts of bilateral vallecular, pyriform sinus, and pharyngeal wall residue from pureed consistency remained after swallows due to reduced posterior tongue elevation, reduced hyolaryngeal elevation, and decreased pharyngeal wall contractions. Chin down posture and alternating thinner consistencies with thicker consistencies helped to reduce but not eliminate this residue. The A-P view revealed reduced bilateral vocal fold adduction, which could also contribute to the penetration observed during the swallows.

## Representation of Problem at the Time of Evaluation

Both prolonged intubation and chemoradiation can result in impaired swallowing. Colice et al. (1989) assessed laryngeal damage in 82 patients who were intubated for more than 4 days. Laryngeal edema and mucosal ulcerations of the vocal folds were found in 94% ($n$ = 77) of the patients. Adequate laryngeal adduction is required to protect the airway from food and liquid during swallows. Postextubation laryngeal damage would suggest impaired vocal fold adduction and hence, impaired airway protection during swallowing. And, as mentioned previously, the videofluoroscopic swallow study documented reduced vocal fold adduction in the A-P view. In addition to prolonged intubation, Janelle had been undergoing chemoradiation, which was found to produce reduced range of motion of oral, laryngeal, and pharyngeal structures, and could explain reduced posterior tongue elevation, reduced hyolaryngeal elevation, and reduced pharyngeal wall contractions (Kulbersh et al., 2006; Rosenthal et al., 2006).

## Treatment Options Considered

Recommendations for a pureed diet, nectar-thick liquids, and swallow precautions were made. Swallow precautions of small bites, liquids by cup sip, chin down posture, and alternating liquids and solids were posted at the head of Janelle's bed and reviewed with the patient, her family, nursing, and Janelle's physicians. The dietician was also contacted because a calorie count, which measures daily caloric intake, was recommended. Because of Janelle's fatigue and reduced endurance from generalized weakness, it was believed that she would not be able to meet nutritional needs orally at the time. Therefore, Janelle would continue to require nonoral supplementation of nutrition.

Maintaining ROM and strength through swallowing exercises during chemoradiation to prevent dysphagia and aspiration has been documented in the literature (Kulbersh et al., 2006; Rosenthal et al, 2006). However, Janelle had never seen a speech-language pathologist prior to beginning her course of treatment. A dysphagia exercise program was developed to help Janelle improve and maintain adequate range of motion and strength of oral, laryngeal, and pharyngeal structures during and after her course of chemoradiation.

The Masako, or tongue-holding maneuver (Fujiu & Logemann, 1996; Fujiu, Logemann, & Pauloski, 1995) was introduced for improved posterior tongue elevation and retraction. The super-supraglottic swallow (Logemann, Pauloski, Rademaker, & Coangelo, 1997) combined with an effortful swallow (Kahrilas, Lin, Logemann, Ergen, & Facchini, 1991) were reviewed and demonstrated. The goals of these maneuvers are to improve hyolaryngeal elevation, tongue base retraction, and pharyngeal contraction. Due to Janelle's reduced endurance and oropharyngeal pain associated with mucositis, she was only able to perform these exercises minimally over the next few days.

## Course of Treatment

Janelle remained hospitalized for 10 more days. During this period, she was followed daily by speech-language pathology services. Sessions included ongoing assessment of diet and liquid toleration, ongoing reassessment of swallow function, and swallowing exercises. Janelle was tolerating the pureed diet and nectar-thick liquids without clinical signs or symptoms of aspiration. She was able to state what her swallow precautions were and followed them independently with 100% carryover. During this time, the pain from the mucositis had almost resolved. Her endurance improved, and her phonatory quality was no longer hoarse and breathy. She was able to perform the prescribed swallowing exercises independently and accurately. Based on clinical examination findings, Janelle exhibited overall improvement in swallow function during her hospital stay. After 7 days on a pureed diet and nectar-thick liquids, she tolerated trials of thin liquids and soft solids without clinical signs or symptoms of aspiration or complaints of pain. Janelle's diet was subsequently upgraded to mechanical soft with thin liquids and it was recommended that she continue her swallowing precautions. TPN was discontinued as Janelle's endurance had improved and she was able to meet nutritional needs orally.

Janelle was discharged from the hospital on May 4. Her pneumonia had resolved and she was tolerating a mechanical soft diet and thin liquids. Discharge recommendations included continuing with the swallow precautions and exercises and returning for a follow-up videofluoroscopic swallow evaluation in 4 weeks, at the completion of her chemoradiation series.

On May 20, she was readmitted to the hospital with a new diagnosis of pneumonia. On May 21, the speech-language pathology service was consulted to assess swallowing and to rule out aspiration. A clinical swallow evaluation was completed that morning. Janelle reported that she had been on a mechanical soft diet with thin liquids at home and that she had been compliant with following her swallow precautions and completing her swallowing exercise program. She complained of increased coughing over the past 4 days with eating and drinking.

The results of the oral-motor-speech examination were WNL, including labial, lingual, buccal, velopharyngeal, and jaw ROM, strength, and coordination. Phonation was also WFL. Oral cavity inflammation secondary to mucositis, which was noted on prior admission, had resolved. Janelle was able to produce timely visceral swallows with adequate laryngeal elevation. Swallow function was assessed at bedside with teaspoon trials of water. No clinical signs or symptoms of aspiration were exhibited with the initial trial. A second teaspoon of water was given. Immediate coughing occurred after the swallow. Immediate coughing also occurred after a third teaspoon of water. Janelle was then given a teaspoon of nectar-thick liquid. Again, immediate coughing occurred after the swallow. Janelle's clinical swallowing presentation was concerning for penetration and/or aspiration. The speech-language pathologist spoke to the physician and nurse, and recommended that Janelle be made NPO. An order for a videofluoroscopic swallow evaluation was obtained and completed that afternoon.

The patient was seated at 90 degrees and lateral views were taken. Swallow function was assessed with thin liquids by teaspoon and cup sip trials. Oral swallow stage was WFL, and characterized by normal bolus formation and control, normal A-P transport, and timely oral bolus transit. Pharyngeal swallow stage also appeared to be WFL. Swallow responses were timely with adequate hyolaryngeal elevation, base of tongue retraction, epiglottic inversion, pharyngeal contractions and upper esophageal sphincter (UES) opening. After 2 teaspoons and 2 small cup sips of thin liquids, there was no evidence of penetration or aspiration. Janelle was then instructed to take consecutive cup sips of the thin barium. After the last swallow, she began coughing markedly and barium was expelled from the trachea. However, the barium was not observed either entering the laryngeal vestibule or being retropropelled from the esophagus. Upon closer examination, it was suspected that the barium was entering the trachea through a fistula in the tracheoesophageal wall. The videofluoroscopic swallow study was stopped and the physician was immediately called. A STAT barium swallow study, or esophagram, and a computed tomography (CT) scan of the chest were ordered to rule out a tracheoesophageal fistula (TEF).

A tracheoesophageal fistula was confirmed that afternoon. Within the mediastinum, there was an air tract connecting the right aspect of the midesophagus to the posterior aspect of the trachea. Aspiration of barium into the right lung and the left lower lobe confirmed aspiration pneumonitis. Unfortunately, the CT scan of the chest also identified blastic osseous lesions of the thoracic spine. As the time in Radiology progressed, Janelle's respirations became more labored and her oxygen requirements increased as a result of the aspiration through the TEF. Janelle was transferred to the intensive care unit, where she had to be intubated for 3 days.

The speech-language pathologist and primary physician met with Janelle and her family and explained the results of the videofluoroscopic swallow study, barium swallow, and CT scan of the chest. It was speculated that Janelle had developed three chloromas, or tumors in the trachea, which are often associated with AML. One of the tumors responded to the chemoradiation, which resulted in the TEF. As noted on the chest CT scan, it was confirmed that Janelle's cancer had metastasized, or spread, to her bones.

## Analysis of Client's Response to Intervention

Further management by the speech-language pathologist was not indicated at this time as the oropharyngeal swallow was WFL, and the reason for the aspiration was a fistula. Medical management was required. It was determined that Janelle was not medically fit for surgery. Instead, a covered, self-expanding metal stent (SEMS) was placed on May 24 in an attempt to palliatively seal the fistula (Fan, Baron, & Utz, 2002). The SEMS successfully closed the fistula, as confirmed by repeat esophagram. However, there was concern that the two remaining chloromas would respond in a similar fashion to the chemotherapy and result in TEFs.

A consult to the palliative care team was made. The palliative care team usually consists of a physician, frequently a nurse, and a social worker. In some settings, a pharmacist and spiritual advisor may be included. Palliative care specializes in medical management and decision making at end-of life. A decision needed to be made regarding the aggressiveness of Janelle's medical care, including whether to consider nonoral nutrition. Several new, and extremely unfortunate, pieces of information regarding Janelle's medical condition had been discovered in the past few days. The presence of two more tumors in the trachea put Janelle at risk for developing more TEFs, which could lead to other episodes of aspiration pneumonia.

Janelle was not expected to live beyond 6 months. She wished to continue with chemotherapy in an attempt to slow down the rate of the spreading cancer. Her endurance was poor due to her illness, and it was expected that she would not meet nutritional needs orally. In consideration of quality of life, she wanted to begin eating and drinking again. Janelle's physicians supported the initiation of oral intake. They explained that at end-of-life the feeling of hunger subsides and that people are often satisfied with a few bites or sips of something they really enjoy (Slomka, 2003).

Janelle's husband and daughters were concerned that Janelle would develop another TEF and develop aspiration pneumonia. They convinced Janelle that she should remain NPO and receive a feeding tube. The palliative care team, and speech-language pathologist conferenced again with Janelle and her family to review Janelle's prognosis and the importance of quality of life in her final days. The team suggested that if Janelle did receive a percutaneous endoscopic gastrostomy (PEG) tube, or feeding tube, oral pleasure feedings should accompany the nonoral nutrition. The speech-language pathologist explained that having a PEG tube did not guarantee that Janelle would not get aspiration pneumonia. With Janelle's history of reflux, it was very possible that she could aspirate refluxed tube feedings. The SLP also reviewed clinical signs and symptoms of aspiration. She suggested that since Janelle had exhibited clinical signs and symptoms of aspiration during her first two bouts with aspiration pneumonia, she would likely exhibit coughing and choking if aspiration due to a new TEF occurred. In this case, the family could immediately contact the physician and Janelle could return to NPO status.

The family was insistent that Janelle receive nothing by mouth to prevent aspiration pneumonia. Against her own wishes, Janelle agreed to receive a PEG tube. The tube was placed on May 25 and Janelle was discharged to home on hospice the following day.

Janelle passed away 1 week later. The feeding tube did not prolong Janelle's life. And, unfortunately, she did not enjoy any foods or liquids that could have contributed to her quality of life. The family, afraid to lose Janelle after a relatively short illness, influenced her to choose aggressive management in light of a very poor prognosis, and focused on quantity of life versus quality of life. Although the medical team can provide information, recommendations, and support, ultimately, end-of-life decisions lie with our patients and their families. Providing the patient and family with education and resources to make these decisions is an important role of the medical team, which includes the speech-language pathologist.

## Author Note

This case study was not based on a single patient. Instead, it was developed from a compilation of patients with similar diagnoses, medical courses, and outcomes. IRB approval was not required.

## References


Colice, G. L., Stukel, T. A., & Dain, B. (1989). Laryngeal complications of prolonged intubation. *Chest, 96,* 877–884.

Fan, A. C., Baron, T. H., & Utz, J. P. (2002). Combined tracheal and esophageal stenting for palliation of tracehoesophageal symptoms from mediastinal lymphoma. *Mayo Clinic Proceedings, 77,* 1347–1350.

Fujiu, M., & Logemann, J. A. (1996). Effect of a tongue-holding maneuver on posterior pharyngeal wall movement during deglutition. *American Journal of Speech-Language Pathology, 5,* 23–30.

Fujiu, M., Logemann, J. A., & Pauloski, B. R. (1995). Increased postoperative posterior pharyngeal wall movement in patients with anterior oral cancer: preliminary findings and possible implications for treatment. *American Journal of Speech-Language Pathology, 4,* 24–30.

Jorgensen, H. S., Nakayama, H., Raaschou, H. O., Vive-Larsen, J., Stoier, M., & Olsen, T. S. (1995). Outcome and time course of recovery in stroke. Part II. Time course of recovery. The Copenhagen Stroke Study. *Archives of Physical Medicine and Rehabilitation 76*(5), 406–412.

Kahrilas, P. J., Lin, S., Logemann, J. A., Ergen, G. A., & Facchini, F. (1991). Deglutitive tongue action: Volume accommodation and bolus propulsion. *Gastroenterology, 104,* 152–162.

Kulbersh, B. D., Rosenthal, E. L., McGrew, B. M., Duncan, R. D., McColloch, N. C., Carroll, W. R., et al. (2006). Pretreatment, preoperative swallowing exercises may improve dysphagia quality of life. *Laryngoscope, 116,* 883–886.

Logemann, J. A., Pauloski, B. R., Rademaker, A. W., & Coangelo, A. (1997). Super-supraglottic swallow in irradiated head and neck cancer patients. *Head and Neck, 19,* 535–540.

Rosenbek, J. C., Robbins, J. A., Roecker, E. B., Coyle, J. L., & Wood, J. L. (1996). A penetration-aspiration scale. *Dysphagia, 11,* 93–98.

Rosenthal, D. I., Lewin, J. S., & Eisbruch, A. (2006). Prevention and treatment of dysphagia and aspiration after chemoradiation for head and neck cancer. *Journal of Clinical Oncology, 24,* 2636–2643.

Sharp, H. M., & Genesen, L. B. (1996). Ethical decision-making in dysphagia management. *American Journal of Speech-Language Pathology, 5*(1), 15–22.

Slomka, J. (2003). Withholding nutrition at the end of life: Clinical and ethical issues. *Cleveland Clinic Journal of Medicine, 70,* 548–552.

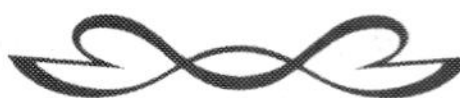



# CASE 57

# Neil: A Holistic Rehabilitation Approach for a Survivor of Traumatic Brain Injury

*Pat Kearns, Janelle Ward, Karen Hux, and Jeffry Snell*

## Conceptual Knowledge Areas

Traumatic brain injuries (TBIs) result from the application of strong, external, physical forces to the skull. Common causes include violent shaking, whiplash injuries, and blows to the head from falls, assaults, sporting accidents, and motor vehicle accidents. The consequent damage to the brain results from a combination of initial or primary mechanisms occurring at the actual time of injury as well as secondary injury mechanisms occurring as aftereffects of the initial insult. Primary mechanisms of injury include cavitation effects and shearing strain causing diffuse axonal injury; secondary mechanisms include events such as the formation of hematomas and the presence of acute cerebral swelling, cerebral edema, and increased intracranial pressure.

Blast injuries represent a special class of TBIs in that they result from any one or a combination of the following primary injury mechanisms:

1. Injury resulting from a primary overpressurization wave (i.e., a blast or percussion wave) impacting the body surface
2. Injury resulting from projectiles (e.g., flying debris, bomb fragments) impacting the body
3. Injury resulting from displacement of the victim (e.g., being thrown into other objects) and/or structural collapse (e.g., crush injuries) secondary to the blast
4. Injury that is a direct consequence of the blast, such as burns, asphyxia, and exposure to toxins

Secondary mechanisms of injury then follow, with the result being diffuse damage throughout the cerebrum.

Treatment for TBI initially focuses on stabilizing the survivor from a medical standpoint, attending to any life-threatening injuries, and preventing or minimizing to the greatest extent possible the occurrence of secondary mechanisms of injury. Physical, cognitive, social, and emotional changes associated with the sustained damage only become evident as the person progresses through the recovery process. Long-term outcome and quality of life following TBI largely depends on the extent to which a survivor has spared abilities, is successful in reestablishing lost or impaired skills, or can learn to compensate for persistent deficits.

Cognitive rehabilitation is the process through which professionals assist survivors in achieving the best outcomes possible. Over time, the focus of a survivor's cognitive rehabilitation program shifts from working to regain lost abilities to mastering compensatory strategies that minimize persistent deficits. The cognitive rehabilitation process often extends over a period of several years and involves the efforts of professionals from multiple disciplines as well as friends and family members.

## Description of the Case

### Background Information

Neil grew up in an upper-middle-class home in a large Midwestern town. Neil's family described him as a "very bright" student throughout high school, in the gifted program, with plans to attend college. He entered college while also working part-time and then reportedly quit school in his first year, because it was "too much like high school." Shortly thereafter, Neil joined the military. His past medical history included a childhood diagnosis of Tourette syndrome with tics that were treated and largely controlled with medication. He also had a history of occasional, though not excessive, alcohol use.

At 21 years of age, Neil sustained a severe traumatic brain injury while serving as an active duty Operation Iraqi Freedom combat soldier in Iraq. His injury occurred when a suicide bomber in a vehicle packed with explosives hit the vehicle Neil was driving and detonated the explosives. Neil was the only survivor of the incident. His injuries included a depressed skull fracture, bilateral subdural hematomas, right lung contusion, open fractures of the mandible, right facial fractures, right humeral fracture, C6 fracture, sternum fracture, clavicle fractures, extensive embedded shrapnel fragments in the right face and neck, and second- and third-degree burns on his right hand, thighs, and knees. Shortly following his initial trauma, he sustained a left frontoparietal stroke.

Neil was initially hospitalized and medically stabilized in Germany and then transported to the intensive care unit of an Army Medical Center in the United States. One month later, he began rehabilitation at the same facility. He had several other inpatient rehabilitation placements over the next year, eventually returning home to live with his mother approximately one year following his injury. He continued to require 24-hour care and supervision at that time. Neil received various home health support and outpatient services while living at home.

### Reasons for Referral and Evaluation Findings

Approximately 3½ years after his injury, Neil entered a postacute residential rehabilitation facility to undergo assessment and intervention for persistent cognitive deficits. His initial assessment included speech-language and neuropsychological evaluations. Neil's hearing appeared adequate for testing purposes. Although he seemed to have some degree of nearsightedness, he compensated for this by placing material close within his visual field. Neil was independent with walking over level surfaces, though he displayed significant ataxia affecting upper extremity use and gait steadiness over uneven surfaces. He demonstrated no bizarre or specifically psychotic thought processes, and his thinking appeared goal-directed and concrete.

The initial speech-language evaluation revealed slowed processing speed and memory impairments affecting performance of lengthy and complex tasks. Neil answered concrete and abstract yes/no questions and followed two- and three-step commands, but he had difficulty with four-step commands. When read a paragraph, Neil immediately answered simple yes/no questions about the story with 80% accuracy. However, when asked to retell the story immediately after hearing it, Neil could not generate either the main idea or details. Further testing revealed that he had stored a portion of the concrete story information in memory but had difficulty accessing that stored information to generate the story retell. His expressive language abilities were largely intact, and he spoke in complete, grammatically accurate sentences. Neil performed sentence completion, object naming, and picture description tasks adequately, and his abstract language comprehension was functional. Given extended time, he generated multiple solutions and solved common as well as novel problems. Neil's speech was slightly imprecise, slurred, and hypernasal. He used several strategies, such as slowing down and taking frequent breaths, to increase speech intelligibility. At times, Neil expressed frustration about the way his voice sounded.

Neil's performance on neuropsychological assessment procedures revealed significant deficits in memory, with performances on immediate recall, delayed recall, and recognition tasks falling within the borderline to impaired ranges. He evidenced substantial decay of information over a relatively brief time (e.g., 20 minutes) and could not retrieve information spontaneously or even recognize target information after that delay. Neil also demonstrated a general slowing of cognitive processing speed, impairments in divided attention, and significant ataxia. Consistent with the speech-language evaluation findings, Neil demonstrated relatively intact language functioning, with average performance on confrontational naming and abstract language reasoning tasks and superior performance on a vocabulary skills task. The only areas of language functioning with suppressed levels of performance were ones requiring rapid responses and verbal fluency. These challenges appeared to stem from slowed processing speed. From a behavioral perspective, Neil demonstrated substantial executive dysfunction, frequently erupting in angry outbursts when frustrated by his inability to perform tasks that were formerly not problematic for him. He was very quick to anger and tended to exhibit behaviors disproportionate to the circumstances, such as yelling, cursing, and fleeing the location. Further complicating Neil's cognitive deficits and difficulty applying compensatory strategies was a general lack of awareness and insight. Neil did not demonstrate accurate insight and awareness "in the moment" when struggling with cognitive tasks or when experiencing an emotional/behavioral escalation and, therefore, did not spontaneously compensate for or initiate strategies to deal with the situation.

Consistently, the most substantial and interfering deficits Neil displayed were those of impaired memory functioning. These deficits limited Neil's independence and hampered his acquisition, mastery, and use of compensatory strategies to minimize the impact of his deficits. As a result, Neil required 24-hour support for initiating and completing all daily activities except dressing himself. Emotional issues, specifically anger, stemmed from Neil's perceived lack of independence and control over his environment. His anger initially resulted in outbursts and actions that compromised his safety. In an attempt to minimize frustration and angry outbursts, Neil's family supported him for all functional deficits, but, after months of providing this 24-hour level of care, his family reported substantial fatigue and discouragement. They described a deteriorating family unit focused only on meeting Neil's needs. Furthermore, constant family support to initiate and complete daily activities prompted Neil to become excessively dependent on others.

Neil expressed a goal of regaining his premorbid level of independent living and purposeful activity, including having his own apartment, engaging in relationships, driving, and working. Neil's family expressed a desire for him to increase independence with daily living skills and, more importantly, to be happy with his life again.

## Treatment Options Considered

A broad range of clinical practice methods exists in the area of cognitive rehabilitation; hence, several treatment options were available to serve as a basis for Neil's program. Options included: (a) *systems of total external support* (i.e., support from family or caregivers) to eliminate decision making and the potential for failure; (b) impairment-specific *cognitive retraining tasks* (i.e., "mental muscle building") using activities such as computer memory games; (c) *academic-type training* using didactic material and homework focused on noncontextual learning and explicit memory; (d) *internal compensatory strategies* such as rehearsal, visual imagery, and organizational techniques to refine self-monitoring skills and teach methods of deficit compensation that could potentially generalize across multiple settings and activities; (e) *external compensatory devices* implementing memory books, planners, and alarms to compensate for specific deficits; and (f) *skill-specific training* focused on contextual learning and use of implicit memory for development of routines.

Neil's treatment team selected the most appropriate treatment option for him by systematically considering the match between his residual strengths and challenges and the skills needed for successful implementation of each cognitive rehabilitation technique. The team rejected the first option, systems of external control, because this was the strategy Neil's family had been implementing and with which they were currently struggling. Next, given the severity of Neil's memory and executive function deficits, the team felt that treatment options dependent on explicit memory and noncontextual learning would not be effective; hence, they also rejected cognitive retraining tasks and academic-type training as the basis for program development. Many practitioners advocate for the provision of compensatory strategy instruction as a "practice standard" for individuals with mild memory deficits who are actively involved in identifying and treating their challenges (Cicerone et al., 2005); however, given the severity of Neil's memory deficits and his limited deficit awareness, the treatment team believed compensatory strategy training requiring self-regulation alone was unlikely to be successful. Evidence exists suggesting that externally directed compensatory devices such as alarms may benefit people with moderate to severe memory impairments if training is incorporated with functional activities and ongoing staff support is provided (Wilson, Emslie, Quirk, & Evans, 2001). Evidence of success also exists for skill specific training with individuals who have moderate to severe memory deficits when the treatment focuses on real-life functional activities, is completed in the context of real-world settings, and involves the use of implicit memory and learning (Burke, Danick, Bemis, & Durgin, 1994; Cicerone et al., 2005; Kime, Lamb, & Wilson, 1996; Schacter, Rich, & Stampp, 1985; Squires, Hunkin, & Parking, 1996).

Based on the above information, Neil's team chose to focus on teaching him specific skill sets that would be functional within his real-world environment of the residential facility and the community. Successful mastery of skill sets relied primarily on implicit memory and the learning of routines through consistent repetitions (Wilson, Baddeley, Evans, & Schiel, 1994; Wilson & Evans, 1996; Ylvisaker & Feeney, 1998). To provide motivation, each routine centered on Neil's interests and goals, and the treatment program included psychology services to address awareness and acceptance issues as well as to deal with emotional issues as they arose. External memory compensation devices were integrated into specific skill sets to the degree they could be included in implicitly learned routines (Sohlberg & Mateer, 1989; Squires et al., 1996; Ylvisaker & Feeney, 1998).

The team hypothesized that helping Neil master a series of implicitly learned routines that included external compensatory devices would allow him to increase his independence regarding management of daily living skills and engagement in purposeful activity. They also hypothesized that Neil's emotional well-being would improve as he developed a sense of hope and optimism for his future through increased independence and control over his day.

## Course of Treatment

Neil began his treatment in an on-site residential facility that provided 24-hour staff support. The setting was a single-story house with eight private bedrooms and community living, dining, kitchen, laundry, and shower areas. Neil's treatment team included a nurse, nutritionist, occupational therapist, physical therapist, speech-language pathologist, life skills specialist, recreational therapist, psychologist, family counselor, case manager, and five residential staff. Neil's treatment program included three components. The first component addressed medical needs as they arose, though these were minimal. The second and primary component was education-based and focused on development of skill sets. The third component was psychological in nature and targeted helping Neil regain hope and optimism for the future and an anticipation of pleasure. Neil's team speculated that addressing the psychological component in conjunction with the medical and education components would lead to optimal participation and maximize outcomes.

Based on the three treatment components, Neil's team identified functional skill sets necessary to meet his goals. In addition to discipline-specific formal evaluations of performance, the treatment team observed Neil closely for all waking hours over three consecutive days to evaluate the functional impact of his impairments on daily living skills. The team also gathered specific information regarding his preferences and natural tendencies. Based on this information, the team developed routines for each skill set. They also considered various external compensatory strategies and devices for implementation with the routines as appropriate. Initially, Neil refused to consider use of any external compensatory devices that he perceived to differentiate him from a "normal" person. Over time and as he became more aware of his deficits through regular counseling and staff encouragement, he agreed to participate in choosing and developing strategies and devices that assisted with increasing his independence for moderately complex and complex routines.

Implementation of the routines focused on providing sufficient support to ensure Neil's success but avoiding excess support that would lead to dependence upon staff. The goal was for each routine to occur successfully (i.e., following principles of errorless learning) and without task failure (Sohlberg & Mateer, 1989; Squires et al., 1996; von Cramon, & Matthes-von Cramon, 1994; Wilson et al., 1994; Wilson & Evans, 1996; Ylvisaker & Feeney, 1998). Therefore, the treatment team continuously and carefully monitored Neil's performance, and, as Neil proved he was implicitly learning a routine by demonstrating initiation of parts or all of it, staff adjusted their support to allow for his increased independence. Each routine was implemented in his real-life environment (i.e., residential and community settings) and with natural support from staff (von Cramon & Matthes-von Cramon, 1994; Ylvisaker, Feeney, & Szekeres, 1998). Because overlap existed in the skill sets on which various team members focused, communication among team members was imperative to ensure consistency across disciplines. Communication with family members and their direct involvement in the treatment program was also important.

## Analysis of Client's Response to Intervention

Neil's team began his course of treatment by developing routines for basic functional skill sets. These basic routines included morning/evening grooming, basic orientation strategies, intake of adequate nutrition, and taking medications. To illustrate the sequence of a basic routine, we describe his morning grooming routine. The team first identified a specific location to keep all items Neil needed for morning grooming along with a written list of specific, sequential tasks to perform during his showering, grooming, and dressing routine. Items on the list included shower, put on clothes from basket, brush teeth, put dirty clothes in hamper. Verbal cues were initially required to retrieve needed items and then to attend to each task on the list. Without the cues and list, Neil completed some items multiple times and did not complete others. Each staff member working with Neil was trained on the exact support to provide the most effective style of interaction and the timing with which to provide the support. Specifically, a staff member was immediately present when Neil woke every day at 6:15 a.m. This was to ensure that Neil started the routine the correct way each day and prevented him from making errors such as starting in the middle of the list. After 5 days, Neil demonstrated that he had learned to initiate using the list, therefore allowing staff to eliminate that cue. With ongoing successful repetitions, staff gradually faded support and Neil showered, dressed, and groomed independently. The team introduced all other basic routines in the same manner; that is, they used a variety of verbal cues and written lists, and the amount of staff support decreased as Neil demonstrated consistent success.

Once the foundation of basic routines was in place, the team addressed skill sets of increasing complexity. These routines included initial management of external memory compensation devices, simple meal planning and preparation, basic home management, and community access focusing on safety, emotional adjustment, and decision making. Although implementation of external memory compensation devices was a routine itself, it also became an important step in other routines within this category. To master this routine, Neil first experimented with several memory compensation devices ranging in complexity from a simple day-planner to a BlackBerry®. Based on his preferences, premorbid strategies, and physical deficits due to ataxia, he settled on using a personal computer with Microsoft Outlook® calendar.

The purpose for using memory compensation devices was twofold. First, they provided Neil with a routine way of preparing for the next day; second, they served as a means of memory compensation to prompt his attendance at daily activities. The memory compensation device routine started with staff providing verbal cues to assist Neil with locating the Outlook icon on his computer desktop, opening the program and calendar, and printing the schedule for the next day. This part of the routine was completed in the evening so that Neil could use the printed schedule to make decisions about planning for the next day (e.g., deciding what clothing to wear and for what time to set the alarm). After completing his next-day planning, Neil placed his printed schedule in a designated spot every evening (i.e., on a shelf near the door along with his watch, wallet, phone, and keys). In the morning, Neil gathered his schedule, watch, wallet, phone, and keys.

After 10 days of successful repetitions, Neil required a cue to initiate the memory compensation routine but independently accessed the program and printed his daily schedule. He also required a cue to put his schedule in the designated spot, but he found the schedule, along with his other items, independently in the morning. Neil continued to require cues throughout the day to look at his schedule. After 2 additional weeks, Neil became independent with placing his schedule on the shelf each evening, but he did not make further progress with using his schedule. To further decrease staff support regarding functional use of his schedule to complete activities, the team considered adding a second external memory compensation device—specifically, a watch with an audible alarm that Neil approved as an acceptable accommodation. After reviewing several options, use of a Timex® Data Link® watch that provided numerous alarm options as well as scrolling written text was implemented. The team's initial intent was to use the watch instead of the paper schedule; however, Neil's tendency to turn off the alarm and then quickly forget what the text cued him to do prevented successful implementation of this substitution. Therefore, the team opted to maintain use of the printed schedule and simplify the watch cues so they only served as reminders about medication times and the need to "check the schedule." With these strategies in place, the number of cues Neil needed throughout the day to use his schedule decreased.

Although Neil became more independent with his memory compensation device routine, after 8 months he continued to need occasional reminders to check his schedule. The team investigated other strategies during this time period, but wearing a "normal" watch and discreetly carrying a paper schedule were the only options to which Neil agreed. Because Neil implicitly learned through repetition routines occurring on a daily basis (i.e., meals, ADLs), the team considered making his entire schedule exactly the same each day. As with most young adults, however, Neil preferred a variety of leisure activities and the opportunity to change or add activities spontaneously to his schedule. Hence, this idea was not put into operation. The team introduced implementation and mastery of all remaining routines included in Neil's rehabilitation program in the same manner with modifications made as appropriate.

As Neil gained independence with activities that met his basic health and safety needs, the team developed additional routines to address his emotional needs and allow him to have a sense of control over his day. Memory compensation devices were again an important component of each of these complex routines. Proposed routines included money management, meal planning and shopping, leisure planning, community access, and medication management. Leisure planning was the most motivating routine for Neil and reinforced previously mastered skill sets. However, Neil required full support for generating ideas for leisure options and filling open time during his day. He frequently refused options offered by others, yet demonstrated anger when his time was not filled. To manage this, staff encouraged Neil to develop lists of options based on prior interests and supported his investigation and participation in similar activities available in the surrounding community.

Leisure activities of particular interest to Neil included dining out, watching movies, and listening to music. To help him master routines associated with these options, team members developed separate written lists for interests Neil could access in his residence (e.g., downloading music, searching the Internet, or playing games online) versus in the community (e.g., going to restaurants, movie theaters, or concert venues). Then, staff assisted Neil with identifying free time in his schedule and choosing activities from his lists appropriate for the time of day and amount of time available. Specifically, each Sunday evening, Neil met with a staff member to identify short periods of free time throughout the upcoming week and then made selections from his list of residential leisure activities to fill those times. Two times per week staff assisted Neil with identifying time slots of sufficient length to allow him to access the community. By again using his written list of choices, Neil selected an activity (e.g., dining out) and then a venue for that activity (e.g., Applebee's®). He then utilized the Internet to find the location, print the menu, and budget for the activity.

Initially, Neil needed maximum support to complete the multiple steps associated with implementing leisure option routines. In particular, Neil required significant encouragement to participate in making choices and following through with selected activities. His reluctance appeared to result from his memory deficits (i.e., he would forget that he chose the activity) and poor acceptance of his deficits (i.e., he appeared embarrassed about his ataxia and the way in which his memory deficits affected his abilities). However, after several successful experiences with community-based activities, Neil became more cooperative with performing leisure option routines and began to demonstrate increased independence with parts of the planning and execution process. Over a period of approximately 6 months, Neil went from maximum staff dependence to only requiring one cue to access and make choices from his list. As Neil gained computer proficiency, the team transferred his written lists to a series of folders that he could access from his computer desktop. The folders were layered, representing the sequence from his areas of interests to category or venue options to specific venue information. For example, if he was planning to access his interest of dining out, he would chose the "Dining Out" folder, then select a food category folder—such as the "American Food" folder—and finally he would choose the specific restaurant—such as "Applebee's®"—which would link him to the restaurant website for further planning. Due to the complexity of the overall routine, Neil persisted in usually needing support to initiate planning an activity for an upcoming evening or weekend, adding the activity to his schedule, and sequencing through the activity planning steps. However, on occasion, Neil independently found community activities to attend.

As Neil gained independence and control over his day, his team consistently observed an overall improvement in his mood that, in turn, appeared to increase his participation in the treatment program. His achievement of complex routines had the greatest impact on his mood, as they allowed for the anticipation of pleasure, a greater sense of control over his life, and increased confidence in his abilities. However, performing complex routines also caused Neil the most frustration, because he could not complete the necessary tasks with the same ease as he had prior to injury. Overall, the team believed the benefits associated with Neil's improved mood and program participation outweighed the periods of frustration and anger. Over time, he responded to redirection with greater ease and acceptance.

With routines in place, Neil was ready to move from the structured rehabilitation setting to a community-based apartment that had 24-hour supervision available as needed. This move provided a means of simulating fully independent living while still ensuring Neil's access to staff support and supervision. Despite replication of all of Neil's previously mastered routines and compensatory devices in the apartment setting, the change of environment resulted in his need for increased staff support. Initially, Neil required maximum support for all routines and 24-hour supervision for safety. With structured repetitions, however, this need for support was gradually decreased to match his previously acquired levels. The team also found that any interruption in Neil's routines necessitated a temporary increase in staff support. For example, after visiting his family for a 10-day vacation during which other activities interrupted his established routines, Neil again required maximum staff support to reestablish his routines in his apartment setting. This support was gradually decreased over a 2- to 4-week period to again match his previously acquired levels.

## Further Recommendations

After 1 year of combined residential treatment and independent living simulation, Neil was independent with all basic routines as long as his environment remained consistent. He was also independent with mid-level routines within his familiar environment if his compensatory strategies were consistently available. Based on his independence with these routines, the support Neil needed decreased from 24 hours to 6 to 8 hours per day. Neil continued to need evening and weekend support to facilitate implementation of complex routines. In conjunction with his family and his funding source, the treatment team decided to discharge Neil from the postacute rehabilitation program and to arrange for him to live in a community apartment close to his family's home. Neil would transition and carry out his daily schedule and all functional skill sets and routines in this permanent environment. Because Neil was not receiving any traditional formal therapies at the time of discharge, the team did not recommend resumption of any such services. Rather, the treatment team recommended (a) continued provision of 6 to 8 hours per week of assistance from a companion to help manage complex routines, and (b) provision of vocational rehabilitation to assist Neil in obtaining a job.

Neil had an extensive support system throughout his treatment including immediate and extended family, childhood friends, and military friends and advocates. Neil's family and friends participated in extensive brain injury education and instruction about how to facilitate his routines successfully. Just prior to discharge, both Neil's mother and father participated in a simulated companion role over a 1-week period. This gave them confidence that they could instruct others in the use of all verbal cues, external devices, and interaction styles to maximize Neil's success.

The accuracy of the team's initial hypotheses about the type of rehabilitation program best suited to Neil's situation allowed for the selection of an effective treatment approach. However, the team did not anticipate that the success or failure of the program would be so dependent on the consistency of Neil's staff interactions, verbal supports, and environments. Specifically, the team did not expect that a simple change of environment or interruption in Neil's daily schedule would lead to a notable decline in his independence with performing basic routines. Despite this setback, the team made accurate predictions about the amount of time that Neil would need support to regain his independence with basic routines after returning to a familiar environment and predictable schedule. Neil's periods of regression when first introduced to a simulated independent living situation and when returning to that environment after a 10-day vacation provided important information for the development of a discharge transition plan. In particular, the team realized that Neil's successful transition to a more permanent independent living setting would require an initial period of increased support as well as exact or nearly exact replication of established routines and devices. Likewise, Neil demonstrated that, given consistency and repetition, he could master both simple and complex routines that allow for decreased reliance on outside supervision and support.

## Author Note

This paper is based on a real case, although names and other identifying information were changed to protect individuals' privacy. Both the Institutional Review Board of the University of Nebraska–Lincoln and the facility's Research Committee and Human Rights Review Committee approved performance of this work. The client and his legal guardian provided assent and consent for participation.

## References


Burke, J., Danick, J., Bemis, B., & Durgin, C. (1994). A process approach to memory book training for neurological patients. *Brain Injury, 8*, 71–81.

Cicerone, K. D., Dahlberg, C., Malec, J. F., Langenbahn, D. M., Felicetti, T., Kneipp, S., et al. (2005). Evidence-based cognitive rehabilitation: Updated review of the literature from 1998 through 2002. *Archives of Physical Medicine and Rehabilitation, 86*, 1681–1692.

Kime, S., Lamb, D., & Wilson, G. (1996). Use of a comprehensive programme of external cueing to enhance procedural memory in a patient with dense amnesia. *Brain Injury, 10*, 17–25.

Schacter, D. L., Rich, S. A., & Stampp, M. S. (1985). Remediation of memory disorders: Experimental evaluation of the spaced retrieval technique. *Journal of Clinical and Experimental Neuropsychology, 7*, 79–86.

Sohlberg, M. M., & Mateer, C. A. (1989). Training use of compensatory memory books: A three stage behavioral approach. *Journal of Clinical and Experimental Neuropsychology, 11*, 871–891.

Squires, E. J., Hunkin, N. M., & Parking, A. J. (1996). Memory notebook training in a case of severe amnesia: Generalizing from paired associate learning to real life. *Neuropsychological Rehabilitation, 6*, 55–65.

von Cramon, D. Y., & Matthes-von Cramon, G. (1994). Back to work with a chronic dysexecutive syndrome? (A case report). *Neuropsychological Rehabilitation, 4*, 399–417.

Wilson, B. A., Baddeley, A. D., Evans, J., & Shiel, A. (1994). Errorless learning in the rehabilitation of memory-impaired people. *Neuropsychological Rehabilitation, 4*, 307–326.

Wilson, B. A., Emslie, H. C., Quirk, K., & Evans, J. J. (2001). Reducing everyday memory and planning problems by means of a paging system: A randomized control crossover study. *Journal of Neurology, Neurosurgery, and Psychiatry, 70*, 477–482.

Wilson, B., & Evans, J. (1996). Error-free learning in the rehabilitation of people with memory impairments. *Journal of Head Trauma Rehabilitation, 11*, 54–64.

Ylvisaker, M., & Feeney, T. (1998). *Collaborative brain injury intervention: Positive everyday routines.* New York: Thompson Delmar Learning.

Ylvisaker, M., Feeney, T., & Szekeres, S. (1998). Social-environmental approaches to communication and behavior. In M. Ylvisaker (Ed.), *Traumatic brain injury rehabilitation: Children and adolescents* (pp. 271–302). Newton, MA: Butterworth-Heinemann.

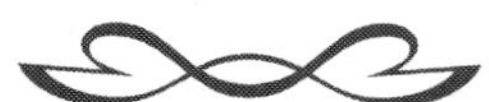

## VELOPHARYNGEAL DYSFUNCTION

# CASE 58

# Emily: Velopharyngeal Dysfunction in an Adolescent Girl: Neurological, Behavioral, or Anatomical in Origin?

*Jeff Searl*

## Conceptual Knowledge Areas

Diagnosis and treatment of individuals with suspected or known velopharyngeal (VP) dysfunction is predicated on a firm understanding of normal speech production and the impact of unintended nasal and oral cavity coupling on speech sound production. The VP mechanism consists of the soft palate and the nasopharyngeal walls (side and back walls of the uppermost part of the throat); clinicians should have an understanding of the usual VP anatomy and physiology as a starting point for diagnosing VP dysfunction. Because the range of what is normal in terms of VP anatomy can be quite large, it is important to have experience examining the mouths of nondisordered speakers, paying particular attention to size, shape, length, relative depth, and movements of the soft palate and pharyngeal walls during speech.

The VP mechanism is not readily visualized during spontaneous speech. Therefore, clinicians who work in this area regularly should have proficiency in conducting or interpreting data from instrumental examinations that can provide anatomical or physiological data (e.g., movement of the palate and pharyngeal walls, aerodynamic recordings, etc.) that inform about VP function. Learning about these types of instrumental assessments may begin in graduate school, but typically, proficiency is gained through self-study, continuing education opportunities, and mentored clinical interactions.

The impact of VP dysfunction on speech production can be predicted, in general, based on an understanding of normal speech sound production. Closure of the VP port is necessary for nearly all sounds in Standard American English with the exception of nasal phonemes (/m, n, ng/). Speech-language pathologists may encounter individuals whose VP port closes inappropriately on nasal phonemes, resulting in hyponasal speech (speech that sounds de-nasal). However, it is more likely that patients seen will have a VP mechanism that does not close (or does not close completely or in a timely fashion) on oral phonemes. The reasons for this deficient VP closure are many, but the most common etiologies include clefts of the palate, neurological disorders that are impacting VP muscles, and mislearning during speech sound development. When VP closure is not attained for oral sound production, the resulting speech may be characterized by hypernasality (too much nasal resonance), audible nasal emission (burst of sound through the nose during pressure consonant production such as stops, fricatives, and affricates), and weak pressure consonants (consonants perceived as imprecise). In addition to the changes in individual speech sound production, loss of air out of the nose due to VP dysfunction can cause an individual to use shorter breath units, have speech perceived as being decreased in loudness, increase phonatory effort, and engage in articulatory compensations. Moving place of production posteriorly is the most common pattern observed.

To diagnose and treat individuals with VP dysfunction, a clinician should be proficient at judging resonance phenomenon (hyper- and hyponasality), completing auditory-perceptual ratings and judgments of speech sound production (articulation inventories, phonological processes analysis, etc.), and evaluating phonatory and prosodic features of speech (voice quality, phrase length, loudness, etc.). Calibration of the ears of the novice speech-language pathologist is primarily done via repeated exposure to the parameters being judged in order to gain a sense of the full range of symptoms being judged. Working alongside a more experienced clinician who can calibrate the novice's judgments, or using standard speech samples against which the productions of a client can be judged may assist the new clinician in making accurate and repeatable judgments more independently.

The differential diagnostic process for VP dysfunction is contingent on a number of pieces of information. However, client history, observation of the pattern of the speech abnormalities, visual inspection of the VP mechanism and its movements, and determination of the client's ability to behaviorally modify the speech are important in narrowing the diagnostic choice. Treatment in this area is largely contingent on understanding the etiology of the VP symptoms, knowing the medical and prosthetic treatment possibilities, recognizing the limits of behavioral intervention for VP symptoms, and understanding typical treatment concepts such as specificity of training, hierarchical structuring of stimuli and tasks, modeling and behavioral modification techniques, and so on.

## Description of the Case

### Background Information

#### Setting and Time of Client Contact

Emily was seen for diagnostic and therapeutic speech services at a university-based hearing and speech clinic housed on the campus of a large teaching hospital. Prior to initiating speech services, she was seen as an outpatient in the Otolaryngology Department at this same hospital to determine whether adenoidectomy would improve her speech. The clinical services described took place within a 4 month time frame during Emily's eighth-grade school year.

## History Information

Emily was 14 years old and in eighth grade at the time of the ENT evaluation that precipitated the speech-language pathology contact. She lived in an urban neighborhood with her mother, father, and one brother who was 2 years older. Both parents had high school educations and worked full-time in the manufacturing industry. They had been married for 16 years. The household was considered to be lower to middle socioeconomic level based on income, parental education, and other measures.

The mother smoked intermittently through the first trimester of the pregnancy, which was normal in all other respects. Emily's birth history was unremarkable. She was diagnosed with moderate pulmonary stenosis within the first week of life and underwent balloon dilation shortly thereafter followed by several years of SBE prophylaxis (subacute bacterial endocarditis prophylaxis). She continued to be followed by a pediatric cardiologist to monitor her heart through the time she was seen for speech therapy. Persistent symptoms of general fatigue, shortness of breath, and a rapid heart rate were attributed to heart issues. Emily had bilateral myringotomy tubes placed at 1 year of age due to frequent middle ear infections that were not responsive to usual antibiotic regimens. Per ENT evaluation hearing now was within normal limits though the tubes were not in place (presumably they had fallen out).

Information about early developmental milestones was provided by Emily's mother. Emily sat unsupported at ~7 months of age, crawled at 9 months, and was walking unsupported by 13 months. Her mother described Emily as being "clumsy" when she ran, threw balls, or did other gross motor activities; Emily herself stated that she remained less coordinated and athletic than most of her peers. Her mother did not feel that Emily was a particularly messy eater as a young child. According to the mother, Emily was a "late talker," not saying her first real words until just under 2 years of age.

Following a preschool screening when Emily was 3½ years old, it was recommended that she receive physical and occupational therapy (PT and OT) to address delayed motor development. Her mother indicated that there was no specific diagnosis offered other than general "developmental delay." There were no reports available detailing the PT or OT treatments, but the mother indicated that Emily continued to be seen by both PT and OT through the end of third grade. She also began receiving speech therapy (ST) near the end of her kindergarten year, reportedly because the teacher was having trouble understanding her. Speech therapy continued through the end of sixth grade. Her mother reported that the reason for the ST was because Emily did not "pronounce" many of her sounds correctly, so teachers and others had trouble understanding her, and she usually only spoke in short phrases or sentences. Mother felt that Emily's speech had always sounded "nasally." At the end of sixth grade, therapy was terminated because, according to the mother, the speech therapist felt that Emily had stopped making progress. Emily's individualized education plan (IEP) involved PT, OT, and ST as well as educational specialists for reading, writing, and mathematics.

Emily was reluctant to talk during the interview. Her responses to direct questions were brief and spoken very quietly. She nodded in the affirmative when asked if her speech bothered her. Her mother felt strongly that Emily's shyness and school performance were impacted by her speech and that she did not raise her hand or speak up in class because she was embarrassed.

## Reason for Referral

Emily was referred for a speech evaluation by an ENT. The reason stated for the ENT visit was "because of her adenoids" and the possibility that removing them might improve her speech (apparently this suggestion came from the speech-language pathologist (SLP) at school). The ENT report described frequent nasal congestion, no known allergies, a family history of chronic fatigue, depression and seizures, cranial nerves II though XII generally intact on cursory examination, no ear issues, mild nasal congestion consistent with a cold, tonsils without erythema or exudates, and "some nasal emissions with plosives." Flexible fiberoptic nasopharyngoscopy was performed. This entailed passing a flexible scope down one side of the nose with the tip positioned superior to the VP port so that soft palate and pharyngeal wall motion during speech could be visualized (see Karnell, 1994) with the following observations: small adenoid pad, inconsistent but fairly extensive palatal elevation during sustained vowel production, intermittent closure of the VP port during productions of plosives and fricatives in syllables and short phrases, and a "very small indentation" in the soft palate near the point of attachment of the hard and soft palate. When VP closure was incomplete (~50% of trials), there was a central gap rather than a lateral air leak. The ENT's ultimate assessment was: "Hypernasality with mild velopharyngeal insufficiency, and history of developmental delays." The ENT recommended a speech evaluation and trial therapy to determine whether Emily could correct the VP insufficiency behaviorally; if not, the ENT was prepared to consider surgical intervention.

## Findings of the Evaluation

Emily's evaluation was completed in one 75-minute meeting. Her mother was present for the entire evaluation.

### Interview

Relevant history obtained during the interview was included in the background section above. Direct observation of Emily during this interview was helpful in gauging the extent of her communication deficit in nonstructured speech tasks and gaining an impression of the impact that her speech had on her. The most striking observations were related to her reticence to speak. She used short phrases, avoided eye contact completely, sat low in her chair with shoulders slumped and arms folded across her chest, and had her body turned slightly away from the table around which everyone sat. This did not come across as defiance, but rather as shyness, embarrassment, or perhaps a lack of self-confidence. Almost without thinking about it, her mother answered all questions, even those that were clearly intended for Emily. In contrast to Emily, her mother was very talkative. Her comments suggested a high level of concern about Emily's speech issues, in particular about how they were impacting school performance. When Emily did respond, her voice was quiet and mouth movements were minimal. The graduate clinician had to request several repetitions because responses were inaudible in some cases and unintelligible in others.

### Articulation Inventory

A single word repetition task was used to sample all consonants in initial and final position of syllables in Standard American English. This particular inventory is not standardized, but was chosen because it allows rapid and complete detailing of a speaker's articulation of all consonants.

The articulation inventory revealed substitution of /w/ for /r/ (when /r/ was a singleton and when it was in a consonant cluster) and /s/ for /sh/. Emily produced the /r/ and /s/ correctly when asked to repeat those words that were initially in error. All stop consonants were produced with perceptually weak bursts, regardless of the position of the consonant within a syllable. These weak bursts were sometimes accompanied by a burst of nasal air flow (nasal emission), but not always (the phenomenon co-occurred ~60% of the time). During a brief speech sample, Emily made similar errors on /r/ and intermittently on /sh/; bursts and frication on stops and fricatives during more spontaneous speech were weak. Speech intelligibility was high (estimated to be at or near 100% during her responses to open ended questions), although careful listening was required because Emily's loudness was reduced.

### Perceptual Ratings of Voice and Resonance

During sustained vowel production, the articulation inventory, and spontaneous responses, Emily's laryngeal voice quality and her habitual pitch were judged to be normal for her age and gender. Pitch range elicited during sustained vowel productions was judged to be approximately 1.5 octaves. As noted previously, she typically spoke with decreased loudness. Emily could increase loudness under instruction (sustained vowel and short phrases), but she did so reluctantly.

Hypernasality was judged on a 5-point scale with 0 = no hypernasality and 4 = severe hypernasality. Hypernasality is a resonance phenomenon defined as excess nasal resonance on oral sound production. It occurs on phonemes that are principally defined by their resonance, namely, vowels and vowel-like consonants such as liquids and glides, and (to a lesser extent) voiced consonants (Bzoch, 2004). She repeated sentences heavily loaded with the vowels /i/, /u/, and /a/ and voiced oral consonants. ("He will read to Lee," "You were rude to Lou," and "Bob had our dollar"). Emily repeated each sentence three times on one breath at a comfortable loudness level while the graduate clinician intermittently closed the nares with her fingers (nasal flutter task, sometimes referred to as the cul-de-sac test; Bzoch, 2004). If air is escaping through the VP port during production of these sentences that should be fully oral, obstructing the nares may result in a perceptible shift in the vowel quality. Before completing this task, Emily blew her nose to clear nasal congestion. If nasal congestion is present it will serve as a confounder to this perceptual test. During this nasal flutter task, Emily's speech was rated as mildly hypernasal (ratings of 2 on the scale). She did have a few trials produced without any obvious hypernasality.

Nasal emission ratings were made during production of sentences heavily loaded with voiceless stop consonants and fricatives (e.g., "Paula paid Perry," "Terry told Teddy," etc.) using the same 5-point scale with 0 = none and 4 = severe. Each sentence was repeated a minimum of 3 times, each on one breath. Nasal emission is a pressure-based phenomenon defined as a burst of air out the nose as an individual attempts to produce an oral burst or frication. This air burst is generally audible, but silent nasal emission can also occur. The nasal emission protocol for this evaluation included assessment of the pressure consonants /p, t, k, f, s, sh, ch/. Voiceless consonants are used because the oral pressure generated for voiceless stops and fricatives is greater than for the voiced counterparts, increasing the likelihood of eliciting nasal emission if a VP gap is present (Trost-Cardamone, 2004). Emily was found to have none-to-mild nasal emission that varied across consonants and across trials of the same consonant. Nasal emission was most consistently present on /p/ and /s/; it was never detected on /t/ or /k/. All other consonants had at least one trial with nasal emission.

Hyponasality is also a resonance phenomenon, but in this case is a reduction in nasal resonance during nasal consonant production. Hyponasality was rated on a 5-point scale (again, 0 = none, 4 = severe) as Emily repeated sentences loaded with nasal consonants. The nose was intermittently obstructed as with the hypernasality speech task. In this case, a change in resonance should occur if the nasal sounds are being produced with nasal air flow and acoustic energy. Obstructing the nares during the nasal sound production causes cul-de-sac resonance; in this manner the nasal flutter serves to facilitate the clinician's ability to detect whether there is sufficient nasal resonance during nasal phoneme production. No hyponasality was observed.

During the limited spontaneous speech productions that Emily offered, hypernasality was more consistently present than during the structured speech sampling. Nasal emission was also more prominent in the spontaneous productions (greater in magnitude and frequency of occurrence).

## Oral Mechanism Examination

When there are concerns about palatal function, a thorough oral mechanism examination is a vital part of the assessment protocol. The information derived is needed to rule out various structural or movement-related factors as influential on the speech that is generated (Peterson-Falzone, Hardin-Jones, & Karnell, 2001). There were no structural abnormalities noted during the oral mechanism examination. The face, lips, tongue, and soft palate were grossly symmetrical and of appropriate size and color. There were no scars on the lip or palate. There was no bifid uvula, notching of the hard-soft palate juncture, or coloration change in the soft palate that might be suggestive of a submucous cleft (Shprintzen, Schwartz, Daniller & Hoch, 1985). Emily did allow the clinician and supervisor to place a gloved finger inside the oral cavity to palpate the hard and soft palate. There were no obvious bony or muscular defects (indentations) in the soft or hard palate that could be felt with the finger tip.

With the mouth open and the tongue resting low in the mouth, Emily was asked to sustain the vowel /a/ for approximately 5 seconds on one breath; she repeated this several times as the clinician and supervisor observed palatal and pharyngeal wall movement. Superior and posterior movement of the soft palate serves as the primary, but usually not the sole movement that results in VP closure (Kuehn, 1976). The posterior and lateral pharyngeal walls need to constrict around the elevated palate in order to fully occlude the VP port. Palatal elevation was consistently rated 2 on a 3-point scale where 0 = no movement, 1 = minimal/slight movement, and 2 = moderate/marked movement. Using the same rating scale, lateral pharyngeal wall movement during sustained vowel production was consistently rated 1. There were no indications of discoordination or poor timing of VP movements during the vowel productions.

Lip, tongue and jaw strength, range of motion, speed of movement, and coordination during rapid alternating movements were all judged to be within normal limits based on subjective observations of nonspeech movements. There were no indications of laryngeal or respiratory abnormalities based on informal observations of Emily at rest and when talking.

## Aerodynamic Assessment

Simultaneous measurement of oral air pressure and nasal air flow were obtained using a Microtronics PERCI-SARS hardware-software arrangement (Microtronics Corporation of Chapel Hill, NC) as Emily produced various speech stimuli. By selecting stimuli appropriately, one can gather information from the aerodynamic recordings that reflect on VP closing. Oral pressure is measured by placing a small tube between the lips with the tip resting above the tongue about a centimeter behind the upper central incisors. The tube is connected to one side of a differential pressure transducer. Nasal airflow was measured by placing a small mask over the nose; the mask was coupled to a pneumotachometer and differential pressure transducer (see Warren, 1979 for a more complete rationale and description of the pressure-flow technique).

Emily produced /p/ in syllable series, words, and short sentences. Syllable series and words with /p/ in a nasal context also were produced (e.g., /pampampam/, "hamper"). The /mp/ context is considered to be particularly challenging for the VP mechanism because it must transition rapidly from an open position on /m/ to a closed position for /p/. Emily's oral pressure on /p/ was, on average, ~2-3 cm $H_2O$ and occasionally ranged up to ~5cm $H_2O$. Her oral pressures were considered to be at or below the low end of normal for teenagers and adults for whom pressures should typically be between ~3-8 cm $H_2O$. For a portion of the recording, the nasal mask was removed so that the nostrils could be manually occluded by the clinician as Emily produced some of the /p/ stimuli a second time. With the nose occluded, oral air pressure increased to an average of 5.2 cm $H_2O$, indicating that she had the respiratory drive and oral articulatory ability to consistently produce adequate oral pressure if the air leakage from the nose is eliminated.

Nasal airflow on /p/ averaged ~150 cc/second (range: 0–230 cc/s). During /p/ production, the expectation is that nasal air flow should be essentially zero (less than ~20 cc/s; Zajac, 2000). There was significant variation in the magnitude of nasal airflow within and across stimuli. For example, during one trial saying /pa pa pa pa pa pa pa/, Emily had nasal air flow on the first, second, and fifth /p/s of approximately 120 cc/s; however, flow on the third and fourth /p/s was ~30 cc/s. On /pi/ stimuli, she always had nasal airflows greater than 110 cc/s. Nasal airflow was also measured on syllable series and sentences constructed with the consonants /t, k, f, s, ʃ, tʃ/ (the oral tube was removed to allow normal oral articulation so only nasal flow is recorded). Flow values ranged from ~60–270 cc/s. Again, these are oral consonants and nasal flow should be generally absent (or at least less than 20 cc/s).

## Stimulability Testing

Emily was asked to attempt manipulations of resonance and oral pressure. Much of the stimulability testing was with the pressure-flow equipment in place for two reasons: (1) changes in nasal air flow and oral air pressure could be quantified, and (2) the visual display of airflow and air pressure could be used as biofeedback to facilitate Emily's ability to change the requested parameters. The target behaviors tracked during stimulability testing with the aerodynamic equipment were: (1) oral pressure on /p/ with a target of at least 4–5 cm H2O, and (2) nasal airflow on all oral stimuli with a target of less than 40 cc/s.

Initially, the stimulability testing was done with the aerodynamic equipment in place, but with the computer display turned away from Emily. Later, the display was adjusted so she could watch the screen to determine whether she could manipulate the targets with just auditory models and instructions, and to assess the impact of visual feedback on behavior. Without the visual feedback, there were no reductions in nasal air flow with any of the following instructions: increase loudness, decrease loudness, increase articulatory precision, instruction to make bursts stronger ("really pop that /p/", "make it stronger with your lips"), and a general command to "get rid of the nasal sound." These types of instruction have been suggested based on clinical experience as possible means of altering VP activity and/or minimizing perceptions of hypernasality, nasal emission, or weak oral pressures, although none have any significant empirical data to bolster the claim. Tomes, Kuehn, and Peterson-Falzone (2004) provide an excellent review of issues related to behavioral intervention approaches for VP impairment. For Emily, oral pressure did increase to ~3–4 cm H2O when she increased loudness, but she could not be prompted to substantially increase her loudness even with significant modeling. This appeared to be reluctance or embarrassment rather than a physical limitation. Emily did whisper with the equipment in place. During the whisper (sentences loaded with /p/), oral air pressure was consistently greater than 6 cm H2O and nasal flow was less than 10 cc/s throughout. When the computer display was turned for her viewing, the same set of manipulations was attempted. In this condition, she was able to increase oral pressure ~30% of the time with the general instruction to "make this peak go higher" and "make the /p/ more strongly." When doing so she appeared to be engaging in exaggerated articulatory activity with slightly prolonged lip closure; there was a perceptibly louder burst under this instruction. When oral pressure increased, nasal flow decreased dramatically, usually down to ~0–10 cc/s, although occasional spikes of flow up to 75 cc/s still occurred. While watching the screen, Emily was able to engage in "negative practice" involving alternating between allowing nasal airflow through the nose on one production, and then eliminating nasal airflow on the next. Sustained /s/ was also elicited. Without instruction, the sustained /s/ had consistent nasal flow of 80–125 cc/s when watching the screen. With the instruction "make it all out your mouth," she could reduce nasal flow below 30 cc/s for 75% of the duration of a given trial.

## Representation of the Problem at the Time of Evaluation

Emily presented with two primary speech issues. The first was persistent articulatory substitution of /r/ and /sh/. She demonstrated the ability to accurately produce these phonemes with limited prompting. Although these errors were not judged to have a large negative impact on intelligibility, they did draw attention to her speech and gave an impression of immaturity.

The second issue was mild hypernasality and none-to-mild nasal emission. A related factor was a general reduction in the strength of bursts and frication that appeared to be linked to nasal air leak when attempting to build air pressure for oral consonants. The aerodynamic recordings of oral pressure were consistent with the clinicians' perceptions of weak pressure consonants; the magnitude of the nasal airflow recordings was somewhat greater than expected compared to the rating of mild hypernasality from the clinicians. Emily's spontaneous speech indicated a fairly constant hypernasality and nasal emission compared to the aerodynamic recording, which suggested greater variability in VP closure for speech.

In addition to describing Emily's VP symptoms, a primary outcome of the diagnostic process for Emily was to help define the reason for the VP symptoms and to develop an appropriate treatment plan if needed. It was clear to the clinicians, the mother, Emily, and the ENT that Emily's speech was not normal and that the VP symptoms were a primary feature that drew listener attention. The problem was of sufficient magnitude that the clinicians had some difficulty both hearing and, at times, understanding Emily. These observations were consistent with her mother's report that teachers complained about Emily's speech. Emily did not volunteer much about her speech, but she did say that she was reluctant to talk in class or with others whom she did not know well. All agreed that the problem was of sufficient magnitude to warrant treatment consideration.

Determining etiology for VP symptoms is critical for treatment planning. Behavioral interventions with an SLP are usually only effective when the cause of symptoms is determined to be functional (rather than physical) or when the severity of the symptoms is limited. Emily presented with pieces of evidence that could support more than one etiology. The diagnostic thinking in this case is presented below with the categories of etiology considered and specific pieces of evidence from the evaluation that seemed to favor one cause over another.

There were two broad categories of etiology considered: functional and physical. Functional origins of VP symptoms imply that a speaker has the physical capability of achieving appropriate VP closure on oral phoneme (and also, opening on nasals), but does not do so, similar to a phonological process of nasalization on oral phonemes. There may be very specific sounds on which nasal air escape occurs; this is referred to as *phoneme specific nasal emission* and is often conceptualized as a specific articulatory error. Physical etiologies for VP symptoms are many and may be neurological or structural in nature. Neurological causes can be any number of diseases or developmental conditions in which impaired innervations or neural control of the VP structure might occur (e.g., stroke, head injury, etc.). Structural causes include clefts of the palate, surgical resections for tumor, adenoidectomy, and accidental injury to the soft palate.

The evidence related to the etiological considerations is given in Table 58.1.

Based on a weighing of the evidence, a functional or neurological etiology seemed most likely. A submucous cleft was also a possibility based on the ENT's nasopharyngoscopy report, but this is not easy to determine definitively unless the defect is quite obvious or the surgeon is able to inspect the soft palate musculature in the operating room. It was not possible based on the diagnostic information to identify the etiology. A combination of causes was considered, including some mild neurological involvement of the VP musculature (or even a structural defect in the form of a submucous cleft) that made closure of the port more demanding

TABLE 58.1 Evidence Related to Etiological Considerations

| Etiology | | Evidence Supporting | Evidence Against |
|---|---|---|---|
| 1. Structural | A. Cleft of the Palate | None. | No reported history or overt clefting. |
| | B. Submucous Cleft | ENT noted a "very small indentation" on the nasal surface of the soft palate during nasopharyngoscopy. | No obvious tactile perception of a defect in the bulk of the soft palate when digitally palpated by the clinician. None of the usual stigmata of submucous cleft were appreciated on the oral mechanism examination. |
| | C. Congenital Insufficiency in Size or Position of VP structures | None. | Length of soft palate was judged to be appropriate relative to the depth of the pharynx during the oral mechanism examination; no other structural insufficiencies noted during this exam. Nasopharyngoscopy showed evidence that the VP port could close at least a portion of the time (50% of trials per ENT) |
| | D. Surgical | None. | No history of surgery on tonsils or adenoids or any other structures in the mouth, nose or throat |

(*continued*)

TABLE 58.1 *Continued*

| Etiology | | Evidence Supporting | Evidence Against |
|---|---|---|---|
| 2. Neurological | A. Acquired condition or disease | She did (and still does) have pulmonary stenosis, which can cause general fatigue and other symptoms. The general fatigue and low energy level might conceivably involve the motor activity of speech. Variability in the speech symptoms, as Emily demonstrated, may be a marker for a neurological cause (D'Antonio & Scherer, 1995). Although not part of Emily's specific history, there is family history of neurological issues (seizure disorders, depression, etc.). | No report from the family of any acquired neurological conditions or diseases. ENT reported cranial nerves 2–12 were intact based on cursory examination |
| | B. Developmental | Early development was worrisome enough ("clumsy," "late talker") that PT, OT, and speech therapy were all initiated in preschool or early elementary school. Variability in the speech symptoms, as Emily demonstrated, may be a marker for a neurological cause (D'Antonio & Scherer, 1995). | No specific information against. |
| 3. Functional | | Nasopharyngoscopy suggests the VP port is capable of closing, at least some of the time. Perceptually, Emily presented with some trials with no hypernasality or nasal emission. She also never had perceptible nasal emission on /t/ or /k/ productions. Aerodynamically, nasal air flow on /p/ was intermittently absent or at least approached the expected range ($<$ 20 cc/s). Stimulability testing indicated that Emily could reduce or eliminate nasal air flow (and increase oral pressure) under certain situations, at least some of the time. | No specific information against. |

and less consistent. It was also possible that Emily had not fully maximized the use of a VP mechanism that appeared to be at least generally structurally sound.

In addition to trying to define the etiology, the evaluation revealed the following:

1. Emily appeared able to exert more control over the VP mechanism in structured speech tasks and with some guidance (auditory, visual feedback) compared to spontaneous speech. This was considered a positive prognostic variable for behavioral intervention, although such variation in performance is not a guarantee of therapy success.
2. Emily's speech might negatively impact her academic and social functioning.
3. Emily did not show or verbalize motivation to work on her speech, although her mother clearly wanted to address the issue.

## Treatment Options Considered

Treatment for VP speech problems is largely dictated by the underlying cause. Physical problems generally require a physical treatment such as surgery or a prosthetic device, while functional problems usually fall to the SLP for behavioral intervention. Magnitude of the VP symptoms should also be considered. Even if a VP problem is known to have a physical basis, a decision may be made to avoid physical interventions if the symptoms are quite limited in severity or if there are extenuating factors that make a speaker a poor candidate for a physical approach (e.g., poor surgical candidate). Conversely, there are situations of a functional VP problem addressed with a physical intervention; usually this occurs when an individual simply is unable to consistently maintain control over VP activity or if the learned pattern of VP dysfunction is extremely resistant to change in behavioral therapy. Treatment options considered for Emily included the following:

- ***Surgical or prosthetic management.*** A number of surgical approaches and prostheses have been utilized to minimize or eliminate symptoms of VP dysfunction, including various pharyngeal flaps (see Peterson-Falzone et al., 2001 for a review), augmentation of the posterior and lateral pharyngeal wall (e.g., Orticochea, 1983), palatal lengthening procedures (e.g., Furlow, 1994), and pharyngeal obturators and palatal lifts (see Rosen and Bzoch, 2004 for a review). There are many studies that document success of surgical and prosthetic management of VP symptoms, the majority of which have focused on individuals with clefts of the palate. In Emily's case, the unknown etiology, variable presence of symptoms, and fairly limited magnitude of symptoms contraindicated surgery or prosthetic interventions. The surgical risks, costs, and potential side effects (nasal airway obstruction, for example) and the costs and time commitment for making a prosthesis and refining it were all weighed against the possibility of improving her speech behaviorally. This was a somewhat difficult choice because the success of various surgeries and prosthetic approaches for reducing or eliminating VP symptoms has a long history, while outcome studies of behavioral management of VP symptoms are less common and less encouraging in terms of positive outcomes (e.g., Golding-Kushner, 2001; Peterson, 1974; Tachimura, Nohara, Fujita, Hara, & Wada, 2001). However, given the serious risks and complications of these physical approaches, any physical intervention must be carefully justified. In Emily's case, she demonstrated enough evidence of occasional VP closure during speech that it was important to determine whether she could do even more.
- ***Behavioral therapy to eliminate articulation errors with no attempt to directly address VP symptoms.*** The /r/ and /sh/ substitutions occur intermittently in Emily's spontaneous speech and give an impression of immature speech. These errors were not considered to be directly related to VP function. For children with clefts exhibiting VP symptoms and compensatory articulation (usually moving the place of production more posteriorly in the vocal tract), some have advocated remediation of the articulation issue as a means of also reducing VP symptoms (Hoch, Golding-Kushner, Siegel-Sadewitz, & Shprintzen, 1986; Ysunza, Pamplona, & Toledo, 1992). However, Emily did

not have a cleft and her articulation errors are not typical of compensatory articulation errors associated with velopharyngeal dysfunction. For these reasons, and because the family was most concerned about addressing the resonance issue (it was the most prominent feature of her speech), therapy to address the residual articulation errors was delayed until behavioral attempts were made at remediating the hypernasality.

- ***Trial behavioral intervention to address hypernasality and nasal emission.*** What was particularly intriguing about trial behavioral intervention for Emily was her demonstration (perceptually, aerodynamically, and endoscopically) of adequate VP closure at times, both under instruction with feedback about aerodynamic events, but also spontaneously in some instances. Others have suggested that individuals presenting with inconsistent "competency" may have the potential to profit from behavioral intervention (e.g., Golding-Kushner, 2001; Karnell, 2000; Kummer, 2001). During stimulability testing, several possible therapeutic strategies were identified that seemed to facilitate VP closure (visual feedback of oral pressure with a set target level; "stronger /p/"; whispering as a means of increasing oral pressure without evidencing nasal flow; sustained /s/) and which could serve as a starting point for behavioral intervention. Trial therapy was considered because neurological causes could not be excluded, raising the possibility that Emily would not be able to exert any more control over VP function. She also had several years of speech therapy and might have reached a plateau and maximized her abilities to control VP activity for speech.

Emily's mother was eager to initiate therapy and was told that within 4–6 weeks Emily's ability to control the symptoms could be noted, but that an additional 4–8 weeks beyond that might be needed to maximize any abilities identified early on. This was based on the clinician's experience rather than any specific guidance from the literature. Emily herself had no questions and no visible reaction to the discussion about trial therapy. When directly asked if she understood the plan, she nodded "yes"; when asked if she was interested in starting the program, she simply shrugged; when asked if she was willing to come back the following week to work on her speech with the graduate clinician, she said "yes."

## Course of Treatment

Trial therapy goals were to identify instructions, strategies, or behaviors that decreased hypernasality and/or nasal emission (ratings of 0–1 in structured stimuli > 90% of the time over 2 sessions); similarly, to identify instructions, strategies, or behaviors that resulted in stronger bursts and frication on stops and fricatives. In addition to the perceptual data set, a parallel set of aerodynamic measures (nasal air flow and oral air pressure) was also logged regularly during the trial therapy to help gauge changes. The specific therapeutic approaches attempted included:

1. Visual biofeedback of nasal air flow on oral consonant productions with associated instructions to manipulate speech. The stated goal for Emily was to generate oral sounds in sentences with nasal airflow less than 40 cc/s greater than 90% of the time. Instructions that were paired with the visual feedback included:
   a. Nondirective instruction to simply "get rid of the air in the nose"
   b. Whispering (based on the observation of essentially no nasal airflow and increased oral pressure when doing so during the evaluation)
   c. Increasing the oral pressure for bursts or frication. In this case, Emily was asked to increase oral air pressure while watching the nasal flow signal.
2. Visual biofeedback of oral air pressure with instructions to elicit increased oral air pressure. The stated goal for Emily was to produce /p/ in sentences with oral air pressure peaks greater than 4 cm H20 greater than 90% of the time. The instructions utilized were:
   a. Nondirective instruction to "make this peak (pressure) go above this level"
   b. Whispering
   c. Increase overall loudness level
   d. Exaggerate the articulation of the consonant

All of the above strategies were also attempted without the aerodynamic feedback. The graduate clinician provided verbal feedback regarding her perception of the strength of the burst/frication or the perception of hypernasality or nasal emission. For the latter, Emily was informed of the 5-point scale described above for perceptual judgments of hypernasality and nasal emission. She was given positive feedback when the clinician rated a production as a 0–1 on the scale. For strength of the burst, a 3-point scale was devised with 0 = no perceived increase from Emily's usual speech, 1 = minimal increase in the strength of the consonant, and 2 = a definite improvement in the strength of the consonant.

## Analysis of Client's Response to Intervention

Emily returned 1 week after the evaluation for her first therapy session. She was compliant and appeared to be fully engaged in the tasks at hand, but remained reticent to talk and did not smile. Her mother watched from an observation room. The first session was structured to sample Emily's performance in each of the conditions noted above. Within each condition, care was taken to record her performance across a variety of speech stimuli allowed by the recording equipment (the oral tube for pressure measurements poses limitations when it is in place). The stimuli were constructed to vary in vowel environment, position of target consonants (syllable initiating vs. terminating position), length and complexity of the stimulus (sustained phoneme in some cases, CV and VC syllable series, short real words in isolation, phrases and longer sentences), and the target consonant itself. The first session was lengthy (nearly 90 minutes with frequent breaks), but Emily did not appear to fatigue or disengage. The data at the end of the first session revealed the following:

1. Visual feedback for nasal airflow and for oral pressure appeared to facilitate meeting the target behaviors. Reductions in nasal air flow were more consistent using the visual feedback than were reductions in hypernasality or nasal emission ratings when auditory-verbal feedback alone was presented. This appeared to be the case across all instructions.
2. Instruction designed to increase oral air pressure resulted in the greatest change in both parameters of interest (nasal air flow and oral air pressure during aerodynamic recordings; nasal emission and burst/frication strength perceptually). Several instructions were attempted to increase pressure, but simply asking for a "stronger" consonant, word, or phrase produced the most consistent results. Using the feedback (nasal flow and oral pressure combined) and instruction for "stronger" speech, Emily produced /p/ in the syllable initiating position at or above the 4 cm H2O level 82% of the time in syllables, 70% in real words, and 68% in short phrases compared to baseline measures of 30%, 32%, and 10% for the 3 stimulus constructions. In the instructed condition, nasal airflow remained below 40 cc/s 100% of the time when the pressure target was met (i.e., she could increase the pressure without increasing nasal escape—in fact, nasal flow decreased). When /p/ was placed in the syllable terminating position, the percentage of success on the pressure measure was even higher by roughly 10% across the three stimulus types.
3. Emily had greater trouble limiting nasal air flow and maintaining the target oral pressure when using the /i/ as opposed to the /a/ or /u/ contexts. Success rates dropped by ~5–10% for /i/.
4. Emily had greater success on increasing oral pressures (measured aerodynamically or judged perceptually as burst/frication strength) on stop consonants as opposed to fricatives. The stimuli were simplified further by having her sustain fricatives while watching the nasal airflow channel. After a short period of instruction involving negative practice ("put it all in your nose"; "make this line [nasal flow] higher—now lower") and derivation of /s/ from the alveolar stop /t/ (recall /t/ never had nasal air flow in the evaluation), she was able to produce a sustained /s/ with less than 10 cc/s nasal air flow 70% of the time.

Emily was seen 2 days later and work focused on those strategies that seemed most effective from the first session, specifically, those stimuli and contexts that elicited strongest pressures and lowest nasal air flow. Visual feedback was used 100% of the time. This second 45-minute session focused on "stronger" consonants/speech using mainly /p/ (both syllable initiating and terminating position) in the /a/ and /u/ contexts. She quickly met target oral pressure and nasal airflow goals at nearly 100% criterion within this session on these syllable and short word stimuli; performance dropped to ~90% when using /i/ contexts or when shifting to sentence stimuli, but even this represented a gain from the prior session. She still required derivation techniques to generate a sustained /s/ without airflow ("start saying a /t/, but when you let the /t/ go, stretch out the sound"), and she was able to produce this derived /s/ in a CV syllable series only 25% of the time with nasal flow <40 cc/s. However, when the derived /s/ was placed in a VC context, she was 100% accurate in meeting the nasal airflow goal.

Emily was seen 3 times a week for the first 2 weeks and then twice a week for 2 weeks. She was given homework to do 2–3 times a day (7 days a week) that reinforced behaviors targeted in therapy. Her mother reported that Emily did the homework as prescribed (5–10 minutes practice, 2–3 times a day), usually with the mother serving as a helper/judge of performance. Emily made very rapid progress within that first week. By the second week, the visual feedback was faded (still recorded for the clinician's benefit) with a goal of having Emily begin to serve as her own judge. This caused a slight regression in her performance that was made up within 2–3 sessions.

Emily and her mother were updated on the progress. It was at that point that Emily was able to produce the /p/ with adequate oral pressure (at or above 4 cm H2O) nearly 100% of the time in structured phrases and sentences. Nasal flow was maintained below 40 cc/s 85% of the time when she was asked to focus on "stronger" speech/consonants. She also was able to produce /s/ and other voiceless fricatives in syllable series and words with perceptually acceptable strength of frication and essentially no measureable nasal air flow (performance dropped to ~80% in words in longer sentences). At the end of the second week, it had become clear that Emily could manipulate her speech and hit the aerodynamic and perceptual targets with fairly limited input required from the clinician or the visual display. At this point, it was agreed to shift focus from trial therapy to corrective therapy. The trial therapy was completed because specific strategies and behaviors that consistently resulted in positive changes in Emily's speech had been identified. Additionally, she had shown the ability to begin implementing these behaviors in increasingly complex stimuli, although still structured by the therapeutic tasks.

The third week of intervention represented the beginning of corrective therapy. The new stated goal was: Emily will produce spontaneous speech with perceptually acceptable bursts and frication and none-to-minimal hypernasality or nasal emission. The outcome measures shifted exclusively to perceptual events (clinician ratings); for bursts/frication the goal was a rating of 2 on the 3-point scale described previously; for hypernasality and nasal emission the goal was a rating of 0–1 on the 5-point scale.

Over the next several weeks, Emily made rapid progress in all areas. A rather traditional hierarchy of stimuli difficulty was constructed that varied target phoneme, phoneme position within the syllable, stimulus length, and ultimately, level of distracters (environmental, cognitive load). By the end of the fifth week, she was able to offer short monologues (20–60 seconds) on clinician-selected topics with perceptually acceptable pressures > 95% of the time and hypernasality and nasal emission ratings of 0–1 throughout. Most encouraging was the report from the mother that the classroom teacher had recently commented on how much better Emily sounded when called on in class. Although Emily still was reluctant to talk freely in the therapy setting, there were noticeable changes in her communication. The student clinician noted greater eye contact and a more relaxed posture during communication exchanges. The school SLP was engaged at that point to continue on with the therapy plan. Emily returned to the clinic a few weeks later for a repeat of the aerodynamic measures. She was maintaining the progress as evidenced by oral pressure > 4 cm H2O on 100% of samples recorded on /p/ and associated nasal flow <20 cc/s. She also was maintaining nasal flow on other pressure consonants in syllable series and phrases well below the original target level of <40 cc/s. At that point Emily was scheduled for a follow-up visit to coincide with the end of the school semester so that a final check on progress/maintenance could be made. However, when the time arrived, her mother politely refused the follow-up, stating that she (and presumably Emily) was happy with the outcome.

## Author Note

This writing is based on a real case, with certain aspects fictionalized for educational purposes and to protect the identity of the individual. Lorna Moore and Jennifer Flenthrope played important roles in this particular case presentation. The author is grateful for their contributions.

## References

Bzoch, K. R. (2004). A battery of clinical perceptual tests, techniques, and observations for the reliable clinical assessment, evaluation, and management of 11 categorical aspects of cleft palate speech disorders. In K. R. Bzoch (Ed.), *Communicative disorders related to cleft lip and palate.* Austin, TX: PRO-ED.

D'Antonio, L. L., & Scherer, N. J. (1995). The evaluation of speech disorders associated with clefting. In R. J. Shprintzen & J. Bardach (Eds.), *Cleft palate speech management: A multidisciplinary approach.* St. Louis, MO: Mosby.

Furlow, F. T. (1994). Correction of secondary velopharyngeal insufficiency in cleft palate patients with the Furlow palatoplasty. *Plastic and Reconstructive Surgery, 94,* 942–943.

Golding-Kushner, K. J. (2001). *Therapy techniques for cleft palate speech and related disorders.* San Diego, CA: Singular.

Hoch, L., Golding-Kushner, K., Siegel-Sadewitz, V. L., & Shprintzen, R. J. (1986). Speech therapy. *Seminars in Speech and Language, 7,* 313–325.

Karnell, M. P. (1994). *Videoendoscopy from velopharynx to larynx: Clinical competence series.* San Diego, CA: Singular.

Karnell, M. P. (2000). *Endoscopic assessment for voice, resonance, and swallowing disorders* [Video]. Rockville, MD: ASHA.

Kuehn, D. P. (1976). A cineradiographic investigation of velar movement variables in two normals. *Cleft Palate Journal,* 13, 88–103.

Kummer, A. W. (2001). *Cleft palate and craniofacial anomalies: The effects on speech and resonance.* San Diego, CA: Singular.

Orticochea, M. (1983). A review of 236 cleft palate patients treated with dynamic muscle sphincter. *Plastic and Reconstructive Surgery, 71,* 180–188.

Peterson, S. J. (1974). Electrical stimulation of the soft palate. *Cleft Palate Journal, 11,* 72–86.

Peterson-Falzone, S. J., Hardin-Jones, M. A., & Karnell, M. P. (2001). *Cleft palate speech* (3rd ed.). St. Louis, MO: Mosby.

Rosen, M. S., & Bzoch, K. R. (2004). The use of prosthetic speech appliances in cleft palate management. In K. R. Bzoch (Ed.), *Communicative disorders related to cleft lip and palate.* Austin, TX: PRO-ED.

Shprintzen, R. J., Schwartz, R., Daniller, A., & Hoch, L. (1985). The morphologic significance of bifid uvula. *Pediatrics, 75,* 553–561.

Tachimura, T., Nohara, K., Fujita, Y., Hara, H., & Wada, T. (2001). Changes in levator veli palatine muscle activity of normal speakers in association with elevation of the velum using an experimental palatal lift prosthesis. *Cleft Palate-Craniofacial Journal, 38,* 449–454.

Tomes, L. A., Kuehn, D. P., & Peterson-Falzone, S. J. (2004). Research consideration for behavioral treatments of velopharyngeal impairment. In K. R. Bzoch (Ed.), *Communicative disorders related to cleft lip and palate.* Austin, TX: PRO-ED.

Trost-Cardamone, J. E. (2004). Diagnosis of specific cleft palate speech error patterns for planning therapy or physical management. In K. R. Bzoch (Ed.), *Communicative disorders related to cleft lip and palate.* Austin, TX: PRO-ED.

Warren, D. W. (1979). PERCI: A method for rating palatal efficiency. *Cleft Palate Journal, 16,* 279–285.

Ysunza, A., Pamplona, C., & Toledo, E. (1992). Change in velopharyngeal valving after speech therapy in cleft palate patients: A videonasopharyngoscopic and multi-view videofluoroscopic study. *International Journal of Pediatric Otorhinolaryngology, 24,* 45–54.

Zajac, D. (2000). Pressure-flow characteristics of /m/ and /p/ production in speakers without cleft palate: Developmental findings. *Cleft Palate-Craniofacial Journal, 37*(5): 468–477.

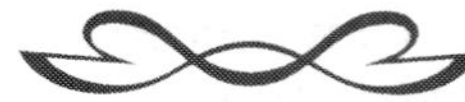

# VOICE

# CASE 59

# Catherine: Finding Catherine's Voice

*Leo Dunham*

## Conceptual Knowledge Areas

Because this case concerns an individual with a disorder of the basal ganglia who demonstrates symptoms similar to those of people with Parkinson's disease, it will be helpful to have some understanding of motor speech problems associated with Parkinson's disease as well as practices appropriate for addressing those problems.

Darley, Aronson, and Brown (1975, p. 195) provide the classic description of the moderately severe hypokinetic dysarthria prevalent in individuals with Parkinson's:

> Significantly reduced variability in pitch and loudness, reduced loudness level overall, and decreased use of all vocal parameters for achieving stress and emphasis. Markedly imprecise articulation is generated at variable rates in short bursts of speech punctuated by illogical pauses and by inappropriate silences. Voice quality is sometimes harsh, sometimes breathy.

The perceptual features of dysarthria in people with Parkinson's reflect the underlying pathophysiology. Yorkston, Miller, and Strand (1995, p. 112) describe the relationship between the pathophysiology and these features in this way:

> Reduced ranges of motion may be reflected in the features of monopitch, monoloudness, reduced stress, and short phrases. Variable rate, short rushes of speech, and imprecise consonants may also be reflective of the reduced range of speech movements. Inappropriate silences may be related to bradykinesia, with its feature of difficulty of initiating movements. The deviant voice dimensions . . . may be the result of rigidity of the laryngeal musculature. Dysarthria in those with Parkinson's affects all components of speech and voice: respiration, phonation, resonance (in a minor way), articulation and prosody. The feature of reduced loudness may indicate that the respiratory system is involved.

Voice disorders in Parkinson's are marked by many of the perceptual features noted by Darley, Aronson, and Brown (1975), primarily those involving pitch, loudness, or changes in vocal quality. Although the vocal folds may appear normal, and the movements of adductor and abductor muscles symmetrical, breathiness may be the result of incomplete vocal fold closure (Aronson, 1985).

Selection of intervention methods for people with Parkinson's has typically been based on physiologic features or on the presence of certain speech characteristics (ANCDS Technical Report No. 3, 2003). The respiratory and phonatory subsystems are critical to speech, the former because it provides the energy source for speaking and the latter because it provides the sound source (ANCDS, 2003). It is these two areas that were the basis for this treatment.

Impairments in respiration and phonation can have a major impact on the production of speech. If functioning is reduced at this level, the impairment likely comes from one of three causes: decreased respiratory support, decreased respiratory/phonatory coordination, or decreased phonatory function (ANCDS, 2003). All three of these areas were incorporated into the treatment plan in the present case: Increasing vital capacity and improving endurance for breathing were addressed by postural changes as simple as sitting upright; phonatory/respiratory coordination was improved by means of cued conversational scripts; and improvement in phonatory function was made by increasing loudness and improving self-monitoring of vocal loudness by means of instrumental feedback.

## Description of the Case

### Background Information

Catherine was admitted to a skilled nursing facility in the Kansas City metropolitan area. She was transferred to the facility from a hospital to which she had been admitted after falling at home. The admission diagnosis was status postfall, with her daughter reporting her admission to skilled nursing was primarily because she could no longer provide the care Catherine needed in her home with numerous other family obligations. Her medical history included the following:

- Progressive supernuclear palsy, a degenerative neurological disease with symptoms similar to Parkinson's disease, including problems with gait and balance, and rigidity. Additional symptoms are mild dementia and problems with voluntary movement of the eyes.
- Congestive heart failure, an inability of the heart to pump blood efficiently, caused by failure of one or both heart ventricles. Symptoms include shortness of breath and circulatory difficulties leading to stasis or edema, and enlargement of the heart itself.
- Chronic bronchitis, or inflammation or swelling of the lining of the airways in the lungs, causing obstruction of the airways.
- Chronic obstructive pulmonary disease (COPD), which is any disorder that obstructs bronchial airflow in a persistent way.
- Atrial-fibrillation, an irregular heartbeat.
- Hypothyroidism, or reduced production of thyroid hormone. Symptoms include depression, edema, increased cholesterol levels, sleepiness, fatigue, weight gain, and decreased concentration.
- Hypertension, or high blood pressure.
- Gastroesophageal reflux disorder, or acid reflux, a chronic condition in which the liquid contents of the stomach are regurgitated into the esophagus, leading to inflammation of the esophageal lining.
- Pacemaker implantation, the installation of an electronic device to control an irregular or slow heart rate.

The original request for orders to evaluate and treat came from the nursing staff, because of difficulty understanding the patient's speech due to reduced loudness and strained voice. The family also found it difficult to understand her speech, making communication a frustrating experience.

#### History

Catherine was a 63-year-old female, widowed, with three children. She lived with one of her daughters for the 2 years prior to admission to the skilled nursing facility, at which time the daughter felt she could no longer adequately care for her mother.

Catherine was a high school graduate and grew up in what she described as a lower-middle-class household in the Kansas City area. Catherine worked for several years as a switchboard operator for local hospitals.

Visual examination of the throat by an ear, nose, and throat specialist indicated dystonia due to hyperfunction of false and true vocal folds, as well as notable dryness of the vocal folds.

Catherine was being treated with Lasix and Albuterol, among other drugs, for the edema caused by her congestive heart failure and for the pulmonary obstructive problems, respectively.

The patient reported that difficulties with speech interfered with relationships with family and fellow residents at the nursing home. Her relationships with other residents in the facility were of most concern to Catherine, as she particularly enjoyed conversations at her table during meals. Her communication problems caused her to withdraw from social situations and made her feel somewhat isolated from her tablemates at meals because she could not participate adequately in conversations.

Family involvement with Catherine was limited to occasional visits by one daughter. Following an initial visit at the skilled nursing facility between the therapist and that daughter, she communicated little to the therapist regarding any interest in treatment or outcomes. The therapist would communicate progress by way of telephone messages or through nursing if necessary.

## Reasons for the Referral

The staff at the skilled nursing facility could not understand Catherine's speech secondary to reduced volume and moderately impaired articulation. Catherine herself reported difficulty with clarity and volume of speech, reporting that at times she "couldn't hear [herself] talking" and felt as though she were "shouting to be heard."

## Findings of the Evaluation

The oral-mechanism examination revealed that Catherine's oral structures were within functional limits, but that lingual and labial functions were impaired slightly. Catherine's face was symmetrical at rest and in movement. Facial sensation was intact. Tone appeared to be increased, with facial expressions slightly exaggerated, and eyes protruded moderately. Both left and right nares were patent. Catherine was primarily a mouth breather, day and night. Her lips were symmetrical at rest and in movement, and sensation appeared intact. Lips were open slightly at rest, but Catherine could close them on request. Lip seal was adequate. The mandible was symmetrical at rest and in movement, and appeared to have an appropriate relationship to the maxilla. Catherine reported no discomfort in her temperomandibular joints. She was able to open her mouth adequately voluntarily and in speech movement. Dental occlusion appeared normal and dentition was complete, with teeth appearing in adequate condition. The tongue seemed relatively small in relation to the size of oral cavity, and was symmetrical at rest and in protrusion. Range of movement for lingual protrusion, retraction, elevation, lateralization, and circular movements was slightly reduced. Width and height of the hard palate appeared to be within typical limits. The soft palate was symmetrical and appeared to move appropriately. The oral cavity appeared typical, including the oral mucosa and saliva. Catherine was able to produce an adequate cough voluntarily and could clear her throat.

Perceptual evaluation results confirmed generally reduced vocal intensity with occasional bursts of increased volume, inconsistent speech rate, poor and inconsistent breath support, intermittent pitch breaks, and poor ability to monitor voice production in terms of rate, volume, and clarity. Findings included: sustained phonation of /a/ sound averaged 3.4 seconds over 3 trials; s/z ratio of 1.16 over three trials and strained voice with reduced loudness.

Poor breath support was demonstrated by labored breathing and short bursts of speech. Breath support was sufficient only for very short phrasing. Respiration was labored, and breathing was shallow with her shoulders in a forward position when sitting. Catherine demonstrated reduced loudness, measuring at or slightly below the 60 dB range as measured with sound level meter. Loudness increased rapidly at times, notably when she tried to complete a vocal phrase as she ran out of breath. Rate in running speech was generally consistent, with rate also increasing as breath supply ran low.

Pitch varied, rising especially at the end of vocalization as breath supply began running out. Pitch range was perceptually adequate. Catherine reported she felt that she could maintain phonation longer when using a higher pitch. Repeated measurement of sustained phonation showed this not to be the case. Oronasal resonance sounded balanced.

Catherine reported she consumed approximately 5–6 glasses of fluids per day (estimated to be about 30–36 ounces). As noted previously, her medications included Albuterol and Lasix. A former smoker, she was diagnosed with gastroesophageal reflux, drank 1 cup of coffee a day, and did not consume any alcohol. She reported no vocal abuse.

Catherine demonstrated few cognitive deficits. Long-term memory appeared intact, but she had a mild impairment of short-term memory. Auditory comprehension was appropriate. She followed all directions, including multistep directions, was able to read and write, and showed no problems with expressive or receptive language skills and had no impulsiveness. Insight and judgment regarding her communication problems were mostly appropriate, but her perception of her respiratory and phonatory deficits was at least moderately impaired, and she asked on more than one occasion during the evaluation, and at various times during treatment, whether she was doing something that caused her to lose her voice. Catherine responded affirmatively to the question of whether the amount or degree of tension in the production of voice varied from day to day.

## Representation of the Problem at the Time of Evaluation

Catherine's progressive supranuclear palsy would cause symptoms including reduced volume and bursts of rapid speech. The chronic obstructive pulmonary disease would compromise breath support for speech, causing her to speak with reduced volume and at times to increase pitch as breath support declined during speech. This rapid burst of speech and reduced loudness combined to impair the articulation of speech sounds as well. If the tension or rigidity in the laryngeal area were contributing to the effort required to vocalize, in combination with variable but generally poor breath support, then a treatment approach designed to address both issues was expected to allow for improved loudness, clarity, and rate of speech.

Progressive supranuclear palsy is often considered to be a form of "Parkinson's plus," a collection of neurodegenerative disorders that share symptoms with Parkinson's disease, such as bradykinesia, rigidity, and tremor. Since the respiratory and phonatory impairments Catherine demonstrated are found in people with Parkinson's disease, treatment options reflected the similarities.

## Treatment Options Considered

Selection of intervention methods for people with Parkinson's disease has typically been based on physiologic features or on the presence of certain speech characteristics (ANCDS Technical Report No. 3, 2002). The respiratory and phonatory systems are critical to speech, the former because it provides the energy source for speaking and the latter because it provides the sound source (ANCDS, 2002). Characteristics of Catherine's speech that would be commonly used as a rationale for intervention included reduced voice production and vocal loudness, and poor coordination of breath support and speech. The choice of intervention strategies was also based on prognostic factors, such as improved phonation when a person is instructed to speak more loudly. A final consideration was to choose treatment options that show some capacity for generalization, a particular problem for those with Parkinson's (ANCDS, 2002).

Impairments in respiration and phonation can have a major impact on the production of speech. If functioning is reduced at this level, the impairment likely comes from one of three causes: decreased respiratory support, decreased respiratory/phonatory coordination, or decreased phonatory function (ANCDS, 2002). Catherine's communication deficits could arguably have been caused by any of these conditions. Hyperfunction of her vocal cords could have caused decreased phonatory function, and chronic bronchitis and COPD could have diminished breath support for speech. Poor coordination of respiration and phonation was apparent.

Treatment options included increasing vocal intensity for its own sake and to aid in slowing speech rate and improving articulation and coordination of breath support for speech. Training in improved vocal hygiene and use of neck and shoulder relaxation exercises was also included. Exercises similar to those used in treatment have been effective in reducing tension

(Dworkin & Meleca, 1997). As Catherine typically reclined in her bed at a 45-degree angle and demonstrated a shoulder-forward posture when sitting, she was encouraged to sit upright with shoulders back when speaking. This is helpful for those with inspiratory impairments in that it allows gravity to aid movement of the diaphragm in breathing (Duffy, 1995). The final component of the treatment plan was improvement of Catherine's ability to perceive variations in breath support and loudness so that she could adjust the length of vocal phrasing to minimize the effects of her respiratory and phonatory deficits on a daily basis.

The treatment plan included both speech and nonspeech tasks, with a preference for using speech tasks to improve respiratory support of speech and to improve phonatory production, in accordance with Duffy (1995), who argued that the use of nonspeech tasks for improvement of respiratory support is not merely unnecessary, it is inappropriate.

Catherine wanted to improve communication skills, particularly with respect to loudness and coordination of breath with speech. Family and caregiver goals were to improve generally the quality of speech communication.

## Course of Treatment

Initially, treatment would be primarily compensatory. The highest priority was to improve Catherine's ability to communicate with staff so she could express her wants and needs more effectively.

The treatment plan included improvement of coordination between speech and breathing, increased loudness of speech, and improved self-monitoring of loudness and clarity. Speech tasks began with Catherine reading out loud, then transitioned stepwise to spontaneous speaking.

Nonspeech treatment tasks in the form of shoulder and neck relaxation exercises were also used, with a gradual increase in endurance and intensity, as rated by the clinician. Treatment began with the goal of improving Catherine's vocal hygiene and providing her with strategies to make communication more effective immediately.

The treatment was provided 5 times per week for 11 weeks. The initial treatment goals were to establish good vocal hygiene, begin relaxation exercises to aid in improved phonation, and begin coordination of breathing and speaking. As Catherine became independent in vocal hygiene and performing relaxation exercises, these activities would be withdrawn from daily treatment sessions to continue progress on coordination of breath support and speech and to begin working toward goals of increased loudness and increased self-monitoring of speech in terms of loudness and breath support.

Catherine needed 2 weeks of training and monitoring with respect to vocal hygiene before withdrawing from sessions. Goals were written to assure compliance with appropriate hydration, minimize vocal abuse by use of natural voice, and improve the effectiveness of her communication by reducing background noise when speaking with others. Daily conversation about these goals led to increased awareness and compliance. Once Catherine gained independence in this area, only occasional discussion about it occurred during the remainder of treatment.

Shoulder and neck relaxation exercises were a part of treatment sessions for 5 weeks. Catherine demonstrated adequate recall of the exercises after nearly 2 weeks, allowing the clinicians to modify short-term goals to increase endurance and quality of the exercises. The number of repetitions and number of sets of each exercise were slowly increased to the point that Catherine performed them consistently and reported that she could pursue the exercises on her own during the day. Acoustic measures such as pre- and post-exercise duration of sustained phonation of the /a/ sound with multiple trials resulted in an increase in duration of approximately 15% during this period, indicating that the exercises reduced stress and tension.

It is noteworthy that the average duration of sustained phonation varied from as little as just over 3 seconds to over 15 seconds across treatment sessions, suggesting significant variability in breath support available to Catherine on a given day. The measure of sustained phonation became for Catherine a reliable daily indicator of breath support and of the relative length of phonation; she might be able to coordinate with respiration.

Treatment to improve coordination of phonation and respiration began with the initial session and continued throughout the course of treatment. Reading tasks were utilized at first, with Catherine progressing eventually to spontaneous speaking tasks. Reading tasks began with single words, which grew quickly in syllable length until she was able to read short phrases. At that point, reading materials were marked with phrase lengths appropriate for her breath support in sustained phonation for a given session. These cued conversational scripts allowed Catherine to anticipate the length of phrase to be spoken, making an effective transition to more independent anticipation of phrase length. She demonstrated a growing ability to coordinate phonation and respiration with use of breath pauses and phrase lengths suitable for the day. At this time, increasing loudness became a component of her speech goals.

Loudness of speech was measured instrumentally with a sound level meter set initially at the 60 dB range, with an analog indication of loudness. The goal was modified after a week to set a target level at 70 dB. As Catherine was still using reading tasks at this stage of treatment, she was given verbal cues to increase loudness when the analog indication fell below the target range. The transition to spoken tasks to coordinate phonatory and respiratory function allowed Catherine to view the analog indication of voice loudness herself. This transition was made quickly, in part for the practical improvement of eliminating interruption of her reading with verbal cues to speak more loudly.

As loudness became more consistent, use of the sound level meter was altered to verify Catherine's accuracy of gauging perceptually the loudness of her voice in various speaking tasks. This phase of treatment, to improve Catherine's reliability in monitoring her own vocal production, began 8 weeks into treatment. To improve her self-perception regarding loudness, Catherine began rating her coordination of speech and breath support. After speaking for a short time, usually no more than 30 seconds, Catherine and the clinician would each give a yes/no rating for loudness (at target level or not) and a scaled rating of phonatory/respiratory coordination between 1 and 10. Catherine's initial tendency was to rate her performance well below the clinician's rating. As the final weeks of treatment passed, her appraisal of her own performance became more consistent with the clinician's for breath support and coordination, and that of the sound level meter in terms of loudness.

## Analysis of the Client's Response to Intervention

Catherine was motivated to improve communication skills, and with consistent effort she made steady progress in meeting treatment goals. Her improved awareness of her ability to coordinate speech and breathing affected the overall quality of her oral communication, to which she responded very positively.

A year after treatment, Catherine reported that she still "had her voice," though she had intermittent episodes in which she demonstrated strained vocalization and reduced volume for a day or so, usually once every 6 to 8 weeks. She continued to participate in group activities and socialized with several other residents. Nursing and therapy staff reported that Catherine's speech communication became more effective and remained clearer and louder.

## Further Recommendations

There are many treatment options available for intervention involving phonatory and respiratory impairments. Some were considered and not chosen, and some were beyond the clinical experience of the therapist or not supported in the facility in terms of equipment needed.

Several treatment options exist for improving respiratory support, including maximum inhalation and exhalation tasks (Ramig & Dromey, 1996), and pushing and pulling techniques (Workinger & Netsell, 1992). Given the severity of Catherine's respiratory impairment and the variability from one day to another, it was felt to be more practical for her to reliably anticipate respiratory support and coordinate phonation to suit.

Various techniques for treatment of vocal fold hyperfunction exist, but were outside the training or experience of the therapist. These include Lee Silverman Voice Therapy, which has been used effectively to treat a patient with progressive supranuclear palsy (Countryman, Ramig, & Pawlas, 1994).

## Author Note

This case is based on the treatment of a real patient. Catherine (not her real name) continues to reside in the nursing facility, and she often calls out exercises and counts repetitions for the restorative therapy group. Catherine has benefited since the original treatment course with a refresher course approximately 1 year later. The facility granted approval for use of the information as it appears here.

## References


Aronson, A. E. (1985). *Clinical voice disorder: An interdisciplinary approach* (2nd ed.). New York: Thieme.

Countryman, S., Ramig, L. O., & Pawlas, A. A. (1994). Speech and voice deficits in parkinsonism plus syndromes: Can they be treated? *Journal of Medical Speech-Language Pathology, 2*(3), 211–226.

Darley, F. L., Aronson, A. E., & Brown, J. R. (1975). *Motor speech disorders.* Philadelphia: W. B. Saunders.

Duffy, J. R. (1995). *Motor speech disorders: Substrates, differential diagnosis, and management.* St. Louis, MO: Mosby.

Dworkin, J., & Meleca, R. (1997). *Vocal pathologies: Diagnosis, treatment and case studies.* San Diego, CA: Cengage.

Ramig, L. O., & Dromey, C. (1996). Aerodynamic mechanisms underlying treatment-related changes in vocal intensity in patients with Parkinson's disease. *Journal of Speech and Hearing Research, 39*(4), 798–807.

Spencer, K. A., Yorkston, K. M., Beukelman, D. R., Duffy, J., Golper, L. A., Miller, R. M., Strand, E. A., & Sullivan, M. (2002). *Practice guidelines for dysarthria: Evidence for the behavioral management of the respiratory/phonatory system* (Technical Report 3). Academy of Neurologic Communication Disorders and Sciences.

Workinger, M. S., & Netsell, R. (1992). Restoration of intelligible speech 13 years post head injury. *Brain Injury, 2*(6), 183–187.

Yorkston, K. M., Miller, R. M., & Strand, E. A. (1995). *Management of speech and swallowing in degenerative diseases.* Tucson, AZ: Communication Skill Builders.


# CASE 60

# Doris: Becoming Who You Are: A Voice and Communication Group Program for a Male-to-Female Transgender Client


*Vicki McCready, Michael Campbell, Sena Crutchley, and Colette Edwards*


## Conceptual Knowledge Areas

Although in recent years more literature about speech-language pathologists (SLPs) serving persons who are transgender (TG) has appeared in journals, at conferences, and in one textbook written specifically for SLPs (Adler, Hirsch, & Mordaunt, 2006), more information is needed, both about this population and about service delivery models. The prevalence reports of TG and transsexual (TS) persons are varied. According to the figures from the sixth version of the Harry Benjamin International Gender Dysphoria Association's Standards of Care

(Meyer et al., 2001), TS persons from the Netherlands number 1 in 11,900 males and 1 in 30,400 females. Although these figures are frequently cited, Meyer et al. (2001) and others (Olyslager & Conway, 2007) point out that current figures are probably much higher than those from the Netherlands. Reports do agree that far more people fall under the larger umbrella term of transgender than transsexual and that male-to-female (MtF) TS persons far outnumber female-to-male (FtM).

As male individuals transition to females, the services of a qualified speech-language pathologist can help them develop a female vocal pitch and range as well as a feminine communication style. One of their main concerns about "passing" as females is that their typically low-pitched male voices can give them away instantly. Some of these individuals try to change their pitch by themselves or through tapes and various materials developed by other transgender people. The problem with this approach is that often the person strains and misuses the voice, increasing the risk for vocal pathology. A trained speech-language pathologist can help the person develop her desired voice characteristics without vocal abuse (Adler, 2006; Davies & Goldberg, 2006a).

In addition to voice as a gender indicator, communication characteristics, both verbal and nonverbal, can lead observers and listeners to an undesired perception. It is important not only for transgender clients but also for speech-language pathology students and practicing clinicians to know that no intervention program for this population is complete without considering these communication components (Hirsch, 2006a; Hooper, 2006; Mordaunt, 2006). As Davies and Goldberg (2006a) point out, it is also important for the clinician and transgender client to determine the "best fit" between the client and her desired characteristics instead of automatically conforming to society's stereotypes of femininity.

The purpose of this chapter is to present an actual case of a male-to-female transgender client who was enrolled in a voice and communication group in the spring of 2008. The group, which served as part of the clinical education program at The University of North Carolina at Greensboro (UNCG), involved 8 clients and a clinical team of 4 graduate students and 4 faculty members (who are also the authors of this chapter) of the Department of Communication Sciences and Disorders.

## Basic Information about Transgenderism

Knowledge about the population to be served is crucial before any assessments or treatment programs are begun. The following definitions of selected concepts from various professional sources are a first step in this process:

- ***Gender:*** "a social, symbolic construction that expresses the meanings a society confers on biological sex. Gender varies across cultures, over time within any given society, and in relation to other genders" (Wood, 2009, p. 320).
- ***Gender identity:*** "an individual's internal sense of his/her gender" (Girshick, 2008, p. 203).

## Gender Identity Disorder

According to the *Diagnostic and Statistical Manual of Mental Disorders*, Fourth Edition (DSM-IV), the following is a medical diagnosis of a mental disorder with two required components: "evidence of a strong and persistent cross-gender identification . . . and of persistent discomfort about one's assigned sex . . . there must be evidence of clinically significant distress or impairment in social, occupational, or other important areas of functioning" (American Psychiatric Association, 2000, p. 576). As pointed out by Girshick (2008), "many challenge the diagnosis as stigmatizing since it implies the individuals are disordered" (p. 203).

The Harry Benjamin International Gender Dysphoria Association (HBIGDA)[1] is "the international organization that establishes standards of care within medical, psychological, and other parameters in the area of Transsexual Medicine" (Adler, 2006, p. 4). "The major purpose of the Standards of Care (SOC) is to articulate this international organization's professional consensus about the psychiatric, psychological, medical, and surgical management of gender identity disorders" (Meyer et al., 2001, p. 1). The SOC include "vocal expression skills" as an option to help male-to-female TG individuals "find more personal comfort" (Meyer et al., 2001, p. 3).

- ***Passability:*** "being perceived by others as a man or a woman. The desire to pass is a complex feeling that may be influenced by the client's self-defined gender; community norms; beliefs and expectations of friends, family, co-workers, community peers, or others who are close to the client; internalized transphobia; degree of social support; and experiences of mistreatment (as individuals who are visibly transgender are often more vulnerable to harassment, discrimination, and violence)" (Davies & Goldberg, 2006a, p. 173).
- ***Sex:*** "a personal quality determined by biological and genetic characteristics. Male, female, man, and woman indicate sex" (Wood, 2009, p. 324).
- ***Sex reassignment surgery (SRS):*** "surgery that allows the body to be more in line with an individual's gender identity, such as surgery that creates a neovagina out of a penis and scrotum" (Girshick, 2008, p. 205).
- ***Transgender (TG):*** "individual who feels that her or his biologically assigned sex is inconsistent with her or his true sexual identity" (Wood, 2009, p. 324).
- ***Transition:*** "the process that an individual goes through to change his/her gender identity to the opposite sex; may or may not include cosmetic surgeries and sexual reassignment surgery; usually includes hormone therapy, psychiatric/psychology visits, endocrinology, electrolysis, voice and communication training, fashion, makeup, and beautician consulting, and consultation regarding legal issues" (Adler, 2006, p. 4).
- ***Transsexual (TS):*** "individual who has had surgery and/or hormonal treatments to make his or her body more closely match the sex with which he or she identifies" (Wood, 2009, p. 324). "After surgery, transsexuals may describe themselves as post-transition males to females (MTF) or females to males (FTM)" (Wood, 2009, p. 28).

In addition to understanding the above terminology, the reader is encouraged to read selections from the reference list at the end of this chapter.

## Male and Female Voice and Speech Differences

Societal norms between males and females are reported for speaking pitch, vocal quality, vocal intonation, resonance characteristics, and articulation patterns (see Table 60.2). Speaking fundamental frequency (SFF) refers to the habitual speaking frequency for an individual. A higher SFF is generally associated with the perception of a feminine voice (Wolfe, Ratusnik, Smith, & Northrop, 1990). In Spencer's study (1988) of the speech characteristics of 8 transsexuals, all subjects identified as female had an average SFF above 160 Hz while all those identified as male had an average SFF of 160 Hz or less. Although pitch levels assist in identification of gender, a higher SFF alone is insufficient for a person to be perceived as a female (Carew, Dacakis, & Oates, 2006; Hirsch, 2006b; Mount & Salmon, 1988).

Women tend to have more inflection and use more pitch variation than men (Addington, 1968; Crystal, 1975; Oates & Dacakis, 1997). In addition to intonation, the voice may be perceived as having various vocal qualities. Breathiness is the only vocal quality that appears to be associated with gender. A breathy voice quality often identifies a speaker as being feminine (Andrews & Schmidt, 1997).

Resonance refers to the quality of a sound that is generated at the level of the vocal folds and then passes through the vocal tract. There is a range of vocal resonance patterns associated with the male and female voice. High front vowels and their formant frequencies can be associated with the perception of female voice (Coleman, 1971; Mount & Salmon, 1988; Pausewant-Geilfer & Schofield, 2000). Differences in vowel formant frequency values between men and women are too great to be due to structural differences alone (Günzburger, 1995). Functional differences, such as forward tongue carriage and lip spreading, increase vowel formant frequency and fundamental frequency (Carew et al., 2006).

In addition to pitch and resonance, rate of speech and articulation affect the listener's perception of gender. Günzburger (1995) reported that "male speakers who were judged to exhibit effeminate speech had a slower speaking rate than speakers who were judged to use normal masculine speech (185 words/min as compared to 194 words/min)" (p. 342). Boonin (2006b) found that women generally pronounce words with greater clarity and elongate their vowels more than men. Conversely, men tend to distort or omit sounds. Gender perception can also be attributed to male and female vocal tract physiology and dimension variations that impact articulation (Simpson, 2001).

## Male and Female Nonverbal and Verbal Communication Differences

Although anywhere from 60 to 90% of a message is transmitted through nonverbal communication (Hirsch & Van Borsel, 2006; Wood, 2009), human beings in general are far less aware of their nonverbal behaviors than they are of their verbal behaviors. According to Hirsch and Van Borsel, many transgender clients "initially have no idea of the communicative power of their biological gender habits" (p. 285).

Nonverbal communication (NVC) refers to "any nonverbal behavior that may be interpreted as having meaning for a receiver, even if not intended as such by the sender" (Hirsch & Van Borsel, 2006, p. 284). Extensive research in this area has demonstrated that there are indeed differences in how men and women engage in NVC and that these differences are related to a particular culture's views of masculinity and femininity. If a client who is TG wants to learn female NVC, the clinician needs a basic knowledge of these characteristics. Some of these differences are listed in Table 60.3.

Verbal communication, according to Hooper (2006), involves "a rule-based, brain-based, socially shared code or system for representing thoughts" (p. 254). It is through this language system that individuals express gendered identities from culture to culture (Wood, 2009). Male and female language behaviors are typically socialized in different, subtle ways (as cited in Wood; see also Campbell, 1973; Coates, 1986, 1997; Coates & Cameron, 1989); these "gendered styles" of verbal communication should be considered when working with transgender individuals (Wood, 2009). Please refer to Table 60.4 for a listing of those choices a TG client has in terms of language use.

## The Role of a Speech-Language Pathologist

### The Scope of Practice and Code of Ethics

According to the Scope of Practice in Speech-Language Pathology from the American Speech-Language-Hearing Association (ASHA, 2007), clinical services delivered by SLPs include "providing services to modify or enhance communication performance (e.g., accent modification, transgender voice, care and improvement of the professional voice, personal/professional communication effectiveness)" (p. 8). ASHA states that "it is both ethically and legally incumbent upon professionals to determine whether they have the knowledge and skills necessary to perform such services" (p. 4). SLPs working with TG clients must possess clinical and cultural competency to work effectively with this population. In addition, ASHA's Code of Ethics (2003) states that "Individuals shall not discriminate in the delivery of professional services or the conduct of research or scholarly activities on the basis of race or ethnicity, gender, age, religion, national origin, sexual orientation, or disability" (p. 13).

### Necessary Clinical Skills

The SLP needs a strong understanding of voice and speech science, including theory, therapy techniques, and speech and voice disorders (Davies & Goldberg, 2006a, Goldberg, 2006). The

SLP should be knowledgeable also of culturally based gender differences and gender-based norms in both verbal and nonverbal communication (Davies & Goldberg). Training need not specifically come from communication sciences and disorders programs. For example, to teach feminization of spoken language, a background in linguistics, gender studies, or anthropology may be immensely valuable (Hooper, 2006). Training in the theater, including such aspects as movement, makeup, and costumes, can be invaluable to teach nonverbal feminine characteristics (Hirsch, 2006a). The clinician has the responsibility to determine his or her competency to serve the TG population.

### Cultural Competency

The SLP should be sensitive to the needs and challenges of TG persons (Davies & Goldberg, 2006a). One should be cognizant of the gender pronoun and name by which the client wishes to be identified. The path that TG persons take as they transition from living in a male role to a female role is complex and varied. There are unique psychosocial issues (as cited in Davies & Goldberg; Goldberg & Lindenberg, 2001). The transition sometimes involves sexual reassignment surgery as well as hormone therapy. TG clients vary in their sexual orientation. TG MtF persons may begin this journey at a point in their lives when they are married to a biological female and have children. Some may stay married, while others may divorce. Others may begin this journey at a much younger age. Clearly, the TG population is heterogeneous.

## The Voice and Communication Group at the Speech and Hearing Center of UNCG

### Grant Funding

In the fall of 2007, the UNCG Speech and Hearing Center received funding from the Guilford Green Foundation in Greensboro, NC, and The Adam Foundation in Winston-Salem, NC (both local organizations that promote diversity throughout the lesbian, gay, bisexual, and transgender community) to offer a voice and communication group for male-to-female transgender individuals in the region at a considerably reduced price. These grants were the first to be awarded by these organizations for transgender services. The receipt of these monies from two respected community foundations helped in recruitment efforts of clients for the new group beginning in the spring of 2008 and continuing through the fall of 2008. Only MtF TG individuals were selected for this group because they were easier to locate due to their higher prevalence rate than FtM TG persons, and because the latter typically do not require voice intervention due to their pitch being adequately lowered as a result of hormone therapy alone (Adler & Van Borsel, 2006).

### Recruitment of Clients

Brochures about the program were distributed through e-mail announcements sent to various organizations in the area such as The Triad Gender Association and The Triangle Transsexual Support group. Brief presentations about the new group and about feminization of voice and communication style were made at both these support groups. A total of 8 individuals including Doris, the client featured in the case study in this chapter, enrolled for the group that began in the spring of 2008.

### Description of the Group Program

The group met weekly for 2 hours over 14 weeks and included primarily small group work in the areas of vocal hygiene, voice, spoken language, and nonverbal communication. Four clinical faculty with expertise and background in theatre, voice, and language supervised four CSD graduate students assigned to this group as part of their clinical practicum experience. Two of the clinical faculty had previous experience with transgender clients.

## Description of the Case

### Background Information

Doris (pseudonym) was a 55-year-old, male-to-female transgender individual practicing medicine in a small town in North Carolina. She was born Daniel in 1953 to a mother whose first five pregnancies ended in spontaneous miscarriages. When pregnant with Doris, her mother was taking diethylstilbestrol (DES), a synthetic estrogen; according to Doris, there is a high prevalence of "trans circumstances" in "DES sons." Daniel realized in his early years that he was different; he played with girls and was attracted to stereotypically female activities ("I was the only boy taking tap, ballet, and jazz."). He eventually married a good friend from high school, and they went on to have two children. He went to medical school and became a family physician in his hometown. (As Doris pointed out: "We transsexuals become overachievers; we are the doctors, the lawyers, the black belts, the Navy SEALS. We do whatever we can to take the thoughts out.")

### Reasons for Referral

Although Daniel had wanted to transition in his 20s, he postponed the decision until his two children had graduated from high school. And so, 30 years later, at the time of his 25th wedding anniversary, after much anguish and depression, he "came out" to his wife and children and began the transition process. His wife was initially devastated, but his children were supportive and told him, "You will always be my dad." Daniel, now Doris, had to meet the Harry Benjamin International Gender Dysphoria Association's eligibility requirements before undergoing hormone therapy or sex reassignment surgery (SRS). One letter from a mental health professional was required before Doris could begin taking hormones, and two letters were required before genital surgery. In addition, Doris had to live full-time as a woman prior to the SRS. Although psychotherapy is not an absolute requirement for SRS, hormone therapy, or the real-life experience, mental health professionals may recommend it (Meyer et al., 2001).

Doris began the transition process with hormone treatment, psychotherapy, and her first facial feminization surgery. Her SRS took place in 2004 in Scottsdale, Arizona, after which Doris described herself as "extremely happy." Doris estimated that the total cost of her transition including hair removal, electrolysis, facial feminization surgeries, breast augmentation, ongoing hormone treatment, psychotherapy, and SRS was $150,000.

As a result of her transition from Daniel to Doris, Doris was forced to resign from her group medical practice, was asked to leave a financial board on which she served with old friends from high school, and was "kicked out of the church" where she had been a member for 35 years. Eventually after being asked by the town manager as well as former patients and friends to stay in town and not relocate, Doris borrowed money and opened her own private practice in which she sees many TG patients. She remained married to her wife of over 30 years.

### Chief Complaint at Time of Referral

An e-mail from client Doris on 12/18/07: "I am a post-op MtF physician in Smallwood [pseudonym], NC. I am currently practicing family medicine in Smallwood which is also my hometown. All is well except for my voice. I am constantly outed when calling in prescriptions or conversing with out-of-town physicians. Can you help me?" Wanting to "pass" as a female in all contexts, Doris was highly motivated to begin the group.

### Findings of the Evaluation

#### Evaluation Results

The evaluation included an assessment of voice, spoken language, nonverbal communication, and hearing. The voice evaluation involved an acoustic assessment and an assessment of laryngeal coordination. Measures of fundamental frequency ($F_0$) were recorded with the KayPENTAX Visi-Pitch IV, Model 3950, and vocal intensity was measured using a Radio Shack Digital Sound Level Meter. Timed tasks, such as maximum phonation time (MPT), were measured using a digital stopwatch. Voice measures were as shown in Table 60.1.

Doris's mean $F_0$ on vowels and in individual sentences was in the gender-neutral range of 150 to 185 Hz. Her mean $F_0$ in connected speech was consistent with male norms. Measures of shimmer and RAP were both high. Doris's MPT was reduced.

Doris also completed the Transgender Self-Evaluation Questionnaire (TSEQ), developed by Davies and Goldberg (2006c). She reported that her voice was "very male" and that her ideal voice would sound "somewhat female." The TSEQ is comprised of 30 questions that are answered on a 5-point Likert scale (1 being "never" and 5 being "always"). Doris rated 23 of the 30 items with a 4 or 5, indicating some level of impairment or dissatisfaction with her voice.

Because Doris failed the initial hearing screening, she was referred for an audiological evaluation. Findings indicated a "notch-shaped" mild hearing loss at 3,000 and 4,000 Hz in the left ear and a moderate loss at 4,000 Hz in the right ear. Overall, her hearing was adequate for participation in the group.

Due to the lack of standardized measures of verbal and NVC behaviors, the authors compiled checklists of the feminine behaviors described by numerous researchers in the literature (see Tables 60.2, 60.3, and 60.4). Doris's use of 10 verbal and 16 nonverbal behaviors was assessed through an analysis of a 13-minute videotaped sample of a conversation between Doris and a clinician. Conversational topics included gender-neutral subjects such as movies and books as well as background information about her transition.

The 13-minute language sample analysis revealed that Doris used 3 out of 10 (30%) feminine spoken language behaviors, that is, adjectives and adverbs (13 times), inclusive pronouns (5 times), and connectors/conjunctions (6 times) when conversing with the clinician. Feminine verbal characteristics not observed (70%) were the use of tag questions, tentative language, questions rather than statements to express wants/needs, adverbial clauses following sentences, socially polite phrases and apologies, empathetic phrases, and stereotypically feminine vocabulary.

An analysis of 3 minutes of the videotaped sample revealed numerous examples of NVC such as fluid, continuous movements; smiling; side-to-side head movements; self-touching; eye contact; and responsive movements. Although the frequency of use was difficult to determine, at least 1 occurrence of 6 out of the 16 behaviors (37%) was observed. Behaviors not observed

TABLE 60.1 Voice Evaluation

| Measures | Doris /a/ | Doris /i/ | Female Norms* | Male Norms* | General Norms* |
|---|---|---|---|---|---|
| Mean $F_0$ (connected speech) | 113.27 Hz | | 217 Hz | 116.65 Hz | |
| Mean $F_0$ (vowels) | 161.5 Hz | 170.96 Hz | 179 Hz /a/, 191.8 Hz /i/ | 118 Hz /a/ | |
| Pitch Range | /a/ 80 Hz to /i/ 485.4 Hz | | 165–255 Hz | 85–155 Hz | |
| Shimmer | 25.8% | 19.0% | .33 /a/, .23 /i/ | .47 /a/, .37 /i/ | <5% |
| Relative Average Perturbation (RAP) | 5.1% | 2.4% | .89 /a/, .54 /i/ | .38 /a/, .42 /i/ | <1% |
| Maximum Phonation Time | 12 seconds | | 13–18 sec. | 15–20 sec. | |
| s/z Ratio | .97 | | | | <1.2 |

* Information from Baken, R. J., & Orlikoff, R. F. (2000). *Clinical measurement of speech and voice* (2nd ed.). San Diego, CA: Singular Publishing Group.

TABLE 60.2 Some Stereotypical Gender Differences in Voice and Speech

| Aspects of Voice, Resonance, and Articulation | Females | Males |
|---|---|---|
| **Speaking Fundamental Frequency (SFF)** (Baken & Orlikoff, 2000; Dacakis, 2000) | Speak in SFF range from 188 Hz–221 Hz and demonstrate a pitch range of up to 275 Hz. | Speak in SFF range from 100 Hz–146 Hz and demonstrate a pitch range up to 165 Hz. |
| **Vocal Quality** (Coleman, 1983; Davies & Goldberg, 2006c; Gorham-Rowan & Morris, 2005) | Display higher formant frequencies due to smaller vocal tract dimensions; use slightly breathy onset. | Display lower formant frequencies due to larger vocal tract dimensions. |
| **Resonance** (Gorham-Rowan & Morris, 2005) | Use more lip spreading and anterior tongue carriage; use higher overtones. | Do not incorporate more lip spreading and anterior tongue carriage; use lower overtones. |
| **Intonation** (Davies & Goldberg, 2006c; Mordaunt, 2006; Oates & Dacakis, 1997; Wolfe et al., 1990) | Use more varied pitch and inflection; exhibit more upward glides (sing-song); use intonation to express meaning. | Are more monotone; have more downward glides, especially at the end of a sentence or statement. |
| **Duration** (Fitzsimons, Sheahan, & Staunton, 2001; Günzburger, 1995; Simpson, 2001) | Prolong vowels and phonemes; use more pauses between words, phrases, and sentences. | Use a more staccato style speech (words and phrases produced separately); use significantly shorter vowel durations in oral reading of words, phrases, and sentences. |
| **Rate and Volume** (Andrews, 1995; Günzburger, 1995; Mordaunt, 2006; Norton, 2000; Oates & Dacakis, 1983). | Have softer utterances; pause more often for lengthier periods; speak in short bursts followed by pause. | Are 2 to 3 dB louder than females; use loudness for emphasis; speak at a more steady and rapid rate. |
| **Articulation** (Andrews, 1995; Boonin, 2006a) | Use softer onsets; incorporate more precise speech sounds that are light; use more forward tongue position and a wider mouth opening. | Use harder onsets; drop and delete phonemes, slurring words. |

(63%) included expressive eye/facial movements, expressive use of fingers, S-shaped posture, self-referential touching, small personal space, and head movements that mimicked the conversational partner.

### Observations

The clinical team agreed that Doris exhibited some typically feminine nonverbal and verbal language characteristics. Her pitch sounded more masculine than feminine, her voice quality excessively breathy, and her resonance hypernasal.

### Interview Revelations

During the face-to-face interview, Doris appeared extremely motivated, friendly, talkative, and open to sharing all aspects of her male-to-female transition. She appeared healthy, although sometimes fatigued due to long hours at her medical practice. For other pertinent information, refer to the Description of the Case earlier in the case.

## The Hypothesis

The clinical team hypothesized that by the end of the first 14-week group program Doris would demonstrate a gender-neutral pitch range or higher with minimal cueing and increased

TABLE 60.3 Some Stereotypical Gender Differences in Nonverbal Communication

| Aspects of Nonverbal Communication | Females | Males |
|---|---|---|
| **Facial Expression** | Are more responsive and smile more often; communicate with all senses in order to pick up details and listen empathically; use more and varied facial expressions; nod head when listening. | Smile less often; are more likely to use facial expressions aggressively in social and business contexts; frown more often when listening. |
| **Touching** | When young, are touched more often and more gently by parents; initiate hugs and touches to express comfort and affection; use self-referential touching. | When young, are touched less frequently by parents; more often use touch to assert power and express sexual interest. |
| **Gestures and Body Movements** | When talking, stand or sit closer together; are more likely to give up their space; tilt and move heads more and condense bodies to take up less space; mirror the movements of partner in conversation; use gestures that are more fluid and toward the body with open, fluid finger motions; lean in while talking or listening. | Take up more space when sitting or standing and use more personal space; enter women's spaces more often than they enter other men's spaces and more often than women enter men's spaces; listen with head in static position; use gestures farther away from the body; maintain a more backward position when listening; use closed fingers in horizontal or vertical gestures. |
| **Use of Eyes** | Engage in more eye contact; use eye contact to respond/relate to others or to express submission; are more comfortable using eye contact. | Use eye contact to establish dominance; do not sustain eye contact in conversations; look at people from an angle. |

*Sources:* Davies & Goldberg, 2006c; Hirsch & Van Borsel, 2006; Wood, 2009.

use of feminine nonverbal and verbal communication behaviors in the clinical setting. The team expected that it would take at least another 14-week program in order for Doris to generalize these new behaviors across settings.

## Intervention Options Considered

### Knowledge/Scientific Evidence

According to ASHA (2004), evidence-based practice (EBP) involves integrating the best available research evidence with clinician experience and expertise and client/caregiver values. Although there are numerous published studies on communication therapy with the TG population, the strength of evidence garnered from those studies is greatly limited (Oates, 2006). According to Oates, based on an extensive review of the literature published from 1977 to 2005, there are "no published RCTs [randomized controlled trials] or large experimental studies in the field of voice therapy for TG/TS clients" (p. 31). Most studies involve few subjects or are case studies (Hooper, 2000). Ultimately, it is incumbent upon the clinician to critically analyze available research and glean from those studies what is most appropriate for the client(s) and what correlates best with clinical experience and expertise.

Although the evidence from the most recently published studies is not strong, one may identify potentially useful information about clinical practice with TG clients. For example, oral resonance therapy can successfully feminize the resonance characteristics of MtF TG persons (Carew et al., 2006). An appropriate target pitch range for MtF TG persons appears to be within a gender-neutral pitch range of 150 to 185 Hz (Mordaunt, 2006). In a literature

TABLE 60.4 Some Stereotypical Gender Differences in Verbal Communication

| Components of Verbal Communication | Females | Males |
|---|---|---|
| **Syntax** | Use inclusive pronouns, adverbial clauses, conjunctions between sentences, and tag questions; use questions rather than statements to indirectly express a want or need. | Are less likely to ask questions in a public situation; use adverbial clauses at the beginning of sentences; end sentences without connectors or subordinate clauses; use more contractions; use shorter sentences. |
| **Semantics** | Use descriptive adjectives and adverbs and feminine vocabulary and topics; use the word "so" more frequently; use nurturing phrases, e.g., "I know how you feel"; use more terms of affection. | Use more "I" references; use more swearing and taboo language; use less descriptive words and fewer qualifiers. |
| **Pragmatics and Discourse** | Use more tentative language, apologies, socially polite and empathetic phrases; use interactive conversations, invitational exchanges, responsive comments, and personal disclosures; offer more compliments and encourage responses through acknowledgements such as "uh-huh" and "mmm"; pause longer for another person to speak. | Avoid disclosing personal information; tend to give advice; use problem-solving to get information and give solutions; interrupt more frequently; use direct, authoritative language; communicate through abstract terms; portray less emotion; try to control the topic. |

*Sources:* Davies & Goldberg, 2006b; Hannah & Murachver, 1999; Hooper, 2006; Hooper & Hershberger, 2006; Wood, 2009.

review, McNeill (2006) reported that subjective measures may be more appropriate in determining success in speech therapy than objective measures for the TG population. Davies and Goldberg (2006a) provide a thorough review of the literature and expert opinion related to clinical practice with communication in TG individuals. They are in the process of evaluating their new treatment program and acknowledge that further evidence is needed to demonstrate its effectiveness adequately. Group therapy has been found to be an effective approach to communication feminization for TG clients, particularly when followed by individual intervention (Mordaunt, 2006).

In terms of the evidence base related to nonverbal and verbal communication in the TG population, according to Byrne, Dacakis, and Douglas (2003), "Despite the implication that components of speech and language other than voice should be considered when treating male-to-female transsexuals, research in this area is scant" (p. 16). Gender differences in verbal and NVC have been described in the literature, although these are often based on social stereotypes that are inextricably related to cultural norms, generational differences, and social class (Davies & Goldberg, 2006a). TG clients must be involved in the process of selecting which communication skills fit their individual lives.

### Client Preferences

Doris reported early in the process her desire to improve her pitch, intonation, resonance, and nonverbal cues. She had the freedom to select which nonverbal and verbal behaviors she felt comfortable integrating into her daily communication. The clinical team regularly sought Doris's feedback about the process and about her progress toward her communication goals.

## Course of Intervention

Doris was one of eight MtF TG clients who began the UNCG Voice and Communication Group in the spring of 2008. Based on her evaluation results and individual preferences, her long-term yearly goal was for her to use a habitual pitch that would be equal to or exceed the gender-neutral pitch range during conversation while maintaining characteristics of a natural female voice, that is, varied intonation and stress. The goal also included use of feminine verbal and nonverbal language characteristics that would consistently portray her as female. Five short-term objectives for the first semester targeted the following outcomes:

- Maintaining a gender-neutral pitch range or higher with less than 3 visual or verbal cues during a 5-minute conversation over 2 consecutive sessions
- Using appropriate breath support and laryngeal coordination to sustain a vowel 15 to 20 seconds 3 times over 3 consecutive sessions
- Using at least 6 of 15 feminine nonverbal behaviors with comfort and fluidity 2 times each during a 5-minute conversation over 3 consecutive sessions
- Using 6 of 10 feminine spoken language characteristics 2 times each during a 5-minute conversation over 2 consecutive sessions
- Using at least 5 feminine nonverbal behaviors and 5 feminine spoken language behaviors during a 5-minute conversation over 2 consecutive sessions.

The group met weekly for 2 hours over 14 weeks. After completion of initial evaluations, the weekly format of the group included an opening circle for the session's agenda and an exercise in a selected area, for example, vocal hygiene; rotation through three small groups focusing on observation and use of feminine voice, spoken language, and NVC; and finally, a closing circle with the entire group sharing any feedback or reflections on the completed activities. Eventually the small group work integrated voice, nonverbal, and spoken language.

Voice work, which included Resonant Voice Therapy (RVT) developed by Verdolini (1998), consisted of "voice production involving oral vibratory sensations, usually on the anterior alveolar ridge or higher in the face in the context of easy phonation" (Stemple, Glaze, & Klaben, 2000, p. 340). RVT aids in the reduction of laryngeal tension and, thereby, minimizes the likelihood of damage to the vocal mechanism (Verdolini, 1998).

## Analysis of Client's Response to Intervention

Doris made excellent progress over the 14-week program, achieving 4 out of the 5 short-term objectives. She often exceeded expectations for use of feminine nonverbal and spoken language characteristics. In addition, she safely maintained a gender-neutral pitch range and incorporated typically feminine, varied inflection in structured conversations in the clinical setting. Doris did not meet the objective for sustaining a vowel 15 to 20 seconds because this task was not measured over 3 sessions; however, as her postintervention assessment indicated, she clearly made progress toward this objective.

The RVT approach helped Doris to safely maintain gender-neutral pitch levels. Breathing and stretching exercises completed during a 3-week period created an awareness of appropriate airflow and abdominal muscle support. By the end of the program, Doris no longer exhibited an excessively breathy vocal quality or hypernasal resonance. She completed weekly homework to begin generalization of her newly learned skills.

In addition to performance on short-term objectives, a comparison of pre- and post- voice and communication measures indicated Doris's progress. As noted during initial assessment, her mean fundamental frequency of 113.27 Hz in conversation was lower than the recommended gender-neutral pitch range. During final assessment, Doris maintained a mean fundamental frequency of 159.74 Hz. Initially Doris's RAP and shimmer percentages were higher than normal limits. During final assessment, these values were within normal limits with the exception of perturbation during phonation of /i/, which was abnormal at 1.23% (normal is below 1%). Doris's maximum phonation time doubled from 12 seconds to 24 seconds, well within normal limits.

Doris completed a written evaluation of her progress on 3 different measures: the TSEQ; a 5-point Likert scale questionnaire of 12 items; and final interview questions. Doris's responses on the TSEQ were quite different from those she gave initially. She rated her voice overall as "somewhat female," while on the first measure she rated it as "very male." On all 30 items she indicated that her voice was more female, reliable, natural, and less tense than she reported 3 months earlier.

On the 12-item questionnaire asking her to rate on a 5-point scale (5 = strongly agree; 1 = strongly disagree) the overall group experience as well as the components of the program, Doris indicated that she strongly agreed with all parameters. For example, she strongly agreed that she learned about vocal hygiene, her appropriate pitch range, and female communication behaviors. She found the interactions with other group members extremely helpful ("I think this is key."). She gave an overall rating of "outstanding" to the group, and she strongly agreed that she would recommend the program to other TG persons. Doris's responses to the open-ended interview questions were very positive and helpful to the authors, who will use clients' feedback in planning the next group. One of Doris's comments was as follows: "Other than my SRS and facial feminization, this group has been the most important aspect of my transition."

## Further Recommendations

As expected, Doris achieved the objectives for the 14-week program. In addition, she reported that she was beginning to apply what she had learned about voice production and female nonverbal and spoken language behaviors in her daily life. In order to help her continue the generalization process, it was recommended that she continue in the Advanced Voice and Communication Group in the fall of 2008.

Not only did this group have an impact on Doris and the 7 other transgender clients, it also affected the 4 young graduate clinicians assigned to them. At the beginning of the semester, the students were nervous, apprehensive, and uncomfortable about working with the transgender population. At the end of this experience, when asked to compare their reactions to this group at the beginning and end, all 4 students expressed the personal and professional impact of this clinical assignment.

It seems fitting to end this chapter with one student's comments:

> Being assigned to this group has been a blessing in disguise to me. It has made me step back and realize that the thoughts that I had prior to meeting this population were stereotypical and quite shallow. The transgender population is just as human as the rest of us; they just are struggling with different issues than most people. . . . It's a speech-language pathologist's responsibility to serve clients in a nonjudgmental way, regardless of the circumstances.

## Author Note

The case presented in this chapter is real; IRB approval (IRB #078326) was received on April 4, 2008, from the Office of Research Compliance at The University of North Carolina–Greensboro (UNCG). The authors would like to thank Doris (pseudonym) for her willingness to share her story in this chapter and the entire transgender group for their motivation, hard work, and support. The authors acknowledge the sensitive and competent work of the four UNCG graduate student clinicians assigned to this group: Jillian Bauman, Elizabeth Davis, Elizabeth Frye, and Kara Tietsort. The authors are also grateful for the awards from the Guilford Green Foundation in Greensboro, NC, and The Adam Foundation in Winston-Salem, NC, that reduced the cost of the group program. Finally, gratitude is extended to Dr. Celia Hooper, Dr. Robert Mayo, and Mr. David Arneke at UNCG for their support and encouragement.

## Endnote

1. Now called the World Professional Association for Transgender Health (WPATH).

## References

Addington, D. W. (1968). The relationship of selected vocal characteristics to personality perception. *Speech Monographs, 35,* 492–503.

Adler, R. K. (2006). Vocal misuse and vocal hygiene. In R. K. Adler, S. Hirsch, & M. Mordaunt (Eds.), *Voice and communication therapy for the transgender/transexual client: A comprehensive clinical guide* (pp. 127–138). San Diego: Plural Publishing.

Adler, R. K., Hirsch, S., & Mordaunt, M. (2006). *Voice and communication therapy for the transgender/transsexual client.* San Diego: Plural Publishing.

Adler, R. K., & Van Borsel, J. (2006). Female-to-male considerations. In R. K. Adler, S. Hirsch, & M. Mordaunt (Eds.), *Voice and communication therapy for the transgender/transexual client: A comprehensive clinical guide* (pp. 139–167). San Diego: Plural Publishing.

American Psychiatric Association. (2000). *Diagnostic and statistical manual of mental disorders* (4th ed., text rev.). Washington, DC: American Psychiatric Association.

American Speech-Language-Hearing Association. (2003). *Code of ethics* [Ethics]. Available from http://www.asha.org/docs/html/ET2010-00309.html.

American Speech-Language-Hearing Association. (2004). *Evidence-based practice in communication disorders: An introduction* [Technical report]. Available from http://www.asha.org/docs/html/TR2004-00001.html.

American Speech-Language-Hearing Association. (2007). *Scope of practice in speech-language pathology* [Scope of Practice]. Available from www.asha.org/policy.

Andrews, M. L. (1995). *Manual of voice treatment: Pediatrics through geriatrics.* San Diego: Singular Publishing Group.

Andrews, M. L., & Schmidt C. P. (1997). Gender presentation: Perceptual and acoustical analyses of voice. *Journal of Voice, 11,* 307–313.

Baken, R. J., & Orlikoff, R. F. (2000). *Clinical measurement of speech and voice* (2nd ed.). San Diego, CA: Singular Publishing Group.

Boonin, J. (2006a). Articulation. In R. K. Adler, S. Hirsch, & M. Mordaunt (Eds.), *Voice and communication therapy for the transgender/transexual client: A comprehensive clinical guide* (pp. 225–236). San Diego: Plural Publishing.

Boonin, J. (2006b). Rate and volume. In R. K. Adler, S. Hirsch, & M. Mordaunt (Eds.), *Voice and communication therapy for the transgender/transexual client: A comprehensive clinical guide* (pp. 237–251). San Diego: Plural Publishing.

Byrne, L., Dacakis, G., & Douglas, J. (2003). Self-perceptions of pragmatic communication abilities in male-to-female transsexuals. *International Journal of Speech-Language Pathology, 5*(1), 15–25.

Campbell, K. K. (1973). The rhetoric of women's liberation: An oxymoron. *Quarterly Journal of Speech, 59,* 74–86.

Carew, L., Dacakis, G., & Oates, J. (2006). The effectiveness of oral resonance therapy on the perception of femininity of voice in male-to-female transsexuals. *Journal of Voice, 21,* 591–603.

Coates, J. (1986). *Women, men, and language: Studies in language and linguistics.* London: Longman.

Coates, J. (1997). *Language and gender: A reader.* London: Basil Blackwell.

Coates, J., & Cameron, D., (1989). *Women in their speech communities: New perspectives on language and sex.* London: Longman.

Coleman, R. O. (1971). Male and female voice quality and its relationship to vowel formant frequencies. *Journal of Speech and Hearing Research, 14,* 565–577.

Coleman, R. (1983). Acoustic correlates of speaker sex identification: Implications for the transsexual voice. *Journal of Sex Research, 19,* 293–295.

Crystal, D. (1975). *Prosodic systems and intonation in English.* London: Cambridge University Press.

Dacakis, G. (2000). Long-term maintenance of fundamental frequency increases in male-to-female transsexuals. *Journal of Voice, 14,* 549–556.

Davies, S., & Goldberg, J. M. (2006a). Clinical aspects of transgender speech feminization and masculinization. *International Journal of Transgenderism, 9,* 167–196.

Davies, S., & Goldberg, J. M. (2006b). *Gender transition: Changing speech.* Retrieved January 27, 2008, from http://www.vch.ca/transhealth/resources/library/tcpdocs/consumer/speech.pdf

Davies, S., & Goldberg, J. (2006c). *Transgender speech feminization/masculinization: Suggested guidelines for BC clinicians.* Retrieved January 27, 2008, from http://www.vch.ca/transhealth/resources/library/tcpdocs/guidelines-speech.pdf.

Fitzsimons, M., Sheahan, N., & Staunton, H. (2001). Gender and the integration of acoustic dimensions of prosody: Implications

for clinical studies. *Brain and Language, 78*(1), 94–108.
Girshick, L. B. (2008). *Transgender voices.* Lebanon, NH: University Press of New England.
Goldberg, J. M. (2006). *Recommended framework for training in speech feminization/masculinization.* Retrieved June 30, 2008, from http://www.vch.ca/transhealth/resources/library/tcpdocs/training-speech.pdf
Goldberg, J. M., & Lindenberg, M. (Eds.). (2001). *Trans-forming community: Resources for trans people and our families.* Victoria, BC: Transcend Transgender Support & Education Society.
Gorham-Rowan, M., & Morris, R. (2005). Aerodynamic analysis of male-to-female transgender voice. *Journal of Voice, 20,* 251–262.
Günzburger, D. (1995). Acoustic and perceptual implications of the transsexual voice. *Archives of Sexual Behavior, 24,* 339–348.
Hannah, A., & Murachver, T. (1999). Gender and conversational style as predictors of conversational behavior. *Journal of Language and Social Psychology, 19*(2), 153–174.
Hirsch, S. (2006a). Nonverbal communication: Assessment and training. In R. K. Adler, S. Hirsch, & M. Mordaunt (Eds.), *Voice and communication therapy for the transgender/transsexual client: A comprehensive clinical guide* (pp. 317–343). San Diego: Plural Publishing.
Hirsch, S. (2006b). Resonance. In R. K. Adler, S. Hirsch, & M. Mordaunt (Eds.), *Voice and communication therapy for the transgender/transexual client: A comprehensive clinical guide* (pp. 209–224). San Diego: Plural Publishing.
Hirsch, S., & Van Borsel, J. (2006). Nonverbal communication: A multicultural view. In R. K. Adler, S. Hirsch, & M. Mordaunt (Eds.), *Voice and communication therapy for the transgender/transsexual client: A comprehensive clinical guide* (pp. 283–315). San Diego: Plural Publishing.
Hooper, C. R. (2000). Voice treatment for the male-to-female transsexual. In J. C. Stemple (Ed.), *Voice therapy: Clinical studies* (2nd ed., pp. 274–284). San Diego: Singular Publishing Group.
Hooper, C. R. (2006). Language: Syntax and semantics. In R. K. Adler, S. Hirsch, & M. Mordaunt (Eds.), *Voice and communication therapy for the transgender/transsexual client: A comprehensive clinical guide* (pp. 253–267). San Diego: Plural Publishing.
Hooper, C. R., & Hershberber, I. (2006). Language: pragmatics and discourse. In R. K. Adler, S. Hirsch, & M. Mordaunt (Eds.), *Voice and communication therapy for the transgender/transsexual client: A comprehensive clinical guide* (pp. 269–282). San Diego: Plural Publishing.
McNeill, E. J. M. (2006). Management of the transgender voice. *The Journal of Laryngology & Otology, 120,* 521–523.
Meyer, W. III, Bockting, W., Cohen-Kettenis, P., Coleman, E., DiCeglie, D., Devor, H., (February, 2001). *The standards of care for gender identity disorders—sixth version.* IJT 5, 1. Retrieved January 27, 2008, from http://wpath.org/Documents2/socv6.pd
Mordaunt, M. (2006). Pitch and intonation. In R. K. Adler, S. Hirsch, & M. Mordaunt (Eds.), *Voice and communication therapy for the transgender/transexual client: A comprehensive clinical guide* (pp. 169–207). San Diego: Plural Publishing.
Mount, K. H., & Salmon, S. J. (1988). Changing the vocal characteristics of postoperative transsexual patients: A longitudinal study. *Journal of Communication Disorders, 21,* 229–238.
Norton, A. (2000). *Voice therapy helps transsexuals.* Reuters Health. Retrieved January 27, 2008, from http://www.moss-fritch.com/VoiceTherapy.htm
Oates, J. (2006). Evidence-based practice in voice therapy for transgender/transsexual clients. In R. K. Adler, S. Hirsch, & M. Mordaunt (Eds.), *Voice and communication therapy for the transgender/transsexual client: A comprehensive clinical guide* (pp. 23–43). San Diego: Plural Publishing.
Oates, J., & Dacakis, G. (1983). Speech pathology considerations in the management of transsexualism: A review. *British Journal of Disorders of Communication, 18,* 139–151.
Oates, J., & Dacakis, G. (1997) Voice change in transsexuals. *Venereology: Interdisciplinary, International Journal of Sexual Health, 10,* 178–187.
Olyslager, F., & Conway, L. (2007, September). *On the calculation of the prevalence of transsexualism.* Paper presented at the WPATH 20th International Symposium, Chicago, IL. Retrieved January 27, 2008, from http://ai.eecs.umich.edu/people/conway/TS/Prevalence/Reports/Prevalence%20of%20Transsexualism.pdf.
Pausewant-Geilfer, M., & Schofield, K. J. (2000). Comparison of acoustic and perceptual measures of voice in male-to-female transsexuals perceived as female versus those perceived as male. *Journal of Voice, 14*(1), 22–33.

Simpson, A. (2001). Dynamic consequences of differences in male and female vocal tract dimension. *Journal of Acoustical Society of America, 109*(5), 2153–2164.

Spencer, L. E. (1988). Speech characteristics of male-to-female transsexuals: A perceptual and acoustic study. *Folia Phoniatrica, 40,* 31-42.

Stemple, J. C., Glaze, L. E., & Klaben, B. G. (2000). *Clinical voice pathology* (3rd ed.). San Diego: Singular Publishing Group.

Verdolini, K. (1998). Resonant voice therapy. In K. Verdolini (Ed.), *National Center for Voice and Speech's guide to vocology* (pp. 34–35). Iowa City, IA: National Center for Voice and Speech.

Wolfe, V. I., Ratusnik, D. L., Smith, F. H., & Northrop, G. (1990). Intonation and fundamental frequency in male-to-female transexuals. *Journal of Speech & Hearing Disorders, 55,* 43–50.

Wood, J. T. (2009). *Gendered lives* (8th ed.). Boston: Wadsworth Cengage Learning.

# CASE 61

# Teresa: Voice Therapy for an Elementary School Teacher with Vocal Fold Nodules

*Judith Maige Wingate*

## Conceptual Knowledge Areas

Vocal nodules are benign lesions of the vocal folds, which may appear as small blisters or calluses, usually on both folds. They result from acute phonotrauma or hyperfunctional voice use (Stemple, Glaze, & Gerdemann, 1993). The lesions have a threefold effect on vocal fold mechanics. The weight of the nodules increases the mass of the vocal folds, resulting in slower vibration and a lowering of the fundamental frequency. The nodules increase the stiffness of the folds, making it harder to initiate quiet voice and interfering with vocal fold closure. This leads to air escape and an increasingly breathy voice quality. Other vocal characteristics include increased roughness, loss of flexibility and vocal range, and voice breaks (Boone, McFarlane, & Von Berg, 2005). Teachers, with their high vocal demand, are at risk for developing vocal nodules.

## Description of the Case

### Background Information

The client, Teresa, was a 38-year-old Caucasian female teacher with a history of vocal problems that began when she started teaching and that had grown progressively worse over the last several years. She complained of hoarseness, increased effort to speak, difficulty being heard by her students, pitch breaks, and deterioration of voice quality throughout the day. She reported that her voice became increasingly hoarse as the week progressed and that she often lost her voice by the end of the week. Typically, her voice improved on Monday after a weekend of rest and by Friday her voice was almost gone. She also noted improvement of her voice during summer vacation with voice loss occurring every year after the first week of school. She was seen by a laryngologist and was diagnosed with bilateral vocal fold nodules. The nodules were described as moderate in size with a typical hourglass closure pattern. There was also slight erythema of the vocal folds. The client was referred to the Speech and Hearing Clinic for voice therapy.

## Reason for Referral

Further information was obtained from Teresa during her voice evaluation. She had been a kindergarten teacher for 15 years. Teresa recalled that she had had intermittent problems with her voice throughout her career, but that they had become more persistent in the last 5 years. Her problems had become severe enough for her to consider a change to a job that did not require her to use her voice. Teresa was the mother of 3 children, ages 5, 7, and 12. The children were involved in a variety of sports and Teresa described herself as their biggest fan. She admitted to yelling and screaming at their sporting events several times a week.

Teresa indicated that she wanted to improve her voice quality. She stated that she was willing to participate in therapy and to make any changes necessary to change her voice.

## Findings of the Evaluation

Perceptual evaluation revealed a breathy, rough voice quality. Teresa was able to sustain phonation for a maximum of 6 seconds and was able to sustain exhalation for 25 seconds. Excessive tension of the strap muscles of the neck was noted during loud talking. Frequent throat clears were also noted, averaging 2 per 5 minutes. Harmonic-to-noise ratio was 1.25, consistent with a rough voice quality and incomplete vocal fold closure. Average fundamental frequency during speech was 145 Hz, significantly lower than the average fundamental for an adult female. Phonation frequency range was 15 semitones, less than the expected of 24 semitones. Frequent pitch breaks were noted during pitch glides and conversational speech. All of these characteristics may occur with vocal fold nodules.

Teresa completed the Voice Handicap Index (Jacobson et al., 1997). This measure quantifies the impact of a voice problem on the client's quality of life. Her score on this measure was a 70 out of a possible 150, indicating that her voice problem had a severe impact on her quality of life.

## Treatment Options Considered

Following completion of the voice evaluation, it was hypothesized that the vocal fold nodules occurred as a result of high vocal load and high vocal fold collision forces that occurred both on the job and while yelling at sports events. In order for Teresa to meet her vocal demands on the job, she needed to be able to produce a clear, audible voice in the classroom without undue strain and effort. However, in order to accomplish this, she first needed to reduce her loudness demand and vocal load to allow the vocal fold nodules to resolve. Several behavioral treatment options were considered, including the following:

- ***An exercise-based program utilizing vocal function exercises.*** (Stemple, Lee, D'Amico, & Pickup, 1994). Exercises are easily learned by clients and offer a consistent program of home practice that is purported to strengthen the three subsystems of voice (respiration, phonation, and resonance).
- ***Resonant voice therapy.*** This therapy method has been demonstrated to produce efficient voice production while reducing vocal fold collision forces (Verdolini, Druker, Palmer, & Samawi, 1998). The method is easy to learn and focuses on sensory feedback.
- ***Classroom amplification.*** The use of amplification has been reported to reduce the perception of vocal strain for teachers (Roy et al., 2003; Sapienza, Crandell, & Curtis, 1999). Additionally, the use of amplification reduces the amount of loudness the teacher must produce. Some clients do not want to consider amplification as they feel that it is artificial and cumbersome.
- ***Easy onset of phonation.*** The easy onset technique is one that reduces vocal fold collision to allow the vocal fold edges to heal while ensuring that the client produces voice with adequate air flow. The technique is easily learned and allows for a smooth transition to projecting the voice without straining (Boone et al., 2005; Colton & Casper, 1990).
- ***Projection exercises.*** In order for a teacher to be heard in the classroom without straining the voice, it is helpful to utilize projection exercises such as those used by

actors. The emphasis is on open mouth, increased resonance, crisp production of consonants, and slight prolongation of vowels (Wingate, Brown, Shrivastav, Davenport, & Sapienza, 2007).

- ***Vocal hygiene instruction.*** Vocal hygiene instruction consists of targeting and eliminating behaviors that may contribute to vocal fold irritation. Environmental manipulation may also be undertaken in a vocal hygiene program. This is a useful adjunct to voice therapy techniques (Colton & Casper, 1990).
- ***Voice rest.*** While often recommended for persons with voice problems, voice rest is not an option for a working professional. There are also compliance issues with vocal rest (Benninger, Jacobson, & Johnson, 1994). Although a short period of voice rest might serve to reduce vocal fold irritation, the client will not make any behavioral changes and would return to the work situation using the same vocal behaviors that led to the development of the vocal fold nodules. Therefore, voice rest was not recommended in this case.

## Course of Treatment

For this teacher, an eclectic approach was selected utilizing all of the techniques listed above with the exception of voice rest.

### Therapy Session 1

Teresa was seen weekly for voice therapy sessions over the course of 12 weeks. At the beginning of the session, basic vocal hygiene recommendations were reviewed. Two issues were targeted. The first was the need to reduce the amount of time that Teresa spent yelling at her children's sports events. She was encouraged to use a noisemaker to express her enthusiasm and allow her voice to rest. The frequent throat-clearing behavior was also targeted. It was suggested that Teresa take a sip of water instead of clearing her throat. This, in turn, would help to reduce vocal fold irritation and swelling. She expressed some concern about increasing her water intake as she had few bathroom breaks during the school day. Other alternatives to reduce throat clears were offered, including keeping a piece of hard candy in her mouth or using a silent cough in place of a throat clear. In a silent cough, air is forced through open vocal folds so there is no contact of the vocal fold edges. Teresa agreed to combine these techniques.

The client was given a demonstration of abdominal breathing with an emphasis on prolonged exhalation. This was practiced during sustained productions of /f/ and /sh/ as well as during the vowels /i/ and /a/. The concept of easy onset was then introduced and practiced in words and sentences. The words began with /h/ to facilitate easy initiation of voice. The pitch glides from the vocal function exercises were demonstrated and practiced with the client. These consisted of glides up and down, which were repeated twice. The client was asked to practice all of the above during the next week.

Finally, a personal amplification system was introduced consisting of a speaker worn around the waist, which was connected to a headset microphone. The client was asked to wear this in the classroom at all times and to use a softer, easier voice with the microphone.

### Therapy Session 2

During the second session, the remainder of the vocal function exercises was introduced. The client sustained a warm-up tone using a nasal /i/ sound on F above middle C. Then the upward and downward glides were produced twice each. Following this, the client sustained 5 pitches as softly and for as long as she could on the word "knoll." The pitches used were middle C-D-E-F-G. Each pitch was sustained twice. The client was instructed to practice these twice daily and to record the length of the sustained pitches on a record sheet.

Easy onset was reviewed and practiced. The client used the technique to answer questions and read short paragraphs. She was asked to continue practicing easy onset daily at home.

### Therapy Session 3

The session was begun with a review of the week. Teresa reported some improvement in vocal quality and a reduction in vocal strain since using the personal amplifier. She reported that she had stopped clearing her throat after implementing the alternative behaviors suggested. Vocal function exercises were also reviewed and sustained phonation times were recorded. An increase in phonation time, especially in mid-range pitch levels, was observed. Next the concept of increased resonance was introduced. An emphasis was placed on feeling increased sensation around the lips and nose during production of nasal sounds and a hum. The client was asked to try to maintain this feeling while reading sentences loaded with nasal sounds. Home practice combining resonance materials and easy onset materials was assigned.

### Therapy Session 4

Vocal function exercises were practiced. The client also practiced resonant voice production using sentences containing both nasal and non-nasal words and responded to short questions using resonant voice.

During this session, Teresa was asked to describe her typical voice use in the classroom and then to brainstorm ways to change her activities to help her voice improve. For example, instead of using her voice to get attention, the teacher was able to realize that she could use a hand signal for quiet. She also decided that she could utilize parent volunteers to help give instructions during some activities. She was asked to continue to think of other ways to minimize any unnecessary talking that she might be doing. The clinician suggested that she look at her schedule and try to alternate quiet activities with those that required more talking. She was asked to begin incorporating some of her new vocal strategies at work for short periods of time.

### Therapy Session 5

After reviewing vocal function exercises, the concept of projecting the voice was introduced. This was built on the concept of easy onset. The teacher was instructed to increase the rate of air being utilized while allowing the mouth and throat to be very open. She was then asked to slightly prolong the vowels in short phrases while maintaining the sensations experienced using resonant voice. Next, crisp articulation of consonants was emphasized. Portions of famous speeches (e.g., the speech by Martin Luther King Jr., "I Have a Dream") were used to practice projection. After a brief trial in which she gave her typical classroom directions while using a more projected voice, she was asked to continue this for at least 2 activities per day.

### Therapy Session 6

As in previous sessions, vocal function exercises were reviewed. Practice was continued with resonant voice and projection. Fewer pitch breaks were noted during glides and Teresa demonstrated longer phonation times. She reported that her voice was becoming clearer and that she noticed much less effort to speak at work. She no longer experienced voice loss at the end of the week. A follow-up session was scheduled in 2 weeks. Further instruction on incorporating her new vocal techniques in the classroom was given.

### Therapy Session 7

Teresa reported that she utilized the techniques in the classroom but had to consciously think about using them and/or would forget to breathe. To assist with the transition, Teresa agreed to schedule 2 activities on the day following her therapy session in which she would use her new techniques. She was asked to double the number of activities on the following day and to continue in this manner. Further follow-up was scheduled at a 1-month interval.

### Therapy Session 8

By this session, Teresa reported that she was able to incorporate the techniques in the classroom with little effort and that she felt they had become more habitual. She continued to use the amplifier, especially during noisier periods in the classroom. She reported no voice loss and significant reduction in effort to speak. However, there was some occasional hoarseness at the end of the day. Throat clearing was no longer observed. Repeat measures were taken, which revealed that Teresa was able to sustain phonation a maximum of 25 seconds across her modal pitch range. Her average fundamental frequency had increased to 185 Hz with phonational frequency range increased to 28 semitones. No pitch breaks were noted during pitch glides. Harmonic-to-noise ratio was. 65. Her score on the VHI was 30 out of 150, indicating that her voice problems now had a very mild impact on her quality of life. Subsequent follow-up with the laryngologist revealed that the nodules were almost resolved with only a small amount of swelling visible.

## Further Recommendations

Therapy was discontinued. It was recommended that Teresa continue using amplification in the classroom and continue to practice the vocal function exercises 2–3 days a week. A practice regimen for vocal conditioning was designed, which consisted of reading aloud, using her typical classroom voice, for an increased amount of time daily until she was able to read aloud for 15 to 20 minutes at a time with no vocal strain. She was asked to implement this regimen at least 3 weeks prior to the beginning of school to help condition her voice to meet the vocal demands of a new school year. She was urged to contact her clinician for assistance as needed.

## Author Note

This case is not based on an actual client but is based on a composite of cases seen in the author's clinical practice.

## References


Benninger, M. S., Jacobson, B. H., & Johnson, A. F. (1994). *Vocal arts medicine: The care and prevention of professional voice disorders.* New York: Thieme Medical Publishers.

Boone, D. R., McFarlane, S. C., & Von Berg, S. L. (2005). *The voice and voice therapy.* Boston, MA: Pearson Education.

Colton, R. H., & Casper, J. K. (1990). *Understanding voice problems: A physiological perspective for diagnosis and treatment.* Baltimore, MD: Williams & Wilkins.

Jacobsen, B. H., Johnson, A., Grywalski, C., Silbergleit, A., Jacobsen, G., & Benninger, M. S. (1997). The Voice Handicap Index (VHI): Development and validation. *American Journal of Speech-Language Pathology, 6*(3), 66–70.

Roy, N., Weinrich, B., Gray, S. D., Tanner, K., Stemple, J. C., & Sapienza, C. M. (2003). Three treatments for teachers with voice disorders: A randomized clinical trial. *Journal of Speech and Hearing Research, 46(3),* 670–688.

Sapienza, C. M., Crandell, C. C., & Curtis, B. (1999). Effects of sound field frequency modulation amplification on decreasing teachers' sound pressure level in the classroom. *Journal of Voice, 13*, 375–381.

Stemple, J. C., Glaze, L. E., & Gerdeman, B. K. (1993). *Clinical voice pathology: Theory and management.* San Diego, CA: Singular.

Stemple, J. C., Lee, L., D'Amico, B., & Pickup, B. (1994). Efficacy of vocal function exercises as a method of improving voice production. *Journal of Voice, 8*, 271–278.

Verdolini, K., Druker, D., Palmer, P., & Samawi, H. (1998). Laryngeal adduction in resonant voice. *Journal of Voice, 12*, 315–327.

Wingate, J. M., Brown, W. S., Shrivastav, R., Davenport, P., & Sapienza, C. M. (2007). Treatment outcomes for professional voice users. *Journal of Voice, 21*, 433–449.